TOWARD
THE HEALTH
OF A
NATION

TOWARD THE HEALTH OF A NATION

The Institute of Health Policy, Management and Evaluation – The First Seventy Years

LESLIE A. BOEHM

Published for the Institute of Health Policy, Management and Evaluation at the Dalla Lana School of Public Health
by
MCGILL-QUEEN'S UNIVERSITY PRESS
Montreal & Kingston • London • Chicago

ISBN 978-0-2280-0085-3 (cloth)
ISBN 978-0-2280-0228-4 (ePDF)
ISBN 978-0-2280-0229-1 (ePUB)

Legal deposit fourth quarter 2020
Bibliothèque nationale du Québec

Printed in Canada on acid-free paper that is 100% ancient forest free (100% post-consumer recycled), processed chlorine free

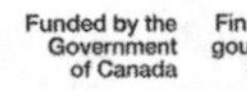

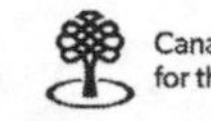

We acknowledge the support of the Canada Council for the Arts.

Nous remercions le Conseil des arts du Canada de son soutien.

Library and Archives Canada Cataloguing in Publication

Title: The health of a nation : the Institute of Health Policy, Management and Evaluation–the first seventy years / Leslie Boehm.
Names: Boehm, Leslie, 1953- author.
Description: Includes bibliographical references and index.
Identifiers: Canadiana (print) 20200271733 | Canadiana (ebook) 20200271962 | ISBN 9780228000853 (cloth) | ISBN 9780228002284 (ePDF) | ISBN 9780228002291 (ePUB)
Subjects: LCSH: University of Toronto. Institute of Health Policy, Management and Evaluation—History. | LCSH: Public health—Study and teaching (Graduate)—Ontario—Toronto—History. | LCSH: Medical policy—Study and teaching (Graduate)—Ontario—Toronto—History. | LCSH: Graduate students—Education—Ontario—Toronto—History.
Classification: LCC RA 395.C3 B64 2020 | DDC 362.1071/1713541—dc23

To department/institute faculty and students, past and present;
also to its new parent, the Dalla Lana School of Public Health

Contents

Foreword

It is my great honour to write this foreword to Les Boehm's fascinating account of the history of the University of Toronto's Institute of Health Policy, Management and Evaluation, including its origins in the School of Hygiene and the Department of Hospital Administration.

Professor Boehm's account is far more than the history of a long academic legacy. His is the history of the development of health care in Canada, and in particular, the history of universal health coverage, from its introduction as publicly funded hospital insurance in Saskatchewan in 1947 through to the Canada Health Act of 1984 and its evolution to the present.

The cast of characters we encounter in this book were academic leaders with intimate connections to governments across Canada in the twentieth century, including J.G. Fitzgerald, Harvey Agnew, Burns Roth, Eugene Vayda, and Peggy Leatt. The legacy continues into the twenty-first century with Louise Lemieux-Charles and Adalsteinn Brown. No ivory tower types, these were practitioner-scholars who always had their eye on how create change to improve the health of Canadians and the state of medical care in Canada.

Because of Saskatchewan's formative work in implementing universal hospital and medical care insurance, scholars such as Burns Roth, Malcolm Taylor, and Fred Mott had worked in Saskatchewan. Originally from Saskatchewan, the author himself was the recipient of a bursary from the Saskatchewan Department of Public Health when he was an MHSc student from 1978 to 1980. I know that he has a conviction (which I share) that Tommy Douglas had a particular affinity for the School of Hygiene and also its Department of Hospital Administration (as it was then called). Indeed, Tommy asked Roth, one of the department's earliest students, to come Saskatchewan to help manage its hospital insurance program and then became its deputy minister of public health.

Through the years this connection has endured. As you will see, the school provided administrators for Saskatchewan's major teaching hospitals. You will also see that two of its grads set up a hospital admin program at the University of Saskatchewan (my alma mater) aimed at smaller hospitals.

I too have had an ongoing connection to the school. Over the years it has been my privilege to meet a number of your graduates and faculty. While I was royal commissioner, some of each of your faculty and graduates submitted briefs and made presentations.

More recently, Greg Marchildon, my former deputy minister and the executive director of the Royal Commission on the Future of Health Care, which I led, left Saskatchewan to become a member of the IHPME faculty as Ontario Research Chair in Health Policy and System Design. Greg and Les have been colleagues and friends for years and share a keen interest in the history of Canadian health care and also of the importance of policy institutes.

Professor Boehm's history touches on a number of important components of health care. These include health systems, including universal health coverage, which is receiving renewed attention in response to to the United Nation's Resolution of December 2012 advocating universal health coverage for all countries, rich and poor.

The history of IHPME in its various manifestations is an important part of our health history and I hope you will enjoy reading about it as much as I have.

Roy Romanow, PC, OC, SOM, QC, former premier of Saskatchewan
and former royal commissioner

Acknowledgments

I gratefully acknowledge the assistance provided by the following organizations at the University of Toronto: Gerstein Library, Institute of Health Policy, Management and Evaluation (IHPME), Robarts Library (Reference Service), and Thomas Fisher Rare Book Library. Sylvia Lassam at the Trinity College Archives was very helpful.

Archival departments at the University of Saskatchewan, University of Montreal, McGill University, and province of Saskatchewan (both the Regina and Saskatoon locations) were helpful.

The Interlibrary Loan Service at Robarts Library needs to be singled out. Their dedication and perseverance is beyond measure in tracking down a number of antiquarian, rare, and esoteric publications from across North America and the United Kingdom. It is my belief that they took it upon themselves never to be defeated in fulfilling a request for such material. Lyle Davis in particular needs to be mentioned.

In addition, the University of Toronto Archives and Record Management Service (UTARMS) needs to be noted. The staff were unfailingly helpful chasing down my hunches and in trying to mitigate the absence of much of the school's (and hence the institute's) records. Tys Klumpenhouwer, recently appointed university archivist, was always ready to suggest sources for my intuitions. Marnee Gamble had a series of recorded interviews digitized, which, almost unbelievably, made hours upon hours of hard-to-understand thirty-year-old reel-to-reel and cassette tapes (which I had been labouring over) crystal clear. Harold Averill filled in gaps with his encyclopaedic knowledge of the university's history. It's said he "knows more about that vast, complex, Victorian federation than probably anyone."[1] Loryl MacDonald would always take time from her hectic schedule to provide me with useful advice on tracking down rare archival material.

At the University of Toronto a number of IHPME individuals willingly gave their time and insights, including John Browne, Rhonda Cockerill, and Eugene Vayda. Raisa Deber, Greg Marchildon, and Julia Zarb read a draft and provided valuable input. IHPME faculty were always ready to answer queries; with Ross Baker, Mark Dobrow, and Paul Williams this happened multiple times. Office staff such as Anita Moorehouse and Rebecca Biason were helpful without exception.

In addition, former director of IHPME and present dean of the Dalla Lana School of Public Health, Adalsteinn "Steini" Brown, took a personal interest in this book project. He was always very supportive, ready to answer my many queries, and he read two drafts of the manuscript.

Another very important source was Paul Bator's work that deals with the School of Hygiene and its constituent departments. His published oeuvre, *Within Reach of Everyone*, provides a very good base upon which to build. His endnotes provide clues on where to go to search for more. His research material housed at the U of T Archives is a source of both further information and clues.

It bears mentioning that the amount of primary material available in the University of Toronto libraries and archives, and the libraries and archives of its federated colleges, is truly astounding and represents a national resource.

If one could say one has a regret it is that, as the result of space limitations, too many dedicated individuals, faculty, and others, have not been mentioned in the work.

Preamble

This book project actually grew out of an idea that occurred independently to Steini Brown and me. In March 2016 he had approached me to develop a *booklet* on IHPME's history to mark its seventieth anniversary the next year.

What Steini did not know was that a year before that, while researching a manuscript on the Department of Public Health in the Tommy Douglas administration, I was finding a number of connections between personnel in the Saskatchewan Department and the School of Hygiene at U of T, and particularly its Department of Public Health and its Department of Hospital Administration (IHPME's forerunner). I said to myself, *Someone should write a book about this*, and promptly parked the idea and continued my work on the Saskatchewan manuscript.

However, even with that thought in mind, I almost said no to Steini, as I was up to my neck in teaching responsibilities and the Saskatchewan manuscript. However, some days later I could not resist heading off to the Gerstein Library and also the U of T Archives to follow a couple of threads that had occurred to me on my initial hunch, and with that I was hooked. I went back and told Steini I would do it. What I did not tell him was that this was never going to be a booklet.

I have been involved with IHPME in one form or another ever since I graduated. My fascination – and admiration – with it, the School of Hygiene, and the Dalla Lana School – the organizations and the people – is total.

Truly, they are this university, Ontario, and Canada at its best.

Les Boehm
August 2019

Abbreviations

ACE	Accessing Centre for Expertise
C3	Converge3
CCMC	Committee on the Costs of Medical Care
CEHIAP	Centre for Evidence in Health in All Policies (later C3)
CHA	Canadian Hospital Association
CHC	Community Health Centre
CHCP	Community Health Centre Project
CJPH	*Canadian Journal of Public Health*[1]
CMA	Canadian Medical Association
CMAJ	*Canadian Medical Association Journal*
DLSPH	Dalla Lana School of Public Health
DHA	diploma of hospital administration, School of Hygiene, U of T
DOHA	Department of Hospital Administration and from 1967 Department of Health Administration, School of Hygiene, U of T
DPE	Department of Political Economy, U of T
DPH	diploma of public health, School of Hygiene, University of Toronto
EHS	Emergency Hospital Service
HSC	Hospital for Sick Children, Toronto
HPME	Health Policy, Management and Innovation (Department of)
HSR	Health Services Research
ICES	Institute for Clinical Evaluative Sciences
IHPME	Institute for Health Policy, Management and Evaluation
MASC	master of applied science
MHI	Master of Health Informatics
MHSC	master of health sciences, Department of Health Administration, U of T
MPP	master of public policy

NAO	North American Observatory on Health Systems and Policies
NGO	non-government organization
NHS	National Health Service (UK)
OHA	Ontario Health Association (formerly the Ontario Hospital Association)
OHSC	Ontario Hospital Service Commission
SAB	Saskatchewan Archives Board
SGS	School of Graduate Studies
SLI	System Leadership and Innovation
TGH	Toronto General Hospital
UHC	universal health coverage
UHN	University Health Network
UTARMS	University of Toronto Archives and Record Management Service
UTM	University of Toronto, Mississauga Campus
UTSC	University of Toronto, Scarborough Campus

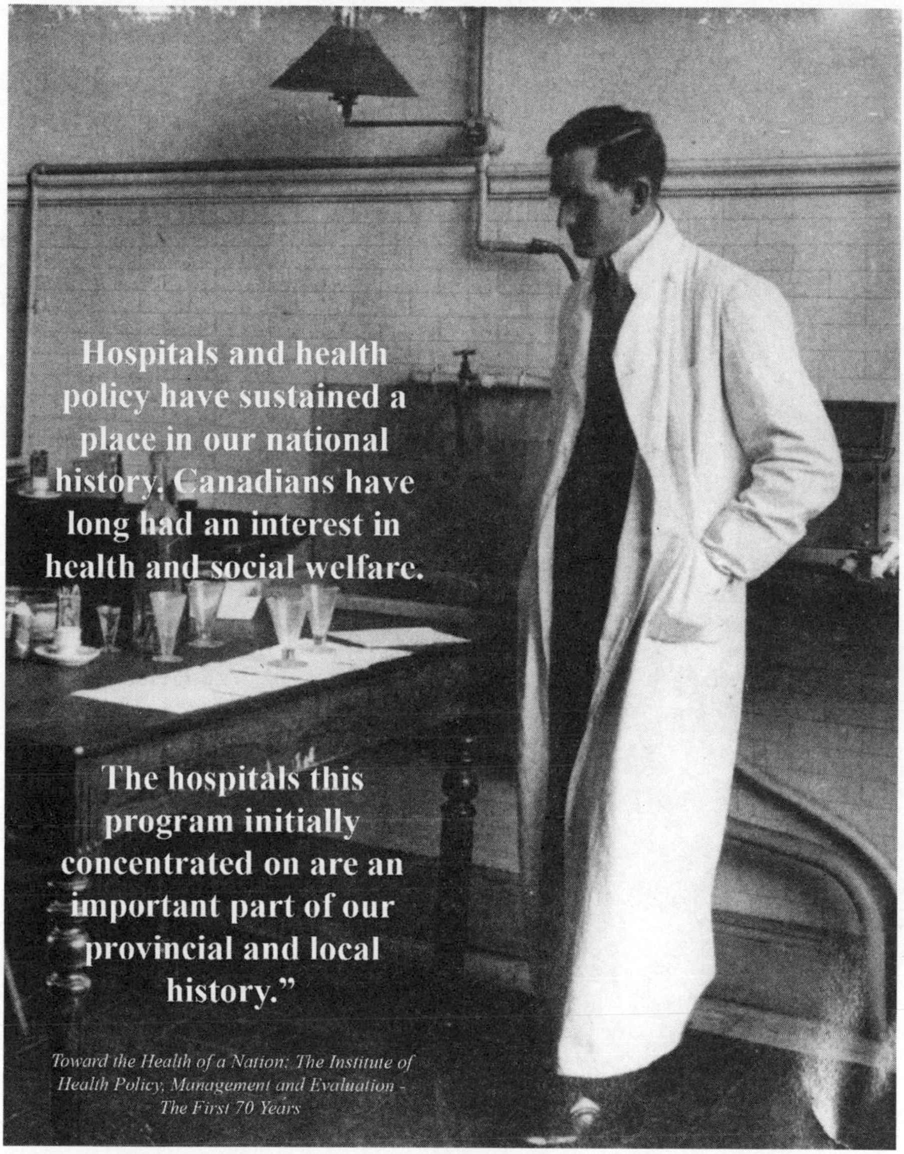

Hospitals and health policy have sustained a place in our national history. Canadians have long had an interest in health and social welfare.

The hospitals this program initially concentrated on are an important part of our provincial and local history."

Toward the Health of a Nation: The Institute of Health Policy, Management and Evaluation - The First 70 Years

J.G. FitzGerald in his lab. A slight variant of this picture, with the quote taken from a draft of this book, was originally used in IHPME, *Our First Seventy Years, 2017 Annual Highlights*.

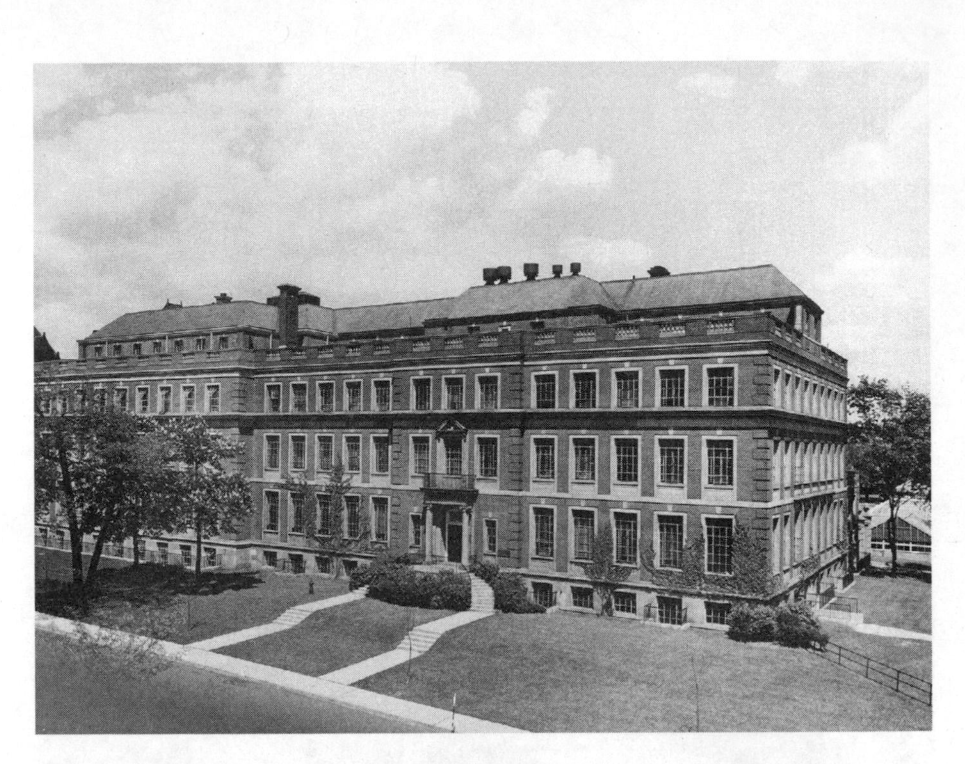

IHPME's first home – School of Hygiene Building, now FitzGerald Building (University of Toronto Archives, A2012-0009/047[06])

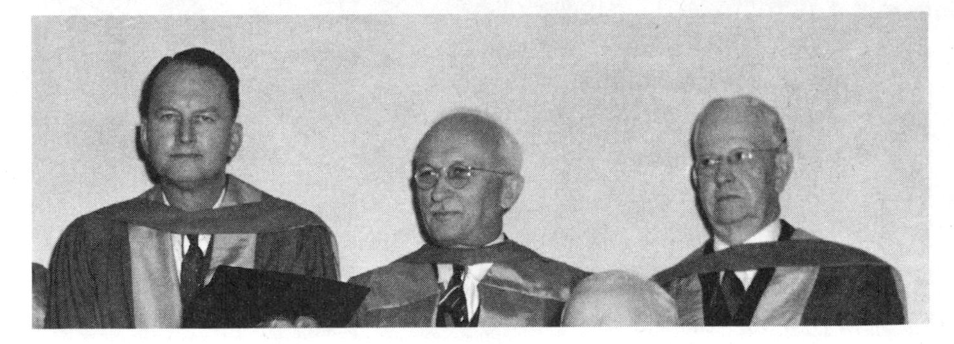

Frederick D. Mott, Harvey G. Agnew, and R.D. Defries receiving honorary LLD degrees, University of Saskatchewan, 14 May 1955. This coincided with the opening of the University Hospital in Saskatoon at which Tommy Douglas presided. Its first CEO was a former DOHA faculty member (University of Saskatchewan, University Archives & Special Collections, Photograph Collection, A-1695)

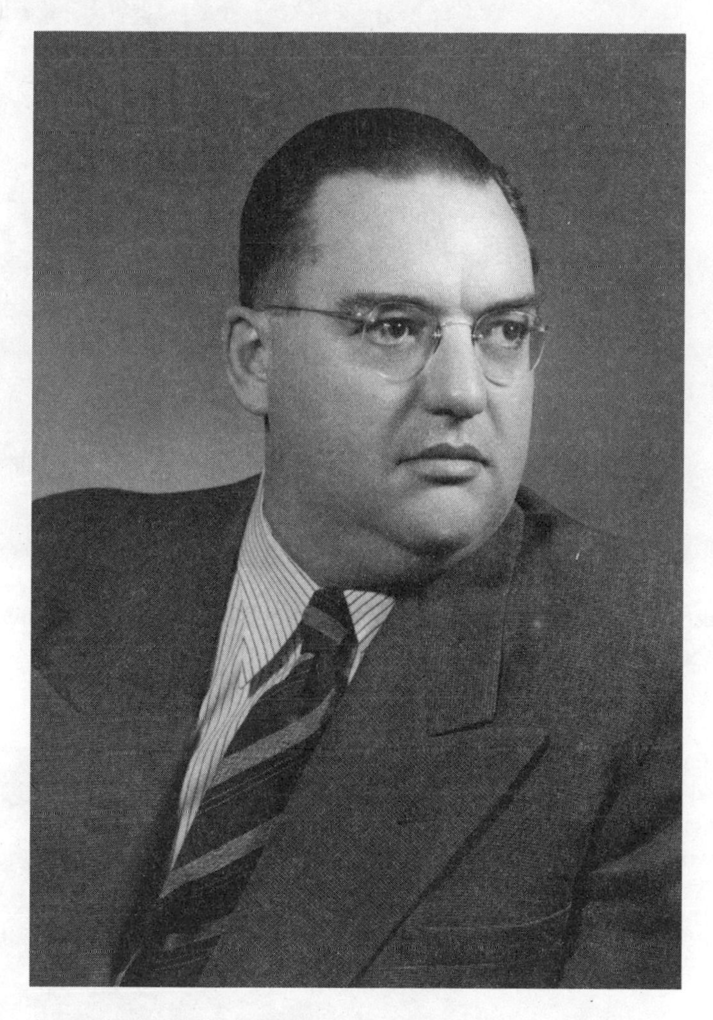

Burns Roth while deputy minister, Department of Public Health, Saskatchewan (Provincial Archives of Saskatchewan, R_A8056)

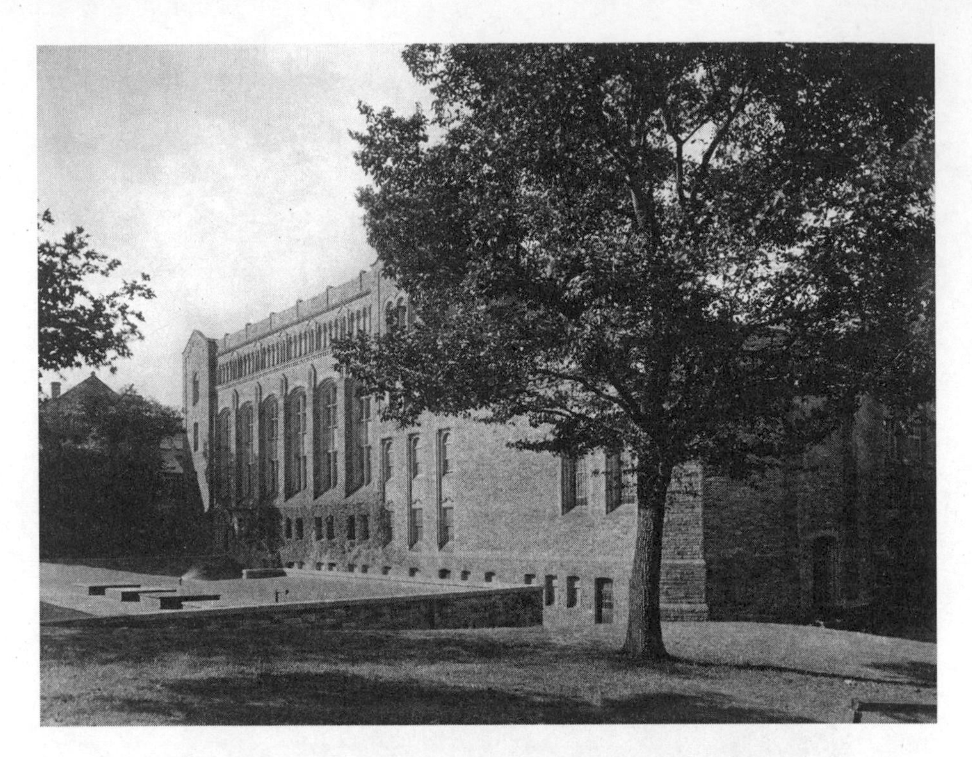

IHPME's second home – McMurrich Building (University of Toronto Archives, A2012-0009/036[08])

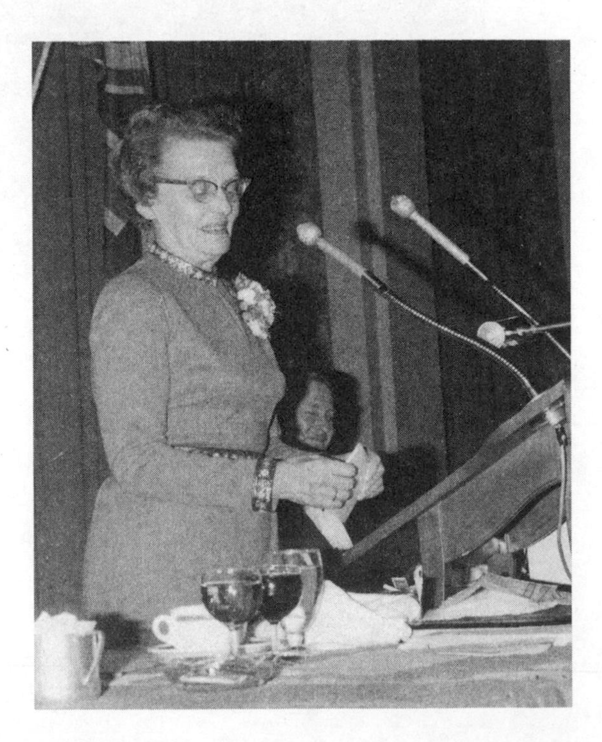

Eugenie Stuart at her retirement, Royal York Hotel, Toronto, 25 October 1971 (University of Toronto Archives, A1998-0023/002)

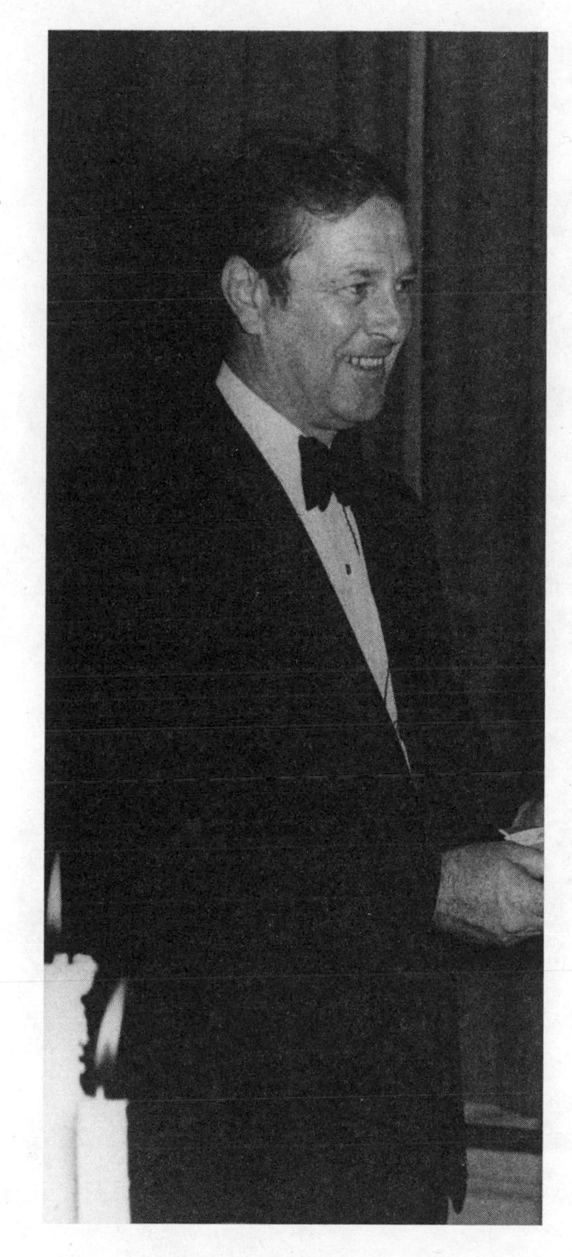

Jim McNab (at the time CEO of TGH) at Eugenie Stuart's retirement (University of Toronto Archives, A1998-0023/002)

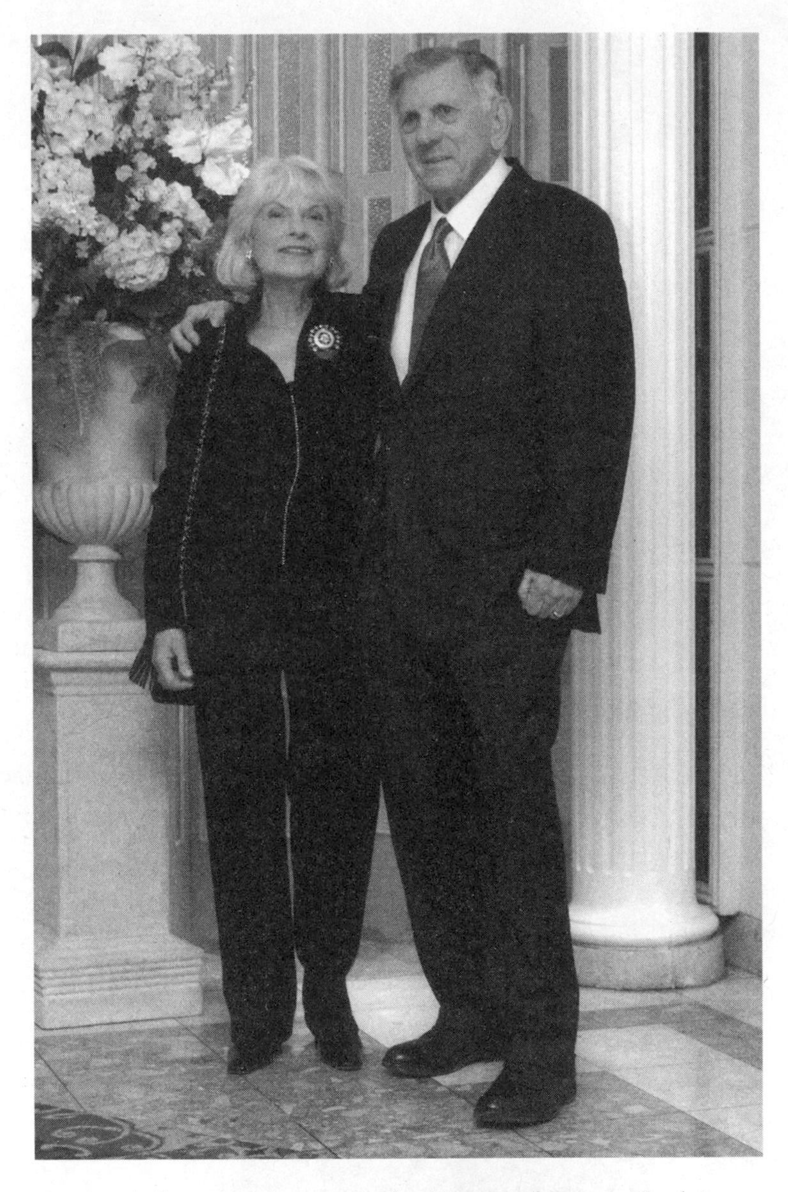

Gene and Elaine Vayda (personal collection of Eugene Vayda)

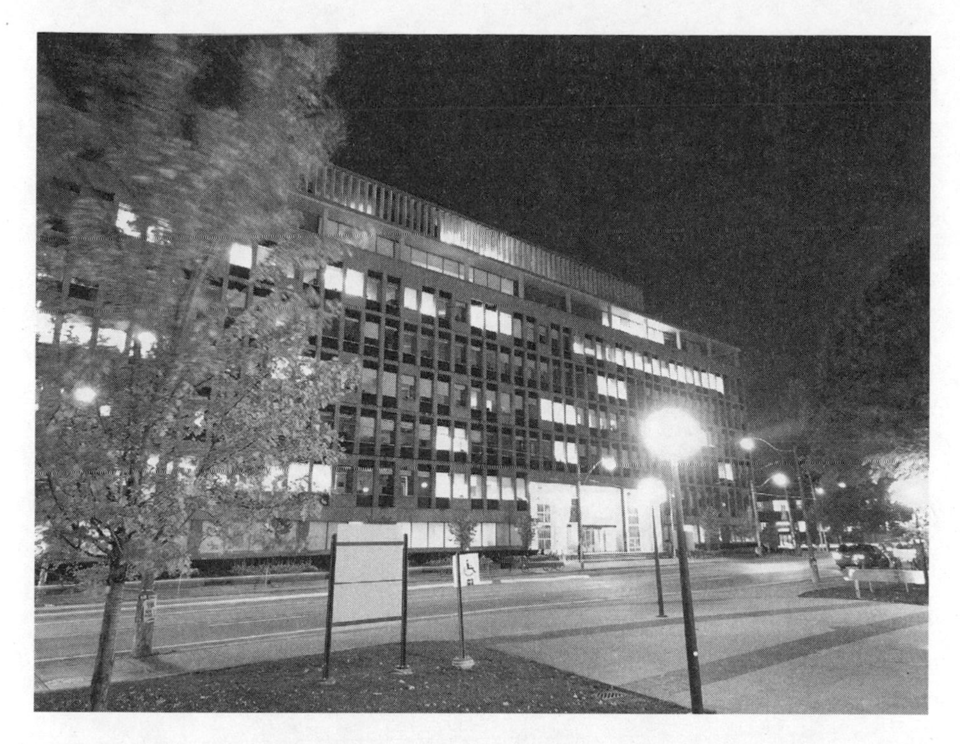

IHPME's third and present home – Health Sciences Building (U of T, Bloomberg School of Nursing photo)

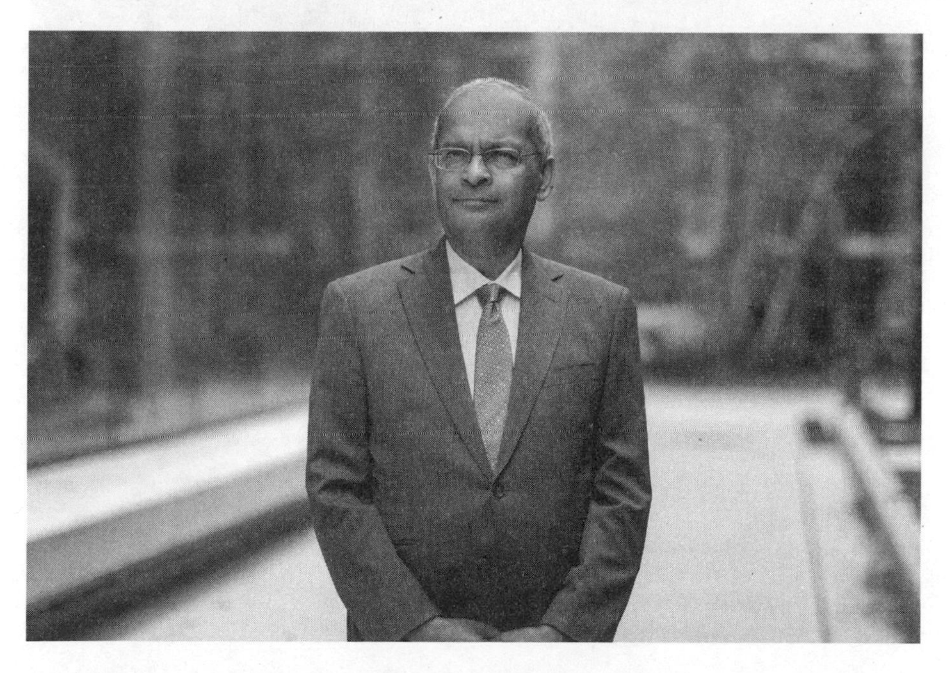

Vivek Goel – on his reappointment as VP, Research and Innovation, U of T in 2019 (U of T, Office of Research and Innovation photo)

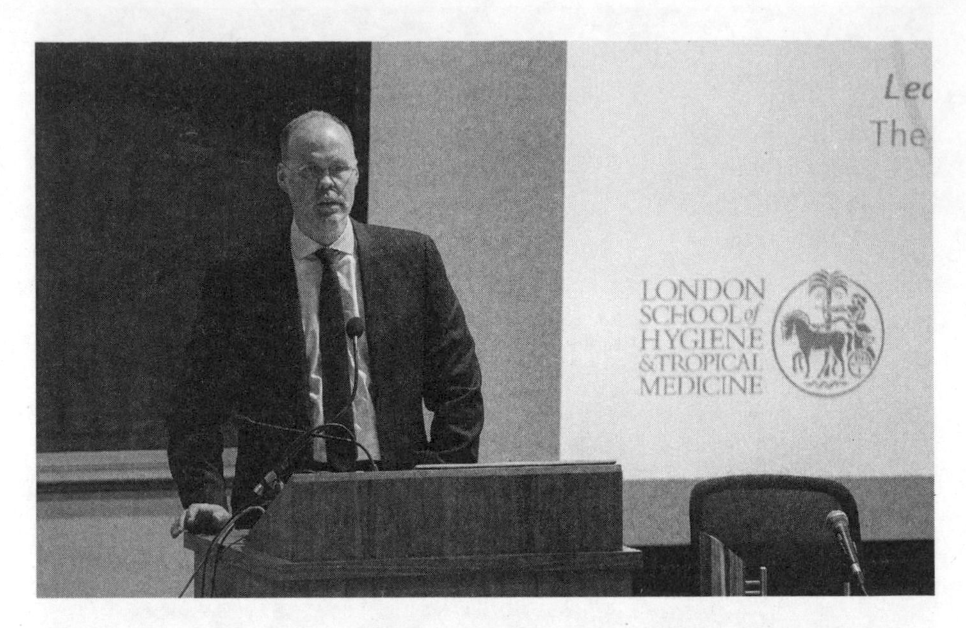

Former IHPME director and current dean of DLSPH, Adalsteinn "Steini" Brown, at the inaugural Boehm Lectures, 29 November 2018 (DLSPH photo)

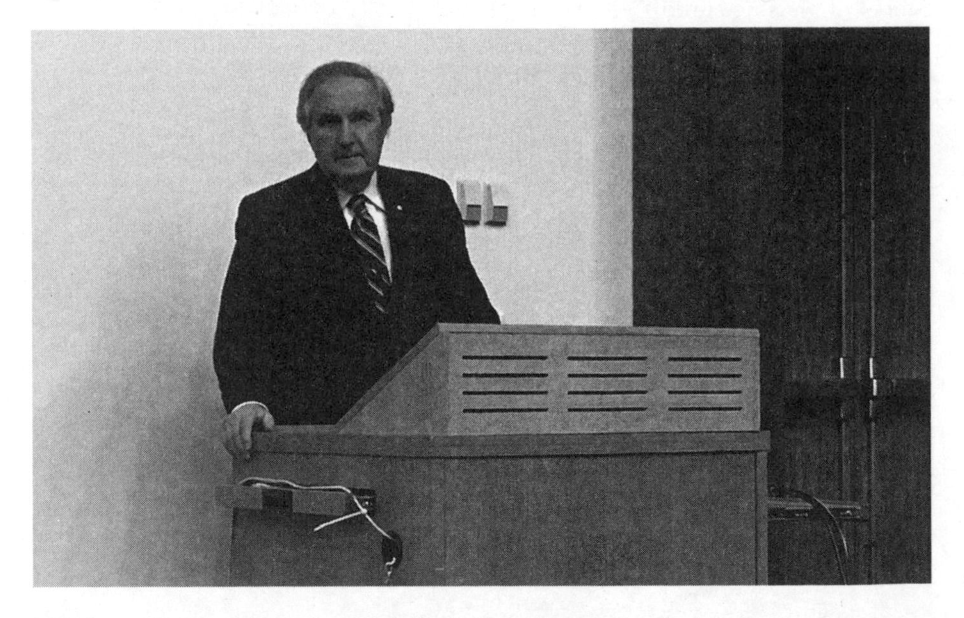

Former premier and royal commissioner Roy Romanow, at the NAO launch, 6 February 2017 (NAO photo)

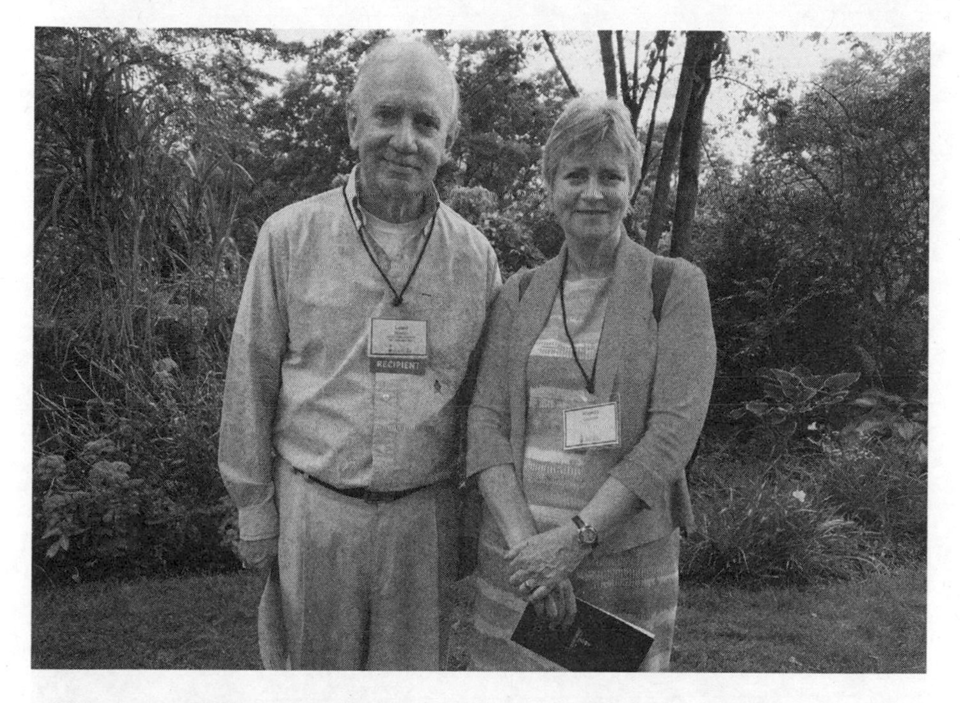

Les Boehm and Rhonda Cockerill, interim director, IHPME, at the U of T Arbor Awards, U of T President's Estate, 14 September 2017 (IHPME photo)

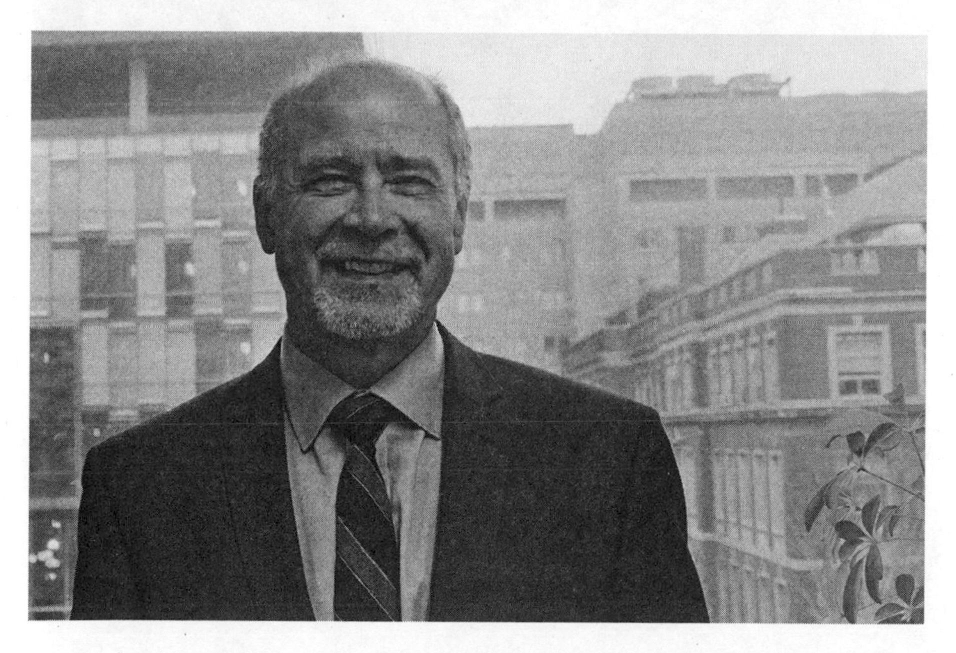

IHPME faculty member and founding director of the NAO Greg Marchildon. The symbolism in this picture is apt as behind Greg (left to right) are the CCBR (medical research), Faculty of Medicine, and FitzGerald buildings (IHPME photo)

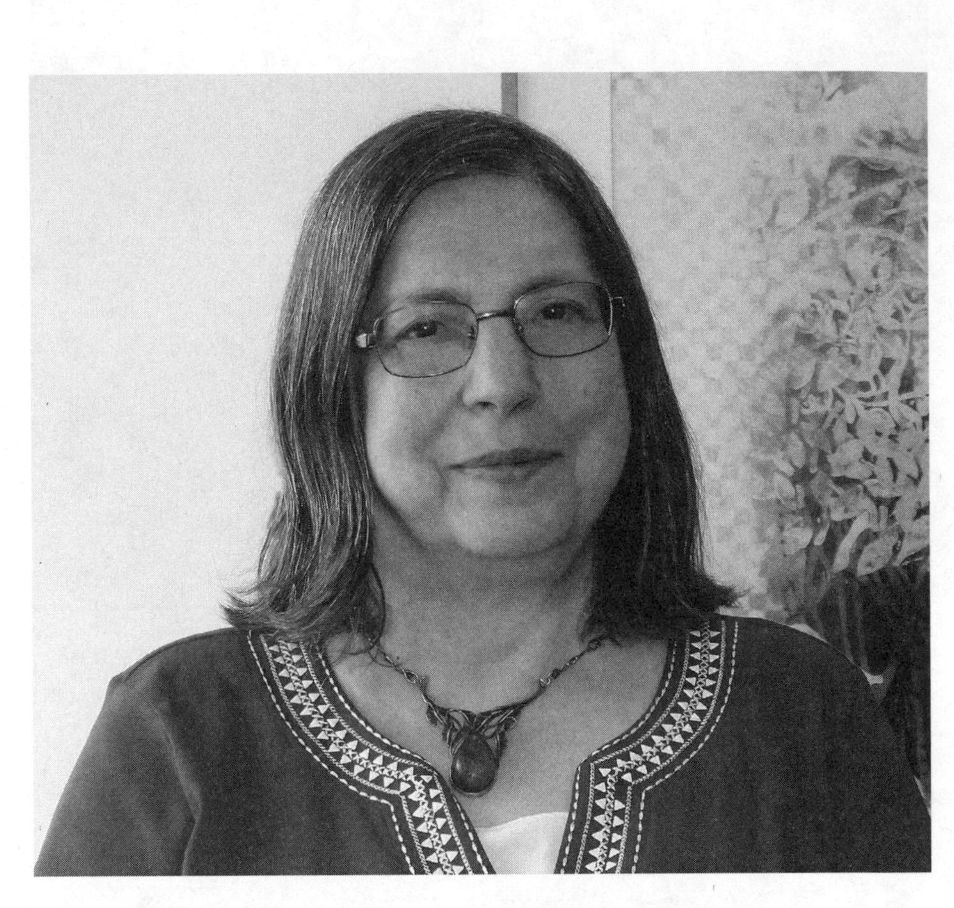

Raisa Deber book launch, 7 February 2019 (R. Deber collection)

PART ONE

Introduction

CHAPTER 1

IHPME's Immediate Context

GENESIS

It was September 1947, and the new Department of Hospital Administration at the University of Toronto was welcoming its first class. The university had chosen to locate this new program within its school of public health – the School of Hygiene – a school of international repute, one of three funded by the Rockefeller Foundation in the 1920s. And its founder, Dr J.G. FitzGerald, enjoyed a similar international reputation.

This new department had a legacy to live up to and it would not disappoint. The reputation of the school attracted the top hospital authority in Canada, Dr Harvey Agnew, another with a reputation that extended beyond our borders.

Through Agnew the new department immediately gained national stature and become known outside Canada. For many years the number of US applicants to the program exceeded Canadian ones. But most important, its graduates assumed leadership positions in hospitals across Canada. Many became community leaders.

Canada has a special feeling for its hospitals and its health-care system. Medicare is said to be part of the Canadian identity, part of the glue that binds this country together.

This new area of health – curative medicine and its companion, health insurance – came to eclipse public health. Through this new department both the school and its university gained an important foothold in this new area.

It was a move that has been given further impetus. In 2012 the United Nations passed a resolution on universal health coverage.[1] The *Economist* in 2018 had a cover story on universal health care.[2] The Oxfam 2019 annual report on economic inequality, released each January before the Davos Conference, concentrated on universal health care and education.[3] In September 2019 the UN convened a special meeting on universal health coverage for heads of state prior to debate of the General Assembly at its seventy-fourth session.[4]

Two of the world's premier policy institutes – the Royal Institute of International Affairs (RIIA) and the Council on Foreign Relations (CFR) – have started health divisions, and health insurance is prominent. The RIIA has convened a Universal Health Coverage (UHC) Policy Forum.[5] Its head notes that universal health coverage is "a potent vote winner." And it notes Canada's implementation of UHC in 1968 and, significantly, mentions Tommy Douglas as "one of the great UHC leaders of the 20th century."[6]

Health care is iconic and its shape in UHC is one of the most magnificent accomplishments of the last century. The mission of IHPME has never been more important.

To keep pace in the ensuing years, the department moved beyond hospital administration to health administration, then beyond professional health education to concentration on research, which involved analysis of health systems and policy. It became the centre of this activity in Canada. Its relevance was underscored by the fact that the RIIA was looking at health insurance programs in both developing and developed countries.[7]

This volume will take you on the journey of this accomplishment. We Canadians tend to be a deferential lot, not ones to boast. Yet in health we have had our moments. However, we have not continued to build on our accomplishments. What is now the Institute of Health Policy, Management, and Evaluation has never been more important.

But let's return now to what was happening that fall 1947. In this young country, just eighty years old, with the world catching its breath on the second anniversary of the end of the most destructive war in history, we see the site of yet another Canadian first: the first program of hospital administration in Canada. This program and these students established themselves almost immediately at the centre of hospital management in Canada.

The creation of this new department was at the forefront of establishing graduate education in health management. It was at the end of the Second World War that the establishment of formal studies in hospital administration in the university really got underway. Many new programs were established in the 1950s so that by 1960 there were eighteen graduate programs in hospital administration,[8] with the U of T program amongst the first.

The Department of Hospital Administration – and the School of Hygiene of which it was a part – were unique Canadian variants on a theme. The defining characteristic of Toronto's school was how seriously it took its mission of having impact, with its intimate link to public health departments across the country and also to a company that produced the fruits of its research. There were also other programs of hospital administration, but none spawned a national network that stretched across a country of continental scale.

That this was possible in Canada was due to the prominence of its first director, Agnew. His national connections reached back to his being head of Hospital Services for the Canadian Medical Association beginning in the 1920s. He was also instrumental in founding the Canadian Hospital Council and its publication, *Canadian Hospital*. Successive classes of graduates formed a strong and involved alumni who established connections to the senior administrators at their former residency hospitals. Most of these administrators were not graduates of the program but became part of the network.

The other defining characteristic of the department and the school was the leaders they produced. In any major event in hospitals or public health there was at least one graduate from the hospital administration or public health program. The same was true regarding the DPH in many ministries across the country.

The hospital administration program was also part of a larger picture. It started in a defining moment of health-care history worldwide. The Western world was debating health insurance and almost every Western country began to implement its own interpretation of this idea. Hospitals were a centrepiece. They were also coming into their own as centres of care and evolving into the most complex of organizations. Canada, along with the United States and European countries, was focused intently on hospitals. The discussion on health insurance, with hospitals as a centrepiece, intensified this focus.

Saskatchewan's Premier Tommy Douglas launched its hospital insurance program, among the first of its kind in the world, in January of the same year the Toronto hospital administration program opened its doors. Douglas took a personal interest in health care; in his first term he was his own health minister as well as premier. During that year, as well, international attention was focused on the United Kingdom, which was feverishly planning implementation of its National Health Service (NHS) the following year.

The implementation of health insurance schemes instantly created a whole new area of major activity. In the United Kingdom, as an example, the NHS immediately became one of the nation's largest employers. The notion of stewardship, of both hospitals and health systems, became important.

These facts necessitated a hospital management program. There was also the prominence of hospitals to Canadians. In many communities they were the largest employer, and source of community pride, emblematic of the spirit of Canadian volunteerism. They came to be at the centre of two of the most iconic social reform schemes at that time.

Years later Saskatchewan pioneered again and launched a medical insurance program. Each Saskatchewan program became a template for a national program. And each was instrumental in the creation of a healthcare system, professionalizing the conduct of health care and initiating organizational infrastructure at government and institutional levels. Health emerged as a centrepiece of government. And the Toronto program was central to the creation of a new profession of hospital and health administrator.

This is the story of the seventy-year history of what today is called the Institute of Health Policy, Management, and Evaluation, more popularly known as IHPME. Founded as the Department of Hospital Administration within the School of Hygiene at the U of T, it very quickly became Canada's national school of health management. First it focused on hospital administration, as hospitals were the pre-eminent health institution of that time, then promptly ramped up to full enrolment. Demand was such that each year it turned away large numbers of qualified applicants. Its graduates were soon found in leading hospitals across the country.

The subject matter of IHPME's predecessor department – health, and hospitals more specifically – was very much in the public mind at that time. The year 1947 was particularly auspicious. It was the second fall since the end of the war and the world had had time to gather its wits. Society was being reoriented toward the goals of peacetime. Reconstruction was the buzzword throughout the Western world.

A HISTORICAL CONTEXT

One cannot separate the inception of IHPME from its historical context.

Generally

The import of what IHPME and the DLSPH do in health is underscored by the fact that health history is becoming a part of our general history. In Canada there are numerous histories of our hospitals, as there are in the United States and the United Kingdom. The United Kingdom also has many books on its welfare state and on the NHS. One by Webster on the NHS and another by Timmins on the welfare state have been directed to the general public to wide acclaim.[9]

Hospitals also form a part of our popular consciousness. There has been a hospital series on television almost since it started. Two popular programs today are *New Amsterdam*, modelled on New York's Bellevue Hospital and based on the book *Twelve Patients*, and *Charité*, based on the iconic Berlin hospital of the same name, ranked number five in the world by *Newsweek*.[10]

Another indication of the import comes from the French historian Fernand Braudel, who suggests that public health is one reason we were able to get ahead in population size and scale up our economy: "Until the eighteenth century, the population was enclosed within an almost intangible circle. Whenever it expanded as far as the circumference, it would almost immediately pull up short and then withdraw."[11]

A major restriction was "a constant stream of diseases."[12] He notes, "These diseases are still encountered today, but yesterday they were apocalyptic scourges.... Infant mortality was enormous ... and health in general was precarious."[13] And "until recent times man's history has implacably been governed by poor health."[14]

Braudel was a member of the *Annales* school of history in France. One of their projects was a five-volume history of the everyday life of people, and health figured in each volume. The last volume covers the need for state intervention in public health and the state's role in making "the medical system accessible to the entire population."[15] It points to the importance of what IHPME and the DLSPH do.

Another facet of this kind of historical treatment of social policy is its inclusion in the historical literature of a country. Britain has a more fulsome experience of it than Canada. It integrates such policy aims into its history. Britain has explored the ground-breaking social policies it developed in education, health, pensions, and the like from roughly 1940 to 1950.[16] Works such as these suggest that our interest in health moves beyond its utility to our everyday lives, beyond policy development, and into our historical consciousness.

And in this there was a notable interaction between government and an intellectual elite. Barnett notes, "There existed ... a constant osmosis between Whitehall and the wider intellectual élite on the topic."[17] There was such an interchange between the School of Hygiene and both levels of government in Canada, especially in FitzGerald's time. We will see the same thing between these levels of government with IHPME and its predecessor departments, which Steini Brown has emphasized as head of IHPME and the DLSPH.

Canada

A part of its history was where IHPME was situated, which was important in two respects. First, and more immediate, was its location within U of T in an internationally recognized school of public health. This school had a culture of excellence and functioned at the highest standards. Its reputation allowed it to look for and attract the top expert on hospitals in Canada. This set the stage for the new department to function at the same high level, and it immediately operated on a national scale. It was able to place its graduates in the top hospitals across Canada, and many became leaders in their communities.

However, though this new graduate program was located in a school of public health, its area of concentration – hospital administration – was not born of public health. It was part of a new, distinct, and parallel activity. Its genesis was in two new and massive movements in health. The first was the rise of medical science in curative modalities, the other the concept of universal social programs, specifically universal health insurance. These led to a concentration on illness care and the centre within which to do it – hospitals.

Tommy Douglas understood this. In a debate in the Saskatchewan Legislature at the same time that discussions were taking place at U of T on the formation of the new hospital administration program, he distinguished between "a program of prevention and hygiene" and "curative services." He said, "The work of my Department can be divided into roughly two categories. On the one hand, there is the work of the established Department: looking after established institutions; providing certain fixed services; carrying on a program of prevention and hygiene. On the other hand, there is the Health Services Planning Commission, whose task it is to ... bring into operation new curative services ... making available to the people of the province the health services which they so urgently need and I think, so greatly desire."[18]

He understood the magnitude of the frontier he was crossing. His commission was separate from his department, and it reported directly to him. Bear in mind that he would implement his hospital insurance program eighteen months ahead of the NHS in the United Kingdom.

This is the second aspect. The hospital administration program was born amidst the most extraordinary social and scientific advances of the last century. While it was not realized at the time, what was taking place was the creation of a new and immense activity in society generally, and health in particular. Hospitals and physician care became an increasing preoccupation of governments worldwide and, in a decentralized federation like Canada, of our provincial governments.

The issues were access and affordability. Provincial governments were grappling with both. Taylor notes that in the eight years since the Second World War, hospital expenditures had increased 250 per cent.[19] Canada had already established a deep tradition in hospital care. Each province had its own initiatives. Saskatchewan had already developed the municipal doctor program to attract physicians to the rural areas, and it had developed the union hospital program for municipalities to band together to build and operate hospitals. As early as 1933 urban and rural municipal associations in Saskatchewan advocated for provincial hospital and medical treatment. However, such ideas proved stillborn, until the inception of the hospital administration program. Tommy Douglas, holding the twin portfolios of premier and health minister, had both the personal commitment and the administrative skill to launch its largest single program, ever. And he would take graduates from both the DHA and DPH programs to help build his system.

The U of T program was launched amidst a rapid acceleration in social thinking. During the Second World War, nations had also been devoting time and energy to reconstruction – the world after the war. Health care was prominent, part of a constellation of social policies that included full employment, pensions, and housing, among others.

After the Second World War all Western nations conceived and pursued certain *universal* programs in one form or another, of which health care was the centrepiece. Nations figured out how to mitigate certain health risks, how to take a principle – insurance – and apply it to everyone. Churchill captured the thinking when he said, "We bring in the magic of averages to the aid of the million."[20] It was less about income redistribution and more about mitigating risk.

Saskatchewan and the United Kingdom led the way respectively with the implementation of hospital insurance on 1 January 1947 and the NHS on 5 July 1948. Other countries soon followed suit. In Canada there was a significant series of events: the introduction of the National Health Grants program (1948), BC's universal hospital insurance program (1949), Ontario's voluntary insurance initiatives (1950s), national hospital insurance (1957), Saskatchewan's universal medical insurance program (1962), the report of the Royal Commission on Health Services (1964), and national medical insurance (1968).

The initiatives of the later 1940s through the 1950s displayed a new focus on hospital and health management. The Second World War had "fostered an unprecedented sense of social unity."[21] The creation of the NHS in Britain was "the result of a new ideological shift toward universalism in welfare provision."[22] "Hospital medicine got a big boost and promotion to centre-stage" and hospital medicine acquired an "elite status."[23] These same sentiments were present in Canada.

Governments became important new players, staffing up and creating new areas of oversight and expertise. Saskatchewan created a new section within the Health Services Planning Commission – the Saskatchewan Hospital Services Plan – which began to staff up in the summer and autumn of 1946, just prior to the inception of the DHA program. Changes were so large and quick that it had trouble securing space and materials, and staff were temporarily housed in converted army huts.[24] BC followed with the British Columbia Hospital Insurance Service in 1949. The major activity was collecting and dispensing funds, but both provinces hired staff consultants to advise on hospital operations. Each also had a division to advise on hospital construction.[25] Ontario created the Ontario Hospital Services Commission (1956).

For each province these were major new activities and the premiers took great care in setting them up. Indeed, each premier – Tommy Douglas in Saskatchewan, Byron "Boss" Johnson of BC, and Leslie Frost of Ontario – is remembered for implementing these programs.

These new divisions within government ministries meant new jobs for DHA grads. For example, Burns Roth went to be the head of a new hospital division in Saskatchewan in 1950.[26] Rod Thorfinnson did the same ten years later.[27] Jim McNab went to the BC Hospital Insurance Service in 1951 and the Ontario Hospital Services Commission in 1961.[28]

With government a new and significant player, the concept of a health system emerged. Hospitals were no longer just a collection of largely independent and uncoordinated voluntary institutions. They began to be organized into primary (local), secondary (regional), and tertiary facilities. There was also an exploration of how hospitals related to other forms of health care, such as physician care and community care. And there were discussions on the scope of health insurance benefits, such as drug, dental, mental health, and home care. All of this taken together was the milieu surrounding this new program.

Health care quickly became iconic. For instance, both the British public and the NHS employees immediately took the NHS to heart; both had very strong feelings about it. In Canada, medicare became part of a national identity, part of what makes us Canadian. Worldwide, health care became a showcase of medical science, of hospitals, of academic health sciences centres, and of research institutes.

Health care showcased government ability to manage such massive programs. It was held in common, by government on our behalf. Everyone – no matter the station – was equally entitled to it. In this sense it was not only about alleviating illness, it was also about nation-building. It epitomized a sense of solidarity, of community. It became a bedrock of citizenship.

These programs were part of a profound transformation in health care, one not limited to Britain and Canada. They were amongst the most ambitious peacetime initiatives ever implemented. They were largely independent of public health, to the extent that when people think of health they think of medicare, not public health. In fact our major challenge today is to integrate them – to integrate a concern with the social and preventive aspects of medicine with curative medicine. Their result was that *individual* health and *illness* care eclipsed *population* health and *prevention*.

When the Department of Hospital Administration was formed, within the School of Hygiene many wondered about its inclusion. They felt it was very much a junior partner. Little did they know that the graduates of this new degree would soon be at the heart of the health system. It would begin as a purely professional school, but by its seventieth year graduate education and research would eclipse professional education. In addition, the location of this new department within the school meant that the school had hedged its bets; it was covering both aspects of health: individual health/illness and population health/prevention.

That said, public health soon enough made its influence felt once again. In the 1950s the United Kingdom queried why dramatic improvements in population health engendered by the NHS had stalled. By the 1960s it established that other non-health factors that figured prominently in health.[29] Canada did important work in this area in the 1970s.[30] And U of T, which lost momentum in public health with the dissolution of the School of Hygiene, still did important work in this area with public health faculty within

IHPME and was back in the fold with important work by Naylor and Goel and the establishment of the DLSPH by the 2000s.

Throughout this work we will look further into the intimate relationship between this educational program and the events surrounding it, how the two evolved in lockstep with each other, and how each shaped the other. The evolving complexity of both entities is fascinating. In its overt activity the IHPME of today bears little resemblance to the original department, yet the values that underpin each – the dedication of the faculty, their commitment to graduate education and to provincial and national health systems – are identical.

International

The war had accelerated several trends in health. In 1938, in anticipation of war casualties, the British government brought all hospitals under its control through the Emergency Hospital Service (EHS). This immediately created a hospital *system.* It then did the same with physicians through the Emergency Medical Service, creating an entire health system.

In 1942 the Beveridge Report (UK) caused an international sensation and amplified hopes for health insurance. Beveridge came to Canada in 1943 to speak at a joint session of two committees of the House of Commons. Canada had its own version of the report written by a former graduate student of Beveridge's, Leonard Marsh.

The post-war reconstruction period in Canada (and the United States) emphasized hospitals, witnessing the growth of hospitals in both countries. Governments on both sides of the border, nationally and sub-nationally, were looking at ways to help build and operate them. In addition, there was pent up demand. In Canada major institutions such as Toronto General Hospital and SickKids had put expansion plans on hold during the war and full energy was now redirected toward implementing them.

In 1946 the Hill-Burton Act ushered in unprecedented levels of hospital construction in the United States, which then spurred rapid advances in hospital design. It also elevated attention on hospitals and increased their profile in the public mind. In December of that year Paul Martin Sr became Canada's minister of national health and welfare. He had an interest not only in health insurance but also in what other countries were doing in that vein. We will see later the interactions former DHA student Burns Roth had with him.

In January 1947 Saskatchewan introduced the first plank of its own health insurance program, which was the first universal hospital insurance plan on the continent. This put more attention on hospitals and, as it would turn out, on graduates of the new DHA program. The Saskatchewan hospital insurance initiative was followed by a federal hospital grants program in 1948 and a hospital insurance program in BC in 1949 – heralding government as an important new player in health. The ensuing need to plan and operate under government mandates added to the skill set required of administrators and expanded the need for this program's graduates (both in hospitals and in government).

On Monday, 5 July 1948, the National Health Service began in the United Kingdom. Its health minister, Aneurin Bevan, had famously called it "the most civilised thing in the world."[31] It alone in the world began providing comprehensive health care to its entire population. It nationalized hospitals and immediately become one of the nation's largest employers. But more importantly the NHS immediately entered the public consciousness as an instrument that made all citizens equal in their right to receive care. It removed a significant risk and expense from the shoulders of the population and put it on the shoulders of the nation. It created a new measure of citizen solidarity with each other and with the nation. On the basis of its unique characteristics from the moment of its inception it came under an international spotlight. It became a pre-eminent national institution, both the public and NHS staff developing strong feelings toward it. Other countries followed suit.

Canada, a young nation, was among them, influenced by Saskatchewan, where a new organization was born. It would quickly staff up, and one of this U of T program's earliest students (Burns Roth) cut short the administrative residency portion of the program out of an acutely experienced urgency to become a part of Tommy Douglas's experiment – Douglas at the time being his own health minister. He would become a part of this grand plan, rise to become a deputy minister in the Douglas government, and eventually return to the U of T DHA program as its director.

As Nicholas Timmins has put it in his award-winning book on the welfare state, "The story of the welfare state is a great adventure."[32] Indeed it is, and universal health care is its linchpin, and the progenitors of each in its gestation period – people like Tommy Douglas in Canada or Bevan and Atlee in the United Kingdom – are to be celebrated for their bold vision and skilful implementation. As an aside, Timmins continued his involvement in health care, working with Sir Chris Ham, the CEO of King's Fund.[33] Chris, in turn, became involved with Steini Brown in Dalla Lana initiatives.

In this work, historical context is important. The type of history just outlined forms its scaffolding. This U of T DHA program was developed within a certain national and international climate. Britain launched the NHS amidst almost crippling war debt and a country still struggling to regain its social equilibrium. The full text of Bevan's observation acknowledged it. He said, "We ought to take a pride in the fact that, despite our financial and economic anxieties, we are still able to do the most civilised thing in the world – put the welfare of the sick in front of every other consideration."[34] Saskatchewan's financial challenges were no less acute. Douglas launched hospital insurance while the province had the highest per capita debt in the nation.

This is the milieu of the department and its early students. This is the legacy they helped to create and uphold.

Meanwhile, the pace of the department's ascendancy was due in part to its placement within the School of Hygiene, its first director and his connections, and the events around it.

EMBEDDED WITHIN A SCHOOL OF HYGIENE

It is because of these interrelationships that a fulsome understanding of the role of IHPME must begin with some understanding of the role of the school and of its founding director, J.G. FitzGerald.

FitzGerald and his colleagues were more than just part of a rapidly evolving health-care scene in Canada; they were among its progenitors, its authors. Moreover, what was remarkable was not just the services they put in place; it was the ideals and the principles that animated them. Further, these principles, their emphasis on public institutions providing a public service and on universality became an integral part of the Canadian identity. There were three parts: health care as an entitlement, the emphasis on public institutions, and availability to all (universal access).

FitzGerald and the school (and Connaught Laboratories) were remarkable, stories in themselves and there are books devoted to each.[35] Their roles were important for IHPME, the university, and indeed this country. For IHPME, the school was a requirement; the Kellogg Foundation was funding four new programs in hospital administration – but only in universities that would locate them within a school of public health.

Being embedded in the school also influenced IHPME through its character or disposition. The ideals and the culture of the school – such as its emphasis on practice and impact, and its national orientation – became aspects of IHPME's predecessor department. Because its influence was powerful, we will begin with a focused outline of FitzGerald and the school. It will also be important in its own right. In its select emphasis of particular facets of each of FitzGerald and the school it will be covering new ground.

Another part to the inclusion of FitzGerald that is particularly relevant to this work is the connections that are made to his administrative ability. That ability was innate in him; however, he recognized the importance of the education of health administrators and supported a nursing initiative in hospital administration before the advent of IHPME's predecessor department. We will see examples of the administrative associations made to FitzGerald and his support of administrative education at various points in this work.

PART OF A DOWNTOWN URBAN CAMPUS

Integral to the department was its location in a downtown campus. There was then, and is even more so today, a vibrancy to having a campus in the city's core. It facilitates the accessibility of faculty and students to related areas such as decision-makers in business and government.

For example, on some days I would hop over to the Legislative Building across from the McMurrich Building to listen to Premier Bill Davis debate with Stephen Lewis. Or Al Rands would allow me to use his office in the Ministry of Health on the tenth floor of the in the Hepburn Block, which made this young graduate student at the time feel very much a part of the system of which he was to become a part.

THE U OF T

There were also qualities of the university itself. A U of T publication at the time noted that a university is "an entire community."[36] Also, "The University of Toronto is *big*," "Size has an excitement of its own," and its library system is "Canada's biggest single intellectual resource."[37] It said, "At the University of Toronto you will enter a tradition of achievement."[38] It is apparent as soon as one sets foot on this campus. This would certainly be so with the hospital administration students of the late 1940s and beyond who would make their mark on major hospitals in Canada.

It was and is a university with a deep history. Mackenzie King was a student of University College (class of 1895).[39] It's said he "cut his political teeth" during the student strike of 1895.[40] Lester Pearson was a student of Victoria College. One need only glance at the alumni rolls of the university to recognize names of intellectual, business, media, or public service achievement of this nation.

One cannot set foot on this campus without a sense of this antiquity. On the one hand one looks around and is very much in the present, students running to class, people in labs doing experiments. And yet, as paradoxical as it seems, ever present is the past, the accumulated contribution of those who have come before – the shoulders upon whom we stand. One especially senses it in some of its oldest buildings, the refectories of Trinity, Victoria, and University Colleges or Hart House; the old wood, built-in bookshelves and huge leather couches of the Hart House Library, or views from the observation deck into the Fisher Rare Book Library. This university is built on their accomplishment.

Another part to the character of the U of T is one of place. We noted the location of its main campus in the heart of the city. It also includes its place in relation to the world at large. This university relates to its city, its province, its nation, and the world – the "global village," to coin a term from one of its more famous faculty. This is absolutely essential for an outward-looking nation like Canada. A university such as this is a conduit to the world at large.

All of this, for this person at least, also evoked a sense of wonder in U of T. The breadth of its collection at Robarts, the number of leather-bound books dating from the early 1800s, that were shelved amongst all the others at Robarts and Sci Med (as the Gerstein Library was then called) was part of this sense of wonder. Another was authors of books this person had read or heard of who were on faculty. Another was people like John Turner, minister of finance, or Pierre Elliott Trudeau, at the time the prime minister, who came to Convocation Hall to speak.

Important as well was that this university was a public university. And it took its public mission seriously. Such public institutions are very important for a nation. They are anchor institutions, institutions of excellence for the nation. This university belongs to Ontario; it also belongs to Canada.

A METAMORPHOSIS FROM A HOSPITAL TO SYSTEMIC FOCUS

The department was inextricably linked to events occurring around it. Provincial ministries of health were moving away from an exclusively public health focus – the health of populations – and becoming concerned with individual health and illness care. Hospitals were the first recipients. As hospitals became an increasing preoccupation of the provincial ministries, it was axiomatic there would be an increasing preoccupation with their management.

This was reinforced roughly ten years after the department began with the introduction of a national hospital insurance program, which would add important new stakeholders (the public, government) to the system. As the hospital sector became more sophisticated, more dependent on the need to plan and operate under government mandates, so too did the need for a different skill set among senior administrators.[41]

Over time the department moved away from its exclusively hospital-centric, practical orientation. Professional education remained an important, even major activity but it reoriented itself to the education of health (not only hospital) administrators.

In addition, two other forces were at work. There was a broadening focus on two other fronts. First was U of T itself, which began in the 1960s to increasingly emphasize research and strong disciplinary studies. It became progressively more research-intensive. Second, within the department the focus broadened. It is no longer just upon management. It now also entailed analysis – of systems, practice, processes of delivery, outcomes. It also included knowing which interventions were needed to improve them, as well as how best to implement them. The department followed the university's lead and placed greater emphasis on research.

THE UNIVERSITY AVENUE MEDICAL CLUSTER

As all of these forces were at work, another phenomenon was at work – a concentration of hospital – or, more accurately – health sciences activity. After the Second World War there emerged what I call "the University Avenue medical cluster." At that time it involved three large teaching hospitals, the faculty of medicine, and some of the departments of the School of Hygiene. Today it is much more than this and we will explore it in more detail later.

HISTORICAL TIES

On 1 July 2017 Dr Adalsteinn Brown formally relinquished his role as chair of the Institute of Health Policy, Management and Evaluation (IHPME) to become the interim dean of the Dalla Lana School of Public Health. His transition from this institute to a public health school was but the latest iteration and emblematic of an almost inextricable relationship between two such organizations. Whilst 2017 marked the seventieth anniversary of IHPME it also marked the ninetieth anniversary of the formal opening of the School of Hygiene, the precursor to the Dalla Lana School and also the faculty where IHPME was initially housed.[42]

In addition, 2017 was the hundredth anniversary of the founding of Connaught Laboratories. It was intimately connected to Hygiene and involved in an area (the application and commercialization of health research) that IHPME would later study. IHPME would also teach courses in this area at the undergraduate and graduate level.

In October 2017 U of T President Gertler, in his welcoming remarks to a packed audience gathered to hear US Senator Bernie Sanders, pointed to just how pivotal IHPME had become in the history of Canadian health care. He noted that the School of Hygiene had "laid the foundation for the development of universal health care" through "former faculty member" Dr Burns Roth.[43] We noted earlier that Burns Roth was an (almost) graduate of the School of Hygiene's Department of Hospital Administration (more on this later). What President Gertler was referring to was that some fifty-five years earlier, on 1 July 1962, Saskatchewan implemented a medical insurance plan that he noted would be "the template for Canadian Medicare." It was also the date that Roth, who had been deputy minister of public health in Saskatchewan and in charge of developing Douglas's program, became a U of T faculty member and director of the Department of Hospital Administration (IHPME's predecessor department) within the School of Hygiene.

President Gertler also alluded to another important contribution of IHPME when he said he saw "the Senator's initiative as part of an important global effort ... the rigorous comparative study of different healthcare systems" and that "the University of Toronto is a global leader" in this endeavour. This activity is exactly the mandate of the North American Observatory on Health Systems and Policies (NAO), which he also mentioned in his introduction.[44] The NAO, through its founding director, Greg Marchildon, a faculty member of IHPME, has been housed at IHPME ever since its inception.

The position of hospitals in that era – what they were and what they should be – was captured by Frederick Mott, at the time a medical student at McGill University who went to Saskatchewan to implement the first hospital insurance program in North America and became a faculty member at IHPME's predecessor department. In an early article he said, "The general hospital should be the organised health center for its area." But, interestingly, he saw it as more than a diagnostic and treatment centre, to also include prevention, public health, health education, social service, and dental hygiene.[45]

There is a certain leitmotif, a certain ethic that is inherent in the School of Hygiene, IHPME, the university, and its major teaching hospitals. All are public institutions, and all are dedicated to a public purpose. All take seriously the fact that they are a public trust. One of these, Toronto General Hospital (which has always had strong connections to IHPME) was rated number seven in the world in a 2019 *Newsweek* ranking.[46] One can add Connaught Labs to this mix, a private institution but, through its ownership by U of T, in public hands, and one that took its public mission very seriously, one that made an indelible mark on the public health of this nation.

But it goes beyond this. A certain theme starts to become apparent. Long before the advent of medicare we see a fundamental ideal emerging, one that became a fundamental tenet of Canadian health care, and that is a principle of inclusion. Bator titles his book *Within Reach of Everyone*. It is an apt phrase, one coined by a *Maclean's* journalist in 1915 when talking about FitzGerald's activities (more about this later in the book).

Toronto General echoed a similar theme. For a time in the 1920s it titled its annual report *For the Common Good*.[47] These annual reports began with a short notation that touched on inclusion and the public trust. It said in part, "Healing all manner of sickness and all manner of disease, for the common good, the Toronto General Hospital, as a public institution, has enjoyed public confidence."[48]

It is a theme embraced by the great public hospitals of many nations. TGH, Bellevue (New York), Barts (London), and Charité (Berlin) are all public institutions – all noted for never turning anyone away. I have been part of that many times at TGH – at 3:00 a.m., the hospital bursting at the seams, looking for more beds. The history of these institutions is legendary. One can only imagine the challenges Charité – a hospital with probably the largest cohort of Nobel laureates in physiology and medicine – faced during six years of war in a city which was 65 per cent destroyed in the end. It is humanity at its best, coping with its worst.[49] Hospitals as a beacon of hope, a symbol of courage.

This is getting at the why. Why are hospitals and public health important? The need for our quintessential large tertiary facilities like a TGH, a Bellevue, Charité, or Barts, or our great public health schools like Dalla Lana, Hopkins, or Harvard, is summed up in the quote by Pulitzer Prize author Oshinsky talking about "The Great Ebola Scare of 2014": "History assures us that Ebola will be fully tamed," but "the next 'fatal strain' is also bubbling up somewhere – in a bat cave, a pig farm, an open-air poultry market. That's the nature of the war between humans and microbes. There is never a truce."[50]

And so there never is. These great public institutions – hospitals, city departments of public health, or the university schools of public health and health administration – stand as beacons of hope and as bulwarks against the worst that nature can throw against us.

From a first concentration on hospitals, a very practical emphasis on hospital management, and a course-based professional graduate degree, it expanded to include thesis-based graduate degrees. The latter included research on health care, health systems, policies, and outcomes. To reflect this, in 2001 the university's governing council approved a name change to the Department of Health Policy, Management and Evaluation (HPME) to include the word *institute* (IHPME). This institute continues to broaden its scope with now also looking into new areas such as the health systems of other countries, an exploration of patient involvement in care and research, and health informatics, to name only a few.

We noted it was a department uniquely positioned to be at the centre of such activities. It was initially nested within an internationally renowned School of Hygiene, which for many years was Canada's only school of public health. IHPME soon established its own national profile, the result, in no small part, of the hospital connections that its first director, Harvey Agnew, had across the country. Also it was next door to the country's largest faculty of medicine. It was physically located (and remains) across from the provincial seat of government. And it is adjacent to one of the larger concentrations of tertiary hospital care.

While initially formed to train people to manage hospitals, after 1967 its program also included the training of public health professionals as the school's Department of Public Health was merged into the Department of Hospital Administration and the Department renamed to *Health* Administration. After a time when this merged department was moved from the school to the Faculty of Medicine, it is today nested again within a reconstituted school of public health.

What is now an institute has a rich heritage in the health care of our country. Its focus on hospitals, public health, and health policy put it at the centre of the Canadian health scene. It began as health was establishing itself as an important national and provincial theme in the country's affairs and evolved as the scope and range of health evolved.

This adaptation and evolution is representative of the institute, constantly at the vanguard, constantly pushing at the frontiers of knowledge of its rapidly evolving discipline. Its faculty has consistently been a part of every major health policy initiative in this province and country with involvement in Royal Commissions and specialized task forces and committees.

The importance of this history is that it is not that this is just a history of a prominent institution – a department that is now an institute. One cannot separate the fact that it is also bound up in a history within a prominent sphere of Canadian activity. Canadians have long associated medicare as a part of the Canadian identity. And we are not alone; the British also feel very strongly about their national health system. What this work will show is that in Canada medicare is but the most recent manifestation of this identity.

IHPME AND ITS BROADER CONNECTIONS

Its Connections to a School of Public Health

For the greater part of its history, IHPME has been nested within a prominent school of public health. The School of Hygiene, its first home, was one of the first three such schools funded by the Rockefeller Foundation in the 1920s. Its present home, within the Dalla Lana School of Public Health, was ranked fifth in the world in a 2017 survey (more on this later).

When the Kellogg Foundation was looking to fund a degree in hospital administration in Canada, one of its requirements was that the program be located within a school of hygiene. The profile of the Toronto school and its standing with the Rockefeller Foundation reflected favourably. Indeed, would Kellogg have funded the first program in Canada had it not been for the School of Hygiene, its reputation, and that of the University of Toronto?

There is also IHPME's own strong connection to public health. While its predecessor department was initially exclusively hospital oriented, that soon changed. Its first director, Harvey Agnew, was a hospital expert. However, its second, Burns Roth, had equal expertise in hospitals and public health. Moreover, during Roth's time the departments of hospital administration and public health merged. The third director, John Hastings, was a public health expert, as was its fourth, Gene Vayda. Indeed, Vayda once remarked to me that for a time IHPME was public health at U of T. We'll talk about this in a bit more detail in the section on his leadership. Suffice to say that after the dissolution of the School of Hygiene and until the DLSPH, a strong argument could be made to support Vayda's statement, that after the School of Hygiene was dissolved the department was the centre for teaching and research in public health at the university until the Dalla Lana School.

There is also the fact that this school had a major national and international influence, in addition to the fact that "public health had long been marked by the transfer of influences and initiatives from one country to another." During the school's existence and its position in and the import of the British Commonwealth, this also meant "Canada, Australia, and New Zealand had influenced public health in Britain previously, and British influences had also been felt in these countries." Also, "Canada played a pioneering role in new public health approaches" of the 1970s, and we will talk about this further in our section on the Lalonde Report.[51]

It is for reasons such as this that a history of the department needs to begin with a brief history of its immediate environment – the School of Hygiene and Connaught Laboratories – an environment that, as history would have it, the department ultimately preserved.

Today public health and health systems are inconceivable without each other, obverse sides of the same coin. At the time this was not evident. At the inception of IHPME's predecessor department, after the Second World War, the whole idea of illness care and hospitals as a significant activity was new and was obtaining a critical mass. And it was doing so in conjunction with another remarkable post-war social invention, the idea of universal health insurance. No one could foresee where this would go, but today it has resulted in a very large new area of health concentration: individual health and curative (or illness) care. This area is complementary to population health and preventive care.

The Breadth of Impact

There is also the issue of impact. We will find that IHPME has had an impact on health care in Canada, but this is part of a bigger picture. Friedland, in his history of U of T, observes that the Massey Commission noted that universities have been a force in Canadian culture,[52] integral parts of the communities in which they are located, and some have had a wider influence. Farley, writing of the International Health Division of the Rockefeller Foundation, called U of T a "fully national university."[53] One could say the same of the department's program in hospital administration.

IHPME began with an outward focus. A majority of its students came from not the city, but from across the province and the nation (and other countries). It was at the leading edge, along with a few US schools, of establishing a new profession. A former head of the department, Burns Roth, noted that the U of T Department in Hospital Administration was one of the first programs established in North America.[54] Its graduates were often found at the leading hospitals of the nation.

IHPME has deep roots in being nested in the university and the School of Hygiene. The sentiment captured by Friedland's quote of the Massey Commission can be said of its faculties. George Beaton, chair of Nutritional Sciences in the School and the school's last director (in an acting capacity), said the school was at the source of a "lot of changes that occurred in Canada, not the least of which were the changes that were happening in health insurance and health care."[55] Such a concern of the school, and its international stature, cannot but have had an effect on IHPME at its beginning.

The original school grew out of an ideal to discover – and then make available to as many people as possible – antitoxins and vaccines that could stop the spread of communicable diseases. Initially called the Antitoxin Laboratory, the Connaught Laboratories was formed out of it, and following that the School of Hygiene. The institute did not escape the influence of being situated within an environment of the labs and school and their international stature. For example, was the fact that Connaught was both research-oriented but research-oriented toward practical solutions, an early influence on the practical orientation of the department?

The people in the labs and the school were at the very top of their field, so when it was decided to form a Department of Hospital Administration it was axiomatic that they would seek the person at the top of his field in this area as well. With Harvey Agnew they found exactly that. Probably there was no one in Canada with a deeper knowledge of hospitals and their operations. It was due to this choice that the department hit the ground running, and almost immediately it became a national program.

It is for this reason, this connection to such excellence, that a history of the department has to begin with some of the qualities of the school in order to provide a context for the atmosphere within which the department was situated. This context is especially important because we have now come full circle. It began within an initial organizational setting, which was within a School of Hygiene, which was dissolved in the 1970s. At that time the department, which now included public health, went to the Faculty of Medicine, where it became one component of the Division of Community Health. It has now once again been placed outside the Faculty of Medicine in a re-established school of public health, one that, within the university's hierarchy, has now been elevated to faculty status.

The department began in response to a need to teach hospital management in Canada. It was the first of its kind in the country, and at the time one of only a few in North America. It has always been at the leading edge. The School of Hygiene, established some twenty years beforehand, was also one of only a few in North America. The school went on to establish a solid reputation in its field, and this would also soon be true of the department as well. Equally important was the international network of which the department and the school became a part. One of the most important was the connection between FitzGerald and the school to the Rockefeller Foundation, which had connections around the world. Indeed, the Rockefeller Foundation's role in supporting ground-breaking institutions and people, such as FitzGerald (and Sigerist, whom we will meet later) is almost legendary. The department also had important links to the Kellogg Foundation (which was an important supporter of department initiatives).

The department was enfolded organizationally and physically within such an atmosphere, which must have had an effect on the department's own milieu, its faculty, and students. And it is this quality of excellence that can be seen as a common thread woven throughout this work, whether it is in the history of the labs, the school, or the department itself.

There were a number of related characteristic qualities of the school. Foremost was an ethos of public service: the school had a strong commitment to making people's lives better – *all* people, not just those who could afford it. It sought to make a difference in tackling the health issues of the day. It had faculty with both strong commitment and outstanding ability.

It was within this setting that the department was founded. It began with a very applied orientation. Conceived and nested academically, it had a very practical emphasis and goal: the establishment of a professional cadre of hospital administrators. Hospitals were emerging as centres of care and rapidly evolving into very complex organizations with multiple specialties and services. This complexity was underscored as hospitals themselves were being tiered into community, regional, and tertiary levels, the last of which also included teaching and research as well as care, another sign of their complexity.

It has often been said that hospitals are the most complex organizations. This is easy to believe when one considers their multiple mandates and stakeholders. In other words, their complexity was not just a function of the organization; it was also a result of their interrelationships.

A Nexus and an Intersection

One question for the reader to keep in mind throughout this work is whether, throughout its history, IHPME has been both a nexus and an intersection. They are not the same thing.

IHPME is a nexus when it brings different people together on a health topic, such as when students, faculty, civil servants, alumni, health professionals, and the public participate in seminars on topical issues. It could be different professions coming together on a panel in HAD 5010 and later the graduate students interacting with the members of that panel. IHPME becomes a nexus promoting dialogue.

An intersection occurs when IHPME (or the school) is a node, such as when different people are working together on a common activity but one outside the institute. One example would be health insurance. Another would be patient engagement. IHPME's role with SPOR on patient engagement is another example.

CHAPTER 2

IHPME's Broader Societal Context

IHPME'S AREA OF STUDY IS DEEPLY FELT

The Import of Health: Linking Health to Nation-Building

We spoke earlier of the iconic nature of some of the health reforms immediately after the Second World War. What also bears mention is just how pervasive and important health care became for nations. Universal health care represented one of the largest peacetime initiatives of any nation, to which the people became almost immediately became strongly attached. Politicians tampered with it at their peril.

As a result, one cannot escape the fact that IHPME has been and is involved in an area that some would put at a nation's very core. Indeed, in recent literature some academics have been very specific about this and have located health care within a perspective of "nation-building."[1] The NHS, for example, was seen as drawing "lessons from global experiences of nation-building."[2] It was the same with Canada, where *Maclean's* called the program Tommy Douglas initiated in Saskatchewan, which spread to the rest of the country, "the most ambitious Canada-building era in our history."[3]

Others see it as very much linked to the "national spirit" of a country.[4] It and social reform are associated with boosting or rejuvenating the national spirit, particularly in times of war or depression.[5] In the United Kingdom the Beveridge Report saw post-war planning to implement health insurance as a morale booster for the populace during the Second World War and an integral part of their reconstruction plans. Some saw the NHS as a result of the "fresh spirit of solidarity and altruism associated with war."[6] In the United States it was planned to be an important part of Roosevelt's New Deal, and he tried repeatedly to have it included.

O'Hara and Gosling note that there was no clamour for a national health service in the United Kingdom prior to the NHS.[7] But almost the opposite occurred in Canada, especially in Saskatchewan, the birthplace of the Canadian system. Here citizens were the drivers, and government action was as a result of citizens (generally through their rural municipalities) asking for the legislation for them to carry out their plans. Saskatchewan innovated in the municipal doctor program (which FitzGerald wrote about) and its union hospital system. And BC repeatedly attempted to implement health insurance in the interwar period. A former director of our Faculty of Social Work was an integral part of this (Harry Cassidy in the Pattullo government). Canadians, both lay and religious, were dedicated in establishing local hospitals. It is easy to see how Canadians see health as linked to our national identity.

We will return to this theme later in this work. In the meantime the reader might consider whether the accomplishments of the School of Hygiene, the Departments of Hospital and Health Administration, IHPME, and the Dalla Lana School have been a part of nation-building.

There is also the link between health care and citizenship. In post–Second World War Britain, the NHS was seen as bolstering an idea of communal citizenship based on the writings of intellectuals such as T.H. Marshall and Richard Titmuss and an idea of a class fusion in which "equality of status was more important than equality of income."[8] Titmuss believed that the Emergency Hospital Service in the United Kingdom demonstrated the benefits of centralized government planning in health delivery and also brought the people and practitioners closer together. In the United Kingdom the war and its fusion of classes in activities directed to the war effort gave rise to an idea (and the climate to enact the idea, at least in part) that there are social rights as well as political rights; that just as citizens had equal political rights, there was an obligation to provide a degree of equity in social rights.

Health is also seen as increasingly integral to the nation state. It is a major economic force. In 2015 it was pegged at 10 per cent of global GDP.[9] The 2013 *Lancet* Commission on Investing in Health estimated that between 2000 and 2011, 24 per cent of total income growth in low- to middle-income countries was attributable to additional years of healthy life.[10] Further, the health sector is slated for rapid growth. "Worldwide, the WHO expects a near doubling in the demand for employment in the health workforce by 2030."[11] This is augmented by additional jobs in health support areas. The number of health workers is estimated to increase globally by 55 per cent between 2013 and 2030.[12] A 1 per cent increase in life expectancy increases economic output by 4 per cent.[13]

And, to further emphasize the import of UHC systems like the NHS, a major report by the Health Foundation in the United Kingdom looks at the NHS as one method to ameliorate a stagnating economy, mitigating economic inequality and supporting community development.[14]

The Emergence of Universal Programs

Concomitant with this expanded ideal of citizenship was the idea of certain benefits being universally available and de-commodified. Health care was prominent among them. Porter notes that the private sector could not provide sufficient common services in areas such as health, nor could it establish a market, because it was difficult if not impossible to price things like public health services. In addition, goods such as public health were seen to be in everyone's interests.[15] In the United Kingdom some said that the implementation of the NHS in 1948 did not result in the building of any new hospitals, training of extra doctors, or evolution of new drugs or treatments. While this point can be argued successfully, there is also the fact that its biggest achievement was in a very different area and that was one of *access*.[16]

There was what had been learned during the war. In Britain the state basically took over health and not only did a credible job but health care was better delivered and integrated through a centralized department and as a whole rather than a series of formerly independent fragments.

Hospitals had loomed large during the war, as they were the first line of contact for civilian casualties. Britain had organized the centralized and state-run Emergency Hospital Service, which most judged to be an outstanding success. It demonstrated the power of state planning, central administration, and integration of service. A Chatham House report recognized this impact as early as 1941. It noted, "Nearly all voluntary hospitals are now working more closely in cooperation with public health authorities than ever before.... It is open to question whether in the period of reconstruction the whole structure of the medical services of Great Britain may not be put on a very different basis to that prevailing before the war."[17]

If we may jump into the present for a moment, this Chatham House statement illustrates a connection to DLSPH and IHPME. The reader will find that later in this work we will deal with policy institutes that have been started by IHPME faculty. These policy institutes are very niche-oriented and do excellent work in their areas. As this volume goes to press Steini Brown has convened a working group to see if DLSPH should start a policy institute and what its purposes might be.

The above quote from Chatham House (itself a policy institute) demonstrates the utility of such an institute, for as early as 1941 its informed opinion was that the post-war UK health system might be very different from anything that had come before. Fifteen months later the Beveridge Report would further support their statement, and seven years later, on 5 July 1948, the start of the NHS would demonstrate that it had been almost prophetic. It demonstrates the utility of such an institute and the need in Canada for one of similar character. At their best they bring learned minds together in dialogue, and conclusions are formed that would not otherwise be made. They also become a part of an international network.[18]

In this case Chatham House took stock of initiatives like the Emergency Hospital Service and the Emergency Medical Service, which came after it. Perhaps they also had in mind that there was a strong undercurrent of popular public sentiment also factoring in, and they correctly intuited that these presaged a radical change in the offing.

Now back to our story. Richard Titmuss noted that the EHS left a legacy of advances in hospital care, and a fund of knowledge and experience in their organization and administration. It had demonstrated what an organized hospital service could be and gave many institutions of varying character and purpose their first real opportunity to work together toward a common goal.[19]

There was also the place of health in the public mind. In Britain the NHS "arguably constituted the single biggest organizational change and greatest improvement in healthcare ever experienced in the nation's history."[20] It "dramatically eliminated all the humiliating disqualifications of the old system" and quickly established for itself a "unique status of esteem among public services."[21]

Almost from inception the public took the NHS to heart. Aneurin Bevan, the Labour minister of health who presided over its development and launch called it "the most remarkable piece of social reconstruction the world has ever seen."[22] Because of it, he said the United Kingdom had "assumed the moral leadership of the world."[23] And though the NHS was far from inevitable, and though its gestation had to be stickhandled amidst a plethora of competing and conflicting interests, Bevan prophesied that the old adage that success has many fathers would hold true in this instance, everyone would take credit for it, and all would own its success.

In his resignation speech of April 1951 Bevan said in the House of Commons, "The National Health Service was something of which we were all very proud, and even the Opposition were beginning to be proud of it. It only had to last a few more years to become part of our traditions, and then the traditionalists would have claimed credit for all of it."[24]

As it turned out, that is exactly what happened. Many years later a Conservative chancellor, Nigel Lawson, would describe the NHS as "the closest thing the English have to a religion."[25] Webster notes that since its inception "the NHS has grown in popular estimation until it has assumed almost unchallenged authority."[26]

Canadians and British Leadership in Health

IHPME's predecessor department's involvement in health was in an area that increasingly preoccupied the people and hence the state. It was an area that is deeply felt by Canadians (as well as the British). Its roots are very much a part of this country. Very early in its history, Canada began to think of health benefit coverage for its people. At that time it could have been in part because of its high proportion of European immigrants, many of whose countries of origin had some sort of health benefits.

And, because at the inception of IHPME, Canada was such an integral part of the British Commonwealth, during much of the twentieth century Canadian politicians were intimately aware of what was taking place in the United Kingdom. The United Kingdom began its journey toward national health insurance with the National Insurance Act of 1911. In 1915 Saskatchewan established the first municipal doctor in North America and a year later passed the first municipal doctor legislation in North America. In 1919 the Liberal Party of Canada made health insurance a plank in its election campaign. There were the British Columbia forays into health insurance in the late 1920s and early 1930s. In 1947 Saskatchewan launched the first hospital insurance program in North America. The United Kingdom would launch the NHS a year later.

The inception of IHPME's predecessor department was a heady time in the development of social insurance. During the Second World War there were rapid developments in this area in both Canada and the United Kingdom. The universalism of a global war was transposed into a universalistic ethos in social welfare. People stood equal in the risk to their life on the front lines. Similarly, in peacetime, initiatives like health insurance saw that "In terms of misfortune's consequences, all who are members of a common risk pool stand equal."[27]

What people like Tommy Douglas and Clement Atlee did in the years surrounding the inception of the U of T program decisively advanced "society's ability to treat each of its members equally" and to create a sense of community and solidarity.[28] "It did so, however, less by redistributing wealth than by reapportioning the costs of risk and mischance."[29]

In the ensuing years the United Kingdom and Canada developed similarly strong feelings for their respective national health systems. In each the people felt it strongly tied to their national identity. In Canada, when the CBC did a poll on the greatest Canadian, Tommy Douglas was chosen for his role in Canadian medicare.[30]

This was so much so in Britain, its centrality so profound, that a segment on the NHS formed part of the opening ceremony for the 2012 Summer Olympics in London, in front of a global audience. Thomas Piketty amplified this message, as he mentioned it in his bestselling *Capital in the Twenty-First Century*: "The National Health Service, established in 1948, is such an integral part of British national identity that its creation was dramatized in the opening ceremonies of the 2012 Olympic games, along with the Industrial Revolution and the rock groups of the 1960s."[31]

It is interesting just how pervasive this sentiment was. It was not limited to the public and patients. The NHS also ranked very high with its employees, of which at inception there were 500,000. Webster noted the staff of the NHS "soon achieved a sense that they were part of a prestigious national service, capable of achieving in peacetime something like the feats of collective action and patriotic service recently witnessed in the special circumstances of total warfare."[32]

Polling company Ipsos MORI ranked the NHS first as the institution that made people "most proud to be British."[33] They ranked it even ahead of the royal family.[34] Webster echoes the same sentiment when he says, "Of all modern institutions of the British state the National Health Service is arguably the most cherished."[35] Boyle noted that he had come under pressure to drop the sequence about the NHS.[36] However, the *Telegraph* noted it was fitting that the opening ceremony pay homage to the NHS as its inception was the year London last hosted the Olympic Games.[37]

And it wasn't only the import of that institution that was being showcased. The *Telegraph* noted another, more subliminal message in the NHS pageantry – and this also illustrates the strength of feeling involved. This choreography was part of a larger message; that producer Danny Boyle (the Academy Award–winning director of *Slumdog Millionaire)* wanted to use the global forum of the opening to give the watching British prime minister and the British Cabinet in the audience a clear message – "Hands Off Our NHS."[38]

This also illustrates the strength of British feeling, as at the time this was a slogan used by thousands of Britons across the country as they protested NHS reforms. And it was also the way Boyle represented the NHS. He drew upon the actual people – hundreds of doctors and nurses involved with the NHS "representing the UK's most cherished institution on a global stage in front of billions of viewers."[39]

British sentiment was tied not just to the service, health care for everyone, but also to the values this represented. It demonstrated a solidarity of Britons; that every British life mattered, that the worth of every British citizen was equally valuable.

Canadians' sentiments are even stronger than those in the United Kingdom. In Canada health care is almost universally loved; 94 per cent of Canadians called it an important source of collective pride.[40] An award-winning Canadian health columnist, André Picard, notes, "Canadians love medicare," they romanticize and mythologize it and say "medicare is what defines us as Canadians."[41]

It all makes for a delicate political issue. He notes Joey Smallwood, the legendary premier of Newfoundland, is purported to have said, "I never had a conversation about health care that didn't lose me votes." Picard says Smallwood's reticence is shared by politicians of all stripes. And this while health care is being consistently identified as the primary concern of Canadians in opinion polls.[42] It's because health care is a complex topic. It is also an emotional one. And this is what makes it a political minefield for Canadian politicians.

The Canadians and British on Hospitals

We tend to underplay the feelings Canadians have about their hospitals and the impact they have had on our communities. They stand as symbols of the resourcefulness, volunteerism, and altruism of the Canadian people. It is much the same with the British. We will explore these sentiments somewhat, for they are integral to helping establish the context of the institutions that DHA grads would administer.

Children's Hospitals

To go back to the London Olympics, Boyle also touched on another theme in his choreography, a health institution as venerated by the British as their health system. It was also the area IHPME first concentrated on: hospitals. Boyle showcased the Great Ormond Street Hospital, more familiarly known by its acronym GOSH, founded in 1852, generally regarded as the most famous children's hospital in the world.[43]

And the symbolism didn't stop there. Boyle had author J.K. Rowling, of the iconic *Harry Potter*, reading from J.M. Barrie's equally iconic *Peter Pan*, the royalties and rights to which Barrie had given to the hospital back in 1929.[44] Peter Pan became forever associated with the hospital and has become "a symbol and champion of children in hospital everywhere," a fact recognized by the British House of Lords when they extended the patent rights to GOSH in perpetuity after their expiration.[45]

Such an association between one of the most enduring children's stories and its proceeds going to support a world-renowned hospital illustrates the depth of feeling health can evoke. Positioning institutions such as the NHS and GOSH, a children's tale like *Peter Pan*, and doing this within its own art form, as part of the choreography of a momentous occasion like the opening of an Olympics connects at an emotive level with the British and indeed the world psyche. It certainly illustrates just how deep the connection of health care and hospitals is to people. And it conveys it through an art form (choreography) and at an occasion that adds to the power.

The depth of feeling the public had for hospitals and how far back it goes is also exemplified by Charles Dickens, who was an "enthusiastic supporter" of GOSH.[46] In 1852, six weeks after the hospital opened, he wrote an article arguing for the necessity of a children's hospital and mentioning the hospital by name.[47] It was the first printed account of the hospital and its effect was immediately apparent. Queen Victoria made a generous donation and became a patron shortly after.[48] It was said Dickens "took up his pen and wrote the hospital into the public's heart."[49]

An 1850 booklet appealing to the British public of the need for a children's hospital noted that of a hundred children born in London, twenty-four die during the first two years of life, and thirty-five before the age of ten.[50] It further noted that there was not a hospital devoted exclusively to children in London or anywhere in the British Empire, despite there being such facilities in a number of European cities (which it listed).[51] It also set out the need and differentiated it from that of a hospital for adults.[52]

Interestingly, it noted the social role of a children's hospital in that era: "The children who have been discharged from the Hospital at Frankfort hang about its gates to see those who tended them when sick."[53] Also, notably, GOSH was to be a teaching centre, and the contribution of the rich would be "twice blessed" in that not only were they helping the poor but they were also facilitating the skill and experience of "junior members of the medical profession" who might well treat their own children in the future.[54]

This points to another more implicit message in Boyle's choice of the NHS and GOSH, which has to do with not just their connection to the British identity or the message regarding NHS reform. These are important but not sufficient to write them into an event as momentous as the opening of an Olympic Games. It goes beyond to the fact that they strike to the British soul, that the British have a love for such public institutions and cherish them deeply. They have, indeed, been written into the British heart

This type of feeling toward a children's hospital is much the same in Canada. In addition, there is also a historic connection between GOSH and SickKids in Toronto. Indeed, in 1986 the chairperson of GOSH laid the first stone for a new hospital on the Toronto site, "taken from the original London hospital, emphasizing the symbolic and historical connection between the two institutions."[55]

This sentiment occurs not just with the feelings evoked by hospitals and health care but in the attraction children's hospitals have to a literary figure. In Canada, acclaimed novelist Max Braithwaite (winner of the Stephen Leacock Memorial Medal) wrote a history of the Hospital for Sick Children (HSC). Each chapter opens with the story of a child's illness. In each he captures, as perhaps only a literary figure can, the vulnerability of the child, the need the hospital serves, its character, and how it weaves itself into the very fabric of the society.[56]

It's an evocative work, a narrative history that captures as well how a hospital could penetrate to people's very core and inspire great acts of voluntarism spanning many years. One such example is the founder of HSC, Elizabeth McMaster. She also represents how such actions became integral parts of our history. She led a group of socially prominent Toronto women to establish the hospital in 1875. Their action was typical of "reform-minded, middle-class women volunteers" of that era who gravitated to "social action."[57]

Another example is an account of how John Ross Robertson (founder of the *Evening Telegram*), one of its greatest benefactors who, from 1881 to 1918, made the hospital his personal ambition. When asked what he got out of it, he said that when on the street "'he is called by name and chatted to'" by one of the formerly maimed and crippled children "'I confess I get dividends which are priceless and above all treasure.'"[58] His bequest to the hospital would amount to over $200 million today.[59] Interestingly, in an appendix Braithwaite lists the executive staff of the hospital, and a DHA grad, Carl Hunt, is the administrator.[60]

One of the children Braithwaite mentions, and one doted on by Robertson, was Josephine Kane. She was admitted in 1880 and not expected to live. However she did. Robertson took a personal interest in her and she remained at the hospital after she recovered. He paid for her schooling and secretarial training and gave her a job at the hospital. She had a room in the nurses' residence.[61] Upon his death she completed a history of the hospital he had begun. Fittingly it ended the year of his death (1918) with a tribute to her benefactor, who, she said, they all missed "more and more, each and every day" and who contributed "far more than the gifts of money that he brought to light at each obstacle." What they missed was "his very self," the person who at each step along the way was behind "the miracle [that] was accomplished."[62]

Braithwaite talks of the kind of sentiment the hospital could evoke. One sees such sentiment in a work by Elizabeth McMaster. In 1888 she wrote a short pamphlet on Christmas at HSC and the excitement of "Tree Day," where the tree was decorated with presents, one for each child, with the larger ones arrayed at its base. Her work captures "the day containing so much excitement as well as joy for the sick little folks," and later "the greater number were fast asleep, each holding one or more of the treasures gleaned that day."[63] It also captures the heart, the deep caring of the staff.

In fact such caring was very much a part of hospitals of the latter nineteenth century. In those days medical science "offered limited treatment; hospitals provided food, care in a clean environment, and 'spiritual nurture.'" HSC, founded in 1875, was "well before hospitals were transformed into institutions of medical science and became the domain of physicians."[64]

General Hospitals

Communities also cherish their local general hospitals. The largest are the urban, academic health sciences centres that epitomize the cutting edge of medicine in teaching, care, and research. Invariably they also capture the civic-mindedness of the rich and powerful, whom they enlist in their insatiable quest for the resources to keep them at the leading edge. These are hospitals like Toronto General in Canada, Massachusetts General in the United States, and Barts (founded 1123) in the United Kingdom.

Some, like Toronto General, are part of the nation's history. TGH grew out of the need produced by a rapidly growing settlement but in particular the need caused by the War of 1812. Its founding was supported through the Loyal and Patriotic Society in the amount of "two hundred and fifty-three pounds, four shillings, and nine pence, New York currency."[65] As Clarke notes in 1913, from its inception it was a centre of medical education, and on "its staff were to be found those whose work has been recognized throughout the world."[66]

No less important were staff whose roles became almost legendary. Among them was Jean Gunn, its superintendent of nurses for many years and a recipient of the Order of the British Empire. Eugenie Stuart of IHPME's predecessor Department of Hospital Administration knew her well. There is a picture of the two of them in a biography of Gunn.[67] Also Stuart spoke at the unveiling of portrait of Gunn by Cleeve Horn.[68]

Hospitals and health policy have sustained a place in our national history. Canadians have long had an interest in health and social welfare. And the hospitals this program initially concentrated on are an important part of our provincial and local history. One need only look at the bookshelves of a major Canadian reference library to see the number of books written about Canadian (and US and UK) hospitals spanning the entire country.

Better yet, one need read only a few pages of these histories to see their pride of place in communities across the nation. To these communities they were places of care and employment, and a source of inspiration that perhaps determined the career path of a future IHPME director.[69] One can delve deeper into the archival collections of these institutions to get a more fulsome sense of Canadians' commitment to hospitals in these communities.

The public sentiment we see on library shelves, or evidenced in the London Olympics, the dedication captured by people like Braithwaite that hospitals like SickKids attracted was the milieu surrounding IHPME. In the case of hospitals, these were the institutions that IHPME grads exclusively went to almost when it was formed in 1947. It is important to note how they could move people (including literary figures) and their place in the public mentality. It points to the fact that the area that IHPME is involved in is as important as the work that it does.

IHPME has attempted to provide the tools to navigate this rich national heritage (and at times political minefield) for some seventy years, initially by educating a new profession and shortly thereafter by an emphasis on evidence-based policy and outcome analysis. Faculty of IHPME have been at the centre of health discussions throughout its history and have also been tapped to lead or make significant contributions to numerous important government studies on health. In many cases, their graduates have become part of that community fabric.

IHPME is a nexus, bringing together faculty, students, outside experts, practitioners, the public, politicians, civil servants, health entrepreneurs, and others in a common dialogue on the health of a nation.

IHPME is about institutions and people. It is an institution but it has also been (and is) at the centre of building important Canadian institutions. And it has been important in building leaders in Canadian health care.

IHPME'S AREA OF STUDY HAS A HIGH PROFILE

In addition, because health is an area that is deeply felt in society, it has built a high profile among governments. It is now the largest single budget item amongst Canadian provinces. It occupies a significant proportion of the GDP among first-world nations and (likely as a result) it garners significant national attention in these countries. Journalists spill a lot of ink on health.

PART TWO

The Deep Roots of "Toward the Health of a Nation"

CHAPTER 3

FitzGerald: Teaching, Research, Practice, Public Service

WHY DID FITZGERALD HAVE SUCH A PROFOUND IMPACT?

IHPME – and the DLSPH – has deep roots in "toward the health of a nation." It traces back to the work of J.G. FitzGerald and a remarkable team he put together. This story in its breadth has already been told in *Within Reach of Everyone* so we won't reprise it here. What we will do is isolate some of these accomplishments and get at the depth of what he was doing and the profound impact of his actions. For what he was doing, what his labs and his school were doing, was inextricably linked to the Canadian health system. And they were wholly aimed "toward the health of a nation."

FitzGerald's impact is due to a number of factors. First was his ability, which was both scientific and organizational. He was able to put together and manage two large and complex organizations. He also had an interpersonal skill; he seemed to have a knack for spotting talent and hiring good people. His skill in administration presaged the department, the subject of this book, that would be established seven years after his death.

He seized onto one of the communicable disease scourges of the day and developed an effective antitoxin. But he did not stop there. He knew it had to be made widely available to individuals and governments. The chief barrier was cost and he set about making it affordable, particularly to governments, as this would give it the widest distribution. He succeeded, and the Ontario and Saskatchewan governments purchased his product for free distribution in their provinces.

He had broken new ground, both in discovery and distribution. He would continue to do so. Royalties for his discovery accrued not to him but to the university.

There were propitious circumstances happening around him. The First World War spawned a need for further antitoxins and vaccines and he proved up to the challenge. His lab at the university was insufficient and a liquor magnate stepped in to remedy the situation, and a new business was established, which, as the result of the war, scaled up rapidly. The university owned the business and this business sold its product at cost. FitzGerald was its director.

The First World War and the large number of conscript rejections made all governments very interested in public health. In the United Kingdom and Canada this meant the initiation of a national department of health in 1919. His boss became the first deputy minister of the Canadian department and he took over as head of the antitoxin lab.

His own interest in public health, which had seen him establish strong ties to local and provincial medical officers of health, carried over onto the national level as well.

How Does This Relate to IHPME?

The need for and the establishment of the Department of Hospital Administration was proof FitzGerald, his two core institutions, and his team had succeeded. They had put together the framework of a Canadian health system. Others in other parts of Canada were doing the same. But FitzGerald and his band were at the core of it. One of them, his protégé Robert Defries, carried his legacy forward. Defries was the head of the school at the inception of the Hospital Administration Department and responsible for its founding.

In FitzGerald there was layering of activity. First was control of communicable disease, then public health organization, at the local and provincial level, then concern with putting in place the policy vehicle (health insurance) to make health available for all, then interest in what other countries were doing.

Fitzgerald died a year after the onset of the Second World War. However, the war greatly accelerated policy development in social security. Particularly from 1942 onward there was intense activity in Canada, the United Kingdom, and the United States.

In the meantime, another need was evolving. The need for training in administration – first public health administration, then medical care administration, and finally hospital administration – was evidence that a health system was emerging, that it was complex and systemic, and that it required professional management. Hospitals emerged as a key component of the total health spectrum and very quickly as distinct institutions in their own right.

There were isolated forays to have hospitals more fully integrated into the public health equation. Miller in the 1950s wrote of ways this might happen. She spoke of an integration of care and the hospital being at the centre of community health services. She noted work underway in Saskatchewan (under Burns Roth) where hospitals were being developed to function as health centres for the district. She pointed out that Reddy Memorial Hospital in Montreal at that time was the first and only hospital to establish a home care department.[1]

None of this was lost on Defries. He initiated lectures in public health administration, medical care administration, and seized on an opportunity presented by the Kellogg Foundation to start the first hospital administration program in Canada. We will touch on all of these historical components to set the context for the inception of the Department of Hospital Administration.

This chapter will begin this focus. It will take us through FitzGerald's activities in the 1910s and 1920s, which were basically internal to the University of Toronto and established a solid reputation for the university in public health internationally. The next chapter will continue to focus on FitzGerald but will look at his involvement outside the university and more on policy and comparative systems.

J.G. FITZGERALD: THE PERSON

We will limit ourselves to aspects of FitzGerald's work that directly concern us here. For a fuller exposition of his life and work, the reader is referred to the book by his grandson, and a brief biography by Defries that appeared in the *CMAJ* after FitzGerald's passing.[2]

His M.O.

FitzGerald had a unique modus operandi, which was aimed primarily at practice and at impact – effective public health. This happened in two ways. There was a professional education program and a research program within his overall U of T program. But research was aimed at an applied end. It was not theoretical and was aimed instead at practical outcomes. This led to another unique aspect of the FitzGerald model in that he created an organizational receptacle to commercialize and scale up his research discoveries so that in the end he had a seamless continuum from conception to product.

The result was a unique educational experience, with an intense focus on practice, aimed at turning out effective public health administrators or developing products that improved public health. Integral to this educational experience was the goal of the latter to make these products available as widely as possible, so there was a focus on not just product development but continual dropping of costs. The final piece was the creation of a virtuous circle, to use royalties to invest in further research.

His Background

For FitzGerald, the idea of an antitoxin lab was to meet an immediate public health need, to develop medicine to combat communicable disease. A school of hygiene met a different need, to educate the people to do the first. What motivated FitzGerald was public service, making a difference. He first needed the physical facility in which to develop the medicine, hence Connaught Labs (initially called the Antitoxin Labs). Next he needed the means of knowledge transmission, hence the teaching, which later, with the assistance of the Rockefeller Foundation, was codified into the school. These were two almost countervailing (but not necessarily antithetical) tendencies, which later became important for the history of not just the School but for the Department as well.

The grandson of J.G. FitzGerald, in his award-winning *What Disturbs Our Blood*, gets at what motivated these early medical pioneers. His grandfather was "a remarkable man of science, an innovator and visionary who transformed the Canadian system of public health between the world wars, a heroic figure who eradicated the disease of diphtheria and made insulin available to the masses, a dynamo who travelled the world for the Rockefeller Foundation, bringing Canada's paragon of preventive medicine to the international community. His singular achievements saved countless lives and earned universal praise."[3]

Later in the book he speaks of the "grandeur, complexity, and impact" of his grandfather's achievement. He was a "bona fide Canadian hero, a medical pathfinder of extraordinary drive and vision," with a career trajectory of "intense, single-minded, self-sacrificing focus." He notes that the organizations he founded (the labs and the school) saved countless lives "nationally and globally." They "rose to become models to the world" yet were essentially unknown in their own country, "typical of our cautious national character – outside praise failing to register at home."[4]

At the time, his grandfather was the youngest student accepted into the medical school of a "fast-growing" university set in the heart of an equally fast-growing city.[5] The university was "a microcosm of national aspirations, determined to test its mettle against its more glamorous European and American cousins."[6] Reflecting these aspirations was the Toronto General Hospital on its southern flank, relocated in 1913 from Cabbagetown to a 670-bed institution with its classical dome that is the largest in North America.[7] A previous location of the hospital had served as the seat of the Ontario Legislature (1824–29) when a fire destroyed the buildings at Queen's Park.[8]

Though the medical school does not have a teaching hospital formally affiliated with it, J.G. regularly travelled to the TGH in Cabbagetown to be trained at patients' bedsides and to be instructed by Dr John Amyot in the chilled basement morgue.[9] Cosbie notes that though J.G. was only indirectly associated with the hospital, he "proved of the greatest value to physicians on the staff of the hospital who were involved in clinical investigations of the prevention and control of certain diseases."[10]

FitzGerald also anticipated what is now taken for granted – the link between research and a clinical site for its application. Cosbie notes TGH served as the site of clinical trials on the value of liver extract suitable for intramuscular injection prepared at the school, and noted that this combined effort involved the research laboratories, the wards of the hospital and its outpatient department, was an "example of a clinical investigative unit at its very best."[11] On 11 January 1922 TGH was the site of the first insulin injection, which had been prepared at the school.[12] It would be an important site for Department of Hospital Administration students (for their practicum rotation). And the idea of a continuum of research, discovery, its trial in a clinical application, and its commercial application would serve many years later as the idea for a graduate course in IHPME.

FitzGerald's grandson notes J.G. had the values of scholar, the drive of an "incisive, cost-cutting" entrepreneur, and a highly developed social conscience.[13] He aptly encapsulates three values that drove his grandfather and would ultimately form an important core of the school. They are also three areas his grandfather ventured into. The entrepreneurial J.G. FitzGerald set up a laboratory that would develop and manufacture vaccines and antitoxins. His social conscience drove him to make them available to the public at cost, and he worked with provincial governments to do the same. The scholarly FitzGerald set up of the School of Hygiene.

FitzGerald originally had looked at a specialty in psychiatry. In preparation he had spent time at the Sheppard and Enoch Pratt Hospital in Baltimore (the equivalent of our Clarke Institute). At the fiftieth anniversary of that institution Clarence Farrar, editor of the *American Journal of Psychiatry* recounted that a number of former students had "later distinguished themselves." One of those he singled out was J.G. FitzGerald who "was probably the most distinguished of our alumni" and, had "he followed his original direction ... would almost certainly have been the leading psychiatrist in Canada."[14]

"The Future of Public Health"

FitzGerald delivered an address at a special meeting of the Ottawa Social Hygiene Council in March 1928.[15] His address contains some of the conviction of the man. He spoke of what was needed in public health for the future. Much of it still holds true today. He traced the history of public health to sixteenth-century England. He touched on the communicable diseases ravaging society in his day.

He emphasized the importance of research. He said, "Research worthy of the name will always be prosecuted where innate intellectual curiosity is given wide scope and generous encouragement."[16] He noted, "Eight years ago many persons in all parts of the world suffering from diabetes knew they had but a brief time to live. The younger the sufferer the briefer the period, generally speaking. Tonight, victims young and old of the disease, scattered in all parts of the world, are no longer in the valley of the shadow of death."[17] He said, "Canada needs more Canadians. Let us keep those we have who now die of preventable causes."[18]

He noted, "The prevention of disease is not, however, itself sufficient. Provision has also to be made for the earliest possible recognition of disease.... This means education of the public and much more practice of preventive medicine. Everyone owes it as a duty to the state to maintain good health. This is a personal and individual responsibility.... Organized society should see to it that scientific truth, now known but to a few, becomes the common possession of all."[19] He also noted, "Present arrangements for the care and treatment of the sick are not altogether satisfactory. Health insurance provided by the individual or by the state, or both, is realizable and would undoubtedly vastly improve the state of public health."[20]

He concluded, "All substantial progress is evolutionary. We learn from past experience ... only through striving do we reach the stars. Progress in the future in public health ... is conditioned only by a desire to learn and to do. Good health and longevity, like other prizes, must be won. In the winning of them we are serving our ... country; no other incentive could be more worthy."[21]

A LAB AND A SCHOOL OF HYGIENE – EACH COMMITTED TO PUBLIC SERVICE

In the Introduction we sketched the influence of the university and school upon the evolution of IHPME. It was at its most profound with the immediate environment of what was then the department, so we will look in more detail into the Connaught Labs and the school, which, while distinct, functionally were a single organization administratively until the 1960s, one combining research, its application, and graduate education.

U of T and the Rockefeller Foundation

The person behind it all was an individual of exceptional ability and drive. He built not just one but two world-beating organizations. His accomplishments were of sufficient magnitude that the Rockefeller Foundation made this school the third place it funded in public health (after Harvard and Johns Hopkins). Such notice helped profile the school and the university at the time and in an ongoing way. Non-Canadian historians writing of the foundation have noted the connection. For example, Farley, in his history of the International Health Division of the Foundation, mentions FitzGerald and the School of Hygiene. Funding for the school "was an indication that the scientific directors agreed ... that Toronto had joined Johns Hopkins to become one of the chief training centers for public health officers on the North American continent."[22] He also noted that the Rockefeller Health Board saw Toronto and London "as model institutions, sharing with Johns Hopkins the distinction of being centers of research with the very highest standards."[23]

It was actually an example of an established relationship between the foundation and the university. And FitzGerald had an important relationship with another prominent Rockefeller institution. At the opening of the Connaught Laboratories in October 1917, Dr Simon Flexner, director of the Rockefeller Institute for Medical Research, delivered a lecture on the activities of the institute.[24]

The foundation had made an earlier grant to the university's medical school (in 1919). The result had been a change to the curriculum and staffing (emphasizing full-time faculty) and an adoption of US and German methods of education. These were centred primarily upon faculty combining teaching and research in order to offer the best learning experience for students (another reason for the need for full-time faculty).

U of T was an early leader in emphasizing the combination of teaching and research in a Faculty of Medicine. It is important for our purposes, because many years later it influenced what the university thought the school and department should be doing. McRae notes the faculty "was distinguished as early as the 1890's by it[s] biological research-oriented approach to medicine."[25] She notes, "This situation of a strong biological group joining a relatively weak medical school and forging an effective programme in scientific medicine was quite unusual in the 1890's, and I believe that this accounts for the extraordinary success of many of the Toronto graduates in biology and medicine who went on to prominent teaching and research careers."[26]

Yet the contribution of Canadian medical schools to medical research has been ignored, for the most part, despite the "important contributions made by Canadian individuals to all aspects of North American medicine."[27] On one of one of our best-known discoveries, she quotes Bliss, who says, "The discovery of insulin is sometimes thought to have caused the first wave of enthusiasm for medical research in Canada. Actually the discovery was in part a consequence of the first wave."[28] One could say more specifically that it was an accomplishment of the faculty, yes, but particularly the school they were a part of, and that financed their research.

It was also something the school and the labs had been doing for years. Fedunkiw notes people like Banting, Best, Collip as providing examples of this ideal.[29] They were all associated with the school and the labs. Four were graduates of U of T.[30] The Connaught Antitoxin Laboratories were involved in teaching and research and McRae mentions laboratory facilities in Hygiene (indicating it is doing research).[31] She is corroborated by FitzGerald's own report for the academic year ended 30 June 1914: "The public service aspect is made to go hand in hand with teaching and research, a combination possible only when the work is being done in connection with the University."[32] And more generally, Fedunkiw notes that the gift "helped certain 'long standing' ideas become realities in Toronto." These included the "scientization of medicine," "establishing the 'research ideal,'" and the "institutionalization of research."[33] FitzGerald took this teaching and research combination to further level. He wanted a practical outcome (a product). And he wanted it available to everyone.

These changes met with considerable opposition. Toronto was not alone in advocating them; there were schools in the United States doing the same thing. However, there was significant opposition in all places, and in Toronto a provincial inquiry (motivated in no small measure by disgruntled part-time physician faculty). The inquiry had a section on the Rockefeller (and also an Eaton) gift and noted that the Rockefeller gift "did have certain conditions" that were, "in the opinion of the Committee, highly undesirable."[34] However, President Falconer prevailed, a new Ontario government was elected that was more amenable to the gift, and the new staffing and curriculum proceeded.

The recognition accorded gifts such as these helped put U of T on the map. And the research ideal infused future departments such as Hospital Administration, which had a thesis requirement very early in its history. The university's relationship to the foundation endured. For example, John Evans, former president of U of T, was asked in 1979 to head the foundation's Commission on the Future of Schools of Public Health, in 1982 to join its board, and from 1987 to 1995 served as its chair, the first Canadian to do so.[35]

COMBINING RESEARCH, EDUCATION, AND PUBLIC SERVICE

One could argue the Connaught Laboratories and the School of Hygiene were an early experiment in linking research and education to public service, because they provided products to the public at cost and in worked closely with local, provincial, and national public health agencies.[36] It could also be argued that they were an early experiment in the commercialization of research, an idea that would initially infuse American universities, with the passage of the Bayh-Dole Act in 1980, and later spread to Canada. It would spawn a whole new area of activity: technology transfer. Yet this was an activity in which the labs were engaging as early as 1913. It involved a very tight relationship between research and application, between intellectual curiosity and public need. These were areas IHPME would study and teach in the early 2000s.

Another focus was public health. It was remarkable that these labs were established within a university, with their concentration on public health and product development, in a country as young as Canada. It is a testimony to the ability of the people involved that U of T and Canada could take their place among countries with much longer traditions and much better intellectual infrastructure. They engaged in activities that are commonplace today but put the U of T and Canada at the leading edge through much of the last century.

Antitoxin Laboratories (1914)

It all started when FitzGerald returned to Toronto in 1913. He had definite ideas about establishing an antitoxin lab. He had been doing postgraduate studies at the Pasteur Institutes in Paris and Brussels, the University of Freiberg, and the New York City Department of Health, as well as teaching at UC Berkeley. He approached the university for funding, but they were reluctant "about linking their academic mission to the commercial production of a drug," so with money from his wife's inheritance he built a small stable near the university (145 Barton Avenue) and began producing serum.[37]

The university came round and the Antitoxin Laboratories were approved by the board of governors in April 1914. They were to meet a need for native-produced antitoxins, especially diphtheria, which were killing up to 12 per cent of young children in the first decade of the twentieth century. Few families could afford the cost of the imported American-made antitoxin.[38] The same was true of the tetanus antitoxin, which was made available by the labs to the First World War troops at a cost of $0.34, as opposed to obtaining it from the United States at a cost of $1.25.[39]

The need for such a lab had been lobbied for some years. An editorial in the *CMAJ* noted that several organizations had been urging the federal government to establish a lab for antitoxins and vaccines. "No country in the world the size of Canada is without laboratories for this purpose."[40]

Sir Edmund Osler, president of the Dominion Bank (now part of TD Bank) and also an MP (until 1917) provided the initial funding. FitzGerald wrote that he expected the work to be self-supporting "within three to six months, probably less."[41]

The labs caught on almost immediately, and in May 1915 FitzGerald was informing President Falconer that Quebec and New Brunswick were interested in their product as well as the French and Russian governments.[42]

FitzGerald wrote an article in 1916 on the work of what was then called the Antitoxin Laboratory. In it he set out the reasons for it. One was already noted: Canada was the only country of its size in the world without laboratories for this purpose. The second was that war was making some products difficult to obtain. The third was economic: those best able to pay were charged the least, and "those whose need was often the greatest and whose purses were slim, were not so favoured." The lab immediately began selling its doses at about one-third of current prices. He noted that J.W.S. McCullough of the Ontario Provincial Health Board, Dr M.M. Seymour (DPH, 1917), commissioner of health for Saskatchewan, and Dr W.H. Hattie, provincial health officer for Nova Scotia, all began to distribute the product through their localities. He also noted the laboratory was to be renamed the Connaught Laboratories, after the Duke of Connaught, then governor-general of Canada, and a friend of liquor-magnate Albert Gooderham.[43] He concluded the article by noting Canada now has an institution comparable in the scope of its activities to the Pasteur Institute in Paris, the Lister Institute of London, and the Research Laboratories of the Health Department of New York City. He noted that proceeds from the sale of the products were being used to further research in preventive medicine.[44]

Dr McCullough was a graduate of Trinity Medical School (run by Trinity College at U of T).[45] He was also received one of the first Diplomas in Public Health from the U of T (in 1914).[46] The Seymour-Saskatchewan connection would presage a relationship with the labs and school that still endures and one in which IHPME would figure prominently (there would be the same close relationship between the province and the Department of Hospital Administration when it was established). Because he believed in the value of postgraduate instruction in public health, Seymour, at the age of fifty-seven, took a special leave from what was then the Bureau of Public Health to attend the U of T program and received a diploma of public health with high standing.[47] He was one of the first recipients of the diploma,[48] in 1917.[49]

What is interesting in the early days of the diploma program is the number of graduates from Saskatchewan. Of fifteen graduates between 1911 to 1920, three were from Saskatchewan.[50] What is also interesting is how well they did. We already know of Seymour. Of the remaining two, Dr Daniel Cameron Lochead (DPH, 1915) was a member of the Saskatchewan Legislative

Assembly. He was a graduate of Trinity Medical School (1905).[51] He later served as deputy medical commissioner (and after that) commissioner for Rochester, Minnesota, where he worked with Dr Charles Mayo (one of the founders of the Mayo Clinic). Malcolm Ross Bow (DPH, 1920) served as the first chief medical officer for Regina and went from there to be deputy minister of health for Alberta. While in Saskatchewan he played running back for the Regina Rugby Club, the forerunner of the Saskatchewan Roughriders. From 1938 until 1956 he combined his administrative duties with teaching public health at the University of Alberta.

The continuity of education at U of T for some of these individuals is striking, some of them having received their medical degree at the university (or one of its federated colleges) and then returning to the university for graduate (DPH) studies.

Connaught Laboratories (1917)

The Antitoxin Laboratories was renamed the Connaught Antitoxin Laboratories in 1917. The fact that the labs were part of a public university was interesting; the fact that they were part of a School of Hygiene even more so. Because of its location within a university it was no ordinary company. One of its distinctive qualities was its large emphasis on basic research, which was unusual for a company. There was a very tight connection between basic research and its application. This was another notable aspect for a company – its output of academic articles. The labs had their own in-house journal, *Studies*, consisting mainly of reprints of articles published in academic journals.[52]

The Profile Accruing to FitzGerald's Work

The profile accruing to FitzGerald's work and the pride of the city were in evidence at the opening of the Connaught Labs on 25 October 1917. Also notable was their location relative to the city at that time. The governor general formally opened the facility "with a significance which impressed itself upon the large gathering of prominent citizens who journeyed out from Toronto." At the ceremony the title deeds to the property were given to the chair of the board of governors, Edmund Walker, by Albert Gooderham.[53]

The *Mail and Empire* noted "the value of the products of the institution in their relation to the efficiency of the men now in the field, to the betterment of public health, and to the welfare of posterity is inestimable." It noted further, "It is the only institution of its kind in the Dominion and has already become a formidable though friendly rival of the Rockefeller Institute and the Pasteur Institute." FitzGerald's work was a prominent part of the opening. Gooderham noted the enterprise began "in the ambitions of Dr J.G. FitzGerald," and the present institution "was but a fulfillment of Dr FitzGerald's idea." The premier of Ontario, Sir William Hearst, also spoke and noted the province was providing a $75,000 endowment to be added to one of $25,000 being raised by Gooderham.[54] This too was an indication of the import and profile being given to FitzGerald's work.

The *Toronto Daily News* reported that FitzGerald had been operating a small facility on Clinton Street, but when war broke out the Red Cross put out a call for antitoxin. It noted the facilities "are on a par with any in the United States or Europe."[55] The *Toronto Daily Star* had a relatively brief article (it noted the role of FitzGerald and his associate, R.D. Defries).[56]

Such media coverage was important, for it acquainted Canadians with the kinds of world-class organizations that were in their midst.

What the Labs Represented

The Labs represented a number of ideals. One would be university outreach: universities had a duty not just in theory but also in practice; in other words they should make things better. Another was that teaching and research and application should be combined and form a continuum. Connaught and the School were doing R&D even before R&D existed as a concept.

And further, had U of T not allowed this, would there have been an internationally renowned vaccine lab in Canada? Is this not exactly what governments and public institutions should do: take the risks private enterprise is not willing to take? Is that not how we got the internet?[57] What Connaught was doing is what IHPME is now teaching in its commercialization of health research classes. Moreover, IHPME is not alone; the Rotman School of Management and the Institute of Innovation Management also highlight principles that Connaught pioneered. One could say it was theory in the service of practice, that the R&D and indeed the teaching were always to serve practical ends, to improve people's health.

There was a very strong connection between the labs and public health. Rutty notes the labs "evolved into the cornerstone of Canada's public health infrastructure and a key player in the national and global control of many infectious and other diseases."[58] In another publication he says it "facilitated and reinforced strong public health connections" and that its uniqueness was "its dual research and biological production capacity within a university setting."[59] He tells us why this is so by pointing out the range of its products: "Connaught is best known for its major contributions to the research and development, and large-scale production of an unusual range of biological products, including diphtheria toxoid, insulin, pertussis vaccine, heparin, penicillin, a variety of combined vaccines, and the Salk and Sabin polio vaccines, as well as its major contributions to the global eradication of smallpox."[60] This intermarriage of research and teaching was noted in its 1953–54 annual report: "Senior members of the Laboratories give direction to several departments of the School."[61]

It is interesting that the Connaught Laboratories, especially given their accomplishments, are relatively unknown[62] – not just as an entity but in what it accomplished. There were a number of important elements afoot here: to have the capability, the capacity, to discover and develop a diphtheria antitoxin, then to be able to produce it in commercial quantities, and finally to make it available to the public at cost. There was also the intent to eliminate the need to import the antitoxin from outside the country (which greatly increased its cost). The illness had been a public health challenge for some time. The *Canada Lancet* had been reporting on it since 1895. In that year it had an editorial on its treatment as well as a request that the government become involved in quality control of serum production.[63]

There was also an issue of how it should be supplied. The *Canada Lancet* reported in 1905 on the results of an initiative of the Chicago Board of Health on a remedy for diphtheria and that "one of the most malignant of diseases has become one of the least dangerous through the discovery of a specific." It noted that some members of the Ontario Medical Association were still "unconvinced" about the antitoxin's life-saving power and that this report "negatives such views effectively." It also noted that a stubbornly high rate of incidence in Ontario was due in part to the expense of the antitoxin and it being out of the reach of poorer patients. It felt that in such instances the municipality should supply it.[64]

A related issue, and one that presaged interest in the commercialization of health research in IHPME about a century later, was captured in an editorial in 1906, "Discovery and Commercialism." It concerned the issue of Von Behring receiving nothing for his discovery of a diphtheria antitoxin while "manufacturers have made millions out of it" and the public are "charged a very long price." It felt that governments should be involved to "reward the one and protect the other."[65] The labs avoided all aspects of this dilemma.

Honorary Advisory Committee on Scientific Work (1917)

The labs also made other important contributions. For example, in September 1917, FitzGerald, in order that the labs "may provide a truly National service," asked that he be allowed to establish an "Honorary Advisory Committee of the Connaught Laboratories." He noted it would have representation from every province. Ontario and Saskatchewan were "providing very largely the financial support" of the labs through their free distribution of antitoxins through their respective boards of health.[66]

He wanted to have a senior member of health from each province and the federal government, "preferably the Chief Health Officer or Commissioner of Health." It was his belief that through the services being provided by Connaught and a forum such as this, "Connaught Laboratories may come ultimately to occupy the position in Canada, that the Lister Institute does in Great Britain and the Pasteur Institute in France."[67]

The committee became important because it is perhaps the earliest evidence that FitzGerald was not limiting his thinking to a university, a city, or even a province. He was thinking nationally – of the health of the nation. The committee became the country's first national forum for health.

He followed up his September letter with another in December further outlining its terms of reference including membership, as well as a draft letter to be sent to each premier asking for representation. In his letter to the president, he said that the chief executive officer in Public Health from each province "would be an especially suitable nominee." He also noted that the director of the labs would serve as secretary.[68] As it turned out, it had representatives initially from seven provinces (soon expanded).[69] In the 1919–20 report to the president, FitzGerald notes, "A very successful meeting of the Honorary Advisory Committee of the Laboratories was held during the year."[70]

The committee's members were all senior officials from the provinces. In New Brunswick it was the minister of health.[71] For Saskatchewan, it was M. Seymour, the senior civil servant in the Bureau of Public Health (he would become deputy minister when the bureau became a department in 1923).

It grew into the Dominion Council of Health in 1920 after the establishment of the Department of National Health.[72] A number of the members of FitzGerald's committee, including FitzGerald himself, became members of the council, and it was felt there was no need to continue with his committee.[73] This would have been a natural evolution, as the head of Hygiene, Amyot, left his position to become the first deputy minister of national health. FitzGerald became the new head of Hygiene, and the two knew each other well.

It is noteworthy that FtizGerald's national orientation was also evident in public health circles in Canada. In issues of the *Journal of Public Health* for 1918 there are multiple calls for the establishment of a department of health at the national level.[74]

It is a quality that would be a significant piece of the character of the labs, the school, and the Department of Hospital Administration. The school and the department would draw students from across Canada. And within this national context, Ontario and Saskatchewan would have a particularly close relationship to all three entities. As one example, Burns Roth, about whom we will learn more later, originated in Ontario, go from the Yukon to be a student in the second class of the department, from there to Saskatchewan, and from there back to the department to be its head.

Dominion Council on Health (1919)

In 1919 Newton Rowell (later of the Rowell-Sirois Commission) became the first federal minister of health and that same year organized the Dominion Council of Health. Its need grew out of the fact that health was a provincial responsibility. However, in that each of the provinces worked independently and none knew what the other was doing, there was a need for communication and coordinated effort. There was also recognition that what Canada needed was a health system.

Interesting, for our purposes, is that increasingly after 1927 membership came from the school's grads.[75] In 1948 all but four of the thirteen members were DPH grads.[76]

FitzGerald played a large role on the council, and the council reflected the concerns of the faculty of the school.[77] It met semi-annually, for a period of three days each time. FitzGerald's membership was a bit anomalous, as the council had the senior health officer of each province, and this meant there were two people from Ontario. The minutes of the council meetings show that FitzGerald was a keen participant.[78]

A Unique Organization

An article in the *Canadian Journal of Medicine and Surgery* in 1915 begins to get at the essence of the context we are trying to sketch. It is important because it illustrates a number of things that were at the leading edge at the time but now would be considered integral to the knowledge-based economy. They include partnerships between government and academia, a scientific evidence-based foundation, a marriage of basic and applied research, and research and knowledge pursued not just for its own sake but to solve a practical issue. It is also illustrative of a certain attitude of government and academia toward citizenship, such as making health available to all and a spirit of public service.

At the outset, the article says,

> Down in an obscure corner of the basement of the Medical Building of Toronto University a great and important public work is carried on. It is great because there is no limit to its expansion. It is important because it is the most outstanding effort of Government organization to stop, with a scientific barrier, the encroachments of disease that claim a high mortality. And it is unique because its service is as free as air and entirely untrammelled with red tape.
>
> The Department of Hygiene of Toronto University, in conjunction with the Provincial Board of Health, is producing and distributing what are known as biological products, such as small pox vaccine, diphtheria antitoxin.[79]

The article went on to talk about how Ontario is distinctive in "the easy manner in which the serum can be obtained" with free distribution that began in February of that year and also in making it available to the Canadian troops.[80]

A 1928 *Maclean's* article noted that prior to 1914 no antitoxins or vaccines were produced in Canada. They were imported from private manufacturers, through middlemen, which further increased the cost. The result was to reduce the amount that government could supply or that people could afford to purchase on their own. The issue was made worse in that diphtheria was a malady more prone to attack the children of poor families. It was all these factors that led FitzGerald to go to the university's board of governors "with a suggestion so unusual as to approach the revolutionary."[81]

The idea was that the university would develop a laboratory to make and sell these materials in commercial quantities at cost. It notes, "The idea of a university laboratory producing public health biological products for general distribution was without precedent. Fortunately, the University of Toronto is not entirely ruled by precedent or manacled by convention."[82] The article also noted that the labs are also "the largest insulin factory in the world" and "one of the greatest achievements in the cause of Canadian public health."[83]

In a 1917 article FitzGerald noted the opening ceremony of 25 October 1917 and the formal presentation of the labs and the fifty-acre farm to the university by Gooderham. He noted as well the premier had stated that $75,000 was to be voted in the next session of the legislature for research in preventive medicine. He indicated the work done at the university was similar to that of the Pasteur and Lister Institutes and added the Rockefeller Institute to that list.[84]

Another article in that volume noted that the labs was publishing a volume of studies presenting the results of experiments. It also noted that the antitoxin division was continuing to grow and that the governments of Ontario and Saskatchewan were distributing the diphtheria antitoxin, smallpox vaccine, and other products for free by their public health departments. In conclusion the antitoxin division was "not only self-supporting, but is able to provide funds for the maintenance of the research division."[85]

FitzGerald noted, "As the first commercial drug firm operated by an academic institution, Connaught Laboratories helped establish Canada as first in the world in preventive medicine and public health. By 1940, the year of FitzGerald's death, Hamilton and Toronto were declared the first cities in the world to be diphtheria-free."[86]

The magnitude of this accomplishment is given in a tribute to FitzGerald by J.W.S. McCullough. He noted that in 1914, while the diphtheria antitoxin had been available for twenty years, its effect on the mortality rate for the disease had been negligible, except where the product had been freely distributed to the public. He recounted conversations with the Ontario minister of health to distribute the antitoxin at first at low cost and later (in 1916) for free. The ministry asked for tenders from six Canadian companies. FitzGerald's from Connaught was the lowest, thirty cents per dose lower than the commercial price of 1914. "The number of deaths in Ontario, instead of being twelve hundred, were last year cut to seven.... This remarkable accomplishment – it is almost miraculous – may be attributed almost wholly to the establishment of Connaught Laboratories."[87]

In an article in *Maclean's* in 1955, June Callwood drew attention to the fact that in the United States their Salk polio vaccination of school children was halted because insufficiently tested vaccine had infected dozens of children with paralytic polio. A U.S. Senator said, "'The Eisenhower administration could learn a lot from our neighbors in Canada.'" She called the labs a hybrid that was part factory, part research laboratory, and part school for public health administrators. She also noted that they produced eighty-four products that ranged from vaccines to insulin to veterinary products to blood fractionation. It had scored a number of firsts, such as being the first in the world to make insulin, heparin, penicillin and combined antigens.[88]

Moreover, its prices for the Salk vaccine were one-third to one-quarter of U.S. prices. It was able to do this because it had very low operating costs and no selling expense. The Institute for Microbiology and Hygiene at the University of Montreal was patterned after it.[89] It established a presence for Canada in its field and built a thriving export market in places as distant as New Zealand, China, and the Caribbean.

Rutty expands on the important role that the labs played in the polio saga: "After World War II, Connaught had become a unique research and production institution."[90] It was able to undertake complex research, mount a large clinical trial, put in place rigorous quality controls, and scale up large production. It attracted much international attention and there was pressure for it to export. "Connaught's vaccine was 'a Canadian prestige item.'"[91] By April 1957 it was allowed to export and by June 1958 more than 5.5 million doses had been sent to Great Britain, with additional vaccine shipped to forty-four other countries. This helped reduce the price charged to governments on three successive occasions. While doing this it continued to supply 87.8 per cent of Canadian vaccine needs.[92] A notable initiative in Canada was "an unprecedented province-wide program in Saskatchewan that vaccinated 82% of the population." This was a major public health challenge, its logistics complicated by the largely rural population.[93]

The labs provide an interesting twist to the idea of the commercialization of research. While it produces a commercial product, it does so at cost. Its aim is not to maximize profits but to make its products available to as many as possible. It raises the question of whether the commercialization of research need not be restricted only to generating profits. It can be to generate a self-sustaining (as opposed to profit-making) company whose main aim is to provide a public service.

FitzGerald's activities were attracting attention. According to *Maclean's*, "Officials at the Rockefeller Foundation began to look at this odd experiment at Toronto where a provincial university was actually running a serum factory!"[94] FitzGerald indicated that what was needed was a facility to house both the research of the labs and the teaching functions of the school all in the same building, a marriage of two activities that we now take for granted. The result was a grant from the foundation to do just that. James FitzGerald describes the foundation as "a charitable trust of unprecedented global scale," which would become "a kind of surrogate government, the largest philanthropic organization in the world, the greatest benefactor of medicine in history," and "a pivotal influence" on his grandfather's destiny.[95]

Rutty has written, "No other university in the world had or has undertaken such an integrated and self-supporting public-health research, manufacturing, teaching, and public service-based biological distribution enterprise."[96] Later he observes, "It has often been suggested that FitzGerald's proposal for the University of Toronto to assume responsibility for his antitoxin production enterprise was a 'revolutionary' one for the university to accept."[97] June Callwood writes, "There was no precedent in the world for a university opening a branch pharmaceutical house."[98]

More recently an article by the head of philanthropic advisory services at Scotia Wealth Management crystallizes the contribution of the labs. It calls them the "greatest impact donation in Canadian history." It notes that the bench to bedside to community health clinic "cycle was exceptionally short." As a result of its success, "millions of dollars of research funding and donation flowed in." U of T became the third-largest medical research centre in North America by the 1920s.[99]

Burrows notes, "This is a philanthropic story that is hard to repeat. There was a rare convergence of independent factors: social need, science, scientist, donor, team, university and governments."[100] FitzGerald was at the centre of it.

All of this points to a nuance in FitzGerald's involvement of the labs, and the school as well: his organizational and managerial abilities. They have never been dealt with directly. We get glimmers when people write about other aspects of his life. For example, according to his grandson, "Former colleagues of my grandfather remember the Connaught as a seamlessly efficient organization demanding selfless service to a collective, missionary ideal."[101] This is an area for future research and one that, once again, points to a link between FitzGerald's activities and the future IHPME. We will see further evidence of FitzGerald's organizational and managerial abilities when we deal with his activities with the Canadian Army in the First World War.

The Discovery of Insulin

FitzGerald's report to the university president for 1921–22 recorded that the Labs were supporting "the very important researches on pancreas extract" by Banting, Best, Collip, and McLeod.[102] The next year it announced the "epoch-making discovery of Insulin" and the formation of an Insulin division of the Labs.[103]

A U of T article in 1922 announced the discovery of insulin: "Probably the greatest discovery in the Medical history of this country, and one of the most important in modern Medical research has been made at the University of Toronto."[104] This work had "been rendered possible through the financial aid generously given by the Connaught Laboratories" and "a discovery of decided importance has been made, the practical applications of which it is difficult to forecast."[105] According to James FitzGerald, "In the early 1920s ... the Connaught Laboratories were manufacturing almost 100 per cent of the Canadian supply of insulin, and its production capacity for its full range of preventive medicines was now comparable to that of the Pasteur Institute in Paris and the Lister Institute in London."[106]

Banting also noted the support of Connaught Labs. He recounted the process of developing a viable extract and Best's role at Connaught in achieving this. His address also mentioned the directorship FitzGerald and, in FitzGerald's absence, that of Defries in relation to Connaught Labs.[107]

Protecting the Availability of Insulin

When insulin was discovered, Banting, Best, Collip, Macleod, and FitzGerald stayed true to the ethos of the labs in making it available to as wide a group as possible. They wrote jointly to the president of U of T, Sir Robert Falconer, proposing that a patent be taken out purely as a defensive manoeuvre. It would not stop anyone else from making the extract. "In fact the point was to stop anyone from ever being in a position to stop anyone else."[108]

The U of T Archives has an interesting summary of the discovery of insulin: a multipage document in the president's papers of a "committee" (likely the Insulin Committee) in the School of Hygiene (FitzGerald was the secretary to the committee). It includes principles of dealing with the discovery, a transcribed letter (undated) to the president from J.J.R. Macleod, J.G. FitzGerald, F.C. Banting, and C.H. Best enunciating them,[109] another from the bursar to J.J.R. Macleod (26 May 1922) noting the board of governors has approved in principle the suggestions of the first letter,[110] and a third transcribed letter (26 May 1922) to Sir Walter Fletcher of the UK Medical Research Council (MRC).[111]

Overall the document sets out the parameters of dealing with the intellectual property aspect of the discovery. The major ones are that licences will be granted, but only to "reputable manufacturers who undertake to conform with such regulations as may be deemed necessary for the safeguarding of the public interest against commercial exploitation." Also that "license fees or royalties be charged only in so far as may be necessary to defray the expenses."[112] The issue of preventing commercial exploitation is evidently very important, as the principles on the administration of patents is "to prevent commercial exploitation on Insulin."[113]

The transcribed letter to the president indicates that the signatories have deemed "it is unsafe for us not to hold a patent" and that failure to take out a patent would open up a risk that others could duplicate the method of preparation of the extract and obtain their own patent, thereby restricting the U of T "continuance of the work."[114] It said, "The patent would not be used for any other purpose than to prevent the taking out of a patent by other persons" and that "the University holds the patent for the sole purpose of preventing any other person from taking out a similar patent, which might restrict the preparation of such an extract."[115]

It notes further the original purpose of the committee is "to protect Insulin against unrestrained commercial exploitation."[116] The transcribed letter to Walter Fletcher asks him to consider what needs to be done in order that "the preparation of 'insulin' may be properly safeguarded, and no one firm, or firms, succeed by patents in securing a monopoly in its production."[117]

There is a subsequent letter from N.W. Rowell (later of the Rowell-Sirois Commission) indicating that the material he has been provided with thus far does not constitute an agreement, though if it had been sent forward to the board of governors and approved, the Insulin Committee would then carry out the recommendations.[118]

Such thinking was all part of a total constellation of ways to use the revenue that was to be generated to help establish self-perpetuating research. In a letter to President Falconer, Fitzgerald proposed a research foundation be set up to administer the patents from insulin and collect a 5 per cent royalty from all companies that it is licensed to.[119]

The U of T report of the board of governors to the provincial government for 1924 notes, "The Insulin Committee has been extending the use of Insulin throughout the world, and has been successful in controlling the quality and price of the output by securing trade-marks and patents in many countries.... It has been a difficult piece of work, partly because there were no precedents for the policy adopted by the University, but happily the results have been good, and the Governors may have the satisfaction of knowing that the great discovery made in its laboratories has been of incalculable benefit at very low cost to sufferers in every part of the world."[120]

The kinds of deliberations of the Insulin Committee, its approach to patents and to their revenues, were farsighted for their time. They represented the same kind of technology transfer that many years later at IHPME would be studied by people like Fiona Miller and taught by people like me.

As important as this discovery was, many years later Dr Charles Hollenberg, a former chair of medicine at the university and head of the Department of Medicine at Toronto General Hospital, observed that the university would probably have been better off if insulin had been discovered someplace else, because he felt that some of the research momentum that had been established in other areas was diverted and perhaps lost.[121]

FitzGerald's Role

FitzGerald was integrally involved in the discussions over protection. Indeed, the principle of making insulin widely available and the proceeds going to support further research were those he had instituted with his own diphtheria products. The minutes of the Insulin Committee for 1 September 1922 note that he made a personal visit to Walter Fletcher, head of the MRC in the United Kingdom. The purpose was to see if the MRC "would be willing to accept the patents for the production of Insulin and use them in England along the same general principles as the University of Toronto." The MRC agreed, and a motion was passed by the committee to offer the patents rights to the MRC under those conditions.[122]

FitzGerald also played other important roles regarding the discovery. The importance FitzGerald placed on Banting's research is evident in Banting's handwritten notes regarding the events leading up to the discovery. Banting writes that he had made a promise to FitzGerald that he would not leave Toronto without consulting FitzGerald.[123] Banting's notes state FitzGerald "forced Dr Collip" to correct a claim made by Collip that Collip had made the first extract that was administered to a human diabetic.[124]

A University-Hospital Link

The discovery of insulin also demonstrated the importance of a teaching hospital as a site of clinical research and clinical trials. Connor notes that in terms of its discovery and efficacy, "Less well known are the contributions of Toronto General Hospital."[125] In January 1922 the first patient was administered the pancreatic extract there. Other patients followed, all with favourable results. In June 1922 the hospital established a diabetic clinic. However, as the word spread, the number of patients increased, and according to the hospital superintendent in his 1923 annual report, "The discovery of Insulin and the very close association of this institution with the early treatment of Diabetes with Insulin, brought to us seemingly all of the City's indigent sufferers from Diabetes."[126]

School of Hygiene (1924)

The roots of the school lay in the establishment of a diploma in public health at the University of Toronto. Robert Defries (DPH, 1914) was the first candidate to take courses for the DPH in the 1912–13 session.[127]

The School of Hygiene was established in 1924 with FitzGerald as its director. That same year the Rockefeller Foundation, as part of a larger international policy to improve health conditions, gave U of T money to construct a building for these purposes. This was the FitzGerald Building, opened in 1927, also (twenty years later) the first home of the Department of Hospital Administration.

Also catching the attention of the foundation was the work of Dr Charles Hastings (a graduate of Trinity Medical School), as medical health officer for Toronto (from 1910 to 1929), who had undertaken innovations that received international attention such as chlorinated water, baby clinics, and the pasteurization of milk. He was an important part of the teaching of preventive medicine in the school. He was the great-uncle of J.E.F. Hastings, the later chair of the Department of Health Administration and the first associate dean of the Division of Community Health.

As a result of Charles Hastings's work, the Rockefeller Foundation had already been sending fellows from different countries to Toronto to gain practical experience. It was also aware of FitzGerald's work in communicable disease. So when it was looking to showcase public health, it was not surprising its representatives paid a visit to Toronto. It would be the third school of public health in North America, the other two being Johns Hopkins (1916) and Harvard (1921).[128] It gave $1.2 million to establish the school. In its day this was a large sum (equivalent to roughly $30 million today). The school soon achieved a record of excellence that would match those of the Connaught Laboratories and the university's earlier efforts in public health.

The Opening of the School of Hygiene Building (1927)

The School of Hygiene was opened with much fanfare on 9 June 1927. As with the opening of Connaught Laboratories ten years earlier, the list of guests was impressive. It was formally opened by Sir George Newman, the first chief medical officer of Great Britain. He was considered a leading authority in public health whose annual reports as chief medical officer were eagerly awaited each year and were widely regarded as authoritative monographs in a variety of aspects in public health. It was felt he had substantial literary skill in always making them understandable to the public. He was the moving force behind establishment of the London School of Tropical Medicine and Hygiene.[129]

The opening was a front-page story in the *Globe*, which called Newman "one of the world's great authorities on public health." He also delivered a lecture "Medicine as a Science to Be Learned in Laboratory and Field."[130] According to a second story in the *Globe*'s "City News" section, Sir George said at the opening, "'The University of Toronto has taken upon itself the honour of having the most complete, advanced and thoroughly organized faculty and equipment of its kind of any similar institution in the world.'"[131]

The *Public Health Journal* (as the *Canadian Journal of Public Health* was called at the time) had a lengthy article on the opening. It reported that Canon Cody said that "Doctor FitzGerald possesses a rare combination of brilliant administrative abilities and an equally brilliant knowledge." He also acknowledged the work of FitzGerald's "Chief of Staff," R.D. Defries.[132]

The Character of the School

The school's three abiding characteristics were innovation, prevention, and inclusion. It constantly sought to innovate, to improve the health of the population. It constantly focused not only on the alleviation of illness and disease but on prevention as well. And it wanted the opportunity of health available to everyone and in this was an early supporter of the principle of health insurance. It was said the school's history is part "of a golden era in our history, when our brightest minds commanded the respect of not just their Canadian peers, but of the world."[133]

Rutty notes the role of the school in the polio saga. Deputy ministers were important in dealing with the epidemic. And Defries had "taught most of them at the School of Hygiene."[134]

In 1972 the University of Toronto sold the labs, and shortly thereafter the multiple divisions within the school were broken up and integrated into the various departments of the Faculty of Medicine. FitzGerald's grandson notes, "Without a forceful personality to sustain it, my grandfather's unique institutional vision had run its course."[135]

The Outcome

Dr G.H. Beaton noted that the "School produced leaders in getting things done," and in health it "was the source of a lot of the things happening in Canada."[136]

One of the strengths of the school was that it was composed of people who "tried to bridge both the development of science and the application of knowledge as it existed.... It may have been possible to do it then and be impossible to do it now with the explosion of knowledge and the drive for research methodology. It is probably more and more difficult for the same person in any country to be involved in the two extremes of quite fundamental research and the fine applications of it. The person in the middle tends to lose respect from the person at either end."[137]

It made for a kind of tension between practical and theoretical knowledge, research and public policy, bridging the differences between research and its application. Beaton was explicit about this tension and debates that took place in the school in regard to it. There was "a difficulty of trying to sort out the purpose, mission, role ... of individual courses. Were they to be academic courses, building theory, building analytical strategies, conceptualizations, which would be appropriate for degree students, or should the courses put a fair emphasis on analyzing practical situations toward practical solutions, which would be much more in keeping with the goal of the diploma programs?"[138]

The school was not necessarily an outlier in this regard. In 1938 Sir Frederick Banting, in his capacity as chair of the Associate Committee on Medical Research of the National Research Council, wanted to establish a research journal, because the two prominent Canadian health journals at the time, the *Canadian Journal of Public Health* founded in 1910 and the *Canadian Medical Association Journal* founded in 1911 both "emphasized papers more closely related to practice."[139]

We have to remember that Beaton made these observations in 1985. It is a discussion that today would not be seen in the same antithetical way. Etzkowitz, in a recent second edition of his landmark work, says that knowledge is polyvalent, more expeditiously translated into practical uses "as simultaneously theoretical and practical."[140]

Beaton also reflected on what made the school what it was and observed that "a real sharing took place in the lunchroom, a real crossing between departments." He sensed a tension between "entering the growing field of the basic sciences, to build the discipline stronger," and that "was a virtual counter-pressure to the concept of becoming global."[141]

Comments such as these suggest the school was facing a real strain in how it delivered on its mandate and in how it organized itself. There was the pull between an academic and practical orientation that Beaton speaks of. He notes the cross-disciplinary discussion that took place in the lunchroom, in other words, on how to properly organize such intellectual energy, on being pulled on the one hand to increasing specialization and on the other to a more generalized, horizontal, open structure. This is analogous to Rockefeller University or the Basel Institute for Immunology, neither of which had departments. Each had a form of organization that facilitated conversation, promoted interaction, the formation of spontaneous networks. Nels Jerne (who would later become a Nobel laureate) in planning the Basel Institute for Immunology's building, tried to maximize opportunities for interaction with numerous staircases between its two floors and a certain overcrowding.[142]

This kind of thinking was carried forward in the present SickKids research institute with the different floors grouped around a succession of three-floor atriums in order to maximize interaction. Staircases were placed to create "connectivity." The aim of the building was to create "free-flowing communities of researchers."[143]

According to Beaton, the "people recruited into, and retained within the old School of Hygiene were a rather unusual, and dedicated bunch of fellows.... It is amazing what that group accomplished both for Public Health and for science in Canada." He observed that the key to the leadership of the school was its "model of teamwork ... a sharing of philosophy as well as a technical level of thinking." He said the scientists in the school "made up a who's who of Public Health in Canada."[144] One only needs to refer to Bator's book and its account of their accomplishments – and not just accomplishments in and of themselves but aimed at improving people's lives – to see evidence of their contributions and how the school came by its reputation. Beaton is a case in point, with service on a number of WHO committees, his contribution to nutrition requirements in developing countries, and his work on vitamin and mineral requirements for populations generally.[145]

In limiting the amount of this work that is devoted to the labs and the school, many other academics associated with each have not been mentioned. But the academic calibre of person involved is borne out by their publication record. And not only was the professional side of these people important; they were also people of a very high level of personal character. One indicator is given in a tribute paid to Dr Donald Fraser, an associate director of Connaught, in whose name a memorial lectureship was set up.[146] Fraser was seen as the third pillar to the building and leadership of the school and labs.[147]

Bator and Rhodes note, "The 'Toronto Group' developed a tradition of teaching, research and public service that distinguished Connaught Laboratories and the School of Hygiene," which they stressed in an interdisciplinary approach to public health. Because of the school, out of twenty-nine institutions, U of T was among the first nine universities in North America, and the only one outside of the United States, accredited for postgraduate teaching in public health by the American Public Health Association.[148]

The school "assembled a remarkable band of men and women" who "combined the roles of stimulating teacher and trail-blazing scientist" who "laid the groundwork for the future development of the school and the Canadian health system after the Second World War ... included in that group were the pioneers of provincial and federal health policies."[149] For example, after 1927, membership of the Dominion Council of Health came from graduates of the DPH course.[150]

In addition, the labs and the school had a major impact on the evolution of health care in the nation and, indeed, internationally. In terms of the latter, Canada, through the labs and school, had a major impact on the international outcome of two diseases: diabetes and polio.

In terms of the nation they were repeatedly involved in eradicating epidemics (diphtheria, TB, polio) "that established new precedents in the free and unconditional provision of public health services." While "the range of specific medical and hospitalization services available ... varied provincially, in an era before universal public health insurance, there was a clear national trend towards their unconditional expansion." Moreover, "despite a tradition of provincial jurisdiction over health matters," such epidemics "led to increased federal intervention and the imposition of national public financing," and such federal intervention was "strongly encouraged if not expected."[151]

In terms of polio, Rutty says that a strong influence in the Canadian state response was the central role played by the labs and school and the leadership of their head, Defries. His national public health connections at the personal, professional, and political levels, coupled with the shared educational experience and values gained through these organizations, established the foundation on which a generation of leaders across Canada approached the complexities of public health and scientific problems, most of whom had been trained at the school. In addition, there was the physical capacity and research experience of the labs.[152]

Comment on the Links between the Labs and School

There are links between the labs and school and the evolving Canadian identity. The labs may illustrate a unique aspect of the Canadian identity: its use of corporations owned either by the government (Crown corporations) or by a public institution. Their distinctive character is that service is as important as revenue and surplus revenue is put to a common good. Connaught Labs is one example, and the Crown corporations of the Tommy Douglas government in Saskatchewan another.

As a further example, Canadian hospitals are private corporations, but non-profit, publicly funded, and with a public (service) mandate. How they are structured matters. A US book on the link between care and the structure of the hospital discusses the commodification of hospital care in that country. It compares three different types of hospitals and notes that, despite certain similarities, "they are in many ways worlds apart."[153]

Rutty notes that the labs influenced public health as well as the evolution of state intervention in health. His dissertation is an account of the major role the labs played in the polio saga. But on a broader canvas, the disease and the labs played a role in the evolution of state involvement in health: "No other single infectious disease had provoked such a broad public response in Canada. While the range of specific medical and hospitalization services ... varied provincially, in an era before universal public health insurance, there was a clear national trend towards their unconditional expansion."[154]

He notes that the strong state-led response to polio was "the clearest feature distinguishing" the Canadian response from that of the American and the Canadian response had "an important historical impact" not only in this country but internationally as well.[155] He adds, "The Canadian Salk vaccine experience dramatically demonstrated the value of government intervention in public health, which resulted ultimately in a fairer, faster, safer and much less expensive program than was the case south of the border ... Ironically, it seems that a tradition and ideology of less state involvement in health care in the United States reinforced more state intervention north of the border."[156]

The labs had demonstrated the same public health spirit in its production and distribution of the diphtheria antitoxin and insulin and in continually driving the price down. It was clear that the Canadian public expected government intervention to help solve public health challenges in areas such as these, as well as diseases such as TB, and emerging ones such as cancer. The role of the labs, owned by a public institution in working with public health officials and influencing public health policy, was unique. It made an international impact in diphtheria, diabetes, and polio. Further, the health systems management aspect of this activity would anticipate the focus of IHPME.

On a more general level, FitzGerald's widow remarked that when her husband showed signs of exhaustion from his frenetic pace, she would say, "Slow down, Gerry. A hundred years from now who will care? It's not that important!" Sometime later she recalled those words: "I guess Gerry knew all along. A hundred years from now, people *will* care. It really *was* that important."[157]

THE SCHOOL'S SUPPORT FOR NURSING EDUCATION: EMPHASIZING PUBLIC HEALTH NURSING

Although today nursing and public health are located in the same building, the School of Hygiene provided important help for what was the Department of Public Health Nursing in the 1920s. Carpenter notes that FitzGerald "gave strong support to the development of nursing education in the University of Toronto."[158] This was important because the university was not entirely sure it had a role in nursing education.[159] A Department of Public Health Nursing was opened in 1920 but its existence was somewhat tenuous. One impediment was adequate office and classroom space. In 1924 FitzGerald offered to accommodate the department in the new building to be erected for Hygiene.[160]

Its integration with the School of Hygiene is evident in a proposal likely seeking funding for a new building and expanded operations of the school. It outlines the activities of the Department of Hygiene and Preventive Medicine, Department of Public Health Nursing, and Connaught Laboratories. It deals with educational responsibilities (at the graduate, undergraduate, and extension levels), present funds available to support operations, and the funds required for a building and endowment (to support further education programming).[161]

This association between the Nursing Department and a school with strong connections to the Rockefeller Foundation brought the department into contact with the foundation.[162] Farley notes that, for the foundation, Toronto's nursing program "became the model nursing institution against which all others were measured." It sent almost 40 per cent of its nursing fellows to Toronto, nine times the number sent to Yale.[163] One reason for its enthusiasm was that the Toronto program emphasized both hospital and public health nursing. It considered the department's director, Kathleen Russell, "the world's finest nurse educator," and its support of her "followed a Health Division pattern of judging a program by the caliber of the personnel involved."[164]

Jean Gunn was another strong advocate of public health nursing and a university-based course. This lent a good deal of support to its establishment because of her position as head of the prominent TGH School of Nursing. Russell was a former student of Gunn's who also considered Gunn a mentor. In 1920 nineteen of the students enrolled in the first program were from TGH.[165] Gunn served with FitzGerald on the board of the Canadian National Council for Combatting Venereal Disease, which was formed in 1919.[166]

There was a close relationship between the U of T Department of Nursing in the School of Hygiene and the TGH School, as the course involved two years of work at the university and two years at either TGH or the SickKids School for Nurses. As well the work at the university for the four-year course also qualified the student for a diploma from either TGH, the SickKids School, or the university.[167]

Gunn was instrumental in the development of public health nursing at U of T.[168] In 1924 she told an audience at the TGH nursing commencement exercises that society's needs were changing, there was unprecedented developments in public health, and graduates had to be prepared to participate in an entirely new field of nursing.[169]

This placed her in a predicament. Her first responsibility was to train hospital nurses. Yet she was keenly aware of the need for her graduates to find work outside the hospital, and public health nursing "was very much a needed commodity in the community." This made for a second responsibility for the nurse to enter this area, which also included a preventive focus.[170]

After the school had been established at U of T, Gunn worked to have nursing education broaden to include prepare graduates for two other areas, noted below. She worked through Sir Joseph Flavelle, who was on both the Board of Trustees of TGH and the Board of Governors of U of T.[171] Flavelle wrote to Falconer indicating that the present mode of instruction at the university "fits graduate nurses for Social Service [meaning public health] work." The result is that "the best graduates are not available for Hospital administration and teaching."[172]

In 1927 the department moved into what is now called the FitzGerald Building. It was a unit of the school but with administrative independence. It would move into its own building when it received its own Rockefeller funding. It is evident Ms Russell had great respect for FitzGerald. On his death in 1940 she inserted a paragraph in her annual report to the university president in which she noted "the loss of a great friend" who helped initiate "formal courses in public health nursing" in 1920, and "the school in its present form owes its very existence to him."[173]

In 1929 in the Gordon Bell Memorial Lecture, FitzGerald singled out the role of the public health nurse in preventive medicine and health education. He noted that the role of the public health nurse in the home, clinic, and school has brought individuals and groups into contact with "the precepts of preventive medicine in its broadest aspects in a manner undreamed of a quarter century ago."[174]

A colleague of FitzGerald's, Donald T. Fraser, described the vital contribution of public health nurses, who played an invaluable role in the delivery of municipal and rural health services. He argued that in a new country like Canada with its wide distribution of population, immigrants from many countries, and limited health resources such as hospitals in certain regions necessitated the adoption of a curriculum that could respond to these conditions.[175]

A short history of the development of public health nursing at the U of T was a part of the first calendar for its School of Nursing.[176] Even when nursing at U of T became its own school in 1933, its emphasis on public health nursing remained. Its relationships with the School of Hygiene, TGH, HSC, the Toronto and Ontario Departments of Health, the Ontario Division of the Canadian Red Cross Society, and others, also remained.[177]

CHAPTER 4

FitzGerald: Health Policy, Comparative Health Systems

HEALTH POLICY

FitzGerald on Health Insurance

Speeches and Writings on Health Insurance

An area that has always been important to both the department and the school is health insurance. At almost every major parliamentary event that debated the issue, the department or the school was either submitting a brief or speaking. It began very early in the school's history. It is another major area of study that it and its predecessor (hospital insurance) would form within the Department of Hospital Administration and later IHPME.

FitzGerald became a proponent of some form of health insurance as early as 1917. At that time he recommended free medical care for university students based on a form of health insurance. He noted the state insurance provided in Britain and similar university schemes at the University of California and University of Wisconsin and said, "The idea is actually the application in the University, of State Medicine."[1]

His support for health insurance continued in the 1920s.[2] In one of his books he wrote, "The state should provide a service for those to whom the cost of complete health supervision is prohibitive" and "no stigma of charity should be attached to its acceptance." He was at pains to assuage those who might be strongly opposed to such measures by saying, "The evolution of such a plan as this does not necessitate the application of principles to which many are opposed, such as the nationalization of the medical profession, or the introduction of national health insurance." He also said the "primary aim should be clearly recognized; it is to provide for all the people … satisfactory provision … which will have as its first aim the promotion of health and the prevention of disease."[3]

In a 1925 address to the annual meeting of the Canadian Life Insurance Officers Association he spoke of the National Health Insurance scheme of Great Britain. He called it an "addition to the provision of adequate central and local public health machinery.... England has, among the great industrial countries, taken the lead in attempting through state aid, as well as by private philanthropy, to cope with the problems on preventable mortality."[4]

In the Gordon Bell Memorial Lecture, presented at the Winnipeg Medical Society in November 1928, he asked, "Is it not desirable to take the next step and make arrangements so that health supervision will be made available for persons of all ages and of any economic or social condition?" In this same address he also noted in such an instance, "curative and preventive medicine shall no longer be separated."[5]

First Conference on Medical Services (1924)

At the meeting of the Canadian Medical Association held in Ottawa in June 1924, it was determined to convene a conference in Ottawa to discuss matters of interest common to all sections of the medical profession in Canada.[6] This was held in December that year. In addition to FitzGerald (and Amyot), other officers who were DPH grads were invited.[7]

Public health received a good deal of attention, and FitzGerald said that determining the "ways and means" of supporting such activities was vital.[8] Dr J.H. MacDermot from British Columbia presented on that province's activities regarding health insurance. As a result, a motion was made to refer the matter to the executive committee of the Canadian Medical Association (CMA).[9] Dr MacMurchy had a lengthy presentation on maternal mortality.[10]

It is interesting for our purposes that, even at this early date, and amongst all the issues discussed, hospital management was a topic. M. Seymour, the deputy minister of public health for Saskatchewan noted it in his presentation.[11] Other topics discussed included the need for full-time local public health organizations, health insurance, and maternal and infant mortality.

Second Conference on Medical Services (1927)

The second conference was convened in Ottawa's Parliament Buildings in March 1927. Among the more prominent topics discussed were public health and "state medicine." FitzGerald and Amyot attended. As with the first conference, other officers who were DPH grads were in attendance.[12]

In the introductory remarks the endowment of the Rockefeller Foundation to create a School of Hygiene at the University of Toronto "under the directorship of Dr FitzGerald" was mentioned. It was noted that there are such schools in cities like Berlin, Prague, London, and the Foundation had established one at Baltimore and Harvard, and said, "It is difficult to overestimate the value of such an institute in the interest of public health activities in Canada."[13]

FitzGerald built on several presentations by suggesting "all-time" services in public health be extended as much as possible from "urban to rural communities." He singled out Saskatchewan in its introduction of maternity benefits, noted that it "is perhaps part and parcel of a larger thing, to which the Deputy Minister of Health made reference." He added that a future conference might consider "how is the community to afford medical, nursing, and hospital service" to the 75–80 per cent of the people who cannot afford them. He noted the wealthy can afford them and the destitute have them provided, but the huge majority are left out. "No one wants to be destitute in order to get good medical and surgical service." He also suggested following the lead of BC in "undertaking a serious study of health insurance." He also advocated for "periodic health examinations" and, interestingly, in the CMA developing the means to carry out "popular health education."[14]

Helen MacMurchy attended and mentioned the Hospital Map of Canada.[15] This was a project Agnew would update with her at the CMA two years later. Her presence linked to FitzGerald's remarks on maternal benefits and the wider issue of maternal and infant mortality, as Canada had much poorer statistics in this area than other countries of the Commonwealth. Because of her work in Ontario, MacMurchy had been hired to direct a national educational campaign to lower infant and maternal deaths. She wrote a number of "Little Blue Books" published by the federal Department of Health, which were printed in dozens of languages and sold millions of copies. Dodd said, "The Blue Books represent the first indication of federal government responsibility for the health of Canadians, and foreshadow later implementation of health insurance."[16]

The second speaker at the Second Conference on Medical Services was J. Amyot. He went from the head of the antitoxin lab at U of T to become the first federal deputy minister of health, and spoke to his medical colleagues on health insurance in that capacity. One section of his address was "Do We

Want State Medicine?" He noted that the wealthy and the poor can each get medical treatment but asked, "What of that great body – the mid-financially placed?" Though he introduced the topic in his remarks at the beginning of the meeting, it was not taken up in any further discussions.[17]

His son, Dr G.A. Amyot, who would become British Columbia's chief medical officer would also be a staunch supporter of the idea. He would be a DPH graduate of the school, would work in the Department of Public Health in Saskatchewan, and be the first deputy minister of British Columbia's Department of Health and Welfare.

Other Articles Supporting Health Insurance

In an article on the future of public health in April 1928 FitzGerald referred to health insurance as "another urgent need [that] must be met" and "Present arrangements for the care and treatment of the sick are not altogether satisfactory." He said health insurance "is realizable and would undoubtedly vastly improve the state of the public health."[18]

Gordon Bell Memorial Lecture (1928)

In the Gordon Bell Memorial Lecture in November 1928 FitzGerald dwelt on health insurance. The lecture was also notable for its treatment of medicine, public health, and prevention, and each was distinctive for the historical overview he provided of their development. What was also notable was his treatment of comparative systems, i.e., the development of these in other countries. He also dealt with other areas that would be considered very current today: mental health and medical education. This was before the era of graduate education and a pool of graduate students to help with the research for the lecture. It is almost certain that this was knowledge FitzGerald had acquired of his own accord.

He devoted a good portion of the lecture to health insurance. It is interesting in that he saw the burden of illness in a society as a public health issue. He said, "It may be fairly asked at the juncture whether the extension of interest of the organized community – the state – into the problem of non-communicable preventable disease or indeed invalidity in general would be in the best interest of the public."[19] He went on, "Satisfactory provision for the necessary requirements in the way of medical and other related services both preventive and curative is for a large part of the population very difficult."[20] What he meant was that cost prevented many people from seeking diagnosis and treatment. The implicit conclusion was that if this cost could be mitigated, the burden of disease on a society would be decreased and the proportion of healthy individuals who could participate in a society could be increased.

He turned to a more detailed discussion of how a good portion of the public could not afford health care and the consequences, health and economic. He asked whether "the present system for the prevention of sickness and the provision of medical care in this country is the best that can be devised" and that, if not, the first essential was "an inquiry into the facts of the situation." The Committee on the Costs of Medical Care in the United States was one example of how such issues might be addressed.[21]

He then went into a detailed account of the voluntary plans in effect in places like Denmark that have been adopted in other European countries. He noted the stance of the International Labour Office of the League of Nations in a 1927 statement on compulsory insurance and the role of the state therein.[22]

What was interesting was that he saw health insurance as an essential tool for public health and prevention. He quoted the chief medical officer for England and Wales as saying the National Insurance Act (1925) brought "a great body of private practitioners into organic relation to our public organization of preventive medicine." A good deal of this was because the patient was encouraged to see the doctor early.[23]

Appearance at a House of Commons Standing Committee (1929)

FitzGerald was asked to speak about sickness insurance at the 14 March 1929 session of the House of Commons Select Standing Committee on Industrial and International Relations. He noted that compulsory insurance against sickness was not new and that since 1884 such a plan had been in effect in Germany and an equally comprehensive plan of voluntary insurance in place in Denmark. He also noted that since 1912 a compulsory plan had been in effect in Britain.[24]

He outlined seven principles that should underlie "social legislation of this sort," such as provision of benefits, free choice of physician, control of the medical service by the medical profession, and provision for education in preventive medicine.[25] It is interesting that he was not necessarily advocating for a state-run insurance system.

He addressed what he termed "valetudinarianism," which suggests that a certain proportion of the insured population may imagine themselves as suffering from some ailment when in actuality they are not and that this could increase costs. He noted that this possibility had not been found to be of significance.[26] He referenced *Medical Benefit*, a study of the experience of Germany and Denmark.[27]

His presentation was very comprehensive, going into proceedings of the Ninety-Second Meeting of the British Medical Association published in the *British Medical Journal* of 1924 and into statements by the chief medical officer of the Ministry of Health of England and Wales. Again as a measure of comprehensiveness he provided the names and page numbers of reports referencing the comments made by these individuals.[28]

He also suggested that it was "highly desirable" that a study be undertaken of the Canadian situation to answer four questions: the volume of sickness and invalidity, provisions to deal with it, the cost of medical care (including dental care), and provisions for insurance against sickness and invalidity.[29]

The famous social democratic MP Mr Woodsworth had several questions for FitzGerald. One was whether the entire bill for medical services would be less under a national system than at present. FitzGerald replied, "The view held in countries where there are systems of national insurance is that the State and the individuals in those countries are better off financially, which probably means that they spend less on preventable sickness than they did before."[30]

FitzGerald was also asked whether the British system could be adapted to Canada. He felt it could. He was then queried about the Canadian demographic condition – scattered population, part of it living in pioneer conditions, a considerable proportion engaged in agriculture – and whether it would make a system more difficult to administer than in an industrialized country like Britain. He replied that the situation in Denmark was not so dissimilar to that of Canada – it was agricultural and scattered, with many people living in isolated communities on islands – and that they had been able to make their system work. He was queried on the case of the Canadian farmer "who is almost on the verge of necessity," and he replied that Denmark had been able to make this work by providing for people below a certain income level. Another social democratic MP, Miss MacPhail, questioned him further on the rural situation and he added information on the Islands and Highlands Medical Service in Scotland as well as an initiative in Kentucky, each of which delivered medical services to those living in remote communities.[31]

Third Conference on Medical Services (1929)

A Third Conference on Medical Services convened in November 1929. Both Agnew and FitzGerald attended.[32] Three of the attendees were DPH grads,[33] and two others (Amyot and FitzGerald) were former and current heads of the antitoxin lab.

One of the first items was in response to a matter "referred by resolution or discussion, for study and action by the Canadian Medical Association" at the Second Conference on Medical Services, a Hospital Service department was set up by the CMA. It was supported by a grant from Sun Life Assurance.[34] Agnew was hired to be its head (more on this later).

The two main topics were health and the state, which included public health and health insurance (also hospitals) and medical education.[35]

Agnew and FitzGerald each supported two amendments to a resolution on the treatment of drug addicts. Agnew asked that the resolution be amended so that hospitals be specifically designated as a place of treatment. FitzGerald took this one step further to ask that judges or courts be empowered to send addicts to hospitals rather than jail.[36]

Agnew was also called upon to provide an interim report of the Medical Survey of Canada.[37]

Article on the Municipal Doctor Program (1933)

Related to health insurance in Canada, many would argue a rural form of it was the municipal doctor program of Saskatchewan, which served 20 per cent of the population.[38] FitzGerald wrote an article on it in 1933 and said that one of the most interesting features of the program was its opportunity for public health work and for preventive medicine.[39]

FitzGerald had more than a passing familiarity with physician practice in Saskatchewan, as he had spent time there on a tour with a postgraduate team that met with small community doctors delivering lectures and clinics.[40]

He also said, "The assumption by the people of a rural municipality of the responsibility of providing ordinary general practitioner services for themselves as they do educational facilities through direct taxation of assessable property possesses at this time [is] a certain novelty."[41]

He also linked what was happening here with the wider issue of health insurance: "Public interest in the question of the provision of medical care at a cost which people can afford to pay is general throughout the United States and Canada at the present time. These experiments in Manitoba and Saskatchewan have their origins in the soil of sheer necessity. Their further evolution and development may be of general interest and importance. As a form of health insurance provided by rural people to meet their own needs and at their expense entirely, it is a radical departure in many respects from the conventional type of private medical practice which has heretofore prevailed."[42]

He called it an "interesting social experiment" and noted, "It is an entirely voluntary effort and in this respect differs fundamentally from the compulsory schemes of health insurance as they exist at present in Great Britain, Germany, France and other European countries."[43]

FitzGerald published the article in the *University of Toronto Monthly*, which had a different and larger readership and was published more frequently than, for example, the *University of Toronto Quarterly*, which had a more academic orientation.

CMA Committee on Economics Report (1934)

In 1931 the CMA Committee on Economics was struck to examine health insurance. DPH grad Grant Fleming served as secretary to the committee, and FitzGerald was a member (he was also the chair of the Committee on Public Health and Medical Publicity). The report was presented to the association at their annual meeting in 1934.[44] For its time it would have easily been one of the best reports on the topic for Canadians and a good referent for provincial governments (a brief outline is provided in the previous footnote). Taylor notes that the report "was remarkably comprehensive and objective."[45] Throughout it noted sources of literature on aspects of the topic (with a bibliography at the end of part 3). It also outlined plans in other countries.

One point very close to the interests of Fleming and FitzGerald was in its concluding statement: "The most serious ill result which could grow out of health insurance would be its being considered as a 'cure all.' At best, it is but a part of what should be evolved – a complete medical service which will secure the fullest application of preventive and curative medicine."[46]

FitzGerald and the Rowell-Sirois Report (1939)

The Rowell-Sirois Report is instructive for what it did not say. This was a major royal commission redefining some of the rules of Confederation to bring them more in line with present realities. One of its "Red Books" was on social insurance and one of its reports was on public health. Each was done by a U of T faculty member, A.E. Grauer.[47] Neither FitzGerald nor the School of Hygiene is mentioned in either.

The report on public health sketched out its role in the nation. Yet the leading graduate program in public health, one with an international reputation, one that has graduated many of the leading medical officers of health it talks about, one that has intimate connections with local and provincial departments of health, is not once noted. And neither is its director, who is a leading authority on the subject, with his own international reputation.

For example Grauer talks of training physicians in public health and notes the role of medical schools in this regard. But he does not mention a free-standing, dedicated school toward this end, one not nested within a medical school, moreover one that is located at his very university.[48]

In the hearings of the commission some of the results of FitzGerald's work were mentioned, though not attributed to him. For example, the presentation of the Health League of Canada noted that at one time diphtheria was the most serious diseases of childhood, causing more deaths between the ages of two and five than any other childhood ailment. However, in Toronto in 1937 there were no deaths, due to the measures taken.[49]

Jean Gunn Presents to the Commission

Jean Gunn, whom we came across earlier regarding her association with FitzGerald and Stuart, presented to the commission. Riegler notes that she had an active interest for a number of years in health insurance,[50] which began as early as 1934 at the Canadian Nurses Association meeting.[51]

She presented to the commission in her role as chair of the Health Insurance and Nursing Service Committee of the Canadian Nurses' Association. The presentation emphasized nursing care and in so doing distinguished between that and physician care. It noted, "A large percentage of ill people can be satisfactorily cared for by a visiting nurse organization."[52] However, "fewer than 38% of the patients who need the services of a trained nurse are able to obtain them" and "only 3 out of 8 people of moderate means who require skilled nursing care, are able to pay for such a service."[53]

It was explicit in the distinction between nursing and physician care in its second recommendation, which she read into the record: "That, if and when legislation for health insurance makes provision for medical service to the insured, nursing service should be included."[54] Miss Gunn explained the reason, which included her emphasis on public health nursing. She noted that "a great many people" think of medical service as being only the service of a physician. However, "Nursing care is an essential part of medical care" and "medical care is not adequate without nursing care."[55] Finally, and this was her implicit statement on public health nursing, "Many patients, if they had adequate nursing care, would not require hospitalization.... The patient is sent to hospital very often when that patient could be taken care of in the home."[56]

She also quoted a recommendation of the Canadian Nurses Association: "That the importance of the preventive aspect be stressed and that it be included under the administrative control of the Health Insurance plan," that any program of health insurance should "dove-tail into the health program of the province or municipality," and that "stressing the preventive side will result in an economy for both the patient and for the state." She went further in saying (and here she was implicitly stressing the need for good primary care), that if people are encouraged to seek advice before they are acutely ill there would be great savings. Also, "Health insurance should not be limited to the people who are ill, if so the chief value is lost."[57]

Contextualizing FitzGerald on Health Insurance

There are striking nuances to FitzGerald's statements on health insurance. That he felt it bore looking at there can be no question. That in many ways he felt it was necessary is most likely. That it was very consistent with his own thoughts of having medicine available to the widest possible group, also not open to question. However, that he felt it should be a state-run system is much less clear. When his thoughts are put against those of people on the League for Social Reconstruction, which was very active in the 1930s and many of whom were U of T faculty, he is not in the same league (double meaning intended).

FitzGerald's views were more in line with those of his colleague and friend at McGill, Grant Fleming. Fleming, who was the witness at the standing committee who preceded FitzGerald, spoke at length about public health. But he also got into the question of health insurance. In his presentation he quoted from the medical secretary of the British Medical Association in listing its benefits to the public and the medical profession.[58]

He actually quoted from a very pragmatic request of the profession that FitzGerald had made at the Gordon Bell Memorial Lecture in November 1928: "To ascertain whether adequate and satisfactory medical service, preventive and curative, is within reach of all persons in need thereof."[59] Dr Fleming also stated that he felt this should include whether the present volume of sickness may be lessened.[60]

Under questioning from Woodsworth on the merits of a public and private system, Fleming noted that one of the things that always impressed him in his experience with the Toronto Health Department was "the whole group were always willing to work Sundays and overtime to give their best services when they know perfectly well that there was not going to be any financial reward ... and my own experience has been that individuals will give everything they have to a public service although their remuneration may be very small, and there certainly would be greater opportunities for gain outside."[61] He was also asked by Woodsworth his opinion about compulsory and voluntary insurance and he came down on the side of compulsory.[62]

Among those more critical of the system, fellow faculty were writing in the *University of Toronto Quarterly* through the 1930s, people like A.E. Grauer and F.R. Scott. They were much more critical of the government's role in areas like unemployment, social insurance, and the Rowell-Sirois Report, and felt that much more needed to be done.

Grauer, for example, criticized the unemployment insurance begun by the Canadian government in 1935 for being not nearly enough. He said, "It does not attack the basic problem, the causes of unemployment." He also said it concentrated "on results, not causes, and by giving people the false feeling that the situation is being adequately met, it tends to obscure the pressing necessity for attacking the causes."[63] He then went on to say, "But as long as the chief causes of breakdown are allowed to operate – as long as the credit mechanism is allowed to get out of hand and our present maldistribution of income allowed to remain – far from having any assurance that the unemployment situation is being adequately met, we cannot even be certain that our industrial system will survive."[64]

Scott, in talking about social reform and the commission, noted, "Reform has been avoided to a degree remarkable in relation to the disclosed need," and "it is the opinion of the present writer that the area in which a progressive democracy must get to work in this Dominion is far wider that that mapped out for consideration by the Royal Commission on Dominion-Provincial Relations."[65]

Bator and Rhodes note, "By the end of the 1920s he [FitzGerald] was a proponent of some form of health insurance."[66] However, he never became as vocal as his colleague at McGill, Grant Fleming (DPH, 1914), whose testimony had preceded his own at the federal Committee on Industrial and International Relations. Fleming wrote about the topic throughout his career.[67]

If one were to construct a spectrum of thinkers, those on the left felt there were endemic problems with capitalism that required state intervention to provide more equal economic opportunity and to mitigate risk, particularly regarding unemployment and health. Others – people like Grant Fleming and Harvey Agnew – felt that "state medicine" was somewhat inevitable and the best way for physicians to have some input into the outcome was to make themselves part of the process. Then for others like FitzGerald, this issue was not central; rather, their life work was all-consuming.

One conclusion one can reach from FitzGerald's approach to health insurance and, in particular, his article on the municipal doctor program, his presentation and comments to the House of Commons Standing Committee (1929), and the Gordon Bell Memorial Lecture, is that he saw illness care and health insurance as a public health problem. He saw the burden of illness of a society as a public health issue, and preventive and curative medicine needed to work together.

It is a most interesting perspective for us in our present era, where illness care consumes most of the health budget of any nation and in the public mind has greatly eclipsed public health. And yet FitzGerald's thinking instructs us, as one of the great public health minds of the last century, that health insurance, that great institutions like medicare in Canada or the NHS in Britain, had its genesis in public health.

His thinking and that of others was that the burden of illness, i.e., the proportion of ill people in a society, needed to be reduced, and to do that there needed to be an available modality for the public – and the public meant everyone – to access it.

What Might Have Been

The ferment of health insurance that was brewing during the latter part of FitzGerald's life was about to become much more active, and the Second World War greatly accelerated its progression. It is interesting to speculate how FitzGerald's thoughts would have evolved and how he might have contended with the issue had he been alive to see the Beveridge Report of 1942, or the Special Committee on Social Security (1943), which he would have almost invariably have presented at (given that Defries did), or the Heagerty, Marsh, and Cassidy reports. Then the Green Book on Health of the Dominion-Provincial Conference on Reconstruction (1945).

Interesting as well would have been FitzGerald being alive to see the election of a young activist premier in Saskatchewan who espoused his ideals in public health and health insurance, a premier who felt so strongly about this he took on the health portfolio himself in his first term. FitzGerald would have seen him make good on the first plank of health insurance – hospital insurance – in 1947. And even closer to FitzGerald's heart, Douglas's personal oversight and emphasis on building a department of health with an emphasis on public health and prevention. In so many ways it would have been a logical progression of FitzGerald's thought. There was also the close relationship that was established between Douglas's department and graduates of the school, both in its departments of public health and hospital administration.

COMPARATIVE HEALTH SYSTEMS

Another area that FitzGerald was involved in that is more mainstream today is comparative health studies. Whether it was dealing with the development of a diphtheria antitoxin, social policies, health insurance, or medical education, FitzGerald always wanted to personally go to other places to seek out other perspectives.

To Denmark to Research Its Social Policies

Fitzgerald made a trip to Scandinavia in 1925 and, importantly, gave media interviews on what he found in regard to their social services. He was most impressed with Denmark, and his media interview focused on it. He noted the number of cooperative societies (4000) in the country that market their agricultural products. He noted the country had old age pensions and sick benefit organizations to which 60 per cent of the people belonged. He said they had "splendid hospitals" and that "they are among the best in the world."

He noted that it was one of the first countries to adopt the manufacturing of insulin after Banting and Best's discovery. Denmark had sent a scientist to U of T to learn how it was made and to get information on their system of public health, medical education, and medical research. In another report he said Denmark was "showing the way to the rest of the medical world in the encouragement of fundamental researches."[68]

Involvement in Global Health

FitzGerald was also an early proponent of what he termed "international public health," today called global health. He was a member of the Permanent Health Committee of the League of Nations, and he presented a synopsis of its activities at the 1933 annual meeting of the Canadian Public Health Association. He noted several issues it was grappling with, the first of which was the repatriation of hundreds of thousands of refugees as a result of the end of the First World War, which "involved migrations of a magnitude probably never previously witnessed."

The committee also studied sanitary conditions in various countries. Another activity grew out of "the present widespread facilities for international intercourse and travel" which gave rise to "new and unforeseen dangers." Preventive medicine was another important activity.[69]

Survey of Medical Schools

FitzGerald resigned his post as dean of medicine at U of T in 1936 in order to undertake a year of travel at the invitation of the Rockefeller Foundation. The purpose was to study the methods employed in the teaching of preventative medicine. It was noted he travelled over 24,000 miles. He visited sixty-four European universities and thirty in the United States and Canada.[70]

Bringing in Foreign Faculty

FitzGerald not only went to other countries. He brought people from other countries to the school. It was important to him that there be cross-fertilization of ideas. An example is in the fall of 1927, just after the opening of the new building funded by the Rockefeller Foundation, when Gaston Ramon, a French scientist from the Pasteur Institute who had been the first to prepare diphtheria toxoid, was working as a guest researcher at Connaught.

During that time he gave a presentation on research and said of the "research man" that it is necessary to move beyond theory to "possible practical applications thereof," that a scientist must "set forth his researches ... to make them known" – in other words, publish. But he also said it was very important was to "discuss problems with those who are working in other places and in other conditions in the same field; he must examine and discuss in conversation with his colleagues the questions which interest them mutually. These meetings, these discussions, these exchanges of ideas are one of the essential conditions for spreading the truth and for scientific progress, towards which all the efforts of the 'research man' must tend."[71]

He next expressed his appreciation "for having permitted me to understand these facts." The visit resulted in FitzGerald being invited to contribute to the *Annales de l'Institut Pasteur.*[72]

PART THREE

The Pressure Builds: An Increasing Profile for Health

CHAPTER 5

Health Increasingly a Provincial and National Concern

Beginning in the interwar period, health began to occupy an increasing profile nationally and in federated countries like Canada and the United States sub-nationally as well. This would continue during the Second World War and the immediate post-war era. This increasing profile for health could not help but have an effect on the profile of the school and its soon-to-be-established Department of Hospital Administration.

The interwar period would see a number of valiant attempts at health care reform in the United States.[1] Canada was also active in this area. Such activity set the stage for an increasing academic involvement in this field. There was successive involvement by the School of Hygiene and the Department of Hospital Administration, and later, on a more intensive scale, by IHPME and the DLSPH.

HOSPITALS EMERGING AS A MAJOR HEALTH INSTITUTION

The founding of the Ontario Hospital Association (OHA) in 1924 was an indicator of hospitals emerging as major health institutions. Agnew was one of the founders.[2]

Agnew an Early Expert on Hospitals

In January 1928 Agnew became associate secretary of the Canadian Medical Association, a post he held until 1945.[3] His position at the CMA illustrated the import hospitals were beginning to assume. His principal duty was to organize and operate a new Department of Hospital Services and administer the Blackader Library – "tasks which he performed so well that he became the acknowledged leader in hospital affairs in Canada."[4] FitzGerald was a member of the CMA committee that developed the program for the new department.[5]

Agnew said that the position was created because a "study had revealed a tremendous need for some central clearing-house for hospital developmental programs." It became the basis for the Canadian Hospital Council, and Agnew noted that it was supported by Sun Life Assurance, who continued to support it when it moved to the council.[6] Bator and Rhodes note that Agnew "was a pioneer in the study, management and planning of hospitals in North America."[7] It speaks to the quality of the school that in setting up their new department they sought out the pre-eminent individual in this new area. Because of his involvement in the CMA and the council he had a national network of hospitals. He quickly used it as a basis for giving the department a national footprint that was similar in scope to that of the school but differed in application because there was a difference in subject matter (public health versus hospitals).

In 1929, while at the CMA, one of Agnew's first contributions was to update a directory of hospitals in Canada, one of the first such publications made. He noted that it "was amazingly difficult to get lists of hospitals" and that some of the provincial data were "very hazy."[8] He worked on the project with Helen MacMurchy from the federal Department of Health who was recognized as a pioneer in public health and one of the first female graduates from the University of Toronto medical school (and the first woman to intern at Toronto General Hospital).[9]

Their hospital directory was forty-four pages long, in three sections, hospitals by province, specialty hospitals (paediatric, orthopaedic, mental, etc.), and a summary. It also had two fold-out maps of Canada with a legend that depicted classifications of hospital in centres across the nation.[10] The 1925 version (that Agnew was not involved in) was a less detailed publication.[11]

In speaking of his study a number of years later, Agnew recollected that the publication had 886 hospitals, with 74,882 beds. He noted the estimated annual expenditure was $35 million, as compared to a 1951 estimate of over $200 million.[12] The comparison showed the growth in hospitals.

In March 1929, as a part of his position with the CMA, he began a regular section in the *CMAJ* on hospitals. In it he said would be discussed "many of the problems which are of interest to the medical profession." It would also abstract from and quote articles appearing in hospital journals not usually available to the members but that expressed "opinions and viewpoints with which the medical profession should be cognizant." He said, "We hope from time to time to quote the viewpoint of our non-medical associates, for we feel that a greater exchange of the medical and the administrative opinions would be of advantage to all parties concerned." He also made an allusion to hospital or health insurance: "The public will insist in the very near future upon some re-arrangement of the burden of hospital expense cannot be denied. Rather than have some ill-considered semi-continental scheme thrust suddenly upon us, we should discuss this timely question ourselves and suggest remedies which would meet the situation."[13]

In 1931 he published in the *CMAJ* the results of a major study on medical practice in Canada. Some 9,000 questionnaires were sent out, with 1,400 returned. The results were organized in two sections: the practice of medicine and medical education. A section on medical economics dealt with the question of health insurance: "Judging by the comments made, many men are of the opinion that the present system of practice is not ideal.... Health insurance and other forms of state medicine are considered by many in their replies, some expressing a doubt as to the wisdom of adopting such a system, while others feel that it would be a panacea enabling the physician to give good service and at the same time minimize the burden to him of the patient who cannot or will not pay."[14]

THE EMERGENCE OF A NEED FOR HEALTH MANAGEMENT

The Interwar Period and Developments in the Health Field

The interwar period was one of an enlarging – and intensifying – profile for health.

Prior to the program's inception, prominent people associated with the school, such as C.J. Hastings and J.W.S. McCullough (the Toronto and provincial medical officers of health respectively) had been interested in hospitals and involved as editors of *Hospital World*, through the 1910s and 1920s (when it was renamed *Hospital, Medical & Nursing World*).[15]

The interwar period saw important reports on health or reports that touched on health in Canada, the United States and the United Kingdom. In the United Kingdom there was the Dawson Report, while in the United States there was the Committee on the Costs of Medical Care.

While in Canada there was no report similar to those of the United Kingdom or United States, one does find in reviewing the debates of the House of Commons that health was becoming an increasing topic of discussion in the House in the 1930s and 1940s. This included discussion on the development of a health system as well as health insurance. For example, in terms of the former, in 1935 an MP raised the issue of a survey of the breadth, efficiency, and cost of medical service to the Canadian people and referred to the work of the Committee on the Costs of Medical Care (CCMC) in the United States.[16] In 1937 one MP noted that the premier of Ontario proposed "there should be a consolidation of health services of the province with that of the dominion."[17] In 1939 an MP noted an article in *Maclean's* entitled "A National Health Program" by the provincial secretary and minister of education in BC.[18]

In the *Maclean's* article the minister, Mr Weir, touched on health issues such as the overall health fitness of the Canadian people and the importance thereof, the difficulty Canadians were having in meeting health costs, and the need for better public health and for health insurance. He noted, "It would appear *preventive* health services are relatively neglected."[19] He said, "Whether we like it or not, if we are going to be healthy we must have more community action – government action if you will. Many types of health protection simply cannot be bought on an individual basis."[20] He spoke out against "present *laissez-faire* methods" of dealing with health issues.[21]

At the time Weir's department was making a major effort to launch a health insurance program in that province and had hired a former U of T faculty member, Harry Cassidy, as director. Cassidy was a former director of the School of Social Work who had also written of the need for health services with a chapter on the topic in the book published by the League for Social Reconstruction.[22] He also wrote a book on the need for social security, including health insurance in Canada[23] and followed up with another on public health.[24] He had delivered lectures in the School of Hygiene (1946–50).[25]

During this era the Royal Commission on Dominion-Provincial Relations of 1940 released the Rowell-Sirois Report with its "Red Books," more than one of which dealt with health. This was followed by the Dominion-Provincial Conference on Reconstruction (1945) with its "Green Book" on health. Between these two, and all occurring in 1943, three very detailed and separate reports appeared that focused in whole or in part on health and narrowed public attention on health generally and health insurance in particular. These were the Marsh Report, Heagerty Report, and Cassidy Report.

The Need for Trained Public Health Administrators

During this time there was also an evolution in the school's approach to public health, which was emblematic of an evolution in the health field. This was the need for a focus on management in health, and management in health was its own distinct form of activity. It could not, for example, be subsumed within business management. At the school this took its first form in public health administration but quickly moved on to a focus on hospital administration.

In public health it was precipitated by the Ontario minister of health approaching FitzGerald in 1939 with his intent to have minimum requirements for public health officers and for the school's help to mount programs to achieve them.[26] This was a very concrete example of the tight relationship between the school and the provincial Health Department.

It was also a recognition that these officers really were public health administrators. Further, it was formalizing the essence of what the school was doing in this regard, which was to focus on administration, in this case public health administration, and provide graduate training for such people. It was a precursor for the department moving into yet another vital area of health administration, that of hospital administration, and the establishment of a whole new department in the school that took place just a few years later.

In raising standards the Ontario department had three areas of concern: full-time medical officers of health, part-time officers in larger municipalities, and part-time officers in small urban or rural municipalities. In order to accomplish this training, and given for the most part these were part-time health officers, it wanted to provide the training without taking too much time away from their regular medical practice.[27]

Defries responded to the minister on FitzGerald's behalf in June 1939. For full-time officers he proposed instruction in four terms, each lasting two months. Training would culminate in a DPH, unlike the next two, neither of which would lead to a diploma. For part-timers in larger municipalities, he proposed tailored, personal instruction dependent on the needs of the individual physician that would involve "suitable field observation visits." To accomplish this, he proposed appointing a physician to the school who had significant "rural and urban health administration." For the part-time officers in small urban or rural municipalities he proposed short courses lasting four or five days. He further proposed the "development ultimately of a field training centre," as in the John Hopkins and Harvard programs.[28]

As a result of this response, the department at Queen's Park moved to establish statutory requirements. In its 1939 annual report in "Public Health Administration," John Phair, chief medical officer of health, stated that requisites had been established "such that a reasonable measure of experience or special training in public health administration is assured all communities irrespective of their size or population." It noted that the School of Hygiene, University of Toronto, had "by arrangement with the department set up short courses of instruction for all those required by the regulations to secure such training."[29] The report included a copy of an Order in Council setting out qualifications for medical officers of health in each of the three areas that the minister had noted in his letter to FitzGerald.[30] It is worth noting that Dr Phair was a 1921 DPH grad, who would later become deputy minister, in another demonstration of the tight relationship between the school and the provincial Health Department.

The next year "Public Health Administration" once again headed up the annual report of the Ontario department. It began, "With the continued increase in the health obligations of the community, there has been an associated increase in the administrative responsibilities of the Medical Officer of Health." It continued, "The day has gone when the Health Department staff consisted of a man with a tack hammer and an arm full of coloured cards.... This type of official health concern has gradually given way ... to a *sustained* interest in such matters" (my italics), which was a direct allusion to public health administration.[31]

It also noted (and here is the reinforcement of the practicum concept), "The interest of the Department in securing for the health officer a background of administrative experience is not limited to supplying academic instruction only. An opportunity to see an effective but unextravagant community health service annually functioning is an essential requisite to any course of training."[32]

This led to the establishment of a health unit near the School of Hygiene to jointly serve the needs of the local population and that of a practical training facility for the school. The East York Health Unit became operational in 1941, headed by William Mosley and supported by the Rockefeller Foundation.[33] It was the first teaching public health unit.[34] It also led to the establishment of a sub-department of public health administration headed by Dr Mosley and involving Phair and Andrew McNabb, director of the Division of Laboratories, Ontario Department of Health, among others.[35]

The Interwar Period and Developments in the Hospital Field

Moving to another area, it is easy to see how during the interwar period a foundation began to be laid for a program in professional hospital management. Hospitals began to emerge as centres of care, and there was increasing expectation for government to take a role in health care.

During this time hospitals also became established centres of the community with the community integrally involved as founders, board members, and fundraisers. This development included some very innovative schemes, such as the union hospital movement in Saskatchewan whereby groups of municipalities joined to create a union hospital district within which they levied taxes to support the building and operation of a hospital. This scheme was given great impetus with the election of the Douglas government in Saskatchewan and its successful implementation of the first hospital insurance program in North America, which resulted in the expansion of the union hospital idea. This occurred at the time of the inception of the Department of Hospital Administration and, as a result, the Department of Public Health in Saskatchewan sponsored a number of people in both the diploma and extension programs. As we will see, the University of Saskatchewan also mounted its own extension program, with DHA graduates heavily involved.

During this time science and medicine were rapidly developing as well and splitting into an increasing number of specialty areas. Medicine was quickly evolving into a leading area of science. Hospitals were emerging as leading centres for the application in patient care, clinical teaching, and research. This rapid evolution of medicine and hospitals was resulting in a disparate and fragmented arrangement, and the need to crystallize this into some sort of health *system* was becoming apparent.

The Dawson Report in Britain (1920) recommended organizing the mode of hospital delivery of care from community hospitals to regional centres, and beyond that, teaching hospitals.[36] The US Committee on the Costs of Medical Care (1928–32), which undertook a very detailed study ostensibly of the costs of medical care but really of all health delivery, observed in one of its reports, "The extensive use of hospitals is a comparatively recent phenomenon."[37] It also noted their complexity, for the hospital is "not a business of the ordinary type" – it was at once a hotel, industrial plant, place for repair and rehabilitation, haven of refuge, educational institution, and "focal point for the concentration and dissemination of knowledge concerning health."[38]

In Ontario the Royal Commission on Public Welfare had a section on hospitals that looked at issues facing them, particularly indigent patients.[39] It recommended the establishment of a provincial hospital for the study of cancer. Harvey Agnew, the first director of the hospital administration program, commented on the report in the *CMAJ*. He focused mainly on the hospitals part of the report. For example, he discussed the merits of concentrating cancer research and treatment in one special hospital as opposed to establishing a separate cancer department in a general hospital.[40]

In terms of hospitals generally, Agnew observed, "The fifty-year period, 1920–70, was the most productive half century in the history of Canadian hospitals."[41] He also noted, "Until the end of the nineteenth century, hospitals in Canada, as elsewhere, were little more than refuges for critically ill indigents and immigrants. Medicine had a limited basis in science and seriously ill patients were treated in the home whenever possible."[42]

His statement tied in to another report of the CCMC, which noted, "Hospitalization is becoming an increasingly common corollary of illness" and that "patients of all social groups" were "seeking hospital care in ever increasing numbers."[43] It was during this time (1930s and 1940s) that Agnew was emerging as an authority on hospitals and wrote numerous articles in the *CMAJ* during this period on the subject.

Studies on the Need for Trained Hospital Administrators

US studies on the need for professional hospital management could have influenced events in Canada. One was a 1922 Rockefeller Commission on the Training of Hospital Executives, which called for a formal training program of two years, including a practicum of six months. In addition it advocated extension courses for existing administrators.[44] It said that any training centre needed also to be doing research.[45]

The Rockefeller Foundation funded a study on the need for professional managers. The result, titled *Hospital Administration: A Career*, published in 1929 by Michael Davis, proposed a two-year graduate degree.[46] It also suggested that such a program needed to be involved in research and proposed that the scope of the program would be research, education, and service.[47]

Davis noted that in the fifty years leading to his book, the population had roughly doubled, while hospitals while had increased from 150 to over 7,500. In addition their range of service was increasing. They now treated more than inpatients. There was also the "clinic." In the thirty years leading to publication, the number of clinics in US hospitals had risen from 100 to over 6,000 and the number of clinic visits from 250,000 to 30 million. He also noted that in the United States and Canada only 23 per cent had over 100 beds.[48]

He observed that the size of the hospital business "needs the kind of management appropriate to large enterprises." It was not just the money that was at issue it was also "higher stakes of ... life and health."[49] In 1934 Davis became the head of the first graduate program in hospital administration in the world at the University of Chicago.

The Committee on the Costs of Medical Care in 1932 also noted the need: "Hospitals and clinics are not only medical institutions, they are also social and business enterprises, sometimes very large ones. It is important, therefore, that they be directed by administrators who are trained for their responsibilities and can understand and integrate the various professional, economic, and social factors involved."[50]

It added, "Definite opportunities should be provided in universities or in institutes of hospital administration connected with universities, for the theoretical and practical training of such administrators. The administration of hospitals and medical centers should be developed as a career which will attract high-grade students."[51]

Agnew was also part of the discussion. In 1940 he wrote an article in *Canadian Hospital* on training in hospital administration. It dealt with the need for training, the training programs taking place around the world (with an emphasis on Canada and the United States), and curricula.[52] One wonders if it was setting the stage for the Toronto program.

The American Council on Education conducted an extensive study on university education for administration in hospitals in the early 1950s, in which the U of T program and Agnew were mentioned. At the time it was one of twelve programs in North America.[53] It also had a chapter on the administrative residency.[54]

INVOLVEMENT OF OTHER U OF T FACULTY/GRADS IN HEALTH POLICY

Another important aspect of the milieu within which the school and IHPME's predecessor department functioned was the involvement of other U of T faculty/grads in health policy – health insurance in particular. Dr

Horace Wrinch, a Trinity Medical College grad (1899), was a well-respected doctor, surgeon, and hospital administrator. In 1904 he built the first hospital in the northern interior of British Columbia. He started a form of health insurance in 1907 in the Hazelton community where he practised. He was later elected to the BC Legislature, where he championed publicly funded health insurance.[55] In 1926 had secured the support of the BC Hospital Association for a health insurance program.[56] In 1929 he made a successful motion for a second BC Royal Commission to assess the merits of a health insurance program.[57]

He said, "Too frequently I have had to deal with people who, had state health insurance been in effect, would have been spared much suffering – people unable to meet the costs of medical care. Dreading the expense of such attention, many do not seek help from doctor or hospital when they imperatively need it. I have long since reached the conclusion that a State health-insurance system would be the solution to the people's health."[58]

There was also Harry Cassidy, who had been a faculty member in the School of Social Work from 1929 to 1934 and would return as dean in 1944.[59] He was hired by the Pattullo government of BC in 1934 to implement a provincial health insurance program. In the 1930s he did important work for the League for Social Reconstruction and published on social welfare in the 1940s.[60]

AGNEW AS PART OF HOSPITALS BECOMING PROMINENT INSTITUTIONS IN SOCIETY

Agnew Proposes Formation of Canadian Hospital Council (1931)

In 1931 Agnew proposed the establishment of a Canadian Hospital Council, suggesting that while there were a number of active provincial associations, there was need for a national body. He also said there was a need "to crystallize and develop the best modern views on hospital administration and organization."[61] He noted that the CMA was sponsoring such an initiative and that it proposed to hold its organization meeting at the convention of the American Hospital Association, to be held in Toronto that year.[62]

The council was formed on 28 September 1931, with all hospital associations and hospital organizations present at the organization meeting eligible for charter membership. An associate membership category was created for the federal and provincial departments of health. Agnew was elected secretary-treasurer of the council[63] and would remain secretary until 1950.

At the 1931 meeting it was determined that the council would meet every two years. One topic proposed for discussion was the relationship of hospitals to the public and to the medical profession with respect to clinics, preventive work, and group hospitalization on a voluntary basis.[64] A second session of the council was held in September 1933.

Agnew Becomes Editor of Canadian Hospital (1938)

In April 1938 Agnew began to be listed as editor of the journal of the Canadian Hospital Council, *Canadian Hospital*, a post he would hold until 1950.[65] Over the years he would publish frequently in this journal, in the *CMAJ*, and in *Hospitals*, the journal of the American Hospital Association. Bator notes that in the 1930s he "established himself quickly as an expert on the Canadian system of hospitals and especially of insurance for hospitalization."[66]

Agnew Part of OHA Board That Forms Ontario Blue Cross (1939)

In 1939 Agnew was a member of the OHA Board of Directors that proposed the OHA create its own province-wide hospital prepayment plan. Ontario Blue Cross was run as a subsidiary of the OHA, was capitalized with a $15,000 loan from the OHA,[67] and grew to be one of the largest health insurance providers in Canada. Agnew notes it was his drive that brought Blue Cross to Ontario at an early date.[68] The major force behind this was Arthur Swanson, who was originally from Saskatchewan. He became administrator of Toronto Western Hospital in 1930 and was asked to become executive secretary of the OHA in 1951.[69]

Later we will learn Blue Cross personnel became integral to the introduction of hospital insurance in Ontario.

THE U OF T PRESIDENT ON HOSPITALS

The president of the University of Toronto, Henry Cody, was a supporter of hospitals. He delivered a wide-ranging address, published in 1940, to the Trustees' Section of the American Hospital Association on the hospital's role in the community. He began, "To-day hospitals form a very important part of what Sir William Osler called 'man's redemption of man.'"[70] He noted, "The hospital today is a city within a city," and "No institution is more dependent on the human element involved."[71] He dealt with many aspects of the hospital, including its role in meeting community needs and as an educational and research centre.[72]

THE NEED FOR HOSPITAL ADMINISTRATION BEGINS TO ASSERT ITSELF

A Prior Course in Hospital Administration at U of T (1938–45)

What is not well known is that the U of T had a prior course in hospital administration before the one the School of Hygiene started. It was run by the School of Nursing (which began as a part of the School of Hygiene but then separated to become its own faculty). It was a postgraduate course and was open only to nursing administrators. It grew from a rather informal extension course to one listed in the calendar as a formal course.

Two journals, *Canadian Nurse* and *Canadian Hospital* reported on the first time it was offered, as a full week course in December 1938. It covered "the legal, physical and scientific aspects of hospital administration" and included observation visits to TGH, TWH, and St Michael's Hospital.[73] It had forty-two registrants, from Winnipeg to Montreal. The organizers were astonished at the response, as the course had been given limited publicity. As a result the decision was taken to continue and expand the course.[74]

The 1938–39 Calendar for the School of Nursing notes a class (two terms) in hospital administration.[75] It also lists extension courses "usually a few days in extent" with topics "selected" from a number of areas, including hospital administration.[76]

The 1939–40 calendar lists it as a specific extension course: "Following the extension course in Hospital Administration given last December, there has been increased demand for further work on this subject." It then notes that a course of three weeks has been arranged and gives the dates. "This will permit the subject to be dealt with in a somewhat fuller manner." In addition, "Authorities in hospital administration" will discuss various topics (which it lists), and lecturers in the course "will include experienced administrators."[77] *Canadian Hospital* in 1940 referred to the three-week course.[78]

The minutes of the Teaching Staff Committee for 26 November 1940 indicate that they were contemplating making the course one year in length.[79] The calendar for 1941–42 lists it as a full-year course, one of four such courses for graduate nurses. The calendar for that year notes it is "for the experienced nurse in preparation for the position of Hospital Administrator." It was an eight-month certificate course with the final two months being "practical work" in a hospital. It covered topics such as economics, business and accounting, hospital organization and management, and public health.[80]

The course in its various formats ran from 1939 to 1945[81] and was discontinued shortly before the diploma in hospital administration started. The last calendar it appeared in was for 1945–46.[82] Students came from long distances to take it. In 1940 it had a student from Greece and another from New Zealand.[83]

Articles Emphasizing the Need for Trained Hospital Administrators (1939)

In 1939, while Harvey Agnew was editor, *Canadian Hospital* published two articles on hospital administration by the foremost authority in the field at that time, an American, Malcolm T. MacEachern. In the first he set out the need for *administration*. He noted "that for the accomplishment of the true purposes of a hospital we must have proper administration."[84]

In the second he focused on the hospital *administrator*, emphasizing the need for trained hospital administrators. He said, "The day is far gone by when any person, regardless of education, training, or experience should accept the responsibility of administering an institution which has to deal with life and death every second."[85]

He made a strong statement to that effect: "Some governing bodies of hospitals still persist in appointing as administrators persons who have neither training nor experience in hospital administration. In so doing, these guardians of hospitals are not discharging their duty in accordance with public responsibility, and in the final analysis are morally guilty of failure to carry out a sacred trust."[86]

CHAPTER 6

The School and the Debate on Health Insurance

AGNEW AND DEFRIES ON HEALTH INSURANCE

Articles by Agnew on the Topic

Agnew had a keen interest in health insurance. While he was editor of *Canadian Hospital* the index always had a section on health insurance, and it was the same at the CMAJ. Because of his role there it is likely that he was influential in ensuring that physicians were informed on the topic.

His interest in health insurance, and particularly its effect on hospitals, went back a long way. He had written an article in 1931 in the *Bulletin of the American Hospital Association* (the forerunner to the well-known *Hospitals)*. In it he noted that twenty-four countries had compulsory health insurance, nearly as many other voluntary plans, and that the United States and Canada were almost the only developed countries without some form of nationwide health insurance.[1] He sketched out several potential issues. For example, "There is a tendency for such a scheme to break down the personal relationship between doctor and patient."[2] The tone of the article was summed up where he said, "I may have emphasized some of the less desirable features of health insurance; it is only fair to point out, however, that much good has been accomplished by these developments and it is noteworthy that no nation has ever abandoned the scheme, once it has been inaugurated."[3]

He had also written an article in the CMAJ in 1932, where he acknowledged that there was much discussion about the possible effects of health insurance on medical practice but relatively little on its effect on hospitals and hospital practice. He noted "profound changes" taking place in western Canada and the attitude of farmer and labour groups. He also recognized that "twenty-four of the leading countries of the world have made health insurance compulsory" and repeated that "Canada and the United States are just about the only important countries which have not adopted some form of nation-wide health insurance."[4]

He noted as well that in Canada several steps had already been taken along this road. He cited hospitalization provided for pensioners and those suffering from war disabilities, psychiatric patients hospitalized by the provinces, union hospitals in Saskatchewan, and Saskatchewan providing care for TB patients.[5] He suggested that any system adopted here would likely include hospital care and that would have profound effect on the operation of hospitals because any "body or organization which foots the bill would feel that it should have considerable say" in the development and operation of such organizations.[6]

He covered a good deal of ground in this article, looking at the possible demands for a uniformity of service (especially in the rural areas), the possible effect on private support, a potential increase in demand for hospital care, and effects on the practice of medicine in hospitals. He also examined the possible effect on university hospitals, querying whether there would be a decrease in the "number of indigent patients available for the demonstration of disease" and whether university hospitals would come "under the government."[7]

In 1934 he wrote once again, this time in *Canadian Hospital* that Canada and the United States were "practically the only leading countries without some national form of health insurance."[8] But he made a distinction between health insurance and what he termed "state medicine."[9]

Agnew Submits a Brief to the Rowell-Sirois Commission (1937)

Agnew presented a brief on behalf of the Canadian Hospital Council to the Royal Commission on Dominion-Provincial Relations (Rowell-Sirois Commission) in December 1937. While referred to as a brief, it was in the form of a four-page letter,[10] which was reproduced in *Canadian* Hospital in February 1938.[11]

It dealt with two topics. The first was requesting government support for the hospitalization for those without the means to pay, including the poor, pensioners, new immigrants, and the disabled, among others.[12]

The second was the CHC's stance on health insurance, and this inserted the resolution passed at the 1936 annual meeting of the CHC. It was quite neutral on what it termed "governmental control and socialization of health services" and recommended explicitly that "various forms of voluntary insurance meeting the needs of the people, without recourse to state control, be fully studied."[13] It also stated that "any form of health insurance which would interfere with the autonomy of our voluntary institutions ... should be strongly opposed."[14]

Agnew's stance on hospital insurance tended always to be supportive of voluntary plans. In a *Canadian Hospital* article in 1938 he suggested that "it is not inconceivable that the present plans may ultimately lead to and may be supplanted by some form of generalized states sponsored or directed plan." However, he said, "one would voice the hope that the voluntary nature of these plans be preserved" and that "direction could best be left to voluntary bodies."[15]

Canadian Public Health Association and School of Hygiene on Health Insurance

Defries, the Canadian Public Health Association, and DPH grads were all active in supporting health insurance in Canada.

At the annual meeting of the Canadian Public Health Association in 1942 a series of resolutions was passed, culminating in a Public Health Charter for Canada. It called for several measures to strengthen public health in Canada, including clean water, adequate housing, control of communicable diseases, immunization, and proper nutrition, among others. But it is particularly significant that the association "endorses the principle of national health insurance as a means to further the nation-wide provision of medical, dental and nursing services." Defries was integrally involved. He was chair of the editorial board, and a number of his faculty were members.[16]

In addition to the charter there was also a specific resolution on health insurance passed at the meeting, which stated that "there is urgent need in Canada for the more adequate provision of general medical, dental, and nursing services." It said that "experience in Great Britain and other countries has demonstrated the value of a system of compulsory contributory health insurance." And it stated "that in any health insurance program, adequate provision for preventive services is essential."[17]

The *CJPH* published a number of articles in 1944 from a variety of sources: the federal minister (June), the past president of the CPHA (February) who would become an MP and finance minister, Henry Sigerist (July), and an editorial on the proposed British program (November). F.W. Jackson, faculty member and DPH graduate, wrote an article in the *CJPH* in March.[18]

Special Committee on Social Security (1943)

Presentation by Agnew

Agnew had echoed similar sentiments in a presentation to the House of Commons Special Committee on Social Security in 1943. His presentation is important for our purposes in that it reveals the personal philosophy about hospitals and health care of an individual who would set the tone of instruction in the hospital administration program for a number of years.

Agnew appeared in his role as secretary of the Canadian Hospital Council, which he had been instrumental in founding. His submission was reproduced in *Canadian Hospital*.[19] He noted that the first hospital in North America had been in Canada, the Hotel Dieu in Quebec, which opened in 1639.[20] He proposed that Canadian hospitals are the equal "class for class, of those found anywhere else in the world" and that the "public hospitals accept patients irrespective of financial status." He also noted that hospitals care for both public and private patients, unlike the United States, where there are "county" hospitals for the poor. He called the Canadian situation "more democratic."[21]

He pointed out some challenges to the present system, chief of which was that the costs of hospitalization were proving to be "a severe strain upon the family with a moderate income." For reasons such as this, he said the Canadian Hospital Council was "generally in favour of the principle of health insurance." He then laid out the principles of its stance.

First among them was the principle of "voluntary hospitals" that are "public hospitals." He said the effort should not be to destroy the "voluntary effort" and replace it "by the more impersonal state support" but to enhance it with a further "cooperative effort in which the individual would be encouraged to supplement the aid and support provided by society as a whole."[22]

He felt everyone should be included under the plan, not just the "breadwinner"; insured persons should have the option of taking higher-priced accommodation by paying the difference in charges; health insurance "should be on a provincial basis but under federal co-ordination"; administration should be "through an independent, non-political commission"; and the health insurance fund "should be a contributory one." He said that although the people would "pay the entire cost in the final analysis," it was "desirable" that the individual have a "feeling of personal responsibility in keeping the operational costs to a reasonable level." He said that contributions should come from four sources: the insured, employers, and federal and provincial governments.[23]

There were further notable aspects to his presentation. He emphasized the importance of preventive medicine, research, teaching hospitals, and the confidentiality of patient data.[24] Under questioning by the committee, he implicitly came out in favour of a compulsory plan by saying that it was desirable that "we should have some plan that would bring in everybody."[25] As a result of other questions from the committee, he further emphasized his beliefs in the importance of the voluntary hospital sector. He noted that in "many European countries" the "state has gradually taken over voluntary hospitals." He said that he felt that "the voluntary hospital contributes something to our life which must be preserved.... Charity should never be entirely lost."[26] He was also quoted in the press on this.[27]

Presentation by Defries

Later R.D. Defries, who at the time was director of the Connaught Laboratories and the School of Hygiene ,also presented to the committee as a member of a special insurance committee of the Canadian Public Health Association. His presentation sets out just how far-sighted the thinking of the school was for its time.

His presentation basically had two parts; one was titled "the purpose of this Submission," which set out an eight-point strategy for the delivery of public health in Canada. His presentation concluded with a nine-point plan for health insurance as outlined by the Canadian Public Health Association,[28] covering everything from health insurance, community health services, regional health, to fellowships for training, and medical research. In essence it was a post-war plan for a Canadian health system.

The presentation started by emphasizing prevention and spoke of a "failure to distinguish between health insurance and sickness insurance" and that what is termed health insurance is really sickness insurance. He said that the "success of health insurance depends ... on the inclusion of public health and preventive medicine."[29]

His presentation also emphasized the total spectrum of health and the importance of organizing services at the local level. He said, "Preventive medicine and public health are directed not only towards the lengthening of life through the prevention of disease and premature death, but also towards all that pertains to health, both physical and mental. Social measures that give security, and free individuals from anxiety, make an important contribution to health."[30] He also pointed out the importance of different professions working together at the local level.

There was a section on local health services and, once again, as evidence of far-sighted thinking, it mentioned forming health districts as well as the municipal doctor plan in Saskatchewan and Manitoba.[31] Another section was on the role of the family physician in conjunction with a local department of health and the local medical officer of health. It emphasized not only physical health but mental health as well and referred to the presentation by the Canadian Medical Association in that regard.[32]

Another interesting section was on the importance of medical research to health insurance. Defries noted that when health insurance was introduced in Great Britain in 1911, provision was made for a small part of each contributor's payment to go toward a fund for the advancement of medical research. Out of this was born the Medical Research Council and the National Institute for Medical Research. Over the years additional funds were made available. He strongly advocated provision be made for medical research to advance knowledge in treatment and prevention in Canada.[33]

THE SCHOOL OF HYGIENE RESPONDS TO THE BROADENING INTEREST IN HEALTH

The School of Hygiene was very involved in responding to this broadening interest. And the Second World War accelerated the growth and evolution of the school. Within the time frame of the war, "the School changed dramatically with the introduction of four sub-departments, three diplomas, a certificate, a field training centre." There was an increase in the number of undergraduate, postgraduate, and graduate students. Special courses were provided for industry, the military, Ontario health officers, public health nurses, and others.[34]

The focus of the school was on the war effort. Facilities in the FitzGerald Building and the Connaught campus were expanded, and the old Knox College building at 1 Spadina Crescent was purchased by the university for

Connaught at the urging of Defries. He recounts these war efforts in his book on the first forty years of Connaught.[35]

Its annual reports note growth in the school. Its report for 1939–40 notes this growth resulting in "an urgent need" for more "teaching and research staff."[36] The report for 1940–41 noted two new sub-departments.[37] In its report for 1942–43 it noted, "The growth of the work of the School of Hygiene and its departments parallels the rapid development of Public Health."[38]

Toward the latter stages of the Second World War, the school was planning for the possibility of moving from an enrolment of twenty-five students to one hundred, and the logistics that were entailed. The new program, indeed the new department of hospital administration, would be part of this growth, though at this point while public health administration is mentioned, hospital administration is not.[39] In 1945–46 enrolment in the school had more than doubled from the previous year, as the result in large measure from returning service personnel.[40]

THE SECOND WORLD WAR AND IMMEDIATELY AFTER

The Second World War ushered in rapid advances in social thinking. Because of its *universal* nature – conscription, whole economies oriented toward the war effort, a blurred distinction between those directly fighting and those indirectly providing the means to fight, a mixing of social classes in a united effort – there arose an expectation that governments would apply this universalist thinking to other areas, such as social services, particularly health.

There was also its *global* nature, an example of which could be called the Beveridge phenomenon. It began with the publication of the Beveridge Report in Britain in 1942, followed by its dissemination around the world. It focused on universal policies in health, pensions, and employment and defined such services as a right. Canada was also at the leading edge of such thinking. Beveridge addressed two committees of the House of Commons that met in joint session.[41] The Rowell-Sirois, Cassidy, Marsh and Heagerty reports all aimed at a publicly sponsored health insurance program.

In Canada a step along that road was the development of the first public hospital insurance program in North America by the Douglas government in Saskatchewan in 1947. It served as a template for a similar program in BC shortly after. Britain established its National Health Service in 1948. The result of all these initiatives was the creation of new and complex provincial or national systems and public agencies to administer them. They focused attention on existing hospitals and the construction of new ones.

The confluence of these factors created a need for a whole new area of management, unlike any other. Hospitals were distinct from industry in its product and the large number of distinct professional groups involved, each of which required years of tertiary-level education. Coordinating the activities and competently managing these organizations created a whole new area of management, one distinctly different from business management, and the need for tertiary-level graduate education for these people. It was a type of management distinct for being highly institutionalized and professionalized.[42] It was this need that drove the development of the first program in English Canada at the University of Toronto.

CHAPTER 7

Setting Context: A Rapidly Evolving Health-Care World

HOSPITALS INCREASINGLY SEEN AS INSTRUMENTAL TO NATIONAL HEALTH

At the department's inception in 1947 it inserted itself into a rapidly evolving health-care world. There was no health system. That would come later. But what did exist, particularly in the United Kingdom and Canada, was growing government involvement in health and hospitals. In hospitals this necessitated new government activity, new bureaucratic mechanisms (divisions with health ministries) to administer hospital grants. And, in the case of Saskatchewan, an additional layer to administer tax dollars to pay for hospital operations.

The focus at that time was hospitals. An article in *Canadian Hospital* in the year of the department's inception was titled "The Hospital: Keynote to National Health."[1] Connor, in his history of TGH, quotes Risse, who said, "Hospital-based medicine formed one of the 'most critical developments' in medical history."[2] Hospitals were important parts of the community as well. And this sense of community existed on different levels. In Saskatchewan the union hospitals drew together different rural districts. In central Canada, hospitals were the community focal point of numerous cities and towns. And at the tertiary level they brought together the elite of business and legal establishments.

A case in point is the involvement of David Fasken, a founder of the Fasken law firm, in Toronto Western Hospital. A donation he made in 1906 was "but the first of many ways in which he would help the hospital, forging a triangular link that would exist for a century between Excelsior Life, Toronto Western, and the Fasken firm."[3] The *Toronto Daily Star* reported in December 1929 that he was one of the earliest supporters of the hospital; his initial donation provided for the main building and later funded other buildings on the site.[4] He poured millions into the hospital.[5]

Hospitals were beginning to figure prominently in the Canadian health-care scene. The first director of the hospital administration program thought they might become even more central to Canadian health care. In a 1947 article about graduate training in hospital administration, he wrote that "there was much evidence" hospitals "will become the community health centre," which would be for prevention, public education, and "community public health activities in general."[6]

Canada was building many hospitals, and it was becoming increasingly apparent that they needed their own specialized brand of management. The School of Hygiene had established a solid reputation in public health, had strong ties to hospitals, and presented a natural fit for this new activity, in a number of respects. The primary one was in the continuous building of a department always at the cutting edge (which mirrored the central characteristic of the school). The chronicle of IHPME shows a successive layering of new activity that mirrors the increasing complexity and breadth of health-care management and delivery.

Throughout IHPME's history the world of health care itself was rapidly evolving. This is what motivated its inception. Health care was no longer being practised out of a physician's office or through a home visit. Physicians were requiring access to sophisticated diagnostic laboratories and specialized diagnostic equipment, which had to be located in specialized facilities. As a result hospitals were emerging as centres of both diagnosis and treatment. At this time, at the apex, they were becoming very sophisticated multipurpose centres of specialized care, clinical teaching, and research.

And their research was distinctly different from that taking place across the street at the medical faculty. It had a much more practical, as opposed to theoretical, orientation. Though all directed to the same end, that at the hospital grew out of and was intimately connected to the patient. It grew out of the dedication of physicians who just could not help but tease out solutions to seemingly intractable problems.

It soon became obvious that institutions of such complexity required specialized professional management, and that these managers required an appreciation of a kind of organizational environment that was very different from that of business. Hospitals were a business, but that was the simplest part of their mandate. Their complexity lay in their diverse stakeholders, professions, and functions. As a result, schools of hospital management emerged that were more often located akin to schools of public health than business administration. This was the case at U of T.

In addition, and as a landmark study of health care in the United States put it, health care itself was no longer an unconnected series of independent doctor's offices. A "system" was emerging, which required management and study. Moreover it observed health care was becoming one of the largest economic activities in the United States (the same could be said of Canada). In addition, its priority and profile were increasing; after the basic needs of a society had been secured, the preservation of health became the next priority. It was being called "an index of civilization."[7]

It is in this complex and evolving environment that IHPME began. There were also uniquely Canadian aspects to its evolution. For about the first thirty years of its existence the institute was part of the School of Hygiene. And this school was joined to a research and biological production facility, the Connaught Labs. The school and the labs were larger-than-life entities, each at the top of its field, each continually achieving new groundbreaking goals. Each was changing the landscape of public health in Canada, and both had strong international reputations.

The department/institute was also intimately bound up with the school. To take one example, FitzGerald's influence on the Canadian Medical Corps in the First World War was a kind of systemic approach coupled with organizational management that was the very definition of IHPME. Further, the tight links between academia, business, and government exhibited by Connaught Labs during this time, and throughout the time it was owned by the university, was farsighted and in line with current thinking on such tripartite partnerships. We will discuss this further later in this work.

There was also another instance of a tight link between department and school. The leaders of each were among the top in their field. This had a trickle-down effect in that the same could be said of the faculty (and the types of students chosen). For example, the first department head was the leading figure in Canada on hospitals and hospital administration. And, as we will see, the heads of the department more than once became heads of the overall entity or were recommended for the position. There were other connections: we will see later that IHPME faculty (Gene Vayda) were very involved in the development of a history of the school.

Very early on we see the progression of events that led to the genesis of the Department of Hospital Administration. First, the proper care of patients was no longer solely between physician and patient; hospitals were becoming important centres of care. In addition, important studies in Britain (Dawson Report, 1920) and the United States (Committee on the Costs of Medical Care, 1932) called for an organized, integrated health system, rather than a group of independent, disparate parts. There was no equivalent report in Canada, but there were somewhat related reports[8] and an increasing interest and debate on health.

It is easy to see that hospitals would become a major concern for both society and government, as their number and budgets increased rapidly. In the United States the number of hospitals almost tripled from 1900 to 1944.[9] In Canada, hospital budgets almost quintupled from 1948 to 1961.[10]

An article in *Canadian Hospital* in 1947 noted that hospitals were a foundation of national health and that hospitals were the medium through which advances in medical science were made available to the public.[11] A somewhat similar thought is advanced in a history of British health care, which alludes that there was a connection "when medicine simply became able to do more," which made it "far more dependent upon the technological capacity of the hospital."[12]

There is another aspect to their import. A recent book on US hospitals in a notation equally applicable to Canada said they are "a place to which we often turn in our moments of greatest physical uncertainty and emotional vulnerability. We have intimate connections to hospitals and strong feelings about them."[13]

From our perspective it is interesting that some of the central figures of our study, namely FitzGerald and Agnew, were very involved in this process.

A RAPIDLY GROWING AND EVOLVING HEALTH CARE SCENE

Just Prior to Inception of the DHA Program

Immediately after the Second World War, perhaps as a redirecting of all the energies and idealism spawned by the war, began the first concentrated push toward making health care accessible. In a number of instances hospital administration faculty of the U of T department (either present or future) and newly minted graduates were at the centre. It would be the same in a second push in Canada in the 1960s.

Sub-Department of Public Health Administration (1941)

In 1941 Defries started a new Sub-Department of Public Health Administration with himself as head.[14] It drew heavily on expertise from the field, utilizing as teachers staff from municipal health departments, Ontario Department of Health, and Department of National Health and Welfare. An indication of the strength of such links was that the deputy minister of health in Ontario, John T. Phair, had been a part-time instructor in the school in the 1930s and included the school in his plans for modern health services. Malcolm Taylor of the Department of Political Economy was a visiting lecturer.[15]

East York Health Unit

A significant feature of the sub-department was the East York Health Unit, which provided a practical setting for students. While such practical instruction was not new to the school – it had been using the Department of Health in the City of Toronto for this purpose for some twenty years – this type of a heath unit created for this specific purpose was new. Also new was combining the practical teaching with practical health studies (in areas such as nutrition and health protection).[16] Another advantage was that East York was a good model for what students might expect in the field. It was comparable in size "to the majority of cities in Canada."[17] Another feature was its link to the School of Nursing and instruction and studies in public health nursing.[18]

William Mosley was appointed medical officer of health for East York and director of field training for the School of Hygiene in August 1940.[19] It brought his experience as a public health administrator to the program.[20] He would later be appointed head of the Sub-Department of Public Health Administration[21] and a faculty member in the merged Department of Health Administration.

The creation of the unit was an example of the school's major emphasis on having a significant component of its curriculum focused on practice. It proved to be a major piece of the program in the Department of Hospital Administration. It was also an example of the school's continual aim to make a difference, as this put in place enhanced staffing and services for East York. Funding from the Ontario Ministry of Health and the Rockefeller Foundation allowed for Mosley's position as well as that of an assistant health officer and a public health nurse. The township continued to provide the funds it had previously been expending to cover the rest of the expenses.[22]

The Ferment Underway in Health in the UK: The Emergency Hospital System

At around the inception of the hospital administration program a ferment was underway in Canada – if anything, one even more profound in the United Kingdom. Hospitals and health insurance were state-of-the-art in health care and it could be argued that the exigencies of the Second World War had motivated Britain to lead in each. Canada had close ties to Britain and followed these developments closely. This much-heightened interest in each spread throughout the developed world.

The first major initiative was the Emergency Hospital Service (EHS) in wartime Britain.[23] Under it the Ministry of Health in London and the Department of Health in Edinburgh organized and assumed responsibility for all of Britain's hospitals in 1938 in anticipation of war- and air-raid casualties. It was deemed a huge success.[24] Webster called it a "great constructive enterprise" and many were so impressed with it that they "called for the immediate conversion into a National Hospital Service."[25] He noted, "The Luftwaffe achieved in months what had defeated politicians and planners for at least two decades."[26] Britain was divided into eleven regions, London into ten sectors.[27] The independence of hospitals was preserved "while combining them into a homogenous whole."[28]

Kinney noted it "laid the groundwork for the NHS."[29] Webster wrote that it was "a springboard for the nationalization of hospitals."[30] Titmuss noted, "It left behind a heritage of huge advances in hospital care and a fund of knowledge and experience in organisation and administration."[31] In addition, "It demonstrated, in its limited field, what a hospital service could be, and it gave many institutions of varying character and type their first real opportunity to work together for a common purpose."[32] Such learning was not lost on other countries.

It had also spurred an unprecedented hospital building boom in Scotland "at a pace scarcely equalled anywhere in Europe before or since." Seven new hospitals were added, along with 20,500 new beds,[33] because Scotland was seen as a refuge if Germany invaded the south of England. It proved its worth at the evacuation of Dunkirk when 28,354 Army and 3,487 Navy casualties were admitted to EHS hospitals.[34]

As noted, it presaged the NHS. The minister of health and secretary of state for Scotland captured this sentiment when in response to a question in the House of Commons on 9 October 1941 he commented on the future of Britain's hospital services: "It is the objective of the Government as soon as may be after the war, to ensure that by means of a comprehensive hospital service appropriate treatment shall be readily available to every person in need of it."[35] The full text of his response makes it evident the government had been doing substantial thinking in this regard. It is instructive that Aneurin Bevan, the future minister of health in the Labour government who would nationalize Britain's hospitals, was part of this interchange of questions.[36]

In a subsequent interchange (21 October) Sir Francis Freemantle (a physician) suggested that hospitals should "become collective centres of all of the services required for health." The medical officer for health should have his offices there, along with clinics, and the "hospital ought to be the centre of research and of private practice and preventive medicine."[37] At that time Dr Edith Summerskill, a Labour MP (and one of the first women to be admitted to a medical school in the UK) said she "would like to see not only the voluntary hospitals taken over by the State, but the profit motive eliminated from the treatment of disease, and every man, woman, and child in this country have an opportunity of availing themselves of State medical services."[38]

Such developments were not lost on Canada. The *Canadian Hospital*, which Agnew was editing at the time, ran a monthly report during the war years, "With the Hospitals in Britain," so its readers could get a sense of the war and the organization of its hospitals into a cohesive unit.[39] The Emergency Hospital Service as a program was featured in a number of such articles.[40]

As a result of such initiatives and their influence on Canada, there was a federal and provincial focus on hospitals and health insurance.[41] But Canada was not alone. There was general concern for better social security measures throughout the developed world, and health was perhaps the biggest piece of it.

To give a further idea of the kind of sentiment afoot, Webster noted that as all-consuming as the war effort was, Britain, as a parallel activity, devoted considerable effort to reconstruction.[42] Titmuss noted that it was somewhat paradoxical that at a time when life was at its cheapest it developed policies that valued it at its fullest.[43] Each of these observations also applied to Canada at that time.

The Beginning of the Welfare State

It was an idealistic time. After the First World War, social security principles became a part of party politics and government policy in many countries. But the breadth of coverage in meeting social risks as well as the people covered were hotly contested items and health, though part of an expanding umbrella of social welfare measures, did not receive wide coverage at that time.[44] To be sure, in a number of European countries concern for social measures and health predated the Second World War.[45]

The post–Second World War era expanded the notion of citizenship, beyond the political realm. It ushered in a concern for social citizenship, which begat the notion of social rights as key elements of universal human rights and on a par with democratic rights. This included social insurance schemes, differing by country, which attempted to treat all citizens equally and to cover all major social risks.[46] It was the Second World War that advanced the notion of social rights as evidenced in things such as the Beveridge Report, the Atlantic Charter, and the British White Paper (National Health Service, 1944). Canada was also a part of this trend. Mackenzie King, in announcing a new series of health grants in May 1948, drew a link between these and other advances in social security legislation in Canada, including unemployment insurance, family allowances, and pensions.[47]

There was also a young, activist premier in Saskatchewan who had very definite ideas about health. There was his involvement as an MP during the 1930s and 1940s, the latter of which had formed in his mind a very definite view of the power of the state to both focus people's energies as well as government policy toward a defined objective. It was a notion he put to positive use covering a whole array of social measures, but particularly in health.

In this there were very definite links to the U of T program in hospital administration as students gravitated to Saskatchewan, which had a lot of health activity (hospital insurance, mental health, public health) underway. Douglas hired one of its earliest students (Burns Roth), one who became his deputy minister of health, and one who, with Douglas's support, launched new initiatives in health care and public health.

Beveridge Report (UK, 1942)

We mentioned earlier that the Beveridge report was released in 1942 and was an immediate sensation, not just in his country but internationally. He had tapped into a deep undercurrent in the nation itself. Barnett notes that there a deep-seated and intense idealism took root around 1940, in which the churches took a prominent part.[48] In 1941 Britain's equivalent to *Life* magazine, *Picture Post*, ran most of an issue on post-war Britain. The cover page said "A Plan for Britain." Julian Huxley wrote an article titled "Health for All."[49] Many articles were by academics: Thomas Balogh, Oxford economist; A.D. Lindsay, master of Balliol; J.B. Priestley, novelist and broadcaster. The special issue itself was the idea of Kenneth Clarke, art historian, museum director, and broadcaster.[50]

The issue sparked discussions about post-war Britain, and while there is no evidence of a direct connection, within six weeks of its release the government had set up a Cabinet committee on reconstruction.[51] It focused attention on this area, one of the outcomes of which would be the Beveridge Report. It is interesting that Britain in the midst of a challenging war was putting its mind to what it might be after it.

In all of this there was also Beveridge himself. In a nod to what Steini Brown and Rob Steiner are presently doing at DLSPH ("communication for impact"), Beveridge was an adept communicator. He had a track record as a journalist and broadcaster as well as an academic and administrator. He could express ideas clearly and could do so in phrases – "six principles," "three assumptions," "five giants" – that lent themselves to print and broadcast media.[52]

His report was highly influential in other countries. Governments in exile were highly influenced by it.[53] It was said to have influenced Henry Gluckman, South African minister of health and his National Health Services Commission report (Gluckman Report) on their health systems done during the same time period (1942–44).[54] There was also the Bhore Report in India (1946). This international influence was helped by the fact that details of the report were broadcast by the BBC beginning at dawn, 1 December 1942, in twenty-two languages.[55]

Webster notes, "Although the government was divided over its response to Beveridge, his report both reflected and released a tide of expectation that could not be stemmed."[56]

Beveridge toured the United States in 1943, stimulating discussion, particularly the matter of the hearings on two US Senate bills (see below).

Beveridge and Canada (1942–43)

Beveridge's prominence was the same in Canada, and Canadians took great interest in his report. A portion of it dealt with health insurance.

Canada's high commissioner at the time, Vincent Massey (future governor general), quickly recognized its international significance. Nine days after it was released, it was the subject of a communiqué by him to Cyril James, chair of the Advisory Committee of Reconstruction (and principal of McGill University). James noted on the communiqué that it was "a scheme of medical treatment of every kind for everybody."[57] From there it was forwarded to the minister of foreign affairs, then to the Ministries of Labour and Finance. Massey noted in a three-page dispatch that it was a subject "of universal discussion" and that "one cannot but feel that this intelligent and courageous attack on the problems of economic insecurity may prove a milestone in the social history of the British people."[58]

Beveridge came to Canada to present to the Special Committee on Social Security in May 1943.[59] None of this was lost on Defries or Agnew. Prior to Beveridge's visit, Defries wrote about the report in the *Canadian Journal of Public Health* in December 1942.[60] *Canadian Hospital* in March 1943 noted the establishment of the Special Committee on Social Security, its mandate, and membership. Interestingly John Diefenbaker, a future prime minister from Saskatchewan, was a member.[61] Defries later wrote about the implementation of the Beveridge Report in the United Kingdom.[62]

Beveridge Tour of the United States (1943)

At the invitation of the Rockefeller Foundation, Beveridge began a three-month tour of the United States in May 1943. Much of it was reported in Canada. He made "over a hundred speeches on his report." He also made "appearances before cine-cameras" and met with "American administrators, trade unionists and philanthropic millionaires."[63]

His tour was regarded as "a spectacular publicity success." It was said, "Everywhere he went he was received with extravagant enthusiasm and praise."

He had "several friendly interviews with Franklin Roosevelt" and was warmly welcomed by the secretary of labour, who was strongly committed to the extension of social security.[64]

Time magazine gave extensive coverage of his tour. It began with a full-page report that he was coming to the US and Canada, and a comparison of his report with the US National Resources Planning Board (NRPB) document.[65] It covered his arrival and a reporter's query about the NRPB document, where Beveridge said it was useful only insofar as showing "'the facts of insecurity in the United States as an argument for doing something.'"[66] A later article reported his comments on the cost for a US Beveridge Plan.[67]

It was during this time that he also went to Ottawa to present to a joint session of two House of Commons committees.

The Beveridge Report: Part of a Wider Movement

We commented earlier that a strong argument could be made that the Beveridge Report, and the reaction to it, was but the most visible manifestation of a deep undercurrent that involved a move to social equality and, in the case of health, access for all.

Fraser notes, "The nearer to a total war, the greater tends to be the degree of social equality involved and so the Second World War tended to reduce social distinctions.... The wider definition of the war effort produced a growing concern for the health and welfare of an ever-widening circle of people."[68] Also, "A people's war had to produce a people's peace."[69] He says it motivated an impulse to universal rather than selective solutions.[70]

Addison notes, "The war effected a quiet revolution" and benefits needed to include the common people.[71] Titmuss says it "developed a measure of direct concern for the health and well-being of the population," which, when contrasted with the role of government in the nineteenth century, "was little short of remarkable." In addition government intervention in social needs needed to be inclusive of all classes rather than targeted.[72]

These are comments about Britain but such thinking could be applied to all countries that fought in the war. But in countries such as the United Kingdom, the United States, Canada, and New Zealand there had been important developments in health during the interwar period. It could well have been that just as the Second World War accelerated progress in social welfare, so did the First World War, just that they were not as far reaching.

The Wider Scope of Social Benefits Regarding Canada

The British sentiments we have outlined about social benefits had a similar and somewhat independent development in Canada. We have already noted the League for Social Reconstruction, the Rowell-Sirois Report, the Heagerty, Marsh, and Cassidy reports, and the Dominion-Provincial Conference on Reconstruction. Even before these activities and even before the Beveridge Report, these sentiments on expanded health benefits were also being expressed by prominent Canadians.

One such was Dr F.R. Davis, minister of health for Nova Scotia. In an address to the joint convention of the hospital associations of New Brunswick, Nova Scotia, and PEI in 1941 he spoke on the importance of group hospitalization and said that it should be combined with group medical care. He noted that ultimate success depends largely on the size of the group and that the "ultimate aim should be a group which would comprise every one of every class in the country."[73] This then "can only be done most effectively by some scheme of health insurance, probably federal in character." He alluded to the war and that "great changes undoubtedly will take place in our social structure." He said that he didn't believe "we will ever be satisfied again to see the present great spread between the poor and the well-to-do." He noted, "There is bound to be a great leveling" and said that when this happens "governments will take on even greater responsibilities than they do at the present time in maintaining the health of the community."[74]

Harvey Agnew, while he was editor of *Canadian Hospital*, was also writing about important reports coming out of Britain. In the January 1943 issue he noted three reports: the BMA Planning Commission report on a comprehensive health policy, a Political and Economic Planning (PEP) report on the same topic, and the Beveridge Report.[75]

All of this created a very fertile environment for the School of Hygiene, playing right into the need for its new department. In fact one could argue that this new department would be but another example of this wider type of thinking in social benefits. One could argue it was a manifestation of such thinking, for it was saying that as a result of this new emphasis, and the new institutions arising as a result, there was a need for a whole new kind of management, one devoted completely to health and not an offshoot of business management.

In addition, we had people like FitzGerald, an early supporter of health insurance, and Agnew of hospitals (and group plans concerning hospitals), who were very much a part of this ferment.

Harvey Agnew on Health Insurance (1943)

A US history of social security said that Beveridge's tour stimulated further discussion of health insurance.[76] There were more articles in 1943 on the topic in the US journal *Hospitals*, of which Harvey Agnew wrote two. He wrote an editorial in the May issue titled "Health Insurance Imminent in Canada,"[77] and a second article on the topic in November, on a health insurance proposal that had hospital support. In it he noted the importance of preserving the voluntary hospital system: "Our voluntary hospitals, lay and religious, have bequeathed to us a heritage of service and of public sentiment that has been one of the finest gems of our civilization."[78] Thomas Parran, the US surgeon general, also wrote an article that year in the journal endorsing health insurance and the important role of hospitals in it.[79]

White Paper, National Health Service (UK, 1944)

History was being made in during that era. Britain had tabled its White Paper, *A National Health Service*, in February 1944. It was a historic document, setting out a new right of citizenship – a new principle of inclusion: "The Government believe that, at this stage of social development the care of personal health should be put on a new footing and be made available to everybody as a publicly sponsored service."[80] It noted that just as people look to the common provision of a clean water supply, or highways, "accepting these as things which the community combines to provide for the benefit of the individual without distinction," so too should health be "a publicly organised service available to all who want to use it."[81]

It set out three main aims. The first was "a comprehensive health service for everybody," meaning a range of services being provided. The second was that health care be organized as an integrated system, and the third that health prevention and promotion be emphasized.[82] An oft-repeated phrase in the report was that the service be "free to all."[83]

Initiatives such as this meant a new import to health. Health would become a significant portfolio (and budget line) for national governments.

Saskatchewan (1944)

Other related events were happening in Canada. The T.C. Douglas government, elected in June 1944, was committed to far-reaching social legislation, and health was perhaps the most significant component of it. His government in October of that year tabled the Sigerist Report by a prominent Johns Hopkins physician.[84]

Hill-Burton Act (US, 1946)

Another important influence was what was happening south of the border.[85] In 1946 the US Congress had passed the Hill-Burton Act, whose legislative title was the Hospital Survey and Construction Act, in response to the first of five proposals of President Truman to improve the health and health care of Americans. It provided an annual US$75 million in federal grants for the construction of hospitals and unleashed an unprecedented building boom, one that resulted in huge advances in hospital design. Grants were processed by a state Hill-Burton Committee.

Agnew noted that he and others in Canada were helping some of the US states as well as the American Hospital Association on the legislative detail because of their experience with "progressive provincial legislation" in Canada.[86] The DHA program would receive a large number of applicants from the US.

What is less well known is that the Act was also a form of provision of hospital service. US states applied for funding. It was administered through the Surgeon General's Office. According to the congressional record, one provision of the Act was "That the State plan shall provide 'for adequate hospital facilities for the people residing in a State, without discrimination on account of race, creed, or color, and shall provide for adequate hospital facilities for persons unable to pay therefor.'"[87] It did two things for the United States: it expressed "a consensus on the centrality of hospitals in health policy" and it allowed hospital interests "to separate legislation for their construction and funding from broader national health programs and health insurance."[88]

Future faculty member Fred Mott presented at these hearings in March 1945. His comments illustrate the kind of faculty the U of T Department would later have. He argued powerfully for strong and equal support for the construction of rural hospitals: "That they should have equal opportunity for health is of the utmost importance to the Nation as a whole."[89] He said, "Failure to achieve the purpose of this bill must not be permitted, for the consequences would not only be felt in rural areas, but throughout the Nation. Our cities would die out, declining about 24 percent in population in a generation, if it were not for the constant flow of young people from the country."[90]

Wagner-Murray-Dingell Bill (US, 1946)

This was an attempt to institute a national medical and hospitalization program, but the bill was not passed. It grew out of a proposal of President Truman for a national health program.[91] Hearings were held on it in 1946. Fred Mott presented in April, alongside the assistant secretary of agriculture and came out strongly in favour of the bill: "There is no question … but that legislation of this kind, and within a very short period of time, would make possible … a kind of medical care that very few of our population have had."[92] He also noted, "The prevention of the future is simply early and adequate medical care.… I think a system which makes medical care accessible and which sets under way forces that will lead to the better distribution of facilities and personnel, will represent the best kind of prevention that we have ever had a chance to know."[93] Mott had also presented at the Senate Committee on the Hill-Burton Act.[94]

What This Meant for Canada

According to Bator and Rhodes, the dramatic rise of private and public medical care programs in the 1940s changed the landscape of Canadian health services.[95] One could add to this equally dramatic developments in health policy and distinguish in this between the early and latter 1940s. In the early part there were dramatic developments in the United Kingdom, the United States, and Canada, the most profound of which was the Beveridge Report. Canada had the Marsh, Cassidy, and Haegerty reports. Marsh had been a graduate student of Beveridge's. In the later 1940s all three governments made attempts at health legislation, but at the national level only the United Kingdom achieved results. However, sub-nationally Saskatchewan and BC were successful.

Bator and Rhodes note that from its inception medical care studies within the DPH relied on a variety of instructors from other departments and schools inside and outside U of T. It was a pattern of teaching that reflected Defries's growing cognizance of the economic, political, and social features of health planning and services, and Defries "displayed a remarkable foresight in introducing social and economic aspects of health care that revealed a growing appreciation of the health needs of ordinary Canadians." They note it is a testament to his willingness, despite the limitations of his own experience in public health administration, to plan for the development of new areas in Canadian health services.[96]

An interesting side note was the appointment of John Hastings in 1953 as a fellow in medical care administration.[97] He, of course, would later become very influential in the Department of Health Administration and the Division of Community Health.

AT INCEPTION

At its inception the department joined the ferment of the rapidly growing and evolving post–Second World War health care scene, not only in Canada but also internationally. The post-war period saw all sixteen countries of Western Europe greatly extend state responsibility for health care,[98] and Saskatchewan was at the beachhead, initiating its state-sponsored hospital coverage a full eighteen months before the United Kingdom began its health coverage. Three national assemblies – Canada and the two countries to which it had closest ties – were all involved in debating major pieces of health legislation.

The situation was accelerated by several factors, including rapid advances in medical science, the cost of accessing them, and increasing public expectation of the provision of medical services. Hospitals were the most visible and potent symbol, for in many communities they were major employers and a primary source of pride. Perhaps they were also a symbol of health security.

In many ways starting a Department of Hospital Administration was a natural next step for the School of Hygiene. Hospitals were growing rapidly in both number and size, and some saw them as a part of the public health constellation. An article in 1939 in *Canadian Hospital* noted, they were seen to be an integral part of public health work in Canada.[99]

Federal Government (1947)

Health and health insurance figured prominently in the debate on the Throne Speech in the Canadian Parliament in 1947, where "questions of national health and health insurance are among the most vitally important questions being faced by Canada today."[100] In Britain the Atlee government was busy preparing for the 1948 implementation of the National Health Service (NHS), having made the commitment in its very first Throne Speech of 1945 "to establish a national health service."[101]

Ontario (1947)

Hospitals were also building an increasing profile with the Ontario government. In March 1947, virtually across the street from the new department, initiatives regarding hospitals were mentioned in the Ontario Throne Speech.[102] Later that month the Budget Speech announced that "for the first time" Ontario would make maintenance and capital grants to hospitals,[103] to encourage the establishment of more hospitals, particularly in rural communities. Later in that legislative session it was noted "Hospital demand is increasing very rapidly" and that "40 percent of all admissions are covered by some plan."[104] They were a growth industry.

Saskatchewan, SHSP (1947)

An early focus of legislators was hospitals. In January 1947 Saskatchewan launched the Saskatchewan Hospital Services Plan (SHSP), the first hospital insurance program in North America. This created a demand for the department's graduates, to manage hospitals and to work within a newly established hospital sector within the Saskatchewan Department of Public Health. The provincial department developed strong ties to the Toronto program, and Saskatchewan financed students in both the diploma and certificate programs.

Commission on Hospital Care (US, 1947)

Also in 1947 the Commission on Hospital Care in the United States published a major study on hospitals (631 pages). The commission had been struck at the request of the trustees of the American Hospital Association.

Its activities had been supported by organizations such as the Commonwealth Fund and the Kellogg Foundation.[105]

Agnew-Swanson Submission to the Dominion Council on Health (1947)

In May 1947 Agnew and Dr A.L. (Arnold) Swanson, while technically not yet part of the U of T hospital administration program, made a submission to the Dominion Council on Health (of which Defries from the School of Hygiene was a member). It was presented under the auspices of the Canadian Hospital Council, calling attention to a "shortage of hospital accommodation" that since 1940 and 1941 "has become very acute." The situation was "now too big for voluntary effort alone to solve" and there was a call for provincial and federal aid.[106]

The matter was discussed at their meeting of 14–16 May 1947, and Defries was in attendance. The submission noted that many hospitals were operating at 130 to 140 per cent capacity.[107] The matter was also discussed at their next meeting (15–17 October), however, only to say that it "would involve very large expenditures" and that they "did not feel in a position to make any recommendation."[108]

National Health Grants (Canada, 1948)

In Canada a federal initiative unwittingly became a huge support to the new U of T program. The National Health Grants program was first mooted in the Green Books attached to the Dominion-Provincial Conference on Reconstruction. The initiative was stillborn because the conference was dissolved with no clear agreement on health insurance. Nonetheless, in 1948, Paul Martin Sr convinced Mackenzie King that the prime minister should not end his career without initiating a national health insurance program. King would agree only to a grants program similar to the 1945 proposals.[109]

These were a series of national grants for activities in health. They were the first plank, a stopgap measure toward national health insurance. Dr G. Donald W. Cameron (DPH, 1928), deputy minister of national health, was instrumental in developing the grants program.

The format followed the 1945 design with two exceptions, one of which was making the hospital construction grant a matching grant rather than a loan. This hugely stimulated hospital construction. Between 1948 and

1953 46,000 new beds were constructed,[110] and the grants continue after that, but the construction piece was reduced.

The implication this had for this new U of T program was an increase in hospital activity, in planning and operations, each of which meant jobs for hospital admin grads.

In 1948 Canada established the National Health Grants program. On 14 May Prime Minister Mackenzie King rose in the House to announce the new series of health grants[111] and closed his remarks by saying, "Of all a nation's resources, its human resources are unquestionably the most precious. The preservation in health and strength of its population is surely the best of all guarantees of a nation's power, of its progress and of its prosperity. Our greatest national asset is the health and well-being of our people."[112]

The grants covered ten areas. Three major ones were for a health survey, hospital construction, and professional training. The health survey Grant would explore the health needs of the province to ensure "the most effective use of the other grants," but also "in planning the extension of hospital accommodation, and the proper organization of hospital and medical care insurance."[113]

Special Meeting of Dominion Council of Health to Discuss Health Grants

A special meeting of the Dominion Council of Health was held on 7–8 June 1948 to outline the terms of these grants. Present and future school and DHA faculty (Defries, Agnew, and Mott) were involved, and the federal minister (Paul Martin Sr) attended, as well as deputy ministers and officers from the federal and provincial health departments. Future faculty member Fred Mott attended from Saskatchewan and was quite vocal in the discussion of the health survey and hospital construction grants. The meeting was to work out the details regarding each of the grants. Defries was quite vocal in the discussion of the public health research grant.[114]

Hospital Construction Grant

The DHA program had not been underway for a year before the federal initiative greatly accelerated the growth of hospitals.

The National Health Grants program included a matching grant for hospital construction.[115] Agnew recounts a call from federal Minister C.D. Howe in early 1948 requesting an immediate figure for what would be required if the government gave grants to hospitals rather than low-interest loans.[116]

An interesting aspect of the program was that a government report on it observed that a hospital can also fulfil public health functions. It noted "a general hospital can often be to a large extent the health centre of a community, and provision is often made therein for public health services."[117]

Agnew's two telegrams to the Dominion Council were entered into the minutes regarding this grant. One expressed the appreciation of the Canadian Hospital Council and noted that it would greatly stimulate hospital construction; however, the result would be the need for more hospital staff and it asked that provision be made for their training. The other asked that consideration be given to hospitals who started construction before the grants were announced.[118]

The grants were important to the growth of hospitals. According to Agnew, a result of the grants was that by the late 1950s more than 40,000 acute, almost 20,000 mental health, 7,000 chronic, and 4,500 TB beds were built with concomitant increases in hospital staffs.[119]

Professional Training Grant

Another feature of the program was provision for professional training. The Dominion Council discussed how it should be awarded. Defries suggested that it should be directed toward public health and hospital services and that it might relate to both professional and sub-professional workers.[120] Mott proposed that it "meet the needs of expanding hospital services, that it be interpreted broadly; for example such workers as hospital administrators."[121]

The School of Hygiene received grants to aid in the establishment of a diploma course in bacteriology and another grant for the diploma course in bacteriology, specializing in virology.[122]

Of more direct relevance to the new diploma in hospital administration was bursaries for hospital administrators. From 1948 to 1961, 147 bursaries were awarded for studies in hospital administration and a further 105 for short courses in this area. The latter almost certainly included the CHA hospital administration certificate course, which utilized faculty from the Department of Hospital Administration at U of T.[123] As for the former, it is reasonable to assume some DHA students benefited from these bursaries; however, no direct reference can be found to corroborate this, especially since until the introduction of a francophone program in Quebec in 1956, this was the only program in Canada, and even after that it was the only program in English Canada for a number of years.

Directorate of Health Insurance Studies

The strong feelings of Paul Martin Sr regarding health insurance led him to form a Directorate of Health Insurance Studies in 1948. He chose the former deputy minister of health from Manitoba, Fred W. Jackson (DPH, 1929), to head it (he would later become federal deputy minister) because of his own strong feelings about health insurance. Jackson, beginning in the fall 1951, went on to study the sickness insurance plans of Norway, Sweden, Denmark, Holland, and Great Britain.

Lectures in Medical Care Administration (1948)

In 1948 Defries wrote to the Rockefeller Foundation to request funding for lectures and studies in medical care administration. It signified his keen cognizance of the rapidly changing landscape of Canadian health care.

The motivation was threefold. First was the rapid growth of prepaid hospital and medical plans in several provinces, many sponsored by associations of physicians. There was also Blue Cross of Ontario (under the OHA), which had enrolled one-third of the province. Many large industries had made provision for medical and hospital services for their employees. Second was the introduction of province-wide hospital insurance plans, with Saskatchewan having implemented one in 1947 and BC signalling their intent to do the same, based on a Saskatchewan template. Third were the health grants announced by the federal government. The foundation gave an award of $17,000 to the school in October that year.[124]

An important feature of the classes was the number of outside authorities who were recruited to give one or more lectures about medical care and health insurance. Even before the award was granted, Defries hired Gordon H.M. Hatcher to teach and study medical problems in Canada. With assistance from the Rockefeller Foundation he conducted studies on the health systems of Newfoundland, Saskatchewan, Alberta, and BC.[125]

Another hire was F.W. Jackson (whom we met in the previous section). Another was Malcolm Taylor, who had been director of research and statistics in the Department of Public Health in the Douglas government in Saskatchewan and taught for a time at the U of T Department of Political Economy.[126]

NHS (1948)

Part of the milieu surrounding the new program was what was taking place with the NHS in the United Kingdom. Agnew and *Canadian Hospital* ensured their readers were aware of what was happening.

Webster noted that the birth of the NHS coincided with "the dawn of a golden age" of medicine.[127] It immediately became the third-largest non-military organization in Britain.[128] Its staff almost immediately developed the sense that "they were part of a prestigious national service, capable of achieving in peacetime something like the feats of collective action and patriotic sacrifice recently witnessed in the special circumstances of total warfare."[129]

The public had similar sentiments. Shortly after leaving his post as Britain's chief medical officer (CMO), Sir George Godber wrote that not long after the inception of the NHS there was "an odd euphoria about what had been done and a tendency to pride ourselves on having the finest heath service in the world."[130] He was eminently qualified to make the statement. The *Guardian* referred to him as a "medical lay saint," one whose name was still recalled "more than 35 years after his retirement" as CMO, "a nostalgic recollection of the halcyon days of the NHS."

He was part of the team that planned it.[131] He worked alongside Aneurin Bevan and William Beveridge, serving as CMO for Her Majesty's Government from 1960 to 1973, and before that as part of the Emergency Medical Service. As with people like J.G. FitzGerald and Robert Defries in Toronto, he was another example of how public health physicians took an active interest in health insurance (having received a DPH from the London School of Hygiene and Tropical Medicine in 1936).

Another fact that underscored the importance of what was happening in Toronto was that the hospital service quickly emerged as the leading institution within the new NHS. According to Webster, they were "in all respects the dominant element" in the NHS and at its beginning accounted for 54 per cent of its budget (a figure that would rise to about 70 per cent in 1975).[132]

ONTARIO HOSPITALS

Hospitals in Ontario were important to communities and the provincial government. The evident pride that communities and the province took in their hospitals is clear in a 1934 illustrated book of almost 300 pages on the subject put together by the Ministry of Health. It noted an almost exponential increase in provincial grants from the 1870s to the 1930s.[133] It was also a large operator of hospitals at that time, mainly in tuberculosis and mental health.

Ontario took advantage of the federal grant money and itself experienced an unprecedented hospital building boom. And its premier teaching hospital was at the leading edge of the advances in hospital design (see the next section). In the 1950s this involved going up. Kisacky notes, "The integrated high-rise facilities of large general hospitals, teaching hospitals, and medical centers stand as the iconic institutional form."[134] It was also said, "High-rise hospitals provided a visible and tangible differentiation" of North American from European development.[135] They were also a "sign of the developing modern, urban, technological culture."[136] The high-rise hospital was "an expression of technological and economic prowess wedded to modern medicine."[137] And at the top of University Avenue, one of Canada's premier promenades, across from the seat of government, stood our own symbol of the pinnacle of hospital design and the potency of academic medicine.

The Beginning of the University Avenue Hospital Corridor

This period also saw the beginning of what would become one of the larger medical clusters.

TGH, SickKids, and Mount Sinai began thinking of expansion toward the latter stages of the Second World War. For SickKids and Mount Sinai it also involved a move to University Avenue. There was also politics involved; it was suggested that the Mount Sinai board agreed to cede the property just south of TGH to the board of SickKids in return for a commitment to support Mount Sinai being granted status as a U of T teaching hospital.[138] In 1948 Mount Sinai began an expansion and construction of a new facility across from the new SickKids site, at the northwest corner of University and Elm.[139]

The TGH redevelopment, which began in 1954, epitomized all this. A new high-rise wing (now called the Norman Urquhart Wing) was built between the College Wing and the Private Patients Pavilion. Associated with it was a large structure housing essential support services and connecting all the major existing buildings on a site that covered approximately three square blocks.[140]

Such redevelopment continued periodically as the University Avenue hospitals constantly strove to be at the leading edge. It required capability and commitment at many different levels – government, voluntary boards, and senior administrators, some of whom were IHPME grads.

And these hospitals stood as a symbol that "academic health centers exert an influence on the health care system that extends well beyond their walls, and affect the average citizen.... They play a pivotal role in applying the fruits of the biological revolution ... to relieving human suffering."[141]

The Evolution of Hospitals Generally

Hospitals figured prominently in the history of other countries as well. A phenomenon that could be called "middle-class medicine" was making hospital medical care available to the masses as a result of the voluntary hospital and health insurance plans of the United States and Canada, and the compulsory national health insurance schemes like the NHS in Britain and those of other European countries.[142] Hospitals figured prominently in the history of health care in many countries.[143]

Many of these same sentiments were to be found in Canadians. Their wish to provide health insurance to all Canadians dates back to the early twentieth century. Their hospitals figure prominently in the history of almost all their communities, ranging from the giant academic teaching centres such as a Toronto General (founded 1829), which now are as much of a world community as a metropolitan community, to places like the Toronto Salvation Army Grace Hospital (founded 1889), to any number of community hospitals across the nation. They were a strong focus of almost all Canadian communities in the twentieth century, and in the major metropolitan centres this can be traced back to the nineteenth century. Building and operating them occupied the minds of civic politicians, prominent business people, and concerned citizens.

It also involved religious orders who saw this as a form of service, a form of missionary work, many of them travelling across the country to found a hospital in a young community. We have noted that municipalities in Saskatchewan banded together co-operatively to form union hospital districts to raise funds to build and operate hospitals – an innovation that attracted international attention.

Gagan and Gagan write that in Canada in the early twentieth century hospitals "underwent a startling transformation." They "became the preferred source of medical treatment and care for people of all classes." They speak of the "invention of the modern Canadian public general hospital" as a "community medical and social institution." Allied to this was a "redefinition of the social objective of Canadian federalism" in making hospital care available to the masses,[144] made possible by the Tommy Douglas experiment in Saskatchewan.

And the strength of this feeling was such that time and effort have been expended to put together histories of this activity. Many, many histories have been written of particular hospitals. In Canada's major medical libraries there are numerous published histories of the proud communities of these institutions:[145] local histories, grassroots histories. They are testaments to the concern communities exhibited to the ill and their ingenuity in finding ways to build and operate hospitals.

There are also separate histories of the schools of nursing associated with many of these hospitals. As the opening to one of them points out, the history of a school for nurses cannot be separated from the general history of the hospital to which it is attached.[146]

And, to jump to the present for a moment, these same communities railed against the government when health care moved beyond inpatient hospital care and the government sought to consolidate and refocus it. Two cases in point are the health reform of 1990s Ontario and in the same period the Romanow government in Saskatchewan closing of many of the rural hospitals that the Tommy Douglas government almost fifty years before had funded in numerous villages to extend health care into the predominantly rural province.

This strong feeling about hospitals persists, and not just at the public level. The Ontario Hospital Association still calls itself just that. The deputy minister of health and long-term care in 2017 noted the strength of hospitals in Ontario and particularly of their volunteer boards, which he called "the best in the world."[147]

PART FOUR

The Need for Professional Hospital *Management*

CHAPTER 8

A Diploma in *Hospital* Administration

EVENTS OF THE FIRST HALF OF 1947 AT U OF T TOWARD PLANNING THE NEW PROGRAM

It is unclear when exactly planning for the program began. An article in *Canadian Hospital* in May 1947 mentioned that the School of Hygiene had been considering such a program for several years.[1]

The memorandum for the council meeting of the School of Hygiene noted that at the last Conference of Professors of Preventive Medicine held in October 1946 at Ann Arbor under the auspices of the Rockefeller Foundation it was stated that schools of hygiene should note the growing need for instruction in hospital administration, "not only for those who may serve as hospital administrators but also for medical officers of health and for the administrators of medical care programmes." It noted as well that the Canadian Hospital Council had expressed the need for such a program. It quoted Harvey Agnew, who said, "'Hospital administration is now an exacting vocation – in many respects it is a profession. Hospitals are an essential part of our social system,'" and training could no longer be on a "learn-as-you-go" basis, that hospital trustees were now asking for trained hospital administrators to fill their postings.[2]

Interest at U of T crystallized in the first four months of 1947, sparked by a letter from the Kellogg Foundation to Defries, dated 6 January 1947. It indicated that the foundation had made a grant to four universities (Columbia, Minnesota, Yale, Washington) for a hospital administration course. It was looking to fund additional programs at four other universities with a school of public health, and the School of Hygiene would be "the logical place to establish such a course for hospital administrators in Canada." It said further that the foundation would be sympathetic to a proposal.[3]

The letter also noted that on "the recommendation of leaders in the hospital field" the foundation's intent was to concentrate on universities with a school of public health. It noted that they were "beginning to experiment with this in Michigan" (the foundation was based in Battle Creek, Michigan) and that the US "Commission on Hospital Care recommends this as a future development." While the letter does not refer to it as an enclosure, included in the U of T president's file with this correspondence is a *Hospital Survey News Letter* from the Commission on Hospital Care, titled "Hospitals and Health Departments," which talks about the need for cooperation between hospitals and public health departments. It outlines the justification for such cooperation and the programs that could be integrated: "Ideally the health department should be located in or adjacent to a hospital" and these should be "branch offices of the official government health department."[4]

This letter set a number of activities rapidly in motion. A series of memoranda were exchanged between Defries and Dr Smith during the four-month period. In addition there is correspondence with Graham Davis, director of the Division of Hospitals at the foundation. The Council of the School of Hygiene discussed the idea at its February 1947 meeting. It noted that over the past ten years courses in hospital administration had been developed in universities in the United States and United Kingdom and, while originally they were in schools of business administration, latterly they had been located in schools of hygiene.[5]

The foundation sent two representatives to Toronto in early 1947 to speak to people in the school and to view its facilities. This was followed by a two-page letter in March 1947 from Sidney Smith to the president of the foundation. It noted the visit, the interest of the foundation in funding such courses generally, and a specific interest in providing the funds to cover the costs for the operation of such a program at U of T for three years, and U of T's intent to establish such a course.[6] This was followed by an 8 April letter to Smith from Defries indicating that the director of the Division of Hospitals for the foundation had agreed to provide the money for the first year of the program as well as to fund five fellowships. This was followed by a 12 April letter from Smith to Mr Davis at the foundation expressing his appreciation.[7]

It culminated in a letter from Emory Morris, president of the foundation, to Smith, dated 22 April 1947, indicating the foundation would provide funding for three years. It included a cheque to fund the first year's operations.[8]

On 11 April the U of T Senate passed statute 1837 enacting establishment of a diploma in hospital administration in the School of Hygiene. It also enacted establishment of a Department of Hospital Administration. Finally, it enacted commencement of the "Course of Instruction" with the 1947–48 session. The statute was signed by the president and registrar and had the imprint of the university seal.[9]

There was an attachment to the statute document providing information on the proposed course in hospital administration. It noted that the Canadian Hospital Council had written to several universities in Canada and addressed a letter to the School of Hygiene "stating that there is a need in Canada for a course in hospital administration to be provided for university graduates." It also noted that the trustees of the Kellogg Foundation "on the recommendation of leaders in the hospital field, have endorsed and are supporting financially the provision of courses in hospital administration in several universities with schools of public health."[10]

It stated "that the hospital administrator should have a suitable background in public health training" and that five such universities in the United States had been assisted by the foundation. It was the foundation's belief "that in the rural areas the hospital and health department be very closely related and that in the urban communities an intimate relationship should be developed.… Hospitals and health department can work effectively in advancing the health of the public." It repeated some of the information in the minutes of the Council of the School of Hygiene relating to the Conference of Professors of Hygiene and Preventive Medicine. It noted that from the standpoint of the School of Hygiene such a course would also be of value "in making possible for adequate instruction in hospital administration" for those enrolled in the Diploma of Public Health.[11]

The attachment also noted that seven universities in the United States were providing or announcing postgraduate courses in hospital administration: Chicago, Northwestern, Columbia, Duke, Yale, Minnesota, and Washington. And the London School of Hygiene and Tropical Medicine was establishing such a course.[12]

On 7 May the president approved and returned publicity material to Defries relating to the course in hospital administration. On 4 June Defries enclosed a copy of a poster announcing the new program as well as a brochure that went into more detail on the program, including an outline the courses involved. Defries noted that these had been sent to hospitals throughout Canada.[13]

On 8 May 1947 the board of governors approved the "Statute of the Senate Number 1837 respecting the Diploma in Hospital Administration and the Course of Instruction leading thereto."[14] On the same day, the board acknowledged receipt of the first instalment of the three-year grant from the Kellogg Foundation.[15] On 29 May the board approved a part-time position for H.G. Agnew at the rank of professor of hospital administration (salary $2,000 per annum), beginning 1 July[16] and a full-time position at the rank of associate professor of hospital administration for L.O. Bradley of $6,500, beginning on 1 August.[17]

The U of T *President's Report* for 1946–47 noted the establishment of the Department of Hospital Administration within the School of Hygiene. The school now consisted of seven departments and two sub-departments. The new degree was established as a postgraduate diploma and the course lasted twenty-one months, with nine months of classes and a twelve-month internship.[18] The department was one of the few in the world at the time. The resolution to the Senate noted that there were graduate courses provided in hospital administration in five schools of hygiene in the United States and one in the United Kingdom.[19] Sidney Smith's handwritten notes (no doubt talking points) attached to a memorandum providing background for the resolution noted there were six US schools, at Johns Hopkins, Minnesota, Michigan, Yale, Columbia, and Iowa.[20]

Milton Brown, former head of the Department of Public Health in the School of Hygiene, noted that at the time it was the only program in Canada. He recounted the pressures that led to setting up the program. As hospitals became larger and more complex, the school felt a person was needed who was "well trained in administration."[21]

We noted earlier that the new department was funded with a grant from the Kellogg Foundation, which also provided scholarships for the first year of the course.[22] This began a relationship with the department that would endure. As with the Rockefeller Foundation and the School of Hygiene, the relationship of the department with the Kellogg Foundation plugged it into a wider network. And being associated with such a foundation helped the new department's profile. The foundation noted its contribution to the U of T in a book on its first twenty-five years[23] and did the same in one on its first fifty years.[24]

Philanthropic organizations played an important role in the establishment of such programs. One could argue that the Kellogg Foundation in regard to hospital administration and the Rockefeller Foundation in regard to public health played an important part in seeding university-based programs in these areas. In doing so, they aided development of these areas of activity, for it was not just in the teaching of professional management, but given their location at a university, the research that would inevitably follow.

Back to the inception of the program itself, according to Andrew Rhodes, at the time there was "quite vigorous objection" from some of the senior staff on the Council of the School of Hygiene on having hospital administration at the university level: it was regarded "as just not quite the sort of thing to do at a university" and not appropriate to be taught at a university level, let alone a school of hygiene. But "we survived the storm," and Defries was usually very able at this sort of thing: he felt we should be teaching hospital administration, and a number of the U.S. schools were doing so. He described Agnew as "one of the greats in that particular field" and he made a major contribution to hospital administration.[25]

Meanwhile, in recognition of developments in the Douglas government in Saskatchewan and also in Manitoba, the director, R.D. Defries in 1947 requested of Sidney Smith, the university president, that a portion of the Rockefeller Foundation grant be used for a study visit to those two provinces for one of the faculty to speak with the deputy ministers of health in each. The request pointed to important developments in each province, "particularly as relating to the provision of medical care." And, to indicate the calibre of people whom the school was attracting as guest lecturers, a second letter to Smith requested payment for the deputy minister from Manitoba for a series of lectures he delivered to students in public health administration.[26]

G. HARVEY AGNEW (1947–62)

His Background

There was probably no one more qualified to lead the new department than G. Harvey Agnew. His role in hospitals with the CMA and with the CHC, as well as being a principal in the hospital consulting firm Agnew Peckham, and his contacts with the American Hospital Association, made him an expert in the field. We have already mentioned him a number of times and in so doing provided information on his background. He was a graduate of the University of Toronto, receiving his MD in 1923.[27] It is said in 1928 he gave up a promising career as a teacher of internal medicine for his Canadian Medical Association position on hospitals. Such a change points back to the reputation of the School of Hygiene and acumen of Defries that Agnew was brought on board.

Agnew had an enduring interest in the move to health insurance and the implications it had for physicians and hospitals. In 1943 he wrote an article in *Hospitals* on health insurance, which included a principle he would repeat many times: health insurance might be a step toward state medicine, but it would be more likely to do so "through a disastrous series of transitions" if "professional bodies and hospitals do not step in at this formative stage."[28] In 1948 he updated and expanded on this article in a book on hospital trends published by the Commonwealth Fund.[29]

He had a wide range of interests. A few months after he started as head of the Department of Hospital Administration, it was reported in the *Bulletin* that he was president of the Royal Canadian Institute and president of the American Physicians' Art Association, and that a reproduction of one of his paintings had been featured in *Life* magazine.[30] In 1947 he delivered a lecture at the Royal Canadian Institute titled "The Romance of Hospital Evolution."[31]

His knowledge of hospitals across the country and his contacts with hospital administrators – begun with his position at the CMA and continued with his association with the CHC/CHA – made him the ideal person to direct the newly established department. His position with *Canadian Hospital* certainly helped profile the department. When faculty and DPH and DHA graduates published in it, their association or diploma from the department was mentioned. While he was editor when the career moves of graduates were included in its "People" section, invariably the diploma and U of T were mentioned.

INCEPTION OF THE PROGRAM

Beginnings

On 22 September 1947 classes began for the first cohort in the diploma of hospital administration.[32] The new department was housed along with the School of Hygiene in the FitzGerald Building.

The courses were very practical in their orientation. There were ten courses. The first was Hospital Organization and Management and others were on departmental management, the legal aspects of hospital administration, personnel management, public relations, planning and construction, public health, and accounting and budgetary control, to name a few.[33]

There were four students, of which two were physicians. The program proved very popular, with thirty applications for the fall 1948. There was course work in the first year (September to May) followed by a twelve-month internship. The internship was an important element in the degree programs that were established at that time, and remain so. The American College of Hospital Administrators noted in 1954 that of fourteen university graduate programs, all had a twelve-month supervised residency.[34]

The residency became an important feature of the Toronto program. Perhaps of equal importance to the practical experience it afforded were the relationships and networks that it spawned. Many endured for years, some for entire careers. Students had strong memories of those who had a big influence on them.

DHA grad Tony Dagnone remembers that his preceptor Dr Bill Noonan in Hamilton offered him a job. The complicating factor was that he had accepted a bursary from Saskatchewan to attend the program, and it had a three-year work clause in it. Noonan offered to buy it out; however, the deputy minister in Saskatchewan would not agree.[35] This was perhaps a good move by the deputy minister, for Tony did return to Saskatchewan and spent the first couple of decades of his career at the Royal University Hospital in Saskatoon. He would eventually make it back to Ontario (to London, more on this later).

Earl Dick makes a similar point when he notes that when he became executive director and was planning for an expansion at what was then known as the University Hospital in Saskatoon, it helped that he and the deputy minister in Saskatchewan had shared an office at the hospital when the latter was an administrative resident.[36]

Two years after the program started, the requirements were revised to include a thesis in order to graduate.[37] In keeping with the orientation of the program, this invariably was on a practical rather than a theoretical topic. The cumulative result was the generation of substantial applied knowledge that others could refer to. They were almost invariably dealing with a topic of practical import to the organization in which they were doing their residency, and when these were provincial departments of health, their thesis could be a component of policy development. Wahn's thesis in the Tommy Douglas Department of Public Health (Douglas was his own health minister for a time) comes to mind. It was on an integrated hospital system for Saskatchewan (more on this later). The theses were all bound, and almost thirty years of them are filed at the Gerstein Library. We will list examples of students, their careers, and their thesis topics at the end of eras of IHPME.

Several students writing the thesis at the time thought they were very theoretical and not practical, while the School of Graduate Studies would have likely had the opposite view. They would have said that the subject matter concerned practical problems, as opposed to advancing the theory of the discipline. Nonetheless, considerable effort went into these theses. And one could argue that in the present knowledge-based society that emphasizes translating knowledge to practice, such an approach by the department did just that.

The department was able to attract pre-eminent individuals in the field to deliver lectures in the first year. These included Dean Conley, executive secretary of the American College of Hospital administrators, and Graham Davis, director of the Division of Hospitals of the Kellogg Foundation; another was Dr Malcolm T. MacEachern.[38] He was originally a Canadian physician (MD, McGill), born in Argyle, ON, and had been superintendent of Vancouver General.[39] He founded the Northwestern University hospital administration program and was author of the landmark work for many years, the 1,000-plus page *Hospital Organization and Management.*

In the department's first annual report Agnew acknowledged the assistance given by the Department of Health of Ontario and hospitals in the Toronto area for field trips and lecture-discussions.[40]

Even before the department admitted its first students, the program was being profiled in *Canadian Hospital.* In its May 1947 issue, in an article almost certainly by R.D. Defries, it noted planning underway for a program at U of T. It said that while the first US programs were established in schools of business administration, the recent trend was to locate them in schools of hygiene. It remarked that the Kellogg Foundation was particularly supportive. It noted information that reiterated some of the information the foundation had transmitted to Defries when it had signalled its interest in funding a Toronto program, that the foundation felt the hospital administrator should have some background in public health, and that in urban communities "an intimate relationship should be developed" and in rural areas they "must be very closely related."[41]

Related to the need for hospital management in May 1947, Agnew wrote an article in the *CMAJ* on the hospital's "rôle of steadily increasing importance in the practice of medicine."[42] He foresaw it would continue to grow.

He noted that 80 per cent of the public hospital beds were operated by voluntary groups and half of these were by Roman Catholic sisters. He felt that this proportion would decrease in favour of more municipally owned hospitals. Overall he saw a continuing increase in hospitals' role.[43]

In the June 1947 issue of *Canadian Hospital* there was a single-page official announcement of the program. It would be a twenty-one-month course with nine months of classes and a twelve-month administrative internship. It also provided an outline of some of the courses.[44] That month also began a series of advertisements for the program that appeared in each month's issue for the balance of that year and into the next.[45]

In its July issue *Canadian Hospital* noted the appointment of Dr Leonard O. Bradley, assistant to the superintendent of the Royal Alexandra Hospital in Edmonton, to the position of associate professor in the Toronto program.[46] Both he and Agnew became regular contributors to the journal. Its offices at the time were located in Toronto not far from the school, and many of the DHA grads were contributors. In October of that year Agnew composed an article on graduate training in hospital administration and why it needed to be at the graduate level. It mentioned the Toronto program.[47]

The US journal *Hospitals* also reported on the Canadian program. It had an article in its February 1948 issue along with a brief bio and picture of Agnew.[47]

In 1948 the department became one of the seven founders of the Association of University Programs in Hospital Administration. By-laws were developed and approved. They stated that members must grant a degree equivalent to a master's degree, they must provide one academic year and one practical residency year, and at least one-third of the curriculum must be devoted to hospital administration.[49]

Also that year Bradley was given a part-time leave of absence to act as director of studies for the Ontario Health Survey Committee initiated by the Department of Health of Ontario with support from a federal health grant. Eugenie Stuart was brought on as an assistant professor in a temporary position to fill in for Bradley's absence.[50]

National Posture and Rapid Growth

The department became fully enrolled almost immediately after it came into being. Each year applications greatly exceeded available spots and US applications greatly exceeded those from Canada.[51] In the second year of the program 20 per cent of the students were from the United States.[52] By

1951–52 it was placing people across the country and in the Health Services Planning Commissions (HSPC) in Saskatchewan and BC, which were dealing with their cutting-edge social policy initiatives in hospital insurance.[53]

According to the school's annual report for 1952–53, "Half of the graduates are occupying senior administrative positions in hospitals in Canada and the United States, and requests for graduates of the course are still in excess of the supply."[54] This was the case for both the diploma and certificate program. In 1954–55 its student cohort came from seven Canadian provinces and four US states.[55]

A SPECIFIC EXAMPLE

Ed Wahn (DHA, 1950) was an early grad who was an example of this national posture. He was at the Saskatchewan HSPC (he began in 1946). He took an educational leave to come to the program (1948–49) and returned to Saskatchewan for his administrative residency. He had several roles in the Douglas Department of Public Health, the Saskatchewan health-care system, and the University of Saskatchewan.

His DHA thesis demonstrated some of the close connections that could be built between an individual on educational leave and the practical needs of a government department. The thesis was on a plan for an integrated hospital system for Saskatchewan and was timely in light of Saskatchewan's hospital insurance program begun in 1947. This initiative, in addition to the National Health Grants Program of the federal government, a major part of which was for hospital construction, meant that Saskatchewan was building a number of hospitals, and that one needed to be mindful of how they would work together. The thesis was also important in referencing another major landmark study: the Commission on Hospital Care in the United States of 1947 (whose survey methods Wahn noted he widely adopted).[56]

His thesis provided a socio-economic overview of the province and a history of its hospitals. It divided the province into a number of districts, indicating what hospitals they had and what they needed. It also demonstrated the access an employee/student in a small province could gain to higher government officials, as he acknowledged both T.J. Bentley, minister of public health, and F.D. Mott, acting deputy minister in his thesis. There is a copy in the Saskatchewan Legislative Library. It complemented the work done under the National Health Grants Program and provided important information for the Saskatchewan department for its very active program concerning hospitals.

WESTERN CANADA HOSPITAL INSTITUTE (1946–1949)

Just months before planning for the DHA program began, the Western Canadian Hospital Institute was formed and held its first conference. Agnew was involved (and would continue his involvement in future institute meetings). It was initially called the Institute on Hospital Administration, which held its first conference from 28 October to 2 November 1946 in Winnipeg and generated substantial interest from the four western provinces.

The institute was remarkable for a number of reasons. First was the commitment of the hospital associations of the four western provinces, and of hospital administrators and trustees. For our purposes it was notable for DoHA faculty (and very soon grad) involvement throughout its lifespan. It was an example of the department building capacity in the system. It was also striking for the extensive reporting *Canadian Hospital* did on it each year and noteworthy for the speakers it attracted, a number of whom came from other countries.

At its first conference Agnew gave the address at the opening dinner sponsored for delegates by the mayor of Winnipeg. Agnew also led some of the round table discussions. Malcolm T. MacEachern from Northwestern University, the doyen of hospital administration, was involved in the planning and also spoke. The Manitoba minister of health and public welfare, his deputy, and the deputy minister for municipal affairs also attended and spoke.[57]

The 1949 institute was held in Regina with both future faculty member F. Mott and DHA grad E.V. Wahn involved. Agnew spoke at the closing session and Premier Douglas was the guest speaker at the banquet.[58] Saskatchewan at that time was two years into its precedent-setting hospital insurance program (the first in North America).

Agnew had a section on the institute in his memoirs. It came into being to provide an educational program for hospital management and trustees for the western provinces and provide "hospital personnel with an opportunity to hear and meet the outstanding leaders in the hospital field." Each hospital association in the four western provinces took turns organizing the conference, which was held in conjunction with the annual meeting of the host association.[59]

It proved to be a highly successful annual educational activity attracting ever-increasing numbers of registrants. Topical issues of the day were discussed and there were sessions on a number of different functional aspects of administration. The conference generally lasted three to five days. That they were organized by hospital associations, which had a large component of voluntary members, illustrated the strong public sentiment regarding hospitals in Western Canada, analogous to that of the country as a whole, and of the United Kingdom, and United States spoken of earlier.

Many DOHA faculty participated for a number of years, and some – Bradley is an example – participated throughout its existence, even after he left the faculty. There was considerable DOHA involvement in the institute each year by faculty, former faculty, and grads.

MAJOR NEW HOSPITAL ACTIVITY: SASKATCHEWAN AND BC, UNIVERSAL HOSPITAL INSURANCE

Shortly after the inception of the DHA program, the provincial hospital insurance plans of Saskatchewan (1947) and BC (1949) created new hospital activity that resulted in new prospects for DHA grads. Both provinces expanded hospital capacity (the number and size of hospitals). In addition, both provinces created Hospital Standards divisions within their ministries, which were staffed by professional experts in hospital inspection, budget analysis, and hospital planning.[60]

WHERE GRADS ENDED UP: I

We will insert a short piece on where some grads ended up at various points along the timeline of the department/Institute. Here is the first instalment. Generally, we will list the name, last known position, and title of the thesis they produced by the end of their administrative residency (bound copies of which are located in the Gerstein Library).

Where possible, we will add further information, such as their native province, undergraduate degree, and other career positions. We will see from these examples, along with those mentioned in other parts of the work, the true national footprint of the program. The program took people from across Canada and placed them in administrative residencies across Canada, then its graduates had careers that took a number of them to places across Canada.

There is a certain complexity to such movement. These individuals have to be attuned to differences in nuance, in two respects. The first stems from the BNA Act, which makes health a provincial responsibility. In a highly decentralized federation like Canada there are distinctions to health delivery in different parts of the nation. Second, the continental scope of the nation makes for different cultures across the nation. It is not just English and French Canada. The Prairies differ from BC, which differs from central Ontario, which differs from the Maritimes. It makes for a highly idiosyncratic milieu where what works in one region will not work in another (either in policy or career advancement).

Here are some examples of graduates in the 1950s:

- Joseph Hornstein (DHA, 1951), appointed assistant administrator of Albert Eibstein Medical Center in Philadelphia. Prior to that he was director of the North Detroit General Hospital.[61] His thesis was "The Hospital Administrator's Responsibility in the Evolution of a Modern Hospital Nursing School."
- John Lee (DHA, 1951) worked in the Saskatchewan Department of Public Health during the Douglas regime and also taught in the extension course program of the U of T department and the Canadian Hospital Council. His thesis was "Collective Bargaining Handbook for Canadian Hospitals."
- James McNab (DHA, 1951), former CEO of Toronto General and North York General hospitals. His thesis was "An Approach to the Determination of Hospital Working Capital Requirements and Methods of Current Financing."
  - He was a native of BC, came to Toronto to do the program, and upon graduation did an administrative residency at Vancouver General Hospital.
  - Following that he was a hospital Inspector and Consultant with the B.C. Hospital Insurance Service. Next, he was the Administrator of the Port Arthur General Hospital.
  - From there he went to the Ontario Hospital Services Commission as director of hospital planning. After that he joined the consulting firm of Woods, Gordon.[62]
- Clifford K. Temple (DHA, 1953) obtained a bachelor of pharmacy degree from the University of Saskatchewan, then went into the DHA program. He was an assistant administrator at Winnipeg

General Hospital and went from there to administrator of the Ontario Hospital in Whitby in 1968.[63] His thesis topic was "Medical Photography."

CHAPTER 9

A Solid Beginning

As we have noted, the program soon found a solid footing and was firmly established within the Canadian hospital scene. The result, primarily, of Agnew's contacts, it was part of a national network of hospital administrators, a fact that served it well in the options it provided its students for administrative residencies as well as employment upon graduation. Both the program and its graduates very quickly began having an impact. We will look at some examples in this chapter. But first a bit of a biography of one of the most beloved faculty – a woman who dedicated her life to the department.

EUGENIE STUART

Throughout her career, Eugenie Stuart was a lynchpin of the faculty. She joined the department in the fall of 1948 and would spend the rest of her career there. She was program director for many years of that time. She quickly became an essential part of the department.

She was born in Palmerston, Ontario. She was one of four girls and her early life was not easy, as the girls lost their parents at an early age. She was a graduate of the School of Nursing of Toronto General Hospital (class of 1925). From there she gained a diploma in hospital and school of nursing administration from the Department of Nursing, which at the time (1929) was an independent division of the School of Hygiene.

Her experience prior to coming to the department included a variety of positions, such as head nurse on Ward A at TGH, which in those days was a seventy-two-bed surgical ward. She had observed her nurses were doing non-nursing duties and had them document their activities in fifteen-minute intervals for two solid weeks. She documented her case and presented it so successfully that she hired the first-ever ward helpers to be engaged by TGH on Ward A. She introduced a card index file for keeping track of doctors' orders on her ward, a system that was almost identical to what became known as Kardex. She startled an OHA convention at that time with the public pronouncement that hospitals were using student nurses as cheap labour, a comment that appeared in headlines in the evening paper.[1]

She became the first clinical instructor at the TGH School of Nursing, service instructor and surgical supervisor at TGH, took courses (in psychology and accounting) at the Ontario College of Education (1931–32), then (1934–37) was a clinical instructor at the University of Toronto School of Nursing (the first undergraduate nursing program in Canada). In 1936 she was awarded a Rockefeller Scholarship to visit teaching centres in the United States.

In 1938 she won a Canadian Nurses Association Exchange Award, which took her with nineteen of her colleagues to South Africa, where she became a staff nurse and tutor at Groote Schuur Hospital in Cape Town, which had just opened that year. There she established a program in clinical nursing. She went on to become director of nursing education at the Kimberley General Hospital in South Africa.[2] She returned to become superintendent of Oshawa General Hospital (1940–46), during which time she completed courses as a special student at the U of T's Department of Commerce and Finance, driving back and forth between Oshawa and Toronto two nights a week to do so.[3] From there she went to McGill University, where she became assistant director and assistant professor of nursing.[4] She came from McGill to the Department.

Eugenie never forgot her nursing roots or important influences like Jean Gunn at TGH. We noted at the outset of this work the picture of her with Gunn. In 1954 she was president of the TGH Nurses Alumni Association.[5] In many ways there was a similarity in their roles, in how important both were to their respective institutions. Eugenie would also continue to publish in the area. In 1954 she wrote an article on a regional approach to nursing administration in small hospitals.[6]

During the time of her arrival at the Department of Hospital Administration she continued her studies by taking summer courses at Northwestern University in Chicago where in 1947 she received a bachelor of science in hospital administration and in 1950 a master of hospital administration.[7] The Northwestern program predated the U of T program (it had been started in 1943).

Harvey Agnew was constantly lobbying for her promotion. Less than two years after her temporary appointment, she was promoted to assistant professor and became the only full-time member of the department.

Comment

Eugenie appeared to have an adventuresome streak. One example was her agreeing to be part of the delegation of nurses to go halfway around the world to Groote Schuur Hospital in Cape Town. The hospital had a position in South Africa analogous to that of TGH in Canada. It had just been completed and had a dramatic location on the slopes of Devil's Peak. It would seem, based on comments by Jean Gunn, TGH nursing superintendent, made to the Royal Commission on Dominion-Provincial Relations (Rowell-Sirois Commission), that Eugenie was part of a somewhat elite delegation. Gunn noted that such an exchange of nurses was planned by the national association of nurses in the different countries, this one by the South African Trained Nurses' Association.[8]

Another adventuresome example was Eugenie's move out of nursing and striking out on a new path, first by moving into hospital administration as superintendent of Oshawa General Hospital, and then to teaching in that area by accepting the position in the new department at U of T. A part of this new direction was her pursuing undergraduate and graduate degrees in that field and at an institution with a profile like that of Northwestern University, which at that time was headed by the pre-eminent leader of the field, Malcolm T. MacEachern. Likely Harvey Agnew had a hand in this, as he knew MacEachern well.

Another point that should be made is that throughout the time of Agnew's tenure she really was the glue that held the department together. Through all of Agnew's time as head, his position in the department was part-time. He maintained his role in the Canadian Hospital Council and in his busy hospital consulting firm. Eugenie's was the full-time position taking care of all the day-to-day operational matters and functioning as the COO of the department.

PUBLICATIONS ON HOSPITAL/HEALTH INSURANCE

Throughout the first twenty-five years of the program there was a close link between it and Canada's major publication on hospitals and hospital management. Faculty and graduates contributed articles. Agnew saw to this in his roles as executive secretary of the Canadian Hospital Council and editor of *Canadian Hospital*. In addition, he ensured that articles on topical issues, what was indexed as "health insurance and social security," appeared regularly in the journal through the late 1940s and into the 1950s. This was only one part of a steady stream of articles throughout the 1950s and 1960s on a variety of topics pertaining to hospital administration.

The emphasis was on policy and practice. In fact, with the inception of the program, a kind of virtuous circle was set up. The faculty, assorted guest lecturers, and very soon the graduates provided a steady stream of authors, and the size of the issues grew. This was also influenced by the degree of activity surrounding health at both the federal and provincial levels. Initially the authors were faculty or guest lecturers of the program and emphasis was on policy, but this changed in the early 1950s. There was the addition of graduates as authors as well as increased focus on hospital management and operations. This led to an emphasis on the practicalities of hospital operations and the implications they had for hospital and health policy in provinces.

The journal also provided an important outlet for graduates who wanted to publish, and they formed an important new source of new ideas for its readership.[9]

Regarding hospital or health insurance, Agnew was careful in his own enunciation of a stance. One is left with the distinct impression that he preferred the private voluntary plans, one of which (Ontario Blue Cross) he helped initiate. Nonetheless he saw a certain inevitability to a state-sponsored program, and he believed strongly that both the physician and hospital sectors needed to be actively involved so that each could make his or her views known and do what each could to be part of the process. He felt equally strongly about the preservation of the voluntary hospital system, that Canada should not follow the UK lead and nationalize hospitals.

Malcolm Taylor (who later taught in the Public Health and Hospital Administration programs), in his role as research director for the HSPC, wrote two articles in 1950 on the Saskatchewan hospital insurance experience. His thesis was that hospitals across Canada were facing rising admission rates and rising costs. BC had followed Saskatchewan and introduced a compulsory hospital insurance program in 1949, and he stated, "It is not now unreasonable to assume that, in due course, other provinces" will follow suit.[10]

His second article dealt with issues of direct relevance to the program and presaged its later concern with health policy and evaluation. He said, "The rates and costs under universal coverage will be higher when compared with the yardsticks of voluntary prepayment plans" (which were prevalent at the time), because the "scope of the task was much greater." The aged, the indigent, and the chronically ill all needed more care, and hospital use increased with the elimination of restrictions for pre-existing conditions. He put it succinctly as "the removal of the economic barrier."[11]

One could argue that Agnew, through the combination of his position as director of the Department of Hospital Administration, combined with his role as editor of the *Canadian Hospital*, and utilizing the kind of academics, sessional lecturers, and graduates this role was putting him into contact with – people like Taylor, Roth, and Mott – was in a very real way helping contribute to the dialogue on hospital and health insurance.

On the one hand one could argue that *Canadian Hospital* was not a journal with high circulation. Yet it was in the hands of almost every hospital administrator in Canada and they, by virtue of the hospital's place in the community, were significant members of their community. Did they help shape discussion? They certainly provided very useful information.

A case in point is an article by Burns Roth in September 1953 on Saskatchewan's hospital insurance plan. Some points particularly relevant to a school of hospital administration was that the Saskatchewan Department of Public Health had set up a kind of consulting service to Saskatchewan hospitals with "the full-time employment of specialists in various fields of hospital administration."[12] Saskatchewan was also finding that "under a comprehensive prepayment plan, and with no limiting factors, the volume of hospital care requested seems to be directly proportional to the number of beds provided."[13]

EXTENSION (CERTIFICATE) COURSE

An area where the department broke new ground was in offering an extension course. The department had not been in operation for even two years when the topic was mooted. The need was clear; it offered instruction in health-care management to those without university degrees and/or those who were interested but who did not have the time or money, or could not forgo their present income to commit to the full-time, twenty-one-month program.

The minutes of the Council of the School of Hygiene for 29 March 1949 include a submission from the Department of Hospital Administration, which noted that regret had been expressed "in many quarters of the hospital field" that people who did not have a university degree could not take the diploma course offered by the department. They stated that Minister of Health Kelly had written to the Ontario Hospital Association suggesting that some action be taken whereby courses could be made available to those who were not university graduates. They also noted that the department had initiated discussions with the university's Extension Department, who were favourably disposed to the idea. They said that another possibility was to offer such a course in conjunction with the Canadian Hospital Council.[14]

They said the department was contemplating a course of four to six weeks. A location had not yet been chosen, but Toronto was under consideration and, if chosen, members of the department would be involved if they so chose. The minutes said it would also involve "leaders in the hospital field," as it did now for its diploma program. They noted the fact that one- and two-week courses were being provided occasionally in various parts of Canada.[15]

Agnew's article in *Canadian Hospital* in July 1950 looked at current facilities for training hospital administrators in the United States, United Kingdom, and Australia. One point he made was that there should be more short courses and that one "body to give leadership" to such a program would be the Canadian Hospital Council.[16]

A meeting was held with Sidney Smith, the university president, on 18 December 1950 at which a seven-page outline of a proposal was circulated. It noted that while the establishment of the graduate course in 1947 was a step toward meeting the demand for trained administrators, the universities offering such programs were not graduating a sufficient number to meet the need. The U of T program had an enrolment of twelve students. A handwritten note on that page of the proposal queried raising this number to eighteen. The extension course would enrol forty students.[17]

The course would extend from 15 September to 15 May of the following year (thirty-four weeks). Students would submit twelve to fifteen assignments. Directed reading lists and areas of study would be given for the preparation of each assignment. There would be a four-week, in-residence summer session in mid-June of each year.[18]

Smith had some misgivings about the proposal, likely over the fact that the instruction was to be done at U of T, yet U of T was not receiving any of the credit nor granting the certificate. A handwritten note attached to the proposal says, "Don't throw out baby with bath water." A letter to Sidney Smith on 28 December 1950 outlined the provisos that the Executive Committee of the school had set out.[19]

The School of Hygiene Council minutes for 1951 note that the Canadian Hospital Council, with financial support from the W.K. Kellogg Foundation, was sponsoring an in-service training program. It said the Canadian Hospital Council would be the body sponsoring the course, would select and enrol the students, and would grant the certificate at the end of the course. All the instruction, curriculum, and examinations would be the responsibility of the Department of Hospital Administration. It would be a two-year course with forty candidates in each year's class. In each of the years one month would be spent on campus, while the rest of the course (thirty-four weeks) would be by correspondence. The subject of the course would be "Hospital Organization and Management."[20] Agnew had close ties to the Canadian Hospital Council, and this could well have been a reason that he strongly supported their role.

The *President's Report* for 1951–52 noted that the department planned and prepared instruction for an extension course in hospital organization in management sponsored by the Canadian Hospital Council. It noted that Mr J.C. Lee (DHA, 1951) was on loan from the Saskatchewan Health Services Planning Commission to help in its development.[21] Saskatchewan had a close association with the department. For example, the minutes of the Council of the School of Hygiene for 1951 noted that graduates of its post-graduate diploma program were "well placed" and singled out the Saskatchewan Hospital Planning Commission as one of the locations.[22]

The Kellogg Foundation noted its contribution as well as a description of the course in a book on its history. A map of Canada showed the communities across the country that had administrators taking the course. It noted that in the 1954–55 school year "there were 197 students from 113 Canadian towns, ten U.S. states and four foreign countries" and that "the lessons are mailed even to remote sections of Canada."[23]

Its Benefits

The extension course was important in increasing accessibility to professional education in this field and thereby as another means to raise the level of training of those involved. It attracted mainly practitioners, people already involved in health-care management who wanted to raise their level of professional qualification.

A benefit of the course was the four-weeks at the university during its off-season (June of each year). It not only provided the opportunity for intensive instruction, it also brought people from across Canada together, many from small cities and towns. It exposed them, even if temporarily, to each other and the atmosphere of a major metropolitan centre and a major university.

In some cases the provincial government supported people taking the course. In another Saskatchewan connection, Andrew Boehm from Prince Albert was one such example. Each of programs such as this, and the support provided for continuing education in health by the Douglas government, gave such people a further option for career building and Canada a further opportunity to build capacity and expertise. Andrew worked at the North Central Regional Hospital Council, which was one of five regional supports to small hospitals in the province that had been set up by the Douglas government.[24] He went on to become administrator of the Holy Family Hospital in Prince Albert and later the Charles Camsell Hospital in Edmonton.[25] His neighbour (and boss) in Prince Albert was Sid Parsons (DHA, 1956). Saskatchewan even had a Hospital Organization and Management Alumni Association that met annually.[26] While at the Charles Camsell, Andrew returned to U of T many years later to take his executive MBA, this time supported by the federal government.[27]

FORGING LINKS

Many asserted that a strength of the department, indeed of the school, was in its use of faculty from other departments from both within and outside the university as well as its use of practitioners from the field. We will speak of Malcolm Taylor in this regard later in this work.

With the Profession

An early and distinguishing feature of the department was the strong links it forged with the profession and its graduates. This was especially evident in the residency portion of the diploma program. Through the 1950s and 1960s, for example, the department had a meeting between the hospital contact for the residency and university faculty. They were called preceptor-staff meetings. The field viewed them as of sufficient import that the administrator or assistant administrator invariably was the preceptor and would attend.

The number of people who came was striking, given how busy such people were and the length of the meeting (three to four hours). Often there were around ten preceptors (a number of whom were DHA graduates) as well as faculty. However, for the years 1967, 1969, and 1970 there were twenty or more attending, with an additional ten to twelve faculty. The meeting dealt with aspects of the residency as well as updating the preceptors on new appointments within the department, trends in education in hospital administration, changes in curriculum content, and the like.[28]

It is also striking is that a number of hospitals took more than one student for the residency. One list notes four students going to Toronto East General, three to Kingston General, three to Toronto Western, and four to Vancouver General, to single out a few. There were fifty residents in total. And another interesting fact was its geographic scope. While concentrated in Ontario, it extended across Canada and the United States. In addition to Vancouver there were residencies in Victoria, Edmonton, Regina, Winnipeg, and Montreal. There were ten US locations such as Denver, Louisville, and Grand Rapids, including US hospitals such as the New England Medical Center (Boston), Jackson Memorial (Miami), Huston Memorial, and Strong Memorial (Rochester, NY).[29] The department preceptors were also included in a preceptors' luncheon held as part the annual Congress on Administration held by the American College of Hospital Administrators.[30]

As noted earlier, almost invariably the hospital CEO was the preceptor, even with the largest hospitals such as Toronto General and Toronto Western. Such high-level contact was deemed very important by the students, and students valued the preceptor–student relationship very highly. Substantial informal learning took place in conversations between the preceptor and student.

Another example of linkages to the field is that there were graduates who taught specific courses in the program, such as Gerry Turner on personnel management and Gerry Turner and Ted Freedman on long-range planning.[31] Both were from Mount Sinai Hospital in Toronto, and it always had very strong links to the department, as did the other University Avenue hospitals: Toronto General and SickKids.

With Other University Departments

The 1950s saw continuing growth of the department. There was the addition of the extension course just noted. The department also began an important and continuing habit of reaching out and forging links with other university departments, because of the interdisciplinary nature of hospital management and the high-quality expertise in other university departments.

An early example was with the Department of Political Economy (DPE). Brownstone notes that School of Hygiene students came over for classes.[32] The records for the DPE list marks for hospital admin students through the 1950s.[33] In 1950–51 it was cost accounting.[34] In 1951–52 it had six students taking an introductory accounting and introductory economics course.[35] In 1952–53 and 1953–54 it had five DHA students take an introductory economics course.[36] In 1954–55 it provided a class in cost accounting to Hospital Admin students.[37] DPE housed the commerce studies of the university until it split into three departments (political science, economics, and commerce). In the 1960s Brownstone co-delivered lectures in public administration with Gerry Turner (his cousin).[38]

Malcolm Taylor, whose primary appointment was in DPE (as assistant professor) had an appointment (as special lecturer) in the Department of Public Health Administration in the school.[39] This department merged with that of hospital administration to form a new department (Health Administration) in 1967. He is listed as one of the faculty in the school's calendar,[40] teaching graduate courses in comparative government and public administration.[41] Bator notes he was an example of the Department of Public Health Administration responding to challenges from many in medical circles who felt that the department had "an archaic preoccupation with the old Public Health" and that his being a political scientist with expertise in medical insurance "represented this new direction in the department."[42]

While it is almost certain that some students from both the Departments of Public Health Administration and Hospital Administration ventured over to DPE to take Taylor's classes, the student records from Hygiene could not be found that would corroborate this. Bator and Rhodes note in a section on the Sub-Department of Public Health Administration that he provided lectures on health insurance.[43]

Outside the University

Forging such linkages was not new to the school. For example in January 1946 the Manitoba deputy minister of health and public welfare delivered a series of ten lectures on national health insurance plans and the integration of health and welfare in the provincial program in that province.[44]

Another type of interchange was a request from the United Nations Relief and Rehabilitation Administration to have two engineers from Ukraine and Byelorussia train in penicillin production at the school's related facility, Connaught Labs. This, of course, was very sensitive at that time. It went to the executive of the board of governors of the university, which was disinclined to comply without direction from External Affairs. The matter went right up to the minister of national health and welfare, who, at the time, was Brooke Claxron.[45]

THE ONTARIO HEALTH SURVEY (1950)

The Ontario Health Survey of 1950 described some of the problems provinces were grappling with in their hospitals. The proportion of hospital income derived from donations had been steadily declining. Donations had actually doubled, but expenses for hospital operations had quadrupled.[46]

An early indication of the program's interface with government was that Agnew and Bradley from the new Department of Hospital Administration were mentioned in the acknowledgements to the report, along with Milton Brown from Hygiene.[47]

THE TORONTO PROGRAM IN CONTEXT IN 1950

Harvey Agnew wrote an article for *Canadian Hospital* in 1950 that put the Toronto program into context in relation to others (notably in the United States). He noted that the seven programs approved by the Association of University Programs in Hospital Administration followed a common pattern of an academic year of instruction followed by a year of administrative residency. In most of the universities the course was associated with a school of public health. However, in the United States there were also programs in schools of business administration, commerce, and medicine. There were others (in the United States) that notably de-emphasized the academic piece on favour of more practical experience. There were no university-directed, full-time programs in Britain. The King Edward's Hospital Fund had set up a "staff college" for the education of hospital administrators, but it did not set examinations or award a degree.[48]

WESTERN CANADA HOSPITAL INSTITUTE (1950–55)

Western Canada Hospital Institute, noted previously, continued to have successful meetings. Agnew delivered more than one address at the 1950 meeting, and faculty such as L.O. Bradley also spoke, while DHA student F.

Silversides was part of the organizing committee. Graham Davis from the Kellogg Foundation and John Storm, editor of *Hospitals*, the main US journal on hospital administration, each spoke.[49] At the 1951 meeting held in Edmonton the premier of Alberta spoke, as did Davis of the Kellogg Foundation and the Mr Storm of *Hospitals*.[50]

L.O. Bradley spoke on hospitals and chronic illness at the 1952 session and on Canadian hospital organizations. The BC minister of health and welfare also spoke.[51] The 1953 session was held in Saskatoon, where T.J. Bentley, minister of public health in the Tommy Douglas administration, spoke at the opening dinner, and former DHA student Burns Roth, deputy minister, delivered the keynote address. Roth also led a discussion on the possibilities of establishing home care programs in Western Canada. Paul Martin Sr, minister of national health and welfare, also spoke. Other notable speakers were Dr E. Crosby, president of the American Hospital Association and Malcolm T. MacEachern. L.O. Bradley (now CEO in Calgary) led a simulated radio program called "Court of Opinion."[52]

The 1954 meeting hosted a debate on compulsory government hospital insurance. Former DOHA faculty member L.O. Bradley and DHA graduate E.V. Wahn were the speakers for the affirmative side.[53] The 1955 meeting also had present and former DOHA faculty involved, such as Dr W. Douglas Piercey, whose topics were "Special Problems in Hospital Administration" and "Who Controls the Doctor in Hospitals." L.O. Bradley presided over the opening session and A.L. Swanson spoke on improving the quality of medical care.[54]

OPENING OF THE UNIVERSITY HOSPITAL, SASKATOON, MAY 1955

On 14 May 1955 Tommy Douglas as premier presided over the opening of the University Hospital in Saskatoon. This was Saskatchewan's first teaching hospital and tertiary-level facility. It was a major accomplishment of the Douglas government and one of the most important events of the health-care history of that province.

What is interesting for our purposes was the number of people involved from the School of Hygiene and its Department of Hospital Administration. The opening of the hospital coincided with a special convocation of the University of Saskatchewan, where Mott, Agnew, and Defries received LLD degrees, presented by A.L. Swanson, Agnew's former colleague in the department.[55] Two graduates were Roth, deputy minister of the Department of Public Health, and Wahn, business administrator of the new hospital (having been appointed in 1953 as the hospital staffed up prior to its official opening).[56]

The opening received wide coverage in *Canadian Hospital*. About two-thirds of its September 1955 issue was devoted to the hospital. As the lead article stated, the opening of a new teaching hospital was an unusual occurrence. The hospital became the "dominating architectural feature" on the University of Saskatchewan campus. It also noted the dietary department was located on the top floor, along with the cafeteria, which gave it "an almost unobstructed view of the ... city."[57]

An all-day symposium was held in conjunction with the opening where both Agnew and Mott spoke, Agnew emphasizing the hospital's research role.[58] Presenters came from across North America, including McGill University, Russell Sage Foundation, and the Massachusetts Institute of Technology.[59]

A RESEARCH PROJECT TO DEVELOP PRACTICAL CASE STUDIES (1955–56)

In April 1955 the department began a two-year research project, "Practical Studies in Education for Hospital Administration," sponsored by the Kellogg Foundation and directed by Harold Dillon (DHA, 1952), who was appointed a research fellow in the department. Since his graduation he was on the staff of the Canadian Hospital Association as an administrative assistant for the committee on education. In that capacity he was closely associated with the development of the extension course that the department and CHA ran in hospital organization and management.

The department noted that the new program was consistent with the department's policy of keeping its curriculum under constant review in order to remain abreast of the latest educational methods. The practical studies were practical situations selected from actual situations in the hospital field and used as a basis for a "case method" of teaching. Hospitals across Canada were canvassed for material.[60] The original manual was published in 1957. It was mentioned in the 1956 annual report of the Kellogg Foundation.[61] A revised edition was assembled by Eugenie Stuart and published in 1960.[62]

It had (anonymous) cases from fifty hospitals ranging in size from 35 to 1,000 beds, and no more than four studies were used from any one hospital.

The cases covered almost all facets of hospital operation, including areas such as administration, board of trustees, business office, by-laws, dietary, legal, medical staff, medical records, nursing, personnel management, pharmacy, plant and maintenance, public health, public relations, and purchasing, among others.

DHA GRAD FIRST DIRECTOR OF MONTREAL PROGRAM IN HOSPITAL ADMINISTRATION (1956)

In 1956 a francophone program in hospital administration began at the University of Montreal, and its first director was a graduate of the U of T program, Dr Gerald La Salle (DHA, 1951), a graduate of medicine from Laval. The format of the Montreal program was quite similar to that of Toronto, with nine months of academic work and a year of residency.[63] One wonders if this was another example of the U of T program seeding another program and whether access to the U of T program in its early years helped Quebec establish its own independent activity in this area.

La Salle was not the only DHA grad in the Montreal program. Sister Jeanne Mance (DHA, 1954) was one of the first professors in the program and its first assistant director. She received a grant from the Kellogg Foundation to study at the DHA program in Toronto.[64] Interestingly, her DHA thesis was on education in hospital administration.[65]

La Salle wrote an article in 1953 on some of the activities taking place in hospital administration in Quebec, in particular a conference held in June that year in Montreal with Canadian and American experts to discuss the topic.[66] The article, in addition to the fact of the program being established in 1956, seems to demonstrate that in the early 1950s Quebec was also wrestling with hospital administration and professionalizing hospital management.

It is illustrative the degree to which Catholic clergy were involved in hospital management at that time. For example, we see from La Salle's article the president of the Comité des Hôpitaux du Québec, and the person who also convened the conference, was a Jesuit. Also instructive is that the journal La Salle's article was published in was the publication of a foundation started by the Jesuits along with the archbishop of Montreal.

The University of Montreal organization, known as the Institut supérieur d'administration hospitalière, was created in 1956, with its mission mainly in the training of administrators to fill high positions in the hospital management following the secularization of Quebec hospitals. It also involved setting up a research program in "organization and medico-hospital economy." The demand for lay managers became an urgent need to be filled after the withdrawal of the nuns who had been responsible for the hospital administration. The Institute was part of their École d'hygiène de l'Université de Montréal until 1969 when, in an interesting precursor to what would happen at U of T, both it and the institute were merged into their faculty of medicine.[67]

Three years after its inception, Agnew reported on the program. It had received funding from the Kellogg Foundation for its first five years of operation (it was expected to be self-sustaining after that) and it was the only graduate program in hospital administration in a French-language university in the world.[68]

DHAS AND CERTIFICATION OF HOSPITAL ADMINISTRATORS FOR SASKATCHEWAN (1956)

In 1956 a future DHA grad (Livergant) was involved in discussions about the certification of hospital administrators in Saskatchewan. It was as a result of a resolution passed at the last meeting of the Saskatchewan Hospital Association that requested the Department of Public Health and the Saskatchewan Hospital Association conduct a study to implement certification for hospital administrative personnel. This would include hospital (corporate) secretaries, secretary-managers, and superintendents. It was aimed primarily at hospitals of fifty beds or fewer, which comprised 80 per cent of Saskatchewan hospitals. A committee was formed with equal representation from the two organizations.

It was felt the Toronto DHA program was more than was required and the extension course run by the Canadian Hospital Association (in conjunction with the Toronto program) could not meet the need within the time frame envisaged. The Department of Public Health, under Burns Roth (class of 1950) as deputy minister, was heavily involved, and, indeed, the Division of Hospital Standards and Administration, where he began at the department, arranged to have a study made with a view to implementing certification program similar to that used by the Department of Municipal Affairs.

Dr I. Gogan, who headed up the division within the department that Roth had headed before he became deputy minister, was advisor to the project. W.C. Hibbert, superintendent of Wadena Union Hospital, was made chair, and Harold Livergant (DHA, 1964) secretary. Gogan toured various education centres in the US and went to Minnesota and Indiana to learn of the licensing of their administrators. The Saskatchewan Department also developed draft legislation with corresponding regulations to govern certification.[69]

MAJOR NEW HOSPITAL ACTIVITY: NATIONAL HOSPITAL INSURANCE (1957)

The Legislation Itself

On 10 April 1957, thirty-eight years since health insurance had appeared as a plank in the Liberal party platform, twelve years since the 1945 postwar reconstruction proposals, and ten years since Saskatchewan pioneered its plan, the House of Commons voted on what was seen as a major decision of national policy, a great new social project affecting the lives of all Canadians, and the largest government expense for any program save defence. It was the Hospital Insurance and Diagnostic Services Act (HIDS).

Paul Martin Sr, as minister of national health and welfare, and his deputy ministers, G. Donald W. Cameron (DPH, 1928) and Fred W. Jackson (DPH, 1929) were instrumental in development of the Act. Martin, however, would not be in office when it was implemented, as the Liberal government was defeated in June 1957. The new Diefenbaker government moved quickly to amend the Act, opening the way for a national plan. We will briefly look at these events.

Implications of HIDS for DHA Grads

The new Act had major implications for DHA grads. However, the major increase in hospital construction and utilization occurred *before* HIDS.[70] The National Health Grants program that began in 1948 and was still in place at the time of HIDS had spurred major new construction. As for utilization, between the advent of the health grants in 1948 and HIDS in 1957, patient days increased by 63 per cent.[71] Over the longer term, the combination of hospital grants and universal hospital insurance resulted in a large increase in bed capacity, more than doubling between 1954 and 1971.[72] Each of these had major positive implications for the job prospects of DHA grads.

OHA Conventions around the Time of the HIDS Act (1956–58)

Beginning in 1955 there was refocused federal attention on hospitals, which culminated in the federal Hospital Insurance and Diagnostic Services (HIDS) Act and the formation on the Ontario Hospital Services Commission.

Health Insurance Initiatives Surrounding These OHA Conventions

Health insurance had been on the federal-provincial agenda since the Rowell-Sirois Report of 1940 and its Red Book, *Public Assistance and Social Insurance* (by a U of T faculty member, A.E. Grauer). It continued with the Dominion-Provincial Conference on Reconstruction of 1945 and its Green Book, *Health, Welfare and Labour.* At a Federal-Provincial Conference of 1950 Premier Douglas kept pressure on the federal government by urging "that a new conference should be convened for the purpose of discussing the whole question of national social security."[73]

At the opening proceedings of the Federal-Provincial Conference of October 1955 Prime Minister St Laurent introduced an important new element into the discussion on health insurance. He stated that his government would be prepared to consider "the provision of universal radiological and laboratory services" and that the "next stage of development ... would appear to be that of hospital insurance." However, a sticking point was that Mr St Laurent stated that for the federal government to become involved, such a program needed to represent "a substantial majority of provincial governments, representing a substantial majority of the Canadian people."[74]

This was followed by Ontario Premier Leslie Frost in March 1956, moving first reading of a bill to establish the Ontario Hospital Services Commission, whose intent was to "ensure the continuance of a balanced and integrated system of hospitals in Ontario" as well as to "provide the power to administer any system of hospital-care insurance."[75] At second reading of the bill he noted the contribution of Malcolm Taylor; his minister of health did the same in his address.[76] Taylor at the time was with the Department of Political Economy at the U of T and lectured in the School of Hygiene.

Premier Frost noted the importance of hospital administration: "Any such insurance plan must be built upon hospital services and administration. This is the foundation. Any structure to be built will only be as secure as its foundation."[77]

As the government drew closer to implementation Premier Frost was not sanguine about the magnitude of the task: "Our commission and its organization will assume a very formidable task – I think one of the most formidable administrative tasks that has ever been attempted in this province."[78]

The federal minister, Paul Martin Sr, introduced federal legislation on 25 March 1957; however, the majority clause proved to be a non-starter.[79] It took another Saskatchewan native, John Diefenbaker, to break the stalemate at the Dominion-Provincial Conference of November 1957, where he announced the intent of his government "to remove the 'six provinces' clause."[80] On 19 May 1958 the amendment to the Act was proposed, with the new program to begin on 1 July of that year.[81]

The Conventions Themselves

The activities at the federal level and particularly in Ontario in March 1956 set the stage for a very energetic OHA convention in the fall. Developments in 1957 and 1958 prior to the OHA conventions of those years continued to focus attention on hospitals. Hospitals, already a prominent community institution, now had even more attention focused on them. The OHA conventions and articles in *Canadian Hospital* reflected this. In reading them one gets a sense of the atmosphere of change and growth as well as a certain excitement about the increasing prominence of hospitals.

If any indication of the status of hospitals in Ontario was needed, the 1956 OHA Convention provided it. The opening address was provided by Sidney Smith, president of U of T. Mayor Nathan Phillips of Toronto took part in the opening session. The speaker at the luncheon on the first day was Leslie Frost, premier (then called prime minister) of Ontario. Malcolm Taylor spoke on "The Hospital Challenge of the Future." Burns Roth, in his role as deputy minister of public health in Saskatchewan, spoke about a functioning public hospital insurance plan.[82] All were reported on in the 1956 report in *Canadian Hospital* but were also followed by articles by Taylor and Roth in early 1957, each of which emphasized the importance of hospitals (see the section below).

The 1957 convention was centred upon "the newly legislated hospital insurance plan." The premier once again addressed the convention.[83] Rhodes from the School of Hygiene presented the Robert Wood Johnson Award to a DHA student Moshe Katz.[84] Agnew spoke on not only planning for the present but also the future.[85] Malcolm Taylor spoke on how the hospital insurance plan would affect hospitals. He noted "a continuing and even greater call for citizen participation."[86]

The 1958 convention reflected the optimism borne of the new Ontario hospital insurance plan, in which 90 per cent of the population was enrolled. Both the premier and Malcolm Taylor spoke at the convention.[87]

Just as an aside, *Canadian Hospital* also reported on the Saskatchewan Hospital Association convention for 1958. It was notable for the number of DHA grads who were involved, which, in order of mention, were E.V. Wahn, Harold L. Livergant, S.J. Parsons, and A.L. Swanson (former faculty).[88]

Eugenie Stuart and Career Talks to Secondary School Students

An interesting feature of these conventions was faculty member Eugenie Stuart, who directed a discussion for high school students on hospital careers. In 1956 this took the form of a panel with members representing twelve hospital careers. They also provided information on their training and the nature of their job.[89] An article in *Canadian Hospital* noted that this was an annual event and, indeed, in the OHA Convention article for the following year there was mention of Stuart speaking on hospital careers to 300 students of secondary schools in Metropolitan Toronto. As in the previous year, there was a panel representing twelve different hospital departments. The career talk also had its own heading in the OHA Convention report,[90] and there was also a report in its own section in the 1958 report. This one took place on the roof garden of the Royal York Hotel and began with a film *Hospitals Are People*, followed by a moderated discussion by Stuart involving employees of various departments.[91]

The New Ontario Initiatives and the DHA Program

DHA students bore personal witness to this charged atmosphere at these conventions, as traditionally those in the first year received passes to the convention through the program and those in second year through the hospital of their residency.

They could also witness other aspects of this charged atmosphere. The source of the change was occurring almost across the street from them. The legislature was across Queen's Park Crescent West from the School of

Hygiene Building where they had their classes. One wonders if any students walked over to the legislature to watch the proceedings. There was also the fact that Harvey Agnew, director of the DHA program, had such a wide range of connections in the hospital field and the CMA so would very much have been in the vortex.

ARTICLES BY BURNS ROTH AND MALCOLM TAYLOR (1957) AROUND THE TIME OF HIDS

Articles by Roth and Taylor were notable for capturing the zeitgeist surrounding the implementation of hospital insurance. The article by Roth was notable for the context in which he placed the Saskatchewan Plan. He talked about the "social dynamics" leading to a specific approach in Saskatchewan that might be different from elsewhere, therefore one should be cautious in considering the transplantation of some of Saskatchewan's particular methods. He talked about the characteristics of the prairies and the necessity for co-operation and social interdependence. In health this was manifest in local programs of prepaid hospital and medical care insurance, which formed a base Douglas built upon.[92]

The article by Taylor captures some of the excitement mentioned earlier: "Never before in our history has so much public attention in the local community, the province and the nation been centered on the role of the hospital."[93] The announcement of the federal cost-sharing arrangement and the establishment of the Ontario Hospital Services Commission were "eloquent evidence of the public's interest in such services" and "concrete evidence that in the last three or four decades the hospital has come to full flower as an indispensable institution of society."[94]

He spoke of "the advance in scientific medicine ... and its concentration in the hospital." Of hospitals he said, "The product is so good that none can be without it." He also noted the hospital had come to occupy a "position of high esteem in contemporary society."[95] He observed, "With the prospect of a national hospital insurance program, the challenge to national leadership becomes even greater." By this he meant leadership in its broadest sense, including administrators and trustees and "the relations of voluntary groups to government in a democratic society." He noted, "This calls for leadership of a new order."[96] As an aside, Harvey Agnew was on the editorial board of the *Canadian Hospital* at the time.[97]

WHERE GRADS ENDED UP: II

Here is a second instalment on graduates of the mid- to later 1950s.

- Donald A. Robertson (class of 1955) was appointed administrator of Cornwall General Hospital in 1962.[98] Prior to that he was administrator of Kitimat General Hospital, and before that on staff of St Mary's Memorial Hospital in Montreal (where he also did his admin residency).[99]
- Gerald P. Turner (DHA, 1955), former CEO of Mount Sinai, whose thesis was "The Control of Medical and Surgical Supplies and Equipment in the Surgical Service."
- George Riesz (DHA, 1957) was the first recipient of the Robert Wood Johnson Award (in 1956). His first position was at New Mount Sinai Hospital in Toronto. He went from there in 1959 to the Lady Minto Hospital in Chapleau, Ontario.[100]
  - He was orphaned at fifteen during the Second World War. He ended up in Canada and completed a bachelor's degree at McGill.
  - He recalled his time in Chapleau fondly, saying the people welcomed him with open arms.
  - He ended his career in the United States, where he worked at the Southern Nevada Memorial Hospital and the University Medical Center (a facility he helped create) in Las Vegas and Cedars-Sinai Medical Center in Los Angeles. He returned to Las Vegas in 1989 and worked at South West Medical Center until he retired.[101]
  - His thesis topic was "Federal Legislation Concerning Hospitals in Canada." His preceptor was Sidney Liswood.
- J.K. Morrison (DHA, 1958), was the first executive director of Sunnybrook Hospital. His thesis topic was "Accidents and Their Prevention in Hospitals."
- Carl A. Meilicke (DHA, 1959). His thesis was "The Economic Feasibility of Using Punched Card Data Processing Equipment for Hospital Accounting and Statistical Procedures." He received a BComm from the University of Saskatchewan, went on to get a PhD, and founded two programs in health administration, as we shall see.

The following more lengthy biographies of a couple of the students provide a more fulsome picture of the careers of some of the graduates and through this of what the program needed to equip its graduates for.

Sid Parsons (DHA, 1956) became director of the North Central Regional Hospital Council in Prince Albert. His thesis was "The Challenge of Long-Term Illness," and his admin residency was at Toronto East General Hospital. The council was one of a group of regional support mechanisms set up by the Douglas government (and under Burns Roth) for the small hospitals in Saskatchewan in particular. It provided support in administration, finance, nursing, pharmacy, and nutrition, to name a few. The division Roth was hired to direct in Regina provided further support from the centre. Sid went from there to become administrator of the Yorkton Union Hospital.

While at Yorkton he served on a three-person committee appointed by the Saskatchewan Hospital Association at the request of the minister of public health to study and report on the closure of two small Saskatchewan hospitals. The committee was headed by a noted jurist, Judge E.N. Hughes, who was chair of the Saskatoon City Hospital Board.[102] Saskatchewan was an early actor in hospital consolidation, and given the strong feelings the public had for their hospitals, issues such as closure or mergers evoked strong public feeling as many provincial governments in Canada would later discover.

Parsons's involvement with Hughes points to another interesting aspect of the lives of graduates: their involvement with prominent citizens on hospital issues. There was also their interaction with volunteer trustees. Some became very involved in the Canadian health-care scene. Hughes went on to become president of the Saskatchewan Hospital Association and the Canadian Hospital Association and the first chair of the Saskatchewan Cancer Foundation. He earned a reputation for his knowledge and support of hospital trusteeship.[103]

Another graduate, Peter Swerhone (DHA, 1957), was a native of Saskatchewan, whose thesis topic was "Job Evaluation in a Hospital."[104] His undergraduate degree was from the University of Saskatchewan (in commerce), he did his administrative residency at Calgary General, and he went from there to the Administration and Standards Division of the Department of Public Health in Saskatchewan.

In 1957 he was appointed assistant administrator of Notre Dame Hospital in North Battleford, Saskatchewan.[105] Eighteen months later he went to Winnipeg General as assistant executive director under former faculty member L.O. Bradley. In 1967 he was made executive director. He later spearheaded the master plan that led to the Winnipeg Health Sciences Centre and became its first president, where he remained until he retired in 1985.[106]

He then went to direct the planning and organizing of the Northern Alberta Children's Hospital for two years. Following that he returned to Winnipeg to serve as the executive director of the Heart and Stroke Foundation of Manitoba. He served as a volunteer on the Board of the Holy Family Nursing Home in Winnipeg. He was a recipient of the Winnipeg Outstanding Achievement Award and the Gold Medal from the American College of Hospital Administrators.[107]

His career demonstrates a number of things. One is the national footprint of the program evidenced in a student from Saskatchewan coming to U of T, to an administrative residency in Calgary, back to Saskatchewan, and then to Winnipeg to work under a former faculty member of the program. There is also the aspect of his community involvement, which is an example of the fact that, by virtue of a position that made them prominent in their community, a number of graduates undertook voluntary work in their community.

To demonstrate the national posture of the program in another way, the class of 1955 had applicants from BC, Manitoba, Nova Scotia, Ontario (five), Quebec, Saskatchewan (two), and Indiana. A missionary from India was also attending as a special student. Residencies were at hospitals across Canada as well as Cincinnati, Ohio.[108]

And to demonstrate the range of connections the program had, there is correspondence between Stuart at the program and Burns Roth (who had been a student in the second class) of the program and who was deputy minister in Saskatchewan at the time. It was regarding a potential job. It shows a continuing connection between a provincial department of health and the U of T department.[109]

In the case noted above, Stuart was asking Roth about a candidate for a job, but one wonders if Roth used the program as a place to send his best and brightest for graduate education. One wonders as well if he used it as a source to recruit from. Not only was there precedent for each of these in the Douglas government, each was an activity its ministries actively engaged in.[110]

In an example of how there could be continuing involvement between the department and its graduates, and even more specifically in how the department could be seen as a resource for graduates in the field, there is correspondence between a graduate and Stuart on a somewhat ticklish issue the graduate was facing regarding medical staff by-laws. The graduate was seeking Stuart's advice. Stuart in turn wrote to Agnew in his capacity as a partner at Agnew, Craig and Peckham, and he provided information which she related back to the graduate.[111]

CHAPTER 10

Continued Growth

INTERPROVINCIAL CONNECTIONS

There were two strong characteristics in the department. One was the interprovincial connections it had and, along this vein, its strong ties to Saskatchewan. Another was an almost seamless interchange between faculty and the field. These are illustrated in the events such as the following.

Burns Roth, a former student who became director of the U of T department, left his studies to work with Tommy Douglas's Department of Public Health in Saskatchewan. But what is even more interesting is while he was working with the Department of Public Health in Saskatchewan, he was a part-time executive director of the University Hospital in Saskatoon while it was in the planning stages (circa 1953).[1] In yet another seamless interchange between academia and the field, one of the first faculty members from the U of T Department, A.L. Swanson, became the first full-time executive director of the hospital in 1954.[2] This was Saskatchewan's first tertiary facility and coincided with the establishment of a full medical school.

INTRAPROVINCIAL CONNECTIONS

Hospital Activity Continues to Grow, Pressure Mounts for a Hospital Insurance Plan

In addition to growth in the department there was an evolving scene across the boulevard at Queen's Park. Through the 1950s hospitals continued to be an important provincial and national topic. Hospital activity continued to grow quickly and it influenced interest in the diploma program. In the eight years since the war and six years since the department began, Ontario hospital expenditures had increased by 250 per cent. Somewhat alarming was the increasing frequency and size of hospital deficits.[3] One of Premier

Frost's closest advisors, George Gathercole across at Ontario Treasury, was involved in sorting out the economics of hospital or health insurance. Malcolm Taylor worked with him, and Taylor was asked in August 1954 to analyze the economics of hospital and medical care and providing for such care.[4]

Steps Taken to Develop a Hospital Insurance Plan for Ontario

Taylor's report was submitted in December of that year to Gathercole and the premier with two foci: immediate imperatives and health insurance. One of the former was the creation of a health service planning body, a recommendation the premier acted upon a year later. On the latter it said, "Health insurance, whether private or governmental, increases the amount of money spent on health services by increasing the demand from an amount that can be *afforded* to an amount more closely approximating what is *needed*" (my italics). He noted a government plan would increase demand more than a voluntary plan because it would cover everyone, including those who could not afford private insurance.[5]

It is evident that also across from the department, Premier Frost was taking an active interest in hospital finances and the public's ability to pay. He moved quickly and continually. One can sense the action behind the scenes in his remarks. In a response to a question in the 1955 Budget Debate and the Estimates of the Department of Health the issue of hospital costs was raised. The premier provided a lengthy and detailed response and it was evident he had given the topic some study. Taylor notes that a couple of hours before the evening session of the legislature, Premier Frost had asked Gathercole to prepare a few remarks for him to incorporate into his budget speech.[6] In his response the premier noted, "The question is not one, however, as to whether health insurance will come – because I believe in the course of time on a gradual basis it will come. The question is simply, when is the right time for it, and how is it to be taken care of and financed?"[7]

A year later (5 March 1956) he introduced legislation for a Hospital Services Commission, which had a provision to administer a hospital insurance plan. In moving first reading of the bill he noted, "It permits a very great strengthening of our hospital system, whether or not there is hospital insurance in Ontario."[8]

In addition the premier had his own views. He convened a Standing Committee on Health to look at the issue and it met six times from 14 to 27 March 1956. It involved the heads of property and casualty insurance companies, Ontario Blue Cross, and the Congress of Canadian Women, among others. It is an example of the methodical way in which he tackled issues. In an address to the committee regarding hospital insurance he said, "One of the great difficulties with private insurance is the fact that, first, there is a time limit which does not take care of catastrophes; and secondly that some companies at least have been pretty free with the cancellation clauses in their policies."[9]

There was a very interesting exchange between him and the insurance companies toward the end of the proceedings. A representative of the insurance companies suggested that they insure those who can afford it – the "cream of the crop" as one committee member put it – and the government insure those who cannot pay. Mr Frost famously said, "That sounds like a bad deal for government."[10]

Taylor was also very involved in the committee, offering testimony on a number of days, one example being on the specifics of the plan being offered by Ontario.[11] Also worth mentioning again is that the deputy minister of health, J.T. Phair, was a DPH grad and had taught at the School of Hygiene.[12] W.G. Brown (DPH, 1942), attending for the Department of Health, later became deputy minister.[13]

A year after that (1957) it was mentioned in the Throne Speech that the government had submitted a plan to the federal government and a month later that the provincial government had a tentative date of 1 January 1959 for its introduction.[14] It published an outline of its plan in 1957, which noted important issues in voluntary coverage: gaps in coverage if employment was not continuous, lack of comprehensive coverage (due to waiting periods, waivers, and exclusions), the cost of merchandising individual contracts, and coverage for the aged.[15] With that began feverish activity within the Ontario Hospital Services Commission toward the January 1959 implementation date. Malcolm Taylor's services as consultant to the commission were acknowledged by the commission's chair.[16]

The 1957–58 report of the director of the School of Hygiene noted, "With the implementation of Hospital Insurance Plans in Canada there will be a steady and increasing demand for university graduates trained in this field."[17] The Throne Speech of 1959 announced, "The Ontario hospital insurance plan, a milepost in the history of health and welfare legislation, not only in this province but in Canada, came into operation on January 1."[18] It noted that over 90 per cent of the population was covered.[19] Had vindication of the U of T program ever been required, this passage of successive hospital insurance plans by the provinces across Canada certainly provided it. Without question these plans focused more attention on hospitals and the DHA program.

Taylor was also involved in an interrelationship between the OHA, Blue Cross, and the newly formed government departments. In 1959, with the introduction of a province-sponsored universal hospital insurance plan, it transitioned from being a primary provider to a supplementary provider. Many of the top staff of the OHA and Ontario Blue Cross moved over to the Ontario government to help introduce the government plan. Arthur Swanson, the executive secretary of the OHA, who had been integrally involved in building one of the largest voluntary hospital insurance plans in the country (Ontario Blue Cross), was asked by Premier Leslie Frost to became the first chair of the Ontario Hospital Services Commission.[20] In turn he asked the board of the OHA for the transfer of the director of Blue Cross, David Ogilvie, to become the director of the Ontario Hospital Insurance Plan.[21] Agnew notes that it was Swanson's skill, and of those he recruited, that led to its successful implementation and its rapid acceptance by hospitals.[22] Swanson had been a preceptor in the Department of Hospital Administration.[23]

Taylor notes that by the end of 1958 all Blue Cross employees not remaining to administer the supplemental plan were transferred to the Ontario public service as employees of the commission.[24] It demonstrated first, the strong ethic of public service in Ontario's public institutions and the seamless interchange of people between them. Second, as much as Ontario is the bastion of Canadian capitalism, and at that time the manufacturing heartland of Canada, it nonetheless had very important non-profit corporations like its hospitals, the OHA, Blue Cross, and others, and it highly values them.

It was a bold, even courageous move. Ontario, unlike Saskatchewan, was not a tabula rasa. It had a well-established insurance industry. Moreover, already over two-thirds of the population had some coverage for hospital benefits. The industry stood to lose. Also, there was inequity in access to care: the insured were admitted more frequently for care and the uninsured had a length of stay 40 per cent longer, suggesting they had delayed seeking treatment.[25] Ontario's move wiped out this inequity. While the insurance companies lost standard ward coverage, they continued to market semi-private and private hospital coverage, and some years later their revenues exceeded those of 1958 (their last full year before the provincial plan). There were striking improvements in hospital facilities and quality of care, and major savings by municipalities through a sharp decline in non-insured indigent patients.[26]

With the new commission and an expansion in the Ministry of Health, a major step was taken toward building a health system. And a major new outlet was created for diploma graduates. It re-emphasized the centrality of hospitals and underscored the fact that the school had made a sound decision in beginning a program that emphasized their management. Taylor noted in his report to the Frost government the centrality of hospitals when he said, "The hospital is becoming the community 'health centre.'"[27]

What was also evident with Leslie Frost bringing Ontario on board, and had happened previously in Saskatchewan and British Columbia, was a building of capacity in government. Saskatchewan and British Columbia did it essentially from scratch. Ontario, as we have seen, drew heavily upon Ontario Blue Cross staff. But the challenge of building this capacity, of implementing huge, brand new government programs, is not to be underestimated. These were huge accomplishments. And the Department of Hospital Administration was somewhat strategically located. We will see later, with the addition of Fred Mott and Burns Roth they brought on two of the foremost minds on the continent in this area.

Malcolm Taylor

Taylor was also an illustration of how a somewhat porous relationship can develop between academia and government that has interactions on different levels. For example, Taylor was in contact with a British expert (J.R. Simpson) on organization and methods, asking him for material he was using and noting that this could "have some influence on administrative practices" both provincially and federally in Canada, given the lecturing Taylor was doing for civil servants.[28] In another letter he corresponded with a member of Gathercole's staff who wanted to do an MA with him while still being employed.[29] In another instance he linked a student (who was subsequently hired) with A.W. Johnson, deputy provincial treasurer in Saskatchewan.[30] There was also a telegram asking Johnson if he would speak to Taylor's class while he was in Toronto.[31] Taylor and Johnson, of course, knew each other from Taylor's time with the Department of Public Health in the Tommy Douglas government.

There were also relationships between Taylor and the School of Hygiene. Though it wasn't his primary appointment, he was listed as on the faculty of the School from 1952 to 1955.[32] In 1955 he applied for a second Rockefeller grant to continue his studies on health insurance. The first grant, on the administration of health insurance, had resulted in a book published by Oxford University Press.[33] This second one was going to study the social, economic, and political issues. He noted that he had discussed the project with his head, Professor Bladen, and also Defries at Hygiene, and had their support. He signed his letter as assistant professor of political science and special lecturer in the School of Hygiene.[34] He also served on the Council of the School of Hygiene.[35] Many years later, while he was at York University, he served as the PhD supervisor to IHPME faculty member Paul Williams.

Taylor's writing also focused on areas shared by Harvey Agnew. In 1959 he presented a paper on volunteerism in hospitals at the annual conference of the Quebec Hospital Association, subsequently published in *Canadian Hospital*, for which Agnew had been editor. This was an issue Agnew felt strongly about. At that time there was some concern that compulsory hospital insurance would discourage such effort, and Taylor in his article stated reasons why this would not be the case.[36]

Taylor is another example of how the school constantly gravitated to the best in the field. At the time he was probably Canada's foremost expert on public policy as it applied to health, and this formed an important part of the (five) public health admin courses taught by the school.[37] During his career he was involved in every major policy initiative on health insurance. His book *Health Insurance and Canadian Public Policy*, first published in 1978, is still in print, and most regard it as the definitive work in the field. It was awarded the Hannah Book Medal from the Royal Society of Canada, one of the highest honours a scholarly publication can receive. He constantly championed social values in unemployment, health, and education, and here was much aligned with people like Defries and FitzGerald. It was not whether but how we would pay and that the financial was less than the human cost, in his view. In a convocation speech to York University students he exhorted them, as they assumed positions of influence that their education made possible, to come down on "the positive side of the human balance sheet."[38]

Comment

Malcolm Taylor's report to the government brings to mind an important characteristic of the department: it was very practically oriented. The approach was working; it was turning out well-qualified graduates who were achieving prominent positions. However, most of its faculty were not working from a research base. They were practitioners. While the school did have such as base in the Connaught Labs, this was in the physical sciences. It did not have the same base in the social sciences. It would became a debate that surfaced in the years surrounding the school's dissolution.

Taylor was at U of T at the time. However, his interest area (health insurance, public administration) and his research, as opposed to practical orientation, were not really aligned with the department. He was also looking at health policy and health systems, and the department at that time was hospital administration. Thus, he was in the Department of Political Economy, as it was then known. Also Taylor was an academic and researcher, not a practitioner. His interests gravitated to economics and politics, not hospital operations. The department in the school was both too practically oriented and too narrowly focused (hospitals rather than the system itself). Thus, when he left Saskatchewan he did not land at the department (though he had connections to the school). And when the Ontario government went looking for an academic to advise it on hospital insurance, it did not come to the department. A part of that could well have been that Al Johnson knew Gathercole, so it is very possible Gathercole called him and he made a recommendation. A question for the department at the time would have been that it did not have the breadth or the horsepower (i.e., expertise, capacity) to produce such a study for the government.

To be fair, it could well be that the school recognized this limitation, because it could also be argued that Hastings was being groomed as a potential future faculty member. And in the early 1960s, when Taylor was tapped by the Hall Commission, the department did have capacity and Hastings was selected for a study on community services. What can also be said is that the connection between the Department of Hospital Administration and the Department of Political Economy for classes in accounting is an early indication of what became an enduring strength of the department/institute: because of the interdisciplinary nature of its subject matter, it did not hesitate to seek expertise from other university departments.

This seeking of expertise had another nuance. Frost had proceeded in a deliberate, sequential fashion. He was a methodical administrator. The Progressive Conservative government elected in August 1943 had brought a new, managerial perspective to governing, which involved a structured approach to decision making. Frost had begun his career as provincial treasurer, and under him Treasury became the key department of the Ontario state. He created the Department of Economics in 1956 and recruited Gathercole to his position as advisor to both Cabinet and the premier to do the thinking on important issues such as hospital insurance.[39]

What was underway was a professionalization of public administration generally. Frost was building a highly professionalized civil service, just as Douglas was doing in Saskatchewan and the department was doing in hospital administration. A part of this was, at times, reaching into the academy for expert advice. Taylor notes that he would consult to the Hospital Services Commission and an individual would be transferred to it from the provincial economist's office.[40] Also Premier Frost distributed copies of Taylor's book, *The Administration of Health Insurance in Canada*, to all members of the legislature.[41]

What we also see is (the beginnings?) of a government-academia interface. Brownsey notes, "The chief academic advisor to the department was Malcolm Taylor of the University of Toronto" and he "had a singular influence in shaping Ontario's approach to hospital insurance and, later, medicare."[42] Taylor also consulted on hospital insurance to other provinces, such as New Brunswick, Manitoba, and PEI, and taught extension courses to civil servants at all three levels of government while he was at U of T.[43] He had written his PhD dissertation on the Saskatchewan Hospital Insurance Plan[44] and, on graduation, had worked in the Douglas government on the successful implementation of this pioneering initiative.

Taylor had also been research director for the Saskatchewan Health Services Planning Commission, which was an example of the Saskatchewan Department of Public Health actively embracing research in its development of policy. The Douglas government generally had a certain academic flavour about it and had great respect for the product of good research. That it had an effect is evidenced in a memorandum from T.K. Shoyama to the members of the Economic Advisory and Planning Board, which noted that he had several meetings with Mr Taylor discussing four alternative approaches to health insurance.[45]

All of this is to say is that even in these early days of hospital insurance it was becoming apparent that government needed expertise from the academy. It presaged where the department would evolve (into IHPME) and that the need was moving away from an exclusive professional orientation. Indeed, IHPME is precisely in this vein: it has a strong research base, its faculty are consulted by governments, and it has the capacity to respond.

THE HOSPITAL AS MEETING PLACE

In 1957 departmental faculty member W. Douglas Piercey wrote an interesting article on "the hospital as meeting place," i.e., whether the hospital (or its associated nursing school) had a role in providing a meeting place for staff, medical, and community groups. Specifically he meant auditorium facilities for public health and medical education purposes. He noted that if the hospital was to be a true health centre, such facilities were an essential requirement. He stated that Guelph General Hospital was presently doing just this in a proposed new nursing school facility.[46] A separate article noted it would take maximum advantage of the fact that it overlooked a valley and was to have a 100-seat auditorium.[47]

Another example was the construction of a new nursing school and residence at the Holy Family Hospital in Prince Albert, Saskatchewan. The hospital was run by the Sisters of Charity of the Immaculate Conception of St John, New Brunswick, and the residence was a three-storey structure, opened in September 1955. It had a 300-seat auditorium,[48] at that time the largest auditorium in this small city (which had a population 17,149 in 1951).[49] It made the hospital a focal point for a number of civic gatherings. In the 1960s when nursing education in Saskatchewan was consolidated at its universities and technical colleges it served another civic purpose, as the residence was converted and used for a number of years as the city hall.

CONTINUED ENHANCEMENT OF THE PROGRAM

As a Result of Hospital Insurance

The program recognized that with implementation of hospital insurance plans in Canada, there would an increasing profile for hospitals, an increase in government activity relating to them, and with this a growing demand for university graduates in this field. The staff of the Department of Hospital Administration had desired for some time to improve the content and instruction offered in the second year of the course, and in 1957–58 the Kellogg Foundation provided funds for a review of the course with special reference to the second year.[50] K.S. McLaren (DHA, 1958), "one of our own graduates" who also had a MEd, was appointed to direct the project.[51] He completed his project in 1960–61, resigned his academic position, and was appointed administrator of the General Hospital, Cornwall, Ontario.[52]

A Glimmer of the Future Institute?

In the school's report to the president for 1958–59 the director noted a gap in the training of health administration personnel: "Despite the many specialist courses now available in the School, there is still at least one important omission, for no Canadian university offers training in the field known as 'medical care administration,' 'health insurance' or 'health services administration.'"[53] It went on to say, "Workers in this field serve as administrators in prepaid insurance schemes, on pension boards, on workmen's compensation boards, in federal and provincial Departments of Health, in privately operated insurance companies, and on the newly established Hospital Services Commissions. Few holders of senior posts in these organizations have had specialized academic training at the university level for their present positions."[54]

It added that U of T, with its range of faculty in areas such as public health, business administration, and the political and social sciences was in a very strong position to offer this type of training. It also noted that the cooperation of staff in other branches of the university would be necessary and that discussions had been started in that regard.

The 1959–60 report noted progress had been made "with the drafting of a curriculum for a course on the Principles and Practices of 'Health Insurance.'" It noted that a postgraduate course in this field was urgently needed, since all provinces were either operating or considering prepaid hospital insurance programs.[55] It is unclear if the course was ever offered as a review of the calendars from 1960–61 through 1964–65 does not list it.

BURNS ROTH ON THE BROADER IMPLICATIONS OF A HOSPITAL INSURANCE PROGRAM (1959)

As a result of implementation of the hospital insurance program, *Canadian Hospital* had articles by high-ranking officials in the four western provinces on the implications of this new and significant activity. These were taken from papers presented at the Western Canada Institute for Hospital Administrators and Trustees in Winnipeg in September 1958.[56] The article by Burns Roth, in his capacity of deputy minister in Saskatchewan, is instructive in its broad approach, in that even then he was taking a systemic outlook – seeing hospital insurance and hospitals as part of a larger picture. Many of the points made in this article are still relevant today.

Given that he was to be the next director of the Department of Hospital Administration, it gives us an important glimpse of the type of orientation he would bring to his next job. It also gives us a brief look at what one deputy minister of health saw as the type of health system he wanted to build.

What is interesting about his article is that even at that time, while most were fixated on building the hospital sector, he was trying to insert aspects such as prevention into the discussion. He went so far as to say why it was appropriate that government take on this important service, why it should be publicly accountable, and how it was consistent with an overall purpose of government.

While he began his article on a Saskatchewan Hospital Services Plan, he moved on to the broader implications of an important consequent issue. Hospital insurance programs were redefining the role of government in health care. Saskatchewan had already been at this for twelve years and so had some experience in this area. He was going to deal with three areas: the role of hospitals, the role of government, and the interrelationship between the two.

In addition, given his experience in both health care and public health before coming to government, he was also implicitly dealing with the fact that the two were different sides of the same coin and needed to be pursued in tandem. He also dealt explicitly with how the community factored into all this.

He began his broader orientation by providing historical context: hospitals historically had not been a large piece of the health care system. They had "developed pretty much by themselves for a long time," the medical profession "for many centuries had not too much to do with hospitals," but nursing, "on the other hand, developed more in conjunction with hospitals."[57] He added, "In the long history of man's search for health, this modern concept of the hospital is really a relatively new phenomenon."[58] He then went on to say, "Society is now saying – with varying degrees of emphasis – that we must look at the hospital in its total setting, i.e., the community, to see what the hospital's responsibility to the community really is."[59]

Another point was that "we must accept *a priori* that the role of the hospital is to serve the public." He then went on to make a radical statement for the time, "The fundamental goal of all health services should be to make their services unnecessary," then provided further detail: "We must view everything we do in our activities as health workers in light of whether what we do today is leading to a disease-free tomorrow." He cautioned against letting one's interests, ingrained habits, resistance to change, and "unwillingness to be unpopular" come into play when evaluating "whether the course of action we take is in the public good."[60]

He noted that health professionals might have varying responses to his notion of a "disease-free tomorrow." Some may say, "It has nothing to do with our job as hospital people." Others, that in curing people there is a responsibility to help them understand how they became ill in order to prevent the same thing from happening again. Yet others will go still further to examine whether the hospital should be a facility in a community to develop preventive programs and health education. This could also include integrating hospital care with other services for things like rehabilitative care in order that the individual not need continued health care.[61]

He then spoke of the role of government, indicating that the basis for government involvement was twofold: society was becoming increasingly interdependent and complex, therefore society needed to develop the appropriate organizational methods to deal with this development. He said that in addition to setting up a framework that would deal with hospital care and the payment of costs, society has said it wants an interest in how this is done. "And as the chosen agent to provide leadership, co-ordination, and supervision, society has selected its representative – the government."[62]

He noted that many times society can take a pejorative view of government, but government is a tool "by which our society chooses to get things done." And by having a government-run hospital insurance system, responsible to elected officials, in effect society has a "more direct way" to "guide its destiny."[63]

He then spoke of the interrelationship between hospitals and government and suggested it needed to be a partnership, one that recognized that the "sole reason" for each was "to serve the public." It also involved the recognition that "there are certain things that each can do best." In this he advocated the autonomy of hospitals, but within this he also saw that the community may not have "the available information to see properly their hospital's role in the provincial or national picture" and may need "direction, guidance, and indeed, supervision from a larger central agency." Within this framework he wanted "continuous discussion and consultation ... to serve as a medium for mutual education" and "for appropriate decisions based on the information available."[64]

Within this he "was an advocate of strong energetic hospital associations" and was not averse to "honest differences of opinion." But he also wanted "a mutual acknowledgement that nobody has all the answers."[65] It was evident that Roth felt that a strong system was one with healthy dialogue and debate.

The article speaks to how Roth, no doubt the Douglas government as well, was focused well beyond hospitals, describing a health-care *system* and, exciting as it was, hospital insurance was but one part of a much larger picture, one that focused not only on illness but on preventing illness from arising in the first place. The article also speaks to the type of material that another physician, the journal's editor and Department of Hospital Administration faculty member W. Douglas Piercey, wanted to put before the reader.

The article presents a vivid picture of not just the Saskatchewan approach to hospital insurance but of health generally. One gets a sense of the role at the local level, the importance of the community, and of different elements of the system. It is also interesting as Saskatchewan (and Roth's department) was months away from the announcement by Tommy Douglas that the province was moving beyond hospital insurance, to fulfil the premier's dream of health insurance.

DHA GRADUATES INVOLVED IN A SASKATCHEWAN CERTIFICATE COURSE (1960)

An important aspect of the department and its involvement in the extension course it jointly ran through the Canadian Hospital Council was the extent to which it served as a model and in this way helped "seed" other extension courses. Even though this was not its conscious intent it was, nonetheless, an outcome.

As early as 1952 Saskatchewan – through the dean of commerce – was writing to Agnew for information on the U of T course. In 1953 Dean McLeod also wrote to Eugenie Stewart asking for a faculty member to come to Saskatoon to speak to their final-year students about opportunities in hospital administration. There was further correspondence from Dean McLeod and Agnew in 1957 regarding the U of T course.[66]

Through 1959–60 there is a large volume of correspondence between the dean of commerce and Andrew Patullo, director, Division of Hospitals, Kellogg Foundation. One particularly instructive letter notes that the director of the Saskatchewan program is a DHA grad, as is Ed Wahn, and that A.L. Swanson is heavily involved: "As you can see, the Toronto influence is likely to be quite heavy."[67]

The DHA graduate in question was Carl Meilicke, who became the first director of an extension course on the administration of small hospitals at the University of Saskatchewan. It was launched in 1960. In addition to funding from the Kellogg Foundation, he was successful in obtaining funding from the Saskatchewan Health Care Association and the Canadian Hospital Association.

Ed Wahn was teaching in the program and was interim director when Mr Meilicke took an educational leave to pursue PhD studies.[68] Another diploma graduate, Frank Silversides (class of 1951) took over as director in 1964, a position he held until 1985.[69]

The program was established to serve the educational requirements of administrators of hospitals of fewer than fifty beds in Saskatchewan and the other two Prairie provinces. Target enrolment was set at 25. By 1966 enrolment was 120 and included all provinces of Canada as well as several students from outside the country. By the late 1970s it was up to 300 and in the 1980s it levelled off at 350.[70] It was a two-year correspondence course with two weeks of seminars held at the University of Saskatchewan in the spring dealing with health and hospital administration.[71]

An important aspect of this course – and the same could be said of the joint department, Canadian Hospital Council extension course – was not just the education it provided in raising the standards of management in small hospitals or in how such programs helped support the evolution of Canadian hospitals. Nor was it only that such courses did their part in helping build a new profession and in providing a stepping-stone to the extension course run jointly by the department and Canadian Hospital Council under Agnew. It was also the opportunities it provided to young Canadians, and indeed how such programs changed the lives of Canadian individuals (and perhaps those of their children as well).

A case in point is the one of Andrew Boehm regarding the joint extension course noted previously. Another is illustrated by one of the people who attended the 1962 spring seminar at the U of S extension course, a man named Jean-Paul Veillet from the village of Carrot River in Saskatchewan.[72] He was the administrator of the Carrot River Union Hospital, which in 1962 had a rated capacity of twenty beds.[73]

Veillet had recently returned to his home province after working on the gold-mining dredges of the Yukon. His story might not be unlike that of many other Canadians. He had been unable to pursue his education as far as he wished, as the family of seven children had lost their father at a young age to tuberculosis, so he went to work in order to supplement his mother's income. However, he was interested in pursuing further opportunities. Hospitals in Saskatchewan had been expanding at a rapid rate and he was told this might be a promising career. He felt he needed grounding in the discipline, and the U of S extension course fit the bill. He went on to manage successively larger hospitals, ending his career as administrator of the Peace River Municipal Hospital in Alberta. In his case his three daughters went on to post-secondary education and careers in health, including managerial positions in the field, one in hospital administration.[74]

The Saskatchewan small hospital story was important for another reason. These hospitals became the focal point of the community almost invariably and its largest employer. It became part of a massive shift in Saskatchewan moving the economy away from agriculture. There were also the downstream effects of building numerous small hospitals in what remained a predominately rural province. Each of these extension programs provided access to hospital management education that might have been otherwise unavailable to those who took these programs. It also built management expertise for the province for these small hospitals.

WHO TRAVEL FELLOWSHIPS

In something that was reminiscent of FitzGerald's travel to see other systems, and the work of Greg Marchildon, Sara Allin, and Allie Peckham on comparative systems, faculty have sought out grants to do the same thing.

Hastings was awarded a WHO travel fellowship and spent an extended summer in 1960 looking at the organization of public health services and health insurance plans in countries similar to Canada, such as the United Kingdom, Sweden, Denmark, and Norway, all of which were noted for their development of comprehensive programs of health care. His also visited the Soviet Union to view its system of state medicine, and densely populated countries such as India, Pakistan, Ceylon, Hong Kong, Singapore, and Japan.[75] Eugenie Stuart received a WHO fellowship in 1963 to study trends in education in hospital administration in the United Kingdom and elsewhere in Europe.[76]

A REVIEW OF THE SECOND-YEAR RESIDENCY PROGRAM (1961)

In 1961 the results of a three-year study of the second year of the diploma program was published – a 311-page study undertaken by Ken McLaren, noted earlier, that had been supported by a grant from the Kellogg Foundation.

It suggested integrating the residency year "more closely with the academic portion of the program." It recognized that it was no longer teaching students in hospital administration exclusively but was increasingly attracting students from both levels of government and voluntary organizations. It looked to inject new areas of study in "health economics, provincial and federal aspects of administration, and research in administration."[77] To this end it sought "to establish an educational program for the second year more in keeping with current practice in the training of graduate students in the University."[78] The means of doing this were more formal, scheduled class work and a program of supervised reading.

The study also looked at the relationship between its own program and other graduate programs at the university.[79] One sees in the report what could be interpreted as the beginnings of a transition from a purely professional focus to one that still emphasizes the professional but also enlarges it to include an academic and research stream.[80]

LECTURES BY AGNEW OUTSIDE THE UNIVERSITY

Agnew gave guest lectures outside the university throughout his term – most within Canada. However, Agnew also exemplified a school trend, which was its international connections. An example was in the 1961–62 academic year when he delivered lectures at the London School of Hygiene and Tropical Medicine and also at the Hospital Administration Staff College in London.[81] In 1967 he gave the Charles F. Willinsky Annual Lecture at the Harvard School of Public Health.[82]

WHERE GRADS ENDED UP: III

Here is a third instalment on DHA grads.

John R. Haslehurst (DHA, 1960) obtained a bachelor of science in pharmacy from U of T, where he his undergraduate thesis was "The Effect of National Health Insurance on the Practice of Hospital Pharmacy in Canada." He worked at the Education Department of the Canadian Hospital Association, was an executive director of the Saskatchewan Hospital Association and the first executive director of the Regina Area Hospitals Planning Council on its inception in 1965. He went on to be superintendent of the Hamilton General Hospital.[83] His DHA thesis topic was "The Employment of Physically Handicapped Personnel by Ontario Public General Hospitals."

A. Rodney Thorfinnson (DHA, 1960), CEO, Victoria Hospital, London, Ontario, thesis, "Nursing Assistants in Canada: Their History, Training and Place in the Modern Hospital." A native of Saskatchewan, prior to going to Victoria Hospital, he was a consultant with the Saskatchewan Department of Public Health, executive director of the Saskatchewan Hospital Association, and assistant director of services, University Hospital in Saskatoon.[84]

Gary Chatfield (DHA, 1961) was administrator of York Central Hospital. From 1969 to 1971 he was president of Medex Nursing Homes, then joined the Ontario Ministry of Health in 1972 and became an assistant deputy minister there in 1976. In 1978 he was appointed deputy minister in the Alberta Department of Hospitals and Medical Care.[85] He later became president of Extendicare. He received the Robert Wood Johnson Award for 1961. He also served on the board of Trillium Health Centre and Sunnybrook and Women's College Health Sciences Centre. He was board chair of Sheridan College and Canadian Blood Services. His thesis topic was "A Study of Administrative Organization Covering Business Office Activities in Medium-Sized General Hospitals."

Carl Hunt (DHA, 1961), former administrator of SickKids, thesis, "A Study of Acute Hospital Bed Requirements in the Province of Nova Scotia."

Demographic Profile of Student Cohorts

To continue with the demographic profile of student cohorts, for the class of 1959–61 there were students from BC, Nova Scotia, Ontario (six), Saskatchewan, Canadian Armed Forces, California, Illinois (two), and New York. One student went from the program to the US Air Force to be involved in management of an Air Force hospital. One had experience in the US armed forces prior the program, one experience in the Canadian Armed Forces. Two were born in Manitoba, two born in Saskatchewan. One person had Department of National Health and Welfare experience, another hospital insurance commission experience. Two were physicians.[86]

In the class of 1960–62 there were students from Manitoba, Nova Scotia, Ontario (four), Quebec, Canadian Armed Forces (two), California, Texas, and Pakistan. Once again residencies were across Canada was well as Seattle, Washington. Two students were born in Saskatchewan, though not living there at the time.[87] Interestingly a number of classes had a student from the Canadian Armed Forces. It is a practice that continues to this day.

Another source for where grads ended up is a history by W. Harding le Riche.[88]

MORE ON PUBLISHING BY FACULTY AND GRADUATES

An interesting aspect to graduates of the program was the degree to which they wrote articles for publication or, for some, to be involved in running a journal. Some published in a professional journal throughout their careers, primarily in *Canadian Hospital* and *Hospital Administration in Canada.*

Canadian Hospital

Some grads appeared repeatedly in *Canadian Hospital*, the journal of the Canadian Hospital Association, which began publication in the 1920s.[89] Arguably it was the major professional journal for hospitals and hospital management in Canada. Subject matter in the journal was concerned almost exclusively with practical issues. The tables of contents for the journal during the 1950s, 1960s, and 1970s list contributions from many DHA grads. People like Ed Wahn, Gerry Turner, and Ron McQueen published throughout their careers, with many articles in this journal.[90] Throughout these periods a number of present and former faculty also regularly published there.

Hospital Administration in Canada

In addition to *Canadian Hospital*, a number of DHA graduates were also involved in the publication of another hospital journal in an editorial, editorial board, or author capacity. It began in 1959 as *Hospital Administration and Construction* and was renamed many times. In 1962 it was renamed *Hospital Administration in Canada*. It began as a Maclean publication, whereupon Maclean-Southam took over, then Southam Business. In October 1966 it had a monthly circulation of 6,000 with an estimated pass-along readership of 20,000.[91] In October 1978 it was renamed again, this time *Health Care in Canada*.

The people involved included R.B. Ferguson (DHA, 1950), its founding editor,[92] and C.A. Wirsig (DHA, 1968), who became its editor in September 1962[93] even before he entered the DHA program. Perhaps this was what aroused his interest.

The inaugural issue of June 1959 presented comparative information on provincial hospital insurance programs. It called the federal Hospital Insurance and Diagnostic Services Act "unquestionably one of the most far-reaching pieces of welfare legislation ever enacted in this country." It had a table that compared the eight plans then in operation.[94] A DHA grad D.M. McNabb (DHA, 1953) had an article in this inaugural issue.[95] Another interesting issue appeared in 1960, which reported on a panel the journal had convened on progressive patient care. It involved a number of faculty from the department such as Agnew, former faculty like L.O. Bradley, as well as adjunct faculty like Sydney Liswood, graduates such as R.B. Ferguson and John MacKay (DHA, 1952), and other senior administrators like J.T. Law.[96] It would convene these topic specific panels from time to time. Another was on issues facing small hospitals, moderated by DHA grad Gary Chatfield.[97]

The DHA grad who probably holds the record for contributions would be Ron McQueen, who wrote the "Consultant's Page" for many years. Another was Ed Wahn, who wrote "Your Hospital and the Law" from March 1966 onward. Mr Wahn had an LLB in addition to his DHA and was an associate professor at the College of Commerce when the column debuted.[98] Many other graduates composed individual articles.[99]

These were not academic journals and were not peer-reviewed, but they were contributing useful knowledge to the field, playing a role in knowledge transfer and helping to build a health care system. They were also helping to build professions, not just in hospital administration, but pharmacy, dietetics, and physiotherapy (to name just a few), as well as draw attention to the subgroups of others, such as *hospital* accounting, *hospital* human relations, and *hospital* engineering (again to name just a few). They were national in scope and through that helped build national and provincial networks in hospital management.

Important in all this is the place of DHA faculty and graduates. Both were notable for their commitment to publishing, and graduates for their involvement in the editorial side. The journals also said something about Canada, that this relatively young country could mount and sustain journals like *Canadian Hospital* and *Hospital Administration in Canada.*

They also drew attention to the DHA program. In the bio that accompanied an article Ed Wahn co-authored, the Toronto program was noted, so publicity regarding the program was being disseminated to a wide audience.[100]

Hospitals (US)

One interesting publication that faculty and alumni published in was the American Hospital Association journal *Hospitals*, to which Agnew was a notable contributor.

One significant issue for which a number of faculty and graduates wrote was a special edition in September 1961 titled "Canada's Program of Prepaid Hospital Care," which was devoted almost in its entirety to the Canadian program. The introductory editorial noted five papers were requested from "distinguished Canadians" on different "significant aspects" of the program.[101] Malcolm Taylor wrote the lead article. Of the five commissioned articles, two were from DHA faculty or alumni. One was from former faculty member A.L. Swanson and DHA graduate Ed Wahn commenting on the program from an administrator's perspective.[102] The other was by faculty member W. Douglas Piercey looking at provincial plans.[103]

In addition to the five articles, an editor of the journal, "after extensive travelling," prepared a report on the total program. The editor spent a month travelling 12,000 miles, interviewing sixty leaders, and compiling 260 pages of transcript. Among those quoted were former DHA students such as Burns Roth (class of 1950), G.B. Rosenfeld (class of 1955), Peter Swerhone (DHA, 1957), and Douglas Peart (DHA, 1951), all of whom had senior positions.[104] J.E. Sharpe, special lecturer in the program and superintendent of TGH was also quoted.[105]

The Hospital (UK)

The equivalent British journal was the *Hospital*, which first appeared in 1886 and was the journal of the British Hospitals Association, founded in 1884.[106] Agnew was mentioned in the February 1952 issue as having resigned as executive secretary of the Canadian Hospital Council in order to enter the consulting field.[107]

Just to point out one value of such journals, the January and February 1947 issues had an article on the Söder Hospital, a 1,200-bed district hospital in Stockholm. It was striking for the futuristic architecture of the building, as well as insight into the integrated and continuum of care it provided.[108] There was also a 1949 article on a teaching hospital built in Stockholm at the Karolinska Institute.[109] Such knowledge transfer was an important aspect of these journals.

Comment

The involvement of Agnew and Wirsig at two separate journals points to the pervasive influence of the U of T department. We have noted Agnew, its first director, was very involved with *Canadian Hospital*. We noted earlier a number of graduates were involved with *Hospital Administration in Canada*. In other words the two main journals in the field had strong DHA involvement. And, in the case of Wirsig, it led him to the DHA program.

Two comments bear mentioning. First is the profiling of the program and its faculty and graduates in these journals both in Canada and internationally. In all three countries these were not academic journals, but they had their place. Also the circulation of probably all four journals, but particularly journals like *Hospitals* and the *Hospital*, greatly exceeded that of most academic journals, so they were reaching a wide audience.

Second is the fact that the U of T library was getting these journals, which afforded an important resource to the university, particularly the School of Hygiene and the Department of Hospital Administration for faculty and students. Especially in the case of the US and UK journals, they provided excellent comparative information on other health systems, an area that IHPME emphasizes today. The British journal did this by looking at the NHS and the systems of other countries. Such detailed information on other countries provided excellent information for the major paper required of students in their second year.

However, it is questionable whether such a paper could have been written at that time. On the one hand the department was very practice oriented, but practice deriving from other systems was not an emphasis. In the Swedish article, both Stockholm hospitals were advanced in design and function. One was more of a community hospital, the other very much a state-sponsored, research-intensive, academic hospital. This information has been at the library for some seventy years and scores of students had access to it. An article outlining what they were doing in Sweden in hospitals or in hospitals and health insurance generally, and then applying this to Canada, would have been a very interesting project.

Another interesting project would have been what the British were doing with hospitals after July 1948 (when they nationalized them). Had this been an emphasis in the curriculum, there was substantial material in all these journals, but particularly both foreign journals, for students to have been able to concentrate on something IHPME is doing today, which is to focus on comparative systems and this not just concerning hospitals but also areas like health policy.

We started this section discussing the department's involvement in these journals, an important and laudable activity. However, and perhaps it is too easy to say this with the benefit of hindsight, there was a very real opportunity to have taken this one step further. That would have been with a curriculum directing students to delve into this information to develop creative possibilities for Canada. And just to point out that it was possible at that time, Fitzgerald had a focus on comparative systems.

MALCOLM TAYLOR ON THE HISTORY OF PREPAID HOSPITAL CARE (1961)

One contributor to the *Hospitals* issue mentioned above was former U of T faculty member Malcolm Taylor, who wrote a history of the emergence of prepaid hospital care in Canada and singled out two main streams of hospital prepayment in Canada that predated the public universal plan. One was voluntary insurance and the other municipal and (later) provincial plans. His emphasis was on the voluntary plans, the prevalent form of prepaid care in the United States. In Canada he noted, "Both the success of voluntary insurance in proving the worth of prepayment and its failure to bring its advantages to all contributed to the present federal-provincial program."[110]

An interesting point he made was that in the establishment of the national program, "the most important contribution of all was made by the knowledgeable and trained men and women, who were either Blue Cross administrators or hospital leaders."[111]

He then made a statement that is reminiscent of our motif of availability to all: "There was unquestionable reluctance on their part to see their projects 'taken over' by the government, but discussions with these leaders suggest that any unhappiness was heavily counterweighted by the knowledge that government action was merely extending to all what they had struggled to bring to many."[112]

Comment

One wonders if Taylor was playing to his US audience. His article emphasizes the extent of the voluntary contribution to the national program. At the time he was principal of the University of Alberta, Calgary (later to become the University of Calgary). Voluntary insurance had a large following in Alberta[113] and it was the predominant form of prepaid care in the United States. He noted, "In a number of provinces, the Blue Cross Plan became the core of the new agency."[114] Also, "The contributions of the voluntary plans to the success of the nation-wide program, cannot be overestimated."[115] In another section, in writing again of the contributions of the voluntary plans, he noted, "In short, they were the men and women who had fought for the nonprofit, voluntary, humanitarian ideals of the Blue Cross movement."[116]

None of this is incorrect factually. However, a countervailing movement toward the same ends had much greater government involvement (locally or provincially), as epitomized in Saskatchewan. And, as it would turn out, this became the Canadian template. Also, at the time of his article, Douglas was on the cusp of tabling his *medical* insurance bill in the Saskatchewan Legislature. The Thompson Committee charged with obtaining public input had had a rough ride. Tensions were running high.

Malcolm Taylor knew all this. He had worked in Saskatchewan when its *hospital* insurance program was implemented in 1947 and he had remained there until the early 1950s. He then became a faculty member at U of T. He lectured in the School of Hygiene and knew of its ideals. He knew Burns Roth (who was at the Saskatchewan Department of Public Health when

Taylor was there). In other words he knew of the local and provincial government initiatives in that province.

Another point is that Agnew liked the tenor of the Taylor article so much he quoted its final paragraph (which emphasized the Blue Cross contribution) in its entirety in his history of Canadian hospitals.[117] One wonders about his attitude towards publicly funded, compulsory universal hospital or health insurance plans versus voluntary non-profit plans like Blue Cross versus for-profit private plans. Agnew's preference was with the Blue Cross variant.

WESTERN CANADA HOSPITAL INSTITUTE (1956–61)

To conserve space we will look at only selected years for this period. At the 1958 Institute L.O. Bradley, W.D. Piercey, F.B. Roth, A.L. Swanson, and DHA grad Peter Swerhone were involved. "Government-sponsored hospital insurance coloured almost every phase of the program" that year.[118]

DHA grad G.B. Rosenfeld was the organizer for the 1959 Institute. Roth presented on the role of consultants and noted that his department had undertaken this service in Saskatchewan for lack of such services and the need particularly amongst the smaller hospitals. A representative of one of the Regional Hospital Councils (a decentralized consultative service of the Saskatchewan Department of Public Health) outlined their role (DHA grad, S.J. Parsons, head of the Regional Hospital Council for the North Central Region). R.J. McQueen and W.D. Piercey were other DOHA individuals involved.[119]

The federal and BC ministers of health spoke at the 1960 Institute. G.B. Rosenfeld was involved.[120] Agnew and W.D. Piercey spoke at the 1961 Institute held in Saskatoon, as did DHA grads H. Livergant and G.B. Rosenfeld. It attracted people not only from the four western provinces but from the US states bordering on them.[121]

CHAPTER 11

A Solid Education Program with Strong Ties to the Field

The need for professionally trained hospital administrators continued to grow through the 1960s and 1970s, as the expansion in hospital care that we spoke of in the 1950s continued. Hospitals themselves continued to grow. In 1963 Ontario had three hospitals of over 1,000 beds. The largest was Toronto General at 1,397. Next were Hamilton Civic at 1,193, and Ottawa Civic at 1,088.[1] The logistics of running these super-size facilities was daunting. Even in the 1980s with TGH at 1,000 beds, it admitted 100 patients and discharged the same number each weekday.[2] The logistics of meals, lab tests, and treatment in such facilities is daunting.

The number of hospital beds within a kilometre radius of the department was striking, with Toronto Western at 835 beds, St Michael's at 800, Sick-Kids at 646, New Mount Sinai (as it was then known) at 373, Wellesley at 283, and Women's College at 279.[3] And the number of beds kept growing. In 1964 total beds available increased 3.4 per cent over 1963.[4]

The growth is not surprising. Recall that when Leslie Frost announced the introduction of the Ontario Hospital Insurance Plan in 1959, roughly 90 per cent of the people were covered. Those insured by the plan continued to rise, and 99.2 per cent of the population was covered in 1964, a rise of 3.2 percent over 1963.[5]

BURNS ROTH (1962–73)

Burns Roth became the first full-time chair of the department in 1962. His appointment was an inspired choice by the school, as had been Agnew's before him. Harvey Agnew was "Mr Hospital"; there was no one in the country who knew more about hospitals, felt more strongly about them, or had better connections. With Roth the focus changed, as it needed to. Hospitals, while still very important, were recognized as only one component of a health system, and the U of T department needed to keep pace with this evolution. What was unique about him was the variety of roles he'd had in health care.

Roth had been a practising physician, for the most part in Canada's northern frontier, first in northern BC near the Yukon border, then in the Yukon itself. When he moved to Whitehorse from northern BC he combined his practice with hospital administration and then public health. He had been a part of the explosive growth of Whitehorse during the Second World War and the huge public health challenges it presented. When he went to Saskatchewan, while much of his time was spent managing a hospital insurance program and planning for medical insurance, he never lost sight of his ministry's role in public health.

Roth's appointment began a tradition of directors of the department having strong public health credentials combined with actual experience. He came to the department with impeccable qualifications. He had been deputy minister of public health in Saskatchewan under Tommy Douglas. He was part of the rapid expansion of hospitals in the province as a result of Douglas's implementation of the first hospital insurance program in North America in 1947. He had also been part of many public health initiatives. Roth had been instrumental in building what many regarded as the finest ministry of health in the country.

He was also unique in having a firm grounding in both hospitals and public health. He had variety and depth in his involvement in hospitals. He had worked in them as a labourer, then intern; he had been a hospital administrator, but not just in any hospital, in a frontier hospital. He went from there to a student in the program he would now head, and from that to a kind of hospital oversight position with the Saskatchewan government in hospital planning and standards, and involvement in the first hospital insurance program in North America. He then became involved in planning the first medical care insurance program on the continent. Indeed, and as was characteristic of the School of Hygiene, when he was tapped to be the head of the Department of Hospital Administration, there was probably no individual in Canada more qualified for the position.

His appointment constituted a fundamental refocus for the department. No one knew better than Roth the importance of hospitals. But conversely no one knew better than he their limits when speaking of a public health system. Perhaps one of the clearest indicators of the difference in focus of the department was the journal of choice that the heads of the department published in. For Agnew it had been *Canadian Hospital.* For Roth it was the *Canadian Journal of Public Health.* Yet, as we will see, the department still retained a very practical orientation.

Background

Early Involvement in Health

Roth was a native of Ontario. He developed an early interest in hospitals after volunteering with the Woodstock General Hospital during the summer while he was in medical school. He had landed a paying job after his first year of medical school but his father "hit the roof when he found I had a job. He was reasonably well off … and found that there was no place for a young man to be working when there were many married men with families who couldn't find a job. So he told me to go back and quit and that he was perfectly capable of supporting me for my further education. However, he did suggest that there was a very real need for some assistance at the Woodstock General Hospital.… He suggested that I should go up there and offer my services for no recompense and that there were a lot of things that I could do."[6]

He did and worked in the kitchen and helped with cleaning and gardening. However he said he couldn't keep his nose out of the workings of the hospital. He said all of the doctors "accepted my presence" and "with considerable alacrity they went out of their way to take me around with them and show me the interesting cases." He said the result was that he had a pretty close feeling for the attitude the "personnel in hospitals" had toward their patents. He noted the doctors treated him like an "embryo doctor" and the nurses and orderlies treated him like one of the non-professional help. After his second year he went back to the hospital and repeated his experience, though he got a lot more exposure to patients. This was unusual experience, as during the first two years one had very little clinical medicine.[7]

He received his medical degree from the University of Western Ontario. After graduating in 1936 he spent a year practising in Vancouver, and then two and a half years in northern BC, arriving in Atlin, BC (150 miles south of Whitehorse, Yukon) in July 1937.[8]

His Time in the Yukon

Roth went to Whitehorse to relieve "a hard-pressed doctor for two months. He stayed for 12 years." He was there when Whitehorse became a major staging centre for the building of the Alaska Highway, which resulted in a rapid, massive influx of military and civilian personnel. According to a press report, it "turned it from a village to a boom town."[9] In the 1941 census its population was 754; by April 1943 there were 10,000 people in Whitehorse.[10]

He was one of two doctors serving a large area during the Second World War, making many of his calls by air.[11] During this time in Whitehorse he "became interested in hospitals as such, in the administration of hospitals and decided that perhaps this was the field into which I should move. Incidentally my father had always told me that this was the field I would eventually get into while I was in medical school."[12]

He built and was superintendent of the Whitehorse General Hospital (he was elected in August 1940), and medical officer of health for the southern Yukon Territory.[13] An archival insert noted, "In those days the doctor practiced from the hospital and managed the hospital with a hospital board."[14] The home that was supplied to him is considered a heritage building and he is mentioned as one if its occupants. It had been built in 1901–02 and was originally owned by the superintendent of the Whitehorse Hospital. It was purchased by the hospital trustees in 1911 to be used as a doctor's residence and had an office and waiting room in it.[15]

An indication of the challenges he faced, particularly as medical officer of health, appears in publications about the Yukon of that time. Coates and Morrison talk of changes to health care as a result of the massive influx of US Army and Royal Canadian Air Force stationed in Whitehorse, changes that would have had a direct effect on Roth's role there. It "exploded from a sleepy river depot to a major military and construction complex."[16] This had profound public health implications, and they note, for example, "Whitehorse's rudimentary sewage and water system could not contend with the massive invasion."[17]

The US Army built a hospital for their use and in 1942 they provided the building material for a further expansion of the Whitehorse Hospital. In another work Coates and Morrison give us a sense of the time: "There was only one, badly overworked, medical health officer, Dr Frederick Roth, to keep an eye on local public health concerns."[18]

A sense of the challenges he faced is provided by a US Army assessment of the town. The Whitehorse Station Hospital commander for the US Army "described sanitary facilities as 'execrable' and called the town 'one vast cesspool.'" It noted that a modern hospital had been established and a health officer appointed and it mentions Roth by name, but says he lacked assistance "and though he tried to improve sanitary conditions, especially in restaurants, he had not received support." The US Army worked with Roth to improve conditions in the restaurants, given that many of their personnel frequented them.[19]

In actuality in the Yukon he had a direct involvement in two areas that became the focus of the rest of his career: hospital management and public health. It was a very formative and educational time. The range of his involvement as a physician, hospital administrator, and medical officer of health in one of Canada's frontier areas gave him a breadth of exposure to health-care delivery and a wealth of experience.[20] To this was added the unique experience of the public health issues encountered by the explosive growth of Whitehorse during the Second World War and his experience liaising with the public health officers of the US Army to deal with these issues.

He Enrols in the DHA Program

Roth become so intrigued by the problems of hospital management and public health that he contemplated giving up his medical practice and going into health management.[21] He originally looked into the University of Chicago program in hospital administration "in 1940 or 1941," but with "the war coming on" he decided he should abandon these plans although there was some indication he would be accepted.[22] He noted that by the time the war ended, or shortly thereafter, there was now a Canadian program and in 1948 he entered the second class of the University of Toronto DHA program. He said his class was a very mixed group, about five physicians, very young graduates coming directly from undergraduate programs, people who had been hospital administrators, and others who had worked in various other occupations.[23]

He entered the program with very strong primary care, public health, and hospital management credentials, given his time in northern BC and the Yukon. His choice of hospital administration rather than public health administration represented his interest in breadth. He got breadth in spades, given his choice to truncate his time at Winnipeg General and join Tommy Douglas's team in Regina.

He did not finish his second year or his thesis requirement, the result of a combination of circumstances. Harvey Agnew had suggested that he do his administrative residency at Winnipeg General Hospital because the administrator was going to be retiring and that he would be the heir apparent. However, he found the experience to be "a very unhappy one" and felt that the hospital "which had always been one of the notable hospitals in Canada was slowly slipping backward" in the way it was run. He also found he was given so much responsibility that he was working from 8:00 a.m. to midnight almost every day.[24]

Likely a combination of factors was involved. Roth was somewhat older and, given his background in patient care, public health, and hospital administration in the north, he had much greater experience than the normal DHA student. Perhaps he was chafing under the administrator's style as well as the residency requirement. Under these circumstances the Saskatchewan offer would have been irresistible.

Involvement in Health in Saskatchewan

It was during this time that Ed Wahn, a classmate from the School of Hygiene's program, asked him to consider coming to Saskatchewan to be director of the Division of Hospital Administration and Standards within the Department of Public Health. He said about three months into his residency the calls seemed to be coming with increasing frequency about what wonderful things were happening in Saskatchewan and that he "should pack it up in Winnipeg and come to Saskatchewan to take up the position." He said Wahn lured him to Saskatchewan for a visit to see what was going on, where he "was extremely impressed" by the "sense of progress that was being made in the possibilities of developing a new kind of hospital system which had not been seen on this continent."[25]

He said, "The result was that after a number of interviews including one with the Premier, Tommy Douglas, who impressed me greatly," and the fact that they wanted him as soon as possible, he returned to Winnipeg and told them he would not be completing his residency and would be leaving at the end of December 1950. As a result he never graduated from the program. But he felt that he simply could not turn down the opportunity in Saskatchewan because of the excitement about what was going on there and especially so, given his unhappiness in Winnipeg.[26]

Historical documents indicate the new division in the Saskatchewan department was formed through the amalgamation of two previous divisions, those of Hospital Planning and Standards and of Hospital Accounting and Administration. It was a key part to meeting needs due to the scaling up of and increased hospital activity and construction as a result of the provincial universal hospital insurance system established in 1947 by Tommy Douglas. The division's primary purpose was to provide assistance in developing union hospital districts and advice on the construction of new hospitals and the enlargement of existing ones. It also had personnel who could advise hospitals in professional areas such as laboratory, dietary, nursing, and others, and it had three university-trained hospital administrators to provide consultations.[27]

This position had a number of different elements, one of which was running an insurance program. This had a number of important components and, of course, given that it was the first such program, there was no precedent to go on. First was financing the program, through premiums, general revenues, and a sales tax. Another was administering it, as well as improving hospital standards and finding ways to pay hospitals for the services provided.[28]

Roth became part of the inner circle of the department. He was also made a member of the Advisory Committee to the Health Services Planning Commission, chaired by Fred Mott, and included Tommy McLeod, deputy provincial treasurer, and Malcolm Taylor, who at that time was secretary to the commission.[29] One wonders if Roth was recruited with eventual succession planning in mind, as by 1952 he was deputy minister of the department.

A number Tommy Douglas's deputy ministers were prolific in publication, and Roth was no exception, along with Al Johnson and Meyer Brownstone (whose partner Diana Moser would be an IHPME grad). While in Saskatchewan he published in public health as well as hospital administration. One example is an article on the Saskatchewan Hospital Services Plan, an area with which he was intimately familiar. His article outlined the basic principles of the plan and how it was funded and noted important distinctions, such as the lack of co-insurance charges.[30]

Roth saw early an integration between the role of hospitals and public health. In an article he wrote shortly after becoming deputy minister he noted the need for such integration as well as outlining the history of such a movement. In the article he also argues for the regionalization of hospital services and sees that the public health officer could provide leadership to such a process.[31]

He saw an early opportunity to mine the vast databank being accumulated by the provincial hospital insurance plan. In an article he co-authored with what would prove to be other public health leaders – and this was an example of the type of public health leadership that his department spawned – he critiqued the basis on which the need for hospital services was made. He also spoke of great variations in the utilization of hospital care among different communities – one could argue an early foray into the area of health inequalities that emerged many years later.[32] The other authors were M.S. Acker (DPH, 1946), M.I. Roemer (an American leader in public health who worked in the Douglas government for a time), and G.W. Meyers, executive director of the Saskatchewan Hospital Services Plan.

Roth also wrote an article on the experience of funding hospitals under such a plan.[33]

Roth is an early example of the almost seamless interchange between academia, the field, and back again. He went from the program (albeit as a student) to government and back to the program. He is also important in the depth of experience he brought to the program, not just in the policies he had implemented but also, in his case, the close working relationship that the Saskatchewan department had with the federal one. Roth notes this in a University Archives interview.[34] It is also borne out by documentation in Saskatchewan. For example there is correspondence between Premier Douglas and the federal minister, Paul Martin, on both the premier and Mott meeting with Martin regarding health programs.[35]

As Head of the Department of Hospital Administration

The genesis of Roth coming to Toronto to become head of the Department of Hospital Administration grew out of a casual conversation with Rhodes. Roth had stopped in Toronto after a meeting in Ottawa and met with Rhodes. During their conversation Rhodes noted that they were looking for a new head of the Department of Hospital Administration and asked whether Roth would be interested. Roth signalled he might be for it was not his wish to remain in any one position too long and at the time there was no great movement toward medical care insurance in Saskatchewan. The result was an informal agreement for him to come to Toronto.[36]

Rhodes noted that this was a landmark in his first few years as head of the school, appointment of the first full-time professor, head of the Department of Hospital Administration, and a professor of medical care made possible by the Kellogg Foundation. He said Roth would "go down in Canadian health history as one of the pioneers and innovators," a "very able civil servant," and "he came to the Department a very able teacher and general stimulator of people in this field."[37]

However, shortly after Roth's return to Saskatchewan, Premier Douglas declared his intent to implement medical insurance, which put the Department of Public Health on a much different footing, the result being that Roth asked Rhodes if he could delay his move to Toronto for one year, which Rhodes agreed to.[38] He noted that he found the "peace and tranquility of the university very welcome after the hub-hub of Saskatchewan."[39]

By the time he arrived at the university department he had experience in medical practice, hospital administration, and public health in the Yukon. His medical practice was unique, as most of it was in Canada's north frontier. He was a student in the second class in hospital administration at the university, integrally involved in the expansion of hospitals in Saskatchewan, and more importantly, with providing the proper government supports to supporting the management of those hospitals. Then he was the deputy minister overseeing the whole system and a senior official in a government that had an international reputation in policy development (and not just in health) under arguably one of the most dynamic premiers this country had ever seen.[40]

According to a news release from the university on his background, "He is best known in Canada as one of the principal architects of the once-controversial Saskatchewan Medicare Plan." It said he had been president of the Canadian Public Health Association, a vice-president of the American Public Health Association, and a member of the WHO Expert Advisory Panel on Medical Care.[41]

His move to the Department of Health Administration coincided with a rapid hospital expansion that was now taking place in the rest of the country as a result of the hospital insurance program going national with the passage of the enabling act by the Diefenbaker government in 1957. He also had a real affinity for what was taking place in the school, as he had not only been part of implementing a hospital insurance program, he had been at the centre of planning for medical insurance and had built a very strong public health program in Saskatchewan. He had also participated in the implementation of tertiary medicine in Saskatchewan. He was deputy minister when the facilities of the College of Medicine at the University of Saskatchewan and shortly after the University Hospital in Saskatoon were opened. The dean of medicine had been recruited by his predecessor as deputy minister, Fred Mott (Roth subsequently convinced Mott to come to Toronto to teach in the department).

The Department of Hospital Administration had established a solid reputation in professional education. He noted that the general feeling in Canada he found was that the program was very successful and good people were being graduated. Moreover it was inculcating the leadership that was necessary to cope with the increasing demands of institutions as they became more sophisticated.[42] Upon his arrival he began teaching in the program of hospital administration. He was also teaching some classes in medical administration in the public health program. It was felt that his experience in public health in Saskatchewan would be useful in the latter program, as the duties of the public health officer were expanding and an administrative component was necessary. He noted that the program was receiving a large number of applicants but was limited to twenty spaces and that this made selection difficult as more and more well-qualified university graduates became interested in the field.[43]

The same thought was expressed by Andrew Rhodes in an oral history of the school. But one gets a sense not only of the applicant process but of the place of the department in the school. He said, "It was obviously a *program*. There was great competition for entry, they had many, many more applicants each year, and they chose very good students."[44] From the way he intonated the word *program*, an adjectival connotation is evident in that that he meant a "great" program or some such meaning.

In the period surrounding Roth's hiring (the early to mid-1960s) Rhodes noted there was still some debate in university circles on public health and hospital administration. Rhodes noted the separation of the Connaught Labs from the School of Hygiene, and with that a separation between "teaching and research" and "production and research." He noted that this was a new school in that many professional schools like pharmacy and dentistry "had found their feet before public health." He noted that the disciplines of public health and health administration, the delivery of hospital care – "this was just becoming, to use a horrible phrase, academically respectable.... Epidemiology was respectable, statistics was respectable, basic sciences was respectable, but the delivery of health care, the delivery of hospital care, there was some question as to whether that really should be in the university."[45]

Because of his position and background, Roth was sought out for his views on the role of health in society. An excerpt his chapter in the *Canadian Annual Review for 1969* gives an idea of a perspective borne not only from being chair of the Department of Health Administration but also from having been in medical practice himself and the deputy minister of such a progressive department of health; and this at a time when it solidified its program of the only hospital insurance program in North America and planned to introduce the first medical care insurance program on the continent.

He began by saying,

> The decade of the sixties was one of the most dynamic in the history of health care in Canada. The year 1969 ended ten years in which highly significant new developments occurred in the basic sciences, in the treatment, and in the socio-economic aspects of health services. The explosion of new technologies and techniques of prevention, diagnosis and treatment, and the increasing understanding about distribution of health services proceeded at an increasing rate during the decade....
>
> The decade began with the final steps being taken to institute a nationwide hospital insurance program; the decade ended with several provinces and the federal government having reached agreement to share the costs of a medical care insurance program.[46]

He called it "an exciting and progressive decade in the health field."[47]

Roth continued to publish. He had an editorial in *Medical Care* on developments in Canada, which concerned mainly the Hall Commission and the initiation of medical insurance in Saskatchewan. In his view, providing universal services would result in a coordinated network, yet that remained an elusive goal. Perhaps "we have the planning and administrative skills to understand and shape the parts individually but can only theorize about, but not manage, the whole."[48]

He also wrote on the training of administrators, which introduced a new section on administration in the *Canadian Public Health Journal*. In it he noted the distinction between health administration and administration in other fields. He also stressed the importance of experience in this field and thereby of the residency. In most other fields a reasonable product outcome was acceptable, but not in health care, where, for example, one is not satisfied in treating an arthritic so that he can walk with a cane; rather he must be able to play eighteen holes of golf.[49] Roth's articles were always interesting in the nuances such as these he captured.

The evolution of Roth's career is another example of the interchange between the U of T department and the field, as well as links between Saskatchewan and the DOHA. In Roth's case, he cut short the practicum and thesis part of his diploma studies for the opportunity to work in the Douglas government. The chance for him to head up a rapidly expanding division in the health ministry, one growing as a result of Douglas's introduction of hospital insurance, was one he felt he could not pass up. In hindsight it would prove to be a very smart decision, as it was not long before Roth became the deputy minister.

The Douglas government also had strong connections to academia and not just in health. The provincial Treasury was known for seeking out the best and brightest from academia. People in his administration, such as Roth, published in academic journals while in their government roles. Roth's career came full circle because went go from Saskatchewan to head up the very U of T department he had not graduated from.

He was an important addition to the department. His range and depth of experience were almost unrivalled, not only in health systems and public health, but also an early model of some of the subtleties of federal-provincial relations in a young and highly decentralized federation such as Canada. For example, at the time he became deputy minister in Saskatchewan, there was Paul Martin Sr in Ottawa who, as federal minister of health and welfare was making a strong push for health insurance in Canada.

This was a very interesting and challenging undertaking. Martin was trying to influence events in an area that was provincial, not federal jurisdiction. In doing so he was also building up an expertise in his own department. For the nation two things were necessary: knowledge of a health insurance program, and the bureaucratic capacity to administer one. Not only did no provinces have an equal measure of each, few had the administrative capacity for such a program. Martin implemented research on the health insurance systems of other countries (what we today would call comparative systems) that were then made freely available. Hodgetts gets at the intricacies of ameliorating some of the unevenness of provincial capacity in areas such as health.[50]

Martin also initiated health grants to provinces for research or activities in a number of areas of health services. It was described by Mackenzie King in the House of Commons as "the first stages in the development of a comprehensive health insurance plan for all Canada."[51] These initiatives of Martin were meant to help build capacity in the provinces. But Saskatchewan was a different matter. It had the only functioning program on the continent.[52]

Roth was an integral part of the intricacies of federal-provincial relations in an area where the federal government did not have jurisdiction but where several provinces needed help, and where some sort of coordination was needed to foster a national program. Roth's involvement with the federal department was an example of the openness of both departments to learn from each other. It is these types of background that he brought to the program – policy and programmatic knowledge, knowledge of intergovernmental relations, and an early knowledge of the distinction between what we would call today health systems and public health.

ROTH'S ARRIVAL AND THE DOCTOR'S STRIKE IN SASKATCHEWAN

Roth left Saskatchewan just as the historic confrontation between physicians and government peaked. The day he started in Toronto was the day physicians withdrew their services. The School of Hygiene is conspicuous by its absence in the debate at U of T surrounding the strike. It is almost inconceivable, given the school's historic stance on health insurance and Roth's former position, that there were no discussions. However no records of them could be found. This could well be because a sizeable portion of the records did not make it to the archives. Also, the Council of the School of Hygiene met only every six months, in May and November, so there were no deliberations there.[53] There is also nothing in Claude Bissell's files (U of T President) under either the Faculty of Medicine or School of Hygiene.[54]

The same was not true of other U of T divisions, especially the federated colleges. There is a signed telegram addressed to Dr Dalgleish, president of the Saskatchewan College of Physicians and Surgeons, Dr McCharles, president of the CMA, and Mr Woodrow Lloyd, premier of Saskatchewan from a number of signatories in high positions at U of T. These included V.W. Bladen (dean, Faculty of Arts), Charles Hendry (director of Social Work, U of T), Rev. J.M. Kelly (president, St Michael's College), Joseph McCulley (warden, Hart House), Derwyn Owen (provost, Trinity College), Moffat Woodside (principal, University College), and Northrop Frye.[55] Frye at the time was principal of Victoria College and incidentally had spent a year after his ordination as a minister in Saskatchewan.

The letter was reported in the *Globe and Mail.* Their article also noted prominent non–U of T signatories, which included playwright Lister Sinclair, the Anglican bishop of Toronto, chair of the Metropolitan Board of Education, and Toronto Transit commissioner, among others.[56] The *Toronto Daily Star* also listed the other signatories and as well had interviews with a number of them. These included several U of T officials. It noted that George Cadbury, president of the Ontario NDP, and G.M.A. Grube, head of the Department of Classics at Trinity College at the University of Toronto (and a member of the NDP National Executive) helped organize the telegram.[57]

In the Trinity Archives the Grube notes relating to signatures being solicited for the telegram have a notation with the names of Hastings and Rhodes. Very likely they were contacted, as the other names were those noted above who did sign, but there is no actual evidence they were contacted or of any potential response in either the Grube records or those of Hastings or Rhodes.[58] There is also no record of any Hygiene response in the Report to the President for that year.

ROTH INITIATIVES

The strike in Saskatchewan notwithstanding, Roth needed to reorient his attention to a very active department within an equally active school.

During his tenure there several initiatives in the U of T department. It was noted in the *President's Report of 1963–64* that Dr Ken Clute had been awarded a four-year Milbank Fellowship in Law and Public Health. For the first year he would enrol in the Faculty of Law as a full-time student at the suggestion and encouragement of the dean of Law, C.A. Wright. Thereafter he would develop a program of advanced courses and research in a field of joint interest: public health and law.[59]

Also during his time Richard Titmuss from the London School of Economics spoke at the school (in November 1964). The topic was health and welfare in East Africa.[60] The talk was also noted in the President's Report for that year.[61] Titmuss was a foremost authority in the world on social policy and in particular the NHS. He was at U of T to receive an honorary degree. In his Convocation address he touched on a theme that was at the heart of what the school was about and one exemplified by the Douglas government: "Confronted with problems of enormous complexity and urgency in government ... in medicine, in social welfare ... people are increasingly turning for guidance, for research know-how, and for knowledge to scientists and scholars in university faculties."[62]

Another example of this academic-field interface was an initiative undertaken during Roth's tenure: a continuing education course called Advanced Topics in Health Services Administration, one of three courses offered by the school in the summer of 1966. They were taught by faculty, along with visiting specialists. They were open to university graduates with experience in the health sectors and were meant to update the knowledge of those who had studied the subjects before, as well as those who had not previously taken graduate instruction. This particular course was taught by Roth to "senior civil servants and staff members of voluntary health agencies [and] concerned the planning, operation and evaluation of health services at the central level."[63] The department continued it the next year.[64]

The school and department also had an active interest in international health and the health issues of overseas countries. In the 1965–66 annual report to the president it noted studies of the health programs of the United Kingdom, Scandinavia, USSR, Israel, and Holland, among others. John Hastings, Cope Schwenger, and Eugenie Stuart had made personal visits to such countries, often with the financial assistance of WHO and the Pan American Health Organization.[65]

The school and department were also cognizant of wanting to broaden their focus in health services administration which had surfaced in the late 1950s. In the 1965–66 academic year it obtained funding from the Department of National Health and the Ontario Ministry of Health which allowed it to hire Fred Mott. It also allowed for hiring of two other faculty. One was Dr Harry Gear, former assistant director-general of WHO in Geneva who had deep experience in international public health. The other was Ken McLaren, who, we noted, had undertaken a review of the second year of the program and now was returning from a position of director of education for the American College of Hospital Administrators.[66]

In 1966–67 the department enrolled hospital admin students in a MSc degree in hospital administration for the first time. That year it had three candidates, two of whom were physicians.[67] With assistance through the Department of National Health and Welfare it also brought on board Dr

Peter Ruderman in health economics and health administration. He had been on staff at the Pan American Health Organization in Washington.[68]

In 1968–68 the department began a new full-time program to meet the needs for advanced training in health administration of people who held or expected to hold senior administrative posts overseas. It enrolled a physician who was going to occupy the chief administrative position in Trinidad, as well as a professor of preventive medicine from a medical school in India. While it consisted of a full academic year, it did not lead to a diploma.[69] In 1969 at its twenty-first annual meeting in Chicago, Roth was elected president of the Association of University Programs in Hospital Administration, which was a consortium of twenty-seven faculties in hospital and health administration in the United States and Canada.[70]

In 1970–71 the department was preoccupied with attempting "to predict the changes which might be ahead in the health field, so that some idea could evolve as to the skills that would be required." On the one hand there were beliefs that broadly trained generalists were needed. On the other there were equally strong views that there should be more concentration on the development of graduates who had highly specialized qualifications. It was felt that "the health field was moving toward some form of consolidation into a true health service system."[71]

There was a very large number of applicants for the diploma in hospital administration. As of 30 June 1971, there were 168 applications for twenty positions. Many already had advanced degrees at the master's level, coming from fields such as business admin, political economy, nursing, pharmacy, engineering, and theology.[72] Roth noted that a change from when he was in the program was that there was less interest from physicians and "people with much more varied backgrounds" were becoming interested (and he added psychology to the list above). He also noted that there was no single undergraduate program that one would expect to generate the largest number of applicants to the program. He recollected an individual who had a degree in history, got a job in a hospital and decided this would be his career, returned for a graduate degree in the field, and became a very successful administrator.[73]

He also noted that in the 1950s and 1960s the primary emphasis was on hospital administration, as hospitals were the main focus of governments and where "the greatest amount of funds and the greatest amount of effort was being expended." This broadened into training people to administer hospital insurance programs. However, in the 1970s there was discussion about "training a generic health administrator who feels competent to deal with any agency or institution in the health field." This led him into musing whether there was such a thing "as a generic health administrator."[74]

WESTERN CANADA HOSPITAL INSTITUTE (1965–67)

In October 1965 Roth spoke at the Twentieth Annual Meeting of the Western Canada Hospital Institute held in Regina that year. He emphasized the "need for bold and venturesome methods to improve health care in Canada." John Haslehurst (DHA, 1960), executive director of the Saskatchewan Hospital Association, served as chair. It attracted 1,200 participants. The minister of the Saskatchewan Department of Public Health, Dave Steuart, spoke. Former DOHA faculty member A.L. Swanson spoke on the results of a three-year survey on the impact of the Saskatchewan Medicare Plan, which was released at the meeting, and another former DOHA faculty member, L.O. Bradley (now executive director of Winnipeg General), spoke on coordinated planning in hospitals.[75]

DHA grad Jim McNab, a hospital consultant with Woods Gordon and Company, spoke on functional obsolescence many times being the result of poor regional planning. DHA grad Peter Swerhone, administrator of Winnipeg General Hospital, presided over a panel of architects dealing with hospital design.[76]

June 1967 saw the twenty-second and last meeting of the institute, a four-day program that attracted 2,500 delegates[77] and speakers from Canada, the United States, and the United Kingdom. The reason given for winding it down was that with the increasing sophistication of provincial annual conventions, the growth of hospital institutes in both Canada and the United States, and the CHA deciding to offer an annual convention, it was no longer necessary to continue. Since its inauguration it had "done an outstanding job in providing hospital administrators and trustees with the opportunity of hearing and meeting some of the finest speakers and lecturers in the hospital field on this continent." DHA grad Peter Swerhone and former faculty member L.O. Bradley (now president, Minneapolis Medical Center) were involved in the last conference.[78]

The participation of faculty and grads in the institute illustrated the national scope of the program as well as the fact that at major events one invariably finds the DOHA represented.

FACULTY AND DHA GRAD ON MEDICARE

The words of faculty were not lost on legislators. On 4 March 1963, K. Bryden (NDP, Woodbine) spoke at length on health insurance in the legislature and quoted John Hastings: "One in five Ontario residents receives 'hopelessly inadequate' public health protection that 'borders on negligence.'… I would commend those words to the Hon. Minister and to the government. I think they are sensible words. They are the words of a man who has obviously considered the needs of a highly organized and complicated community, such as we have in Canada today."[79]

Former DHA faculty member A.L. Swanson wrote two articles in late 1965 on the effect of medicare on Saskatchewan's hospitals, in yet another example of people associated with the program taking the time to write and publish.[80] It was very timely, as with the Pearson government debating the possibility of medicare for Canada, the topic and its possible effects was on the mind of many people.

There had been a federal-provincial conference in July of that year, and the prime minister stated that "the provision of health services" was the "item of our agenda which is the most important of all."[81] The deputy minister of national health, who attended the conference, G. Donald W. Cameron, was a DPH grad (1928), had done bacteriological research at Connaught, and taught at the School of Hygiene.[82]

The reader will recall we noted Swanson had left the DHA program to become the first full-time executive director of the University Hospital, Saskatchewan's first tertiary hospital. He was a former Saskatchewan colleague of Roth's, as Roth had been the temporary part-time executive director of the hospital (along with his position in the Department of Public Health), and Roth's division was the one that looked after Saskatchewan's hospitals. Saskatchewan, of course, had initiated the first comprehensive, compulsory, government-sponsored medical care program in North America and was the only place with any experience of what might transpire in the rest of Canada.

And there were effects. Swanson noted that in their three post-medicare years nearly twice as many people were hospitalized.[83] Outpatient care had almost doubled, with the greatest increases in the smaller hospitals, some having increases of multiples of their previous number. It was unclear whether these increases were a result of medicare or the addition of outpatient benefits to Saskatchewan's hospital insurance plan.[84]

A few years later DHA grad R.B. Ferguson, who at that time was the executive director of Humber Memorial Hospital wrote an article on hospitals and the Canadian economy. He called the Hospital Insurance and Diagnostic Services Act the "best piece of social legislation enacted in the last ten years." He also noted the "era of the private health insurance carrier has passed."[85]

INITIATIVES OF DHA ALUMNI

DHA Grad Secretary to Woods Royal Commission

In the summer of 1963 back in Roth's old Department of Public Health in Saskatchewan the Saskatoon Agreement had ostensibly resolved the Doctors' Strike. However, as former premier Romanow puts it, this resolution "was only on the surface." Beneath, the "undercurrents were strong and swift moving." They concerned hospital privileges and recurring rulings by the Saskatchewan College of Physicians and Surgeons that physicians who had delivered services during the strike "were somehow not qualified to be granted hospital privileges."[86]

To deal with the issue, two future premiers and a DHA graduate were involved. Premier Lloyd had asked Alan Blakeney to be minister of health in order to stickhandle the rearguard actions of the physicians and protect the nascent legislation (and hence the medicare program) and the individual rights of physicians. Two royal commissions were set up; first the Thomson Commission and later the Woods Commission. DHA graduate Ed Wahn, who had recruited then DHA candidate Roth from the U of T program to Saskatchewan, was secretary to the Woods Commission and future premier Roy Romanow served as assistant secretary to Wahn.[87] Marchildon noted that Romanow was highly influenced by this experience for the rest of his life.[88]

DHA Grad Proposes Health Admin Master's to University of Alberta

In 1966, DHA graduate Carl Meilicke proposed a graduate course in health administration for Western Canada. He approached Walter Mackenzie, dean of medicine at the University of Alberta, to say that the Kellogg Foundation might be interested in funding a master's program in health services administration within the Faculty of Medicine. Meilicke was a recent graduate of the hospital administration PhD program at the University of Minnesota. U of A's proposal was approved by the foundation in 1967 and Mackenzie recruited Meilicke as the first director of the new Division of Health Services Administration, a position he held until 1980. The first students were admitted in 1968.[89]

Meilicke said, "The times begged for better policy research, better planning and better administration at all levels of the health care system."[90] Incidentally, his PhD dissertation was on the Saskatchewan Doctors' Strike.[91]

DHA Alum Initiates Health Admin Specialization to University of Saskatchewan MBA

The same year (1966) that Carl Meilicke was proposing the Alberta program, Frank Silversides (DHA class of 1951) was starting a specialization on health administration as part of the University of Saskatchewan MBA. The program began in September 1967, a year before the Alberta program. They applied to Kellogg for funding but were unsuccessful, likely because Kellogg wanted such programs to be within a school of public health.

There was actually some drama associated with this, as the president of the University of Alberta wrote to the president of the U of S in September 1967 to note that they had received funding to start a program in September 1968 and wondered if the U of S might consider dropping their program.[92] This sparked a flurry of activity between the division of health administration in the College of Commerce, the dean, and the U of S president as they contemplated how to respond.

DHA Alum Forms External Advisory Committee to U of S Certificate Program

In 1968 Frank Silversides proposed reconstituting an Advisory Committee to the U of S certificate correspondence program in hospital administration. Interestingly, there were three DHA alumni (Wahn, Meilecke, and Silversides) as well as a DPH alum (Vince Matthews) on the earlier committee.[93] It had been acting in that capacity but Silversides wanted to reconstitute it into a committee that comprised practitioners primarily. He received approval from the dean and a new committee was struck in February 1968. Its membership was administrators of hospitals of various sizes and from different parts of the province. One member was A.E. Boehm, who was administrator of the Holy Family Hospital in Prince Albert at the time.[94]

We noted earlier that this program had originally been started by DHA grad Meilicke. Over the ensuing years it proved to be quite a success. In 1984 it had 124 graduates, who were not limited to Saskatchewan but were from across Canada, including the territories.[95] In 1987 36 per cent of the students were from Saskatchewan and there was an average of 125 graduates per year since 1982. Enrolment in the program (number of students registered) was 120 students by 1966, increased to 300 by the late 1970s, and to 350 in the 1980s. Students were from all provinces in Canada as well as several from outside the country.[96]

AMALGAMATION OF HOSPITAL ADMIN AND PUBLIC HEALTH INTO DEPARTMENT OF HEALTH ADMIN

In 1967 Roth, "the widely respected head of the Department of Hospital Administration," was chosen to succeed Milton Brown as the head of the Department of Public Health in the school.[97] He was also appointed associate director of the school.[98] He was a strong choice.

Roth headed up the Department of *Hospital* Administration, and perhaps partly as a result of his strong background in public health, the school combined the Departments of Hospital Administration and Public Health Administration into a single Department of *Health* Administration, with Roth as its head. The amalgamation removed overlaps in teaching and recognized the increasing interdependency of the different facets of health-care management and delivery. It merged Public Health Administration people like Clute, Hastings, Langford, Mosley, and Schwenger with existing Hospital Administration faculty into the new department.[99]

Roth noted at the time the general feeling that there was need for some kind of universal health care, that one should discontinue the sharp distinction between public health and hospital administration. This was influenced by the fact that Milton Brown had hoped for an integration, for a total system of health care that had not yet developed, that public health and medical care still remained quite distinct.[100] It is an issue with which we still wrestle.

Roth already had the status of professor of medical care administration in the School of Hygiene, Department of Public Health. With this dual appointment the Public Health and Hospital Administration Departments were combined into a new Department of *Health* Administration. This was proposed by A.J. Rhodes, director of the school, to Dr J.D. Hamilton, vice-president, Health Sciences, for the university in a letter dated 3 March 1967. In the letter Rhodes noted the reasons why such an amalgamation should occur, listing nine reasons for the proposal, including "a common core of academic interest," "much greater possibility of developing research activities which involve the relationship of health services in the community and in hospitals," and "considerable overlap in the teaching responsibilities" of the two departments. Another reason was that the Department of Hospital Administration was a small department, with only three full-time staff (though it had many part-time and sessional lecturers). It said this lack had hindered progress at the graduate degree level and made it difficult to carry out research.[101]

A further reason was that the new department would have approximately twenty full-time academic staff. They would be involved in "teaching 70 or 80 graduate diploma students registered in the School of Hygiene" and MSc students registered in the Graduate Department of the School of Hygiene. In addition there would be teaching of approximately 400 undergraduates registered in the Faculties of Pharmacy and Food Sciences and the Schools of Nursing and Physical and Health Education. A further reason was that "the new department will represent what is often referred to as an 'area of excellence' able to compete even with the larger Schools of Public Health in the U.S.A."[102]

The proposal noted that the amalgamated department would have five sections. Three major sections would be Public Health Administration, Hospital Administration, and Medical Care Administration and the two smaller sections, Social Science in Public Health and International Health Administration.[103] Public Health Administration and Hospital Administration were both headed by John Hastings, Medical Care Administration by Fred Mott, and International Health Administration by Harry Gear.[104] The faculty in Social Sciences were A.P. Ruderman and Ken Clute.[105]

Rhodes noted in his annual report to the president that Ruderman was a "well-known health economist and administrator." Rhodes stated Ruderman had served for many years on the headquarters staff of the Pan American Health Organization in Washington and so had a wide knowledge of health administration in the Americas.[106]

There was also a formal six-page proposal in the president's file that went into much more detail on the assignment of teaching responsibilities, the different graduate diploma degrees being conferred by the school, the graduate degree programs, undergraduate programs, and responsibilities of the various sections. It also noted two changes on the teaching of preventive medicine: the formation of a Committee on the Teaching of Preventive Medicine and an Interdivisional Committee on the Future of Preventive Medicine. The first would report to the director of the school, the second to the vice-president (Health Sciences) of the university.[107] Claude Bissell, president of the university, sent a letter to Rhodes on 6 April 1967, indicating that the board of governors of the University had approved Roth's appointment.[108]

Rhodes in his annual report to the president noted it had "become evident in the last few years that there is a considerable community of interest not only in academic circles but in the field between those who administer hospitals and those who have a wider responsibility for the administration of health services, for example medical care and public health services."[109]

Bator notes that the move to combine the departments "reflected the advent of a common core of academic interests centering on the organization and administration of all health services." In merging the public health and hospital roles, "both ultimately had to serve the needs of the community." He also notes that a distinguishing feature of the school in the 1960s was the extent to which it changed and its openness to change. He said members of the school did not resist change; rather, "they realized the absolute need to modify programs, courses, and departments."[110]

The focus and curriculum also needed to evolve to recognize the different complexion of the system itself. Roth notes that the health care system was becoming much more diverse and complex. What it needed was not just hospital administrators with a specialist education in hospitals but managers with a kind of generalist education that allowed them to move into a multiplicity of roles. These included hospitals, or within government administering a medical insurance program, or home care programs, medical care administration, or public health administration.[111]

One criticism of the department was that it was not doing much research and that its faculty had little inclination to do so. And yet as Roth's department and that of Public Health was being reorganized into one of *Health* Administration, Roth felt he felt he might have been looked upon somewhat pejoratively because he was not a researcher. He found the transition to academia from government challenging and he was not "research oriented." He mentioned that rather than get involved in a research program he got involved in setting up the Metro Toronto Home Care Program and became its president. He observed "'I don't know how I was regarded by my colleagues at the university, I suspect with some disdain,'" in that he wasn't a typical academic.[112]

But that said, he felt there needed to be a "better balance between a practical hands-on approach and academic investigation." He argued they can coexist, and that they involve quite different skills, problems, and ways of accomplishing things. He noted that the school tended to be rather pedestrian, but its emphasis was on trying to equip people to cope with problems out there in the field, in essence to "say to people these are the ways in which this is accomplished" to take "reasonably knowledgeable people and make them [more] reasonably knowledgeable" – people who can deal with a multiplicity of situations, and reason their way through any complex problem. He said it was the issue of generalists versus specialists. There were more and more specialists but there was no cross-fertilization between the two.[113]

One change with the merger of the two departments was a difference in publication activity. Whereas previously faculty and graduates were publishing in *Canadian Hospital*, and graduates and people like Agnew continued to do so, now Roth and others (such as John Hastings) were publishing in more academic journals such as the *Canadian Journal of Public Health*.

Roth was also concerned with two other trends in the field: the separation between public health and "curative medicine" and the increasing fractionation of knowledge. He said that at the same time as the general body of knowledge had increased the response had been a fractionation of the efforts of individuals and the so-called rise of the specialist who has mastered a relatively narrow area of the broad field he worked in. He said this posed organizational problems in trying to make sense of the way in which the total system operates.[114]

There was another aspect to this academic tension. Roth was very much a part of educating doers, giving people the requisite skills to run a hospital, a public health system, or any of the other health care organizations now emerging. However, the department was now part of a larger and emerging constellation of forces, and that was a disciplinary as opposed to a professional commitment. The department and the school needed to be a part of this activity. Indeed some saw this as its singular activity. This tension, and the school's significant commitment to knowledge for practical outcomes, was at odds with an objective of generating new theoretical knowledge. A balance needed to be found.

Along with all this, it was proposed that the degrees granted be changed. The council of the school felt that almost all of the diplomas should be replaced with three new professional master's degrees. It was felt that "the diploma pattern of postgraduate education, based on that offered in the United Kingdom, is now outmoded and little used in Canada" and in the United States. It proposed a master of public health, master of health administration (with one stream in hospital administration and one stream in medical care administration), and a master of public health sciences.[115]

FRED MOTT

Roth in his new role as director was able to convince his former boss in Saskatchewan, Fred Mott, to follow him into the academic milieu and take over his former role in medical care administration. He was there from 1968 to 1972. In speaking of Mott, Bator notes, "A distinguishing hallmark of the University of Toronto School of Hygiene was the presence on the faculty of leaders with a proven track record of accomplishment in Canadian health services."[116] Before coming to the school and in many instances while on the faculty of the school, many of these faculty "pioneered the establishment and development of provincial health systems in Canada." Mott was an "outstanding example of these senior statesmen."[117] The director of the school, A.J. Rhodes, referred to Mott as an "elder statesman" with an "unrivalled knowledge of health administration."[118]

Mott had been hired by Douglas in 1946 to plan and implement the first hospital insurance program in North America. Douglas, in his first term, was also minister of health. Douglas had set up a Health Services Planning Commission (HSPC) and bypassed his own department by having it report directly to him. Mott had been recommended to Douglas, and Douglas had gone to Washington to appeal to Mott. Douglas wanted him to head up the HSPC.

While at the HSPC Mott had involved it in four major activity areas that would have been an important model for students in the DHA and DPH programs. The first was administering the hospital insurance program. Interestingly, at year-end each family received a receipt (which could be used to claim income tax deductions under Canadian tax law) indicating the amount of hospital costs paid on its behalf by the SHSP.[119] The second was the establishment of health regions, which were local government units formed under the Saskatchewan Health Services Act to provide a complete range of public health services. This was an early recognition of a concentration on two areas: individual health and illness care and population health and the prevention of illness from happening in the first place. A third area was involving the HSPC in research functions: on medical programs, health data, personnel requirements, and hospital facilities and operations. A fourth area was providing support and funding for innovative health-care programs. There were two main initiatives here: one a universal tax supported a health insurance project in Swift Current. The second was the municipal doctor program, which involved negotiations between local governments and medical societies.[120]

These were all areas that Roth continued and built further upon when he became deputy minister. He would add regional hospital councils, which would have boundaries different from those of the health regions. However, in sum, it was a real boon to have had Mott and Roth, who were both so integral to the development and operation of the only hospital insurance program on the continent at the School of Hygiene, to have had the benefit of their thoughts in the areas noted above, particularly in what today we would differentiate as health systems and public health.

Some years later the HSPC was positioned in the Department of Public Health and the chair of the HSPC and deputy minister's positions were combined. Mott served in this role in 1950–51. Interestingly, Mott had hired Roth, who in the reorganization became director of the Division of Hospital Administration and Standards and succeeded him as deputy minister.

Mott was also intimately familiar with rural health and had co-authored a book on the subject with Milton Roemer.[121] Mott had been part of the Farm Security Administration program in the United States, part of Roosevelt's New Deal medicine, which had basically implemented a form of health insurance for the rural population in the United States during the Depression years. For part of this time he also concurrently had a commission in the US Public Health Service (a part of the Surgeon General's Office) when it flirted with the idea of health insurance from the mid-1930s to mid-1940s.[122]

He also came by his ideals early. As a medical student at McGill University in 1932 he wrote a paper on state medicine, which he referred to as "a cooperative medical venture with state backing."[123] It sets out a complete health-care delivery template that also recognized the importance of hospitals and preventive medicine, one that a person could see as foundational to his later activities.

In it he noted, "The state is coming to realize that the health of the people is its chief asset, and should therefore be its chief care."[124] He was critical of the European systems, saying, "The principle of spreading the cost of medical care over a large group is in itself excellent, but in a scheme of health insurance there are many shortcomings"[125] because they were focused on the poor and ignored the plight of the middle class. He felt that the medical profession should lead in organizing and planning such a service, which should be administered as an autonomous unit in government.[126]

Mott's expertise in public health and health insurance was undoubtedly recognized. Prior to his coming to U of T he wrote a report for Governor G. Mennon Williams of Michigan, who had convened a conference on health and medical care. The report was very comprehensive, getting into all aspects of care, but also dealing with issues such as strengthening public health organizations and support for research. A large portion of it dealt with health insurance, where he advocated that there "be prompt development of a national policy on health insurance."[127]

While at U of T Mott served on the WHO Expert Advisory Panel on the Organization of Medical Care.[128]

Comment

During the period these two individuals were there, the Department of Health Administration had two of the foremost minds in health insurance and public health. They had been at the cutting edge of health policy, not just in this country but on the continent. They had published widely, and each of them had also been involved in groundbreaking policy development at the highest levels of government.

Mott had successfully implemented the first universal hospital insurance program on the continent. He had done so on a very strict timeline in order that the program be operational well in advance of the next provincial election. His template would serve as the template for the rest of the provinces. Roth had arrived in Saskatchewan shortly after the program was implemented and headed one of its key divisions. He quickly rose to the level of deputy minister and oversaw the operation of the program. He later chaired the Interdepartmental Committee, which developed the blueprint for a medical insurance program, which, as it turned out, also served as the template for the rest of the provinces. Each of these, as a working model, influenced the federal government to provide the legislation and funds for what was a national program, provincially administered.

Roth knew that his era was at the confluence of a number of emerging forces, not just in health management, but in knowledge itself. He clearly understood the distinctions between hospital administration, medical administration, and health system administration. Moreover, he understood the increasing fractionation of knowledge into specialties and educationally the implication this had between specialists and generalists. A further distinction was between a theoretical versus a practical orientation.

THE DEPARTMENT AND THE SCHOOL'S INVOLVEMENT IN THE HALL COMMISSION

Discussion Leading Up to the Hall Commission

It is interesting that the kind of activist agenda that FitzGerald took on providing some sort of universal health insurance was continued. For example, Andrew Rhodes commented on it in his annual report to the president in 1960–61: "Plans for a comprehensive health service in Canada continue to arouse controversy, although there can be no doubt of the increasing public and official interest in a service financed on a prepayment basis." He noted the United Kingdom's program and that "Canada is still a long way from one." He said, "It is the role of an academic institution such as our School, concerned as it is with the maintenance and improvement of the public health, to study the problems of a comprehensive health scheme objectively, to seek for general principles, and to suggest sound practical applications."[129]

The Department and the School and the Hall Commission

The school and the department were very active in a number of Canadian commissions on health. Two of the major ones so far were the Royal Commission on Health Services and the earlier House of Commons Special Committee on Social Security.

Submission from the School (1962)

The School of Hygiene presented a brief to the commission in May 1962. Rhodes, Brown (DPH, 1939), and Hastings were the presenters. Roth had already presented to the Commission in January of that year in his capacity as deputy minister of public health in Saskatchewan.[130] There were a number of similarities to the Saskatchewan presentation to the commission in things like the emphasis on prevention and its accent on community care. Roth was still deputy minister in May, but weeks away from coming to the school to take up his position as head of the Department of Hospital Administration, so one wonders if there was any dialogue between him and its authors, such as its principal author, Andrew Rhodes, head of the school, who had hired Roth. It also had input from John Hastings, a member of the faculty and author of his own report for the commission. It was one, perhaps the only one, from academia to come out in support of a national insurance plan.

It noted, "Our objective is a *Comprehensive Health Service* which will make it possible for all Canadians to have the benefits of modern health care, without regard to means, age, occupation, or place of residence."[131] The brief's major point was the importance of public health. It also noted that hospitals were emerging as the real centre for scientific medical work; that it was only in hospitals or large clinics that the full range of specialized and costly equipment needed for diagnosis and therapy could be provided. In this regard it noted that hospitals needed to be planned on a regional basis and administered by trained managers.[132]

It elaborated on the idea of a comprehensive health service by noting that it had four major components: public health services, hospital services, professional and technical people providing personal health services, and voluntary health agencies. It noted that government already played a major role in the direction of hospital and public health services. It now felt that it needed to move into personal health services: "*This move has been discussed in Canada for over forty years and has been taken in many other countries.* Those who feel it to be unnecessary have had all these years to put forward an effective alternative scheme. *No adequate alternative, which would embrace the principles we have laid down above has in our opinion been put forward.*"[133]

Bator notes that Rhodes's advocacy of health insurance "earned him some bitter criticism from his colleagues in the medical school." The School of Hygiene was tagged with the epithet "the little red schoolhouse." However, given what eventuated with the commission's report, that is, a national plan for health insurance, the school's stance was farsighted, as much of what it advocated came to be accepted by all provinces.[134]

Connaught Laboratories also presented a brief to the commission, one concerned mainly with drugs. It said a medical care insurance plan should cover some but not all drugs. It recommended drug benefits be initiated by "providing only the more expensive drugs needed for long periods" and that over time the scope of service should be enlarged.[135]

Ted Goldberg's Dissertation Quoted in the Ontario Legislature (1963)

By the time of the Hall Commission and prior to the release of its report, there was new leadership in the Conservative party that was much less disposed than Leslie Frost had been to a government plan. The Robarts administration was dead set against a public plan and was equally committed to preserving and growing the business of the private plans.

This stance was creating tensions in the legislature with both opposition parties, but particularly the NDP. The misgivings of the NDP were expressed in detail with the NDP member for Woodbine charging, "The government has capitulated 100 per cent to insurance companies and the medical profession."[136] Interestingly he mentioned the dissertation of Ted Goldberg (future head of the Department of Health Administration), quoted from parts of it, and its comparison of two Hamilton voluntary plans.[137]

Other Citations of Ted Goldberg's Dissertation

Goldberg's dissertation had some interesting inter-loan requests. One was from Ottawa by B.R. Blishen in 1963 while Blishen was research director for the Royal Commission of Health Services. Another was from Saskatoon by W.P. Thompson, former president of the University of Saskatchewan and head of the Thompson Commission, which was the public consultation body for medical insurance under T.C. Douglas.[138] Thompson's request was undoubtedly for material for his book on medical insurance (in which he cited Goldberg).[139]

Thompson had written to Goldberg about Goldberg's work in Hamilton. Goldberg had sent Thompson an abstract of the thesis and provided direction on how to obtain the full thesis. He had also said to Thompson that he was "thoroughly familiar" with Thompson's work on the Advisory Planning Committee and felt that it had "made a tremendous contribution, both to the province as well as to the development of medical care programs."[140]

Also at around this time Ted was corresponding with Andrew Andras, the director of legislation for the Canadian Labour Congress as the Congress was working out its views on the debates on health insurance taking placc in the House of Commons.[141]

Hastings Quoted in the Ontario Legislature

On Health Insurance (1965)

After the Hall Commission Report was released with its advocacy of a Saskatchewan-type plan, the Robarts government continued to work toward a private alternative. In the ensuing debate Hastings was quoted in the legislature as having said to the *Globe and Mail*, "Public schemes are almost more responsive to the needs of subscribers and less expensive to the public than private plans." He also provided facts regarding the Saskatchewan plan premium contrasted to those suggested by the government's Hagey report recommending private carriers. The minister of health took issue with Hastings's figures without providing any of his own to refute them.[142]

On Public Health (1966)

Hastings was quoted as saying that the Hall Report was deficient in its role for public health. Stephen Lewis quoted from a paper by Hastings that public health departments are not given "a particularly active role" in the future development of health services.[143] He was quoted again the next day on regionalization and coordination of health services and his study for the Royal Commission, whose publication was imminent.[144]

The Hastings/Mosley Study (1966)

Though the report of the commission itself received the most attention, a significant strength of the overall report was its subsidiary studies. One by J.E.F. Hastings and William Mosley was published two years after the main report and was on community health services. It recommended comprehensive public health services across the country.

Its main premise was regional coordination of services:

> Scientific, social and economic changes are making the traditional pattern of separately developed and administered community health services less and less efficient. Circumstances have combined to create a rapid proliferation of health services of ever increasing complexity. The resultant overlapping of service in some areas, gaps in service in other areas, and uneconomic use of skilled personnel and complex facilities are hampering the ultimate objective of providing a balanced pattern of modern community health services which work together effectively. Segregated community health service planning and administration should be ended. *Therefore, the main suggestion is for a regional administrative pattern for all community health services.*"[145]

Another area of comment concerned the training of hospital administrators. It noted the University of Toronto and University of Montreal programs along with that offered by the Canadian Hospital Association. Along with this was a recommendation for a course comparable to that offered through the University of Saskatchewan for administrators of small hospitals of fifty beds or fewer. It was suggested this be through an Ontario university in conjunction with the Canadian and Ontario Hospital Associations.[146] It tied this into a recommendation for a regional hospital services organization.[147]

The Hastings/Mosley Report did not receive much attention in the commission's final report and John Hastings was later told by a senior consultant to the commission that it was the result of the commission's decision not to further alienate organized medicine. It was felt that they would already be upset with the commission's proposal for medical insurance and that advocating a major restructuring of the health-care system would greatly add to that alienation.[148]

Comment of the School on the Commission's Report

Rhodes also commented on the report itself. Two recommendations of the commission were "of particular and immediate interest to the School of Hygiene." One was that grants be made available to establish undergraduate and postgraduate courses in health services administration. The other was for training grants to be made available to graduate students proceeding to a higher degree. He said, "It follows that the School of Hygiene, as the oldest-established and most experienced educational institution in Canada in this area should provide such courses."[149]

He also commented on the reception of the report: "The concept of society as increasingly involved in the provision of health services to its members has gained wide acceptance on the part of the general public." But he noted, "Acceptance of this concept by some members of the medical and dental professions has been less than enthusiastic." He cited the events in Saskatchewan in this regard.[150]

He also noted a need to "retread" senior health personnel and educate graduates on the school's programs of the wider concepts in health services administration as "expressed with such clarity" in the report. He noted that the report "stresses the urgent need for well-prepared administrators who can take a broad view of the complex workings of modern health services."[151]

In his last annual report he commented again on the Hall Commission Report: "It is said that Toronto's professional schools tend to be conservative, yet at the time of the Royal Commission on Health Services (Hall Commission), when many of our colleagues in other professional divisions supported the *status quo*, a group in the School supported the concept of state responsibility for the organization and financing of personal health services" a concept since accepted in all provinces."[152]

Rhodes makes an important distinction when he says state involvement in personal health services. State involvement in community health services – whether the community is the locale, province, or nation – has always been accepted, because the costs of not doing so are so high both economically and socially, as the costs of not doing so are big increases in disease or, even worse, epidemics.

COMMENT ON THE TENOR OF RHODES'S ANNUAL REPORTS

Rhodes wrote roughly fifteen annual reports to the president (beginning in 1956–57). They make for very interesting reading as they had greater length and depth than the reports of other faculty and departmental heads. They went beyond the normal reporting of highlights and interwove ideals of public health, the role of the school, and a connection to Canadian political and social movements into his reports. Over time he found a certain style; his first few reports were closer to the norm.

Bator also comments on the latter reports: Rhodes "reported on more than the activities and affairs of the school." He "displayed a keen appreciation of the role of history" and a "keen awareness of the interplay among the social and political principles." Rhodes's reports "represent an articulate statement of the philosophy of Canadian Public Health, rather unique in his time and still unique today."[153]

The following will illustrate some of the character of his reports. In 1960–61 he spoke of plans for a comprehensive health insurance program in Canada and quoted from Winston Churchill on British initiatives.[154] There is also his last report in 1969–70. We noted in the previous section his comment on how the school took a much more activist approach to the Hall Commission. He continued his activist emphasis by noting an address of President Bissell in which Bissell said while the primary purpose of the university was to preserve, disseminate, and expand knowledge, it also had an indispensable, if secondary, social role in which it should be "both active and critical." This included sharpening the social consciousness of the student.[155]

He quoted extensively from material coordinated by Peter Ruderman of the Department of Health Administration for an accreditation visit by the American Public Health Association, where Ruderman spoke of the objectives and ideals of public health. Two principles stressed in the material were the interdisciplinary nature and community basis of its approach.[156]

OTHER GOVERNMENT REPORTS CITING WORKS BY FACULTY

Ontario Committee on the Healing Arts

The Hastings study for the Hall Commission illustrates another way in which the department continued to exert influence on health care: faculty wrote or otherwise participated in major government studies or commissions. Works of department faculty were also cited in government studies and committees. During Roth's tenure the Ontario Committee on the Healing Arts in 1970 is an example. Mott, Clute, and Hastings were cited in volume two of the report.[157]

In volume three, Roth and Clute were referenced. For example Roth was cited for his views on expanding the role of hospitals, i.e., integrating them with other types of medical or social services in the community in something called "progressive patient care." He expressed misgivings about hospitals moving into this area, saying that while attractive conceptually, there were many problems to be surmounted in organizational and executive competence.[158] Hastings also wrote an editorial on the committee's report.[159]

Faculty were also quoted in some of the study volumes of the committee. In the one on the economic aspects of health care, Fred Mott's book on rural health care and John Hastings's study for the commission were noted. Ken Clute's book on the general practitioner was extensively referenced. For example, Clute and Mott were cited on the issues faced by rural physicians in their practices.[160] The School of Hygiene had completed a questionnaire for the committee.[161]

Ontario Health Planning Task Force

Another example is the report of the Ontario Health Planning Task Force. In it the Community Health Centre Project, undertaken by a committee chaired by Hastings (which we will look at in a subsequent section), was mentioned.[162]

LECTURES BY ROTH AND DEPARTMENT STAFF OUTSIDE THE UNIVERSITY

Earlier we noted Agnew's international talks when he was department head. Roth was in high demand to deliver lectures outside the university. As with Agnew, most were in Canada; however, also like Agnew, a number were outside Canada.

Roth's first year was his heaviest for outside speaking engagements. This reflected his previous connection to the implementation of medical insurance in Saskatchewan, which began on the day he started at U of T. Its novelty and the controversy surrounding it with physicians withdrawing services received international coverage. There was a wish to hear Roth's insights. In that year, places in which he spoke included Winnipeg, Miami, Toronto, and at the Quebec Hospital Association and Maritime Hospital Association.[163] Other examples are in 1966–67 he spoke on medicare in Canada to the Medical College of Virginia.[164] In October 1967 he was rapporteur of a meeting of the WHO Expert Committee on Hospital Administration in Geneva.[165]

Mott was also in high demand. In 1966–67 he presented "What More Prepayment of Medical Services Will Do to Hospitals" to the American College of Hospital Administrators District 8 Assembly, and "Current Developments in Medical Service Insurance in Canada" to the Conference of State and Provincial Health Authorities."[166] Also, the same academic year, Hastings spoke in Nagpur, India.[167]

EUGENIE STUART RETIRES

In October 1971 Eugenie Stuart retired. A tribute dinner for her was held at the Royal York Hotel.

Much of her background was contained in a tribute delivered by Jim McNab, DHA graduate and the recently appointed executive director of TGH.[168] He always had great respect for her. For that reason as well as the fact that she received her nursing degree from TGH (which was also the site of her first job), it was probably especially fitting that he delivered the tribute address.[169] Jim was also an example of the success of the program that Eugenie had dedicated herself to, a program that could generate a calibre of graduate to run Canada's premier hospital facilities (the University Avenue hospitals were testimony to this).

Eugenie was notable not only for her contribution to teaching but also her role as a student confidante. Agnew noted that she was a "mother confessor to succeeding classes for more than twenty years until her retirement in 1971." He also noted that she had "considerable administration experience in Canada and South Africa."[170]

She was also dedicated to the Department. The department was her life not only because it comprised the majority of her career but she was also totally committed to it. This was exemplified not only in the countless hours over many years she spent on department activities but also in a very generous bequest she made to the department that became the basis of the Eugenie Stuart Awards.

A memento of pictures and letters regarding the testimonial dinner spoke volumes of the esteem in which she was held by former students. Letters and telegrams were received from across Canada. W.A. Holland, president, Canadian Hospital Association and administrator, Oshawa General Hospital, sent a letter. There were letters from the University of Ottawa and Queen's University. There were telegrams from the United States and overseas; from institutions like Northwestern University (Chicago), Kaiser Foundation Hospital, the American College of Hospital Administrators, and the King's Fund in London. In addition, Frank Reeves from the King's Fund attended in person.[171]

Even after her formal retirement she still attended functions of the department and the Society of Graduates for many years. She was always introduced to the audience when she attended. Jim McNab was always very attentive to her at these functions.[172] Other graduates who achieved prominence in the field, such as Ron McQueen at Agnew Peckham Consultants or Gerry Turner, executive director of Mount Sinai, spoke fondly of her.

WHERE GRADS ENDED UP: IV

Here is a selected list of thesis topics and where grads ended up during Roth's term:

- Harold Livergant (DHA, 1964), first executive director of the Metropolitan District Health Council and co-founder and CEO of Extendicare. His thesis topic was "The Global Budget."
- Tomy Dagnone (DHA, 1967), whose thesis title was "A Study of Multiple Unit Hospital Systems." He received the Robert Wood Johnson Award for 1967. He is former CEO of the Royal University Hospital in Saskatoon (his family emigrated to Saskatchewan from Italy).[173] He was also CEO of the University Hospital in London and London Health Sciences Centre. He noted that a big attractor to the Toronto program was Burns Roth being its director.[174]
- Dieter Kuntz (DHA, 1968), whose thesis title was "A Step-by-Step Procedure to Establish a Preventive Maintenance Program," was a preceptor for students in the University of Saskatchewan and Canadian Hospital Association courses in hospital administration.[175] He was later CEO of Oakville-Trafalgar Memorial Hospital.
- David W. Corder (DHA, 1970), a native of Saskatchewan, studied nursing in Scotland, then Halifax (Dalhousie), then the DHA program. He was a director of nursing at the Victoria Hospital in London. He received the G. Harvey Agnew Award as the top student.[176] His thesis topic was "Operating Room Technicians: Their Role and Functions as Seen by Operating Room Supervisors." He analyzed their role at TGH and recognized its CEO, J.D. Wallace, in the acknowledgements.[177]

- Theodore Freedman (DHA, 1970), former CEO, Mount Sinai, whose thesis title was "A Review of the Experience of the In-Common Laboratory in the Development of Joint Laboratory Services." He received the Robert Wood Johnson Award for 1970.
- Leo Steven (DHA, 1970), former CEO, Sunnybrook Health Sciences Centre, whose thesis title was "A Survey of Medical Audit Programs in Teaching Hospitals in Canada."

Longer Bios on Selected Grads

Gerald Hiebert (DHA, 1966, class of 1964) on leaving the program was appointed assistant administrator (and later administrator) of Saskatchewan Hospital in Weyburn (Tommy Douglas's old riding). When the hospital was completed in 1921 it was the largest building in the British Commonwealth.[178] In 1967 he was appointed administrative assistant to the College of Health Services at McMaster University, where he was involved in the development and building of its new medical school.[179] His thesis topic was "A Survey of Organized Recreation in Acute Treatment Hospitals over 200 Beds."

Another grad during Roth's time was Jeannine Girard-Pearlman (DHA, 1972). She had a series of senior administrative positions at Mount Sinai Hospital culminating in senior vice-president. During her time at Mount Sinai she continued to be involved in the department/institute and remains involved with the university. Her thesis was "The Four-Day Work Week and the Hospital." Interestingly attached to Jeannine's thesis there is a copy of a request from an educational institution in the Netherlands requesting her permission to copy it. So, evidently, even though the theses were sometimes criticized as not being "academic" enough, they had some heuristic value.[180] Jeannine received an Arbor Award from U of T in 2017.

Roth's fellow classmate Edwin V. Wahn returned to Toronto in 1969 as executive director of the Metropolitan Toronto Hospital Planning Council. He resigned in 1971 because he felt the council lacked the power to solve Toronto's hospital planning problems.[181] While in Toronto one project was a 1970 plan to integrate five hospitals in the northwest of Toronto. In it he had an interesting discussion on hospitals as "dynamic institutions" in an environment of accelerating change and another on mergers and the limitation of large hospitals.[182]

What also should not be lost sight of is the fact that there were also people involved in the MSc degree in health administration. The School of Graduate Studies had recognized a Graduate Department of the School of Hygiene since 1963.[183] One example is Phyllis Jones from the Faculty of Nursing, who received such a degree in 1969.[184] She acknowledged Roth in her thesis.[185] She presented a number of papers at the School of Hygiene, one on the Hastings Report (Hall Commission), and one at the Inaugural Symposium of the Division of Community Health.[186] She became dean of nursing at U of T from 1979 to 1988.

An Even Longer Bio

Claus Wirsig (DHA, 1968) was also a Rhodes Scholar (1957–59) and received the Robert Wood Johnson Award for 1968. His thesis topic was "Management Initiative in the Organization and Staffing of the Patient Care Unit." He was born in Manitoba and attended the University of Alberta as an undergrad studying history and politics. He also received an MA from the U of A. He began his career as a journalist in Toronto, where he discovered a passion for health care. He was assistant editor for *Hospital Administration and Construction* from January 1961 to August 1962, then in September 1962 he became its managing editor. He became consulting editor in October 1966, leaving in September as the October issue went to press as his DHA classes began in September.[187]

Wirsig did his administrative residency at the Hospital for Sick Children and remained there afterward. He was executive director of the University Teaching Hospitals Association and of the Hospital Council for Metropolitan Toronto.[188] He ended his career as president of the Hospital for Sick Children Foundation.[189] He was appointed there in October 1977.[190] After his retirement, the foundation established the Claus Wirsig Humanitarian Award. He was also active in the World University Service of Canada.[191] Through them he participated in a study tour of the Soviet Union and Czechoslovakia with seven other Canadian students in 1956, where the group found that 70 per cent of practising doctors were women.[192]

His diploma thesis was notable for its combination of philosophical and practical approaches. He noted at its outset, "From my earliest contact with the hospital field, I was intrigued by the organizational systems and structures through which hospitals and their staffs seek to provide the health care and treatment needed by patients at various points in their lives."[193] He noted that while on the one hand he "marvelled at the tenacity and basic structure at the direct care level" in the face of many challenges, he also became "convinced that these strengths can also turn into weaknesses in the long run." One had traditions that were a mechanism for "continuity and relative certainty" but also an inherent conservatism and a certain unwillingness to change. Yet there was a continual need to absorb medical advances.[194] He set out to reconcile these differences. In his preface he acknowledged Eugenie Stuart and J.T. Law.[195]

John T. Law was the executive director of SickKids. He also started and became first president of its foundation (Wirsig became its second president). The relationship that developed between the two was an example of an important outgrowth of the DHA program. Law was Wirsig's preceptor for the residency piece of the DHA program, and Wirsig's respect for his mentor was evident in the tribute he wrote after Law's passing.[196]

Wirsig became a strong supporter of public health insurance (as did Law). When Wirsig entered the program, Ontario only had a public hospital insurance program. When it was implemented by Premier Leslie Frost there were fears in the hospital field that it would lead to a takeover of hospitals. There certainly were at SickKids[197] and were shared by many hospital administrators. It is important to point out, and this indicates the diversity of Canada, that the atmosphere in Ontario was very different from that of Saskatchewan, where the director of Wirsig's program, Burns Roth, came from.

Saskatchewan had been pioneering health programs for many years, some of which have been mentioned here. An important one was that of union hospitals. Partly as a result of this experience, and partly as a result of Douglas's ability as a politician and his ability to get the public on board with his programs, Saskatchewan implemented its hospital insurance program without the same apprehensions as Ontario, and it did so a number of years beforehand. The Douglas government was also a strong supporter of hospitals, and when Roth went to Saskatchewan after the U of T program, that support increased even further and Roth was very much at the centre of it.

Wirsig had a good vantage point on these developments in his role as assistant editor of *Hospital Administration in Canada*, and his position at the journal was ideal from which to witness the evolution of hospital insurance as well as the debate on medical insurance. Then when he was admitted to the program, it was under a director who had been heavily involved in both hospital and medical insurance in Saskatchewan, which served as the Canadian template in each case. And Wirsig still had the vantage point of being a consulting editor that the journal afforded.

This strong support for public health care remained with Wirsig. After he retired he presented on his own behalf to the Romanow Commission at its public hearings in Toronto on 31 May 2002 (see the section on the commission later in this work).

Demographic Profile of Student Cohorts

The class of 1962–64 had students from the following provinces/countries: Alberta (three), BC (two), Manitoba, Nova Scotia (two), Ontario, Quebec, Saskatchewan (two), Indonesia, and the Philippines.[198]

For the class of 1964–66 the breakdown was Alberta, BC, Manitoba, New Brunswick, Nova Scotia (two), Ontario, Saskatchewan (two), Canadian Armed Forces, New York, and Wisconsin. One of the applicants had an MPH from Harvard.[199]

For the class of 1966–68 it was Alberta, BC (three), Ontario (five), Manitoba, Saskatchewan (two), and Michigan. Two of these from other provinces had their original degree from the University of Saskatchewan.[200]

The Class of 1969

At the time of this writing the class of 1969 was planning a reunion in Toronto for September 2019. This provided an opportunity for me to get some information on the class of '69 from Don Carley, DHA graduate and reunion organizer.

This information, particularly the personal observations made by the individuals, provided a more intimate glimpse of the ensuing lives of graduates after they left the program. While this has been a history of the program, there is a much larger history out there – the individual lives of all the graduates, lives whose unfolding this program set on a new trajectory.

Here are some vignettes:

Don Carley went to Peel Memorial after graduation and stayed ten years. He then went to Queensway Carleton and then to Children's Hospital of Eastern Ontario. From there he returned to Alberta to University Hospital and then to executive director of the hospital in Cold Lake, site of the Canadian airbase. While there he organized a hospital fundraiser that brought the Royal Canadian Air Farce to Cold Lake. He closed out his career where he began it, as a pharmacist.

Al Whiting did his residency at Kingston General. He went from there to Oakville Trafalgar, then to Mississauga General, then to Scarborough Centenary as executive director, where he stayed for twenty-two years. He notes one of the most distinctive features of the Ontario Hospitals Association, its defined-benefits pension plan. He says, "A day doesn't go by that I do not thank the OHA for their great pension plan."[201]

Ken McGeorge (DHA, 1969) is active in New Brunswick. He is interim director of the Alzheimer Society of New Brunswick and vice-chair of the Coalition of Concerned Citizens, a group of long-time residents of New Brunswick who want to have a positive effect on the province by building an informed and empowered electorate. He is former CEO of the Dr Everett Chalmers Hospital and the York Care Centre, both in Fredericton. In 2016 he was picked by New Brunswick Health Minister Victor Boudreau and Social Development Minister Kathy Rogers to co-chair a council on aging. He has served on the Board of Directors of the New Brunswick Hospital Association and has been CEO of the Halifax Infirmary and Kingston General Hospital. He notes that one of the highlights was as CEO of the hospital in Red Lake, Ontario. He noted it was a "great lifestyle, remote, multi-cultural, great rural health strategy, wonderful people."[202]

Richard (Dick) Wall began his career as assistant administrator at the Victoria Union Hospital in Prince Albert, Saskatchewan. He went from there to being a hospital administration analyst with the Saskatchewan Hospital Services Plan in Regina, where he noted "we had constant company," no doubt due to the fact that Saskatchewan continued to pioneer in health. He was later executive director of the Alberta Hospital in Edmonton. While in that position he attended the World Mental Health Conference, which was held in Vancouver in 1977. While there he met Rosalynn Carter (who had chosen mental health as one of her projects as First Lady) and Margaret Mead.[203]

PART FIVE

Transition

CHAPTER 12

Moving on Many Fronts: 1

JOHN HASTINGS (1973–76)

His Background

John Hastings continued the idea, established by the tenure of Burns Roth, of a director with strong public health credentials. Moreover he came from a family steeped in the history, traditions, and philosophy of public health in Canada. His father's side had a medical background, his mother's, political. His paternal great-uncle was Charles Hastings, who had an international reputation as Toronto's medical officer of health from 1910 to 1929. Another great-uncle, Andrew (brother to Charles), was also a physician in Toronto, as was father, Elgin. On his mother's side a great-uncle, James S. Duff, was a minister of agriculture in the Whitney government of Ontario. His maternal great-grandfather, Thomas Roberts Ferguson, was an MPP for twenty years in the Ontario Legislature. A great-great-grandfather, Ogle Robert Gowan, was a federal MP.[1]

Hastings was fascinated by politics and had initially seriously considered studying political science and law but entered the pre-med program in September 1945. At U of T he was an active member in the Young Progressive Conservatives, "with a strong 'Red Tory' perspective." He had strong links with Hart House while at U of T and the wardens Joseph McCulley and Nicholas Ignatieff (brother to George Ignatieff, provost of Trinity College, and uncle to Michael Ignatieff) were said to be influential in his intellectual development. He did his internship at Toronto General Hospital, then arranged a special year with the School of Graduate Studies, taking courses in social psychology, mental health, and the evolution of the social welfare state and NHS in the United Kingdom. He became interested in the sociopolitical and economic bases of social and preventive medicine after hearing

Professor John Ryle, the first Regis Professor of Social Medicine at Oxford, speak at Convocation Hall in 1950.[2]

He then took postgraduate studies in public health at the School of Hygiene, receiving his DPH in 1954. For the next two years he was a fellow in preventive medicine at the school. During this time (1953–55) he was also a don in the men's residence at Victoria College. In 1956 he received the specialty qualification in public health from the Royal College of Physicians and Surgeons of Canada. He was the first person to receive this qualification through formal examination. In 1956 he was named a lecturer in the Department of Public Health Administration in the school. In 1964 he acquired a diploma in international health planning from Johns Hopkins University.[3] His term (noted above) was acting chair of the Department of Health Administration.

He firmly believed in public/community health as "a multi-disciplinary and eclectic discipline drawing together the expertise of a wide range of health-related and other disciplines in partnership with strong community practice links for promoting and protecting the health of the population." In his view, "academic teaching and research function most effectively when a core grouping of disciplines worked regularly together and reached out in collaboration with other areas of expertise in the University in a fully cross-disciplinary manner, according to the requisites for a particular area of investigation." In addition, "a close symbiotic relationship between the academic world and the field of practice was essential, each informing and supporting the other." He "consistently advocated the re-establishment of a modern school of public health as a full member among the health sciences rather than as an academic subdivision within the Faculty of Medicine."[4]

Bator notes that at the school, in the era before the 1970s, Hastings "encountered a vision of public health" that "had 'a kind of missionary quality.'" As a young faculty member he came into contact with a number of people who proved to be mentors, one of which was Milton Brown. Others (and here again a Saskatchewan connection) were Burns Roth and Fred Mott. Bator notes in an interview that took place after Hastings retired that Hastings said Burns Roth was "'one of the shrewdest and most perceptive individuals I ever met in the field'" and that Mott "'had devoted his life to trying to better circumstances of the poor.'" Another was Andrew Rhodes, who Hastings said had "enormous social insight and compassion and concern for society." He told Bator that people such as these made for a very progressive department, one active "for promoting health and preventing disease." He said an example was the stance it took on health insurance, one that was not popular at the time but based on the principles the school stood by.[5]

Hastings was also influenced by other giants in the field. Beveridge and his seminal report in the United Kingdom and its emphasis on social medicine had a big influence on him.[6] Another giant, one who also emphasized social medicine (as well as the importance of health insurance and the interrelationship between teaching and research) was Henry Sigerist from Johns Hopkins. Sigerist had done a study and report of Saskatchewan health care in 1944, a copy of which is in Hastings's personal records.[7] Sigerist was appointed by Tommy Douglas two days after being elected premier. His report was tabled in early October 1944 and served as a blueprint for the reform of health care in Saskatchewan.

Special Field Studies in Western Canada

While Hastings was a fellow at the school he went to the three western provinces in 1954 from the last week in July to the last week in September. He spent about five weeks of that time in Saskatchewan and the balance in Alberta and British Columbia. It is unclear whether this was his idea or that of R.D. Defries, the director of the school. It appeared that Defries provided the funding for the trip.[8] Defries also provided a letter of introduction to the deputy minister of health in Alberta and British Columbia.

Dr Hatcher (DPH, 1947), an assistant professor in public health administration, also wrote a letter to the assistant secretary of the CMA outlining the purpose of the trip. Hatcher notes it was their desire to have Hastings "obtain … first-hand experience of the integration of medical care administration with the administration of a provincial health department."[9]

The trip was to gather data on the health-care systems of the three provinces. But to what end? Whether it was it for curricula development or other purposes is unclear. It might have been to provide an opportunity for growth and development to someone being groomed to be a new faculty member. For Hastings it was educative. In addition to the gathering of information, his notes at various points had the heading "Problem" followed by potential issues he saw with what was being observed.

Alberta and British Columbia

The time spent in Alberta and BC was more observational than participative. In both provinces it involved interviews with people in the Department of Health as well as organizations such as Workmen's Compensation, Cancer Care, and physician-sponsored group health plans. In Alberta his notes make the observation that there is no direct legislative control of public money and that there is no real way to evaluate the quality of the service or manage usage. His notes on the BC visit indicate physician opposition to a government plan.[10]

Five Weeks at the Saskatchewan Department of Public Health

The trip to Saskatchewan had a different complexion. There was also a round of interviews. He not only observed but actually worked in the Medical Services Branch of the Department of Public Health in that province the last week in July until the end of August.[11] The letter from Hatcher noted the intent that Hastings relieve the medical assistant to the Saskatchewan Hospital Services Plan as well as the medical director of the indigent medical care plan.[12]

The time in Saskatchewan was interesting for a few reasons. First, the Saskatchewan Department had a reputation as a leading Department of Public Health. It had been attracting many of the best and brightest internationally ever since Tommy Douglas has been its minister (in addition to his role as premier) in his first administration (1944–48). Irrespective of who made the decision, it is likely that the idea to spend some time in the Saskatchewan department was a stimulating and important occasion.[13]

While Hastings was there, Milton Roemer from the United States was the head of the branch Hastings was in and he spent his first week working in Roemer's office. Burns Roth was deputy minister and Murray Acker was director of research.[14] Hastings later involved a number of the contacts he made in the department in committees or projects that he chaired or was in charge of. The branch Hastings was in was running several innovative programs and this was probably the reason for his placement. It was operating the first and at the time only air ambulance service in North America. It had the first and one of the few hospital insurance programs on the continent.

It had important municipal medical care programs such as the municipal doctor program and the union hospital district program. The department's annual report for the time noted the municipal doctor program had expanded to include not just providing for a portion of physician income but also entering into agreements "ensuring complete coverage of all residents, with a wide range of benefits." It also noted, "Physicians were expected to undertake a certain amount of public health work."[15] The scope of these services and their organization was very much in line with the values of the school. The section of the annual report for the Department of Public Health notes two distinguishing features of the plans: control was by an elected public body and coverage was comprehensive.[16] To this could be added the decentralized nature of the agreements with the physician: the agreements were between the municipalities and the physicians, not Regina and the physicians.

Hastings spent his first week working out of Roemer's office. Roemer was an advocate of social medicine and health insurance. Henry Sigerist had been an important influence on him, and it is likely that it was through Sigerist that Roemer ended up in Saskatchewan. Roemer had come to Canada because his left-wing leanings had put him on Senator McCarthy's radar. He eventually returned to the United States and became one of its leading academics in public health.[17] Hastings also spent time at the offices of the Saskatchewan Hospital Services Plan. He took over the duties of Dr R.G. Merifield, the acting director of the Medical Services Division, while he was on vacation. This was authorized personally by Roth, the deputy minister.[18] Hastings visited the offices of the doctor-sponsored medical insurance plans run out of Saskatoon and Regina. Based on correspondence with Defries, it would appear that the latter was involved in making the opportunity to visit the Saskatchewan Department available to Hastings.[19]

Hastings spent ten days in Swift Current with Dr Vince Matthews (DPH, 1947), the regional medical health officer, to see first-hand the operation of its health insurance program. He got an impression of its range of services, as his notes indicate that among the staff were nine nurses, four dentists, a psychologist, and a nutritionist, among others. It would have given him a very clear impression of its operation, as his notes indicate the level of physician satisfaction with the operation and also the fact that there was a physician who lent others money to start their practice and then expected them to refer patients to him.[20]

His visit to Vince Matthews would have been very stimulating, as Matthews had returned to Saskatchewan after receiving his DPH from the School of Hygiene and was one of its leading grads. The first universal hospital and medicare insurance and comprehensive children's dental programs in North America were pioneered and the first Regional Hospital Council was formed in Swift Current.[21]

Hastings spent time in every major area of the branch headed up by Roemer. He also spent time with Roemer himself, and his notes indicate discussions with Roemer on subjects such as physician capitation, patient choice of doctor, drug costs, what is a necessary service, and a provincial formulary. One note reads, "Any plan must take into account the cupidity of the doctors and the stupidity of the patients."[22]

The Medical Services Branch was at the heart of what the department was doing and would have given Hastings a very good idea of the range of the department's activities. The department also had a strong regional health services branch and it was involved in community-focused and prevention programs that would have been very much in line with Hastings's thinking. The Swift Current Medical Care Program that he visited was one of the branch's major programs.[23]

The objectives of the department were very consistent with Hastings's thinking. Its annual report for the year that included the time Hastings was there noted, "Four main spheres of activity concern the Department of Public Health: these are, the promotion of health, the prevention of illness, curative medical services, and the return to working capacity of the handicapped."[24]

There was also a strong emphasis on coordination between the different branches of the department, and this would have been very much in line with Hastings' later thinking on community health centres. The annual report for the previous year noted, "The organization of ... medical and hospital services into a branch of the Department of Public Health has provided various opportunities for coordination of services among division. Since many of the departmental activities relate to hospitals and since services of physicians and hospitals are obviously closely associated, there are common objectives that can be promoted.... At the same time, coordination between the Medical and Hospital Services and the activities of other branches of the Department of Public Health is actively promoted."[25]

Given the people involved and the innovative programs the department was administering, the visit provided substantial intellectual stimulation and he made a number of important contacts. Almost all the people Hastings spent time with ended up in senior positions, giving some indication of the quality of people with whom he was interacting. There could also have been other potential influences, which have to do with the context within which the Department of Public Health was situated. It was not the only Saskatchewan government department deemed to be innovative and at the cutting edge. The Douglas government was moving on a broad front, innovating in many areas. Its emphasis on planning and its Economic Advisory and Planning Board, its emphasis on budget and objective-setting through the Budget Bureau, and its recruitment mechanisms were all seen to be at the cutting edge. Also Saskatchewan was a bit of an economic hinterland. Many companies simply would not invest there, and Douglas was using Crown corporations as a mechanism to develop new business and diversify the economy. It was also sending its most promising civil servants off for advanced academic work, with many ending up at the Harvard School of Public Policy.[26]

All this gave Regina the reputation of a place of energy and innovation. The word was spreading. One of the people sent to Harvard, who studied under the legendary economist John Kenneth Galbraith, and who was the spouse of an IHPME alumnus (we will talk later of the award he established in her name), was Meyer Brownstone, and he noted that Galbraith and others at Harvard were very interested in what was going on in Saskatchewan.[27] All these could have been additional reasons for Hastings spending some time in Regina. There were also close links between the Department of Public Health and the School of Hygiene, judging by the number of senior staff who had the DPH degree. As well there appears to be a link between Defries and Roth.

System Transition

The tenure of John Hastings as chair coincided with changes in the Canadian health system. Medical care insurance had begun its rollout on 1 July 1968. The scale and complexity of the Canadian health system continued to grow, a process that had begun with the implementation of a hospital insurance program ten years earlier. The last province came on board in 1971. With this, the provincial and the federal health departments emerged as big new players in health. Unlike a US-style system, which had a large number of small players (the private insurance companies), in comparison Canada had eleven public insurers.

This influenced academic departments focusing on health in two ways. One was the need to graduate more professional managers. The other was the emergence of rich new data sources, ripe for the ministrations of researchers as the respective departments of health developed their own statistical divisions. Saskatchewan already had a well-respected statistical and analytical division, an area that had been pioneered when Tommy Douglas was both premier and minister of public health.

With the implementation of medical care insurance, and because health was a provincial responsibility, departments of health in all provinces were gaining a new and very increased stature. They were becoming major players in all governments. They would eventually become the largest cost centre in government. The same was true to a lesser extent with the federal government. In all cases, along with the increased scale and complexity of the departments came an increasing level of sophistication in both the development and management of a provincial health system. Saskatchewan had taken this to the furthest extent, and the sophistication it built up is very apparent in its actions toward the development of its medical insurance system. Its Interdepartmental Committee and the more public Thompson Committee were models of a policymaking apparatus. The same could be said of the government's handling of the Doctors' Strike. It is a very large question as to whether a government with less sophistication could have coped. Another feature of the Saskatchewan department, and one more relevant to our purposes here, is that it sent a steady stream of students to both the extension course and the diploma course in Toronto.

The system was also differentiating itself. A tiered hospital system began to emerge with the large teaching hospitals at its pinnacle. These hospitals became more than centres of teaching and patient care. They added a third mandate, that of research, with many building their own research institutes. The ties of these academic health sciences centres, as they came to be known, grew increasingly close to provincial universities.

In addition, new emphases were emerging. Health care itself was evolving. Prevention and promotion, while always present (especially in public health circles), were receiving new emphasis. Areas like the determinants of health were emerging. Canada was an early leader in this area and played an important role with the publication of the Lalonde Report in 1974.[28] During this time it was becoming increasingly evident that illness care was only a part, and some were arguing a relatively small part, of overall health.

There were other reasons for the Lalonde Report. Former faculty member Browne notes,

> I was in Ottawa 68–70, doing some work at Health and Welfare. I remember clearly the transition from Munro to Lalonde. What I did not grasp at the time was that the Lalonde's principal mandate was to re-

work the cost-sharing formula. The formula then was that Ottawa paid half the cost of all hospital services; as the feds put it, the provinces were spending "50 cent dollars" and taking all the credit. Lalonde had to provide alternatives; hence the "New Perspectives on the Health of Canadians" paper published when he was Minister.[29]

He adds,

I worked on an early draft of that and I can tell you that the introduction was written entirely in the Minister's Office with a view to shifting the debate from funding to outcomes. At the same time, senior persons from Treasury Board were being placed in key roles in Health and Welfare. I now think the Community Health Centre Study was another piece of Lalonde's strategy to create alternatives. All of this caused JH [John Hastings] to rethink the role of the Department in producing administrators who could work in a significantly different system.[30]

Browne noted, and it is not well known, that Lalonde got his material from H.L. Laframboise,[31] who, at the time was director-general of the Long-Range Planning Branch in Lalonde's department.[32] In a *CMAJ* article in February 1973 Laframboise noted that the health field needed to be segmented into four primary divisions: lifestyle, environment, health care organization, and basic human biology and clinical application: "This framework gives a more balanced view of the health field than the traditional divisions of prevention, diagnosis, therapy, and rehabilitation, or, public health, mental health and clinical medicine."[33]

Laframboise was also very concerned with the quality of the federal public service and also issues of public administration that also closely related to what was being taught in the department. In 1971 he wrote that he was concerned with the quality of the federal public servant and the amount of reform being introduced in the federal public service: this might be exceeding the capacity of the system to absorb. The article was also interesting for the historical context within which he situated innovation and a number of the federal public servants who had been known for their competence.[34]

The Lalonde Report was part of a wider movement and had international recognition. A UK academic, Berridge, notes, "Health promotion emerged during the 1970s and 1980s with a 'Canadian-European' focus. Canadian initiatives in public health were important, in particular the publication in

1974 of the Lalonde Report … [which] stressed the non-medical approach and the inadequacies of PHC [primary health care] provision, emphasizing the role of social structures in promoting health."[35]

It formed an important part of the curriculum in the first MHSc classes. I recall it was much discussed and referred to in the core courses of the 1978–80 cohorts. This meant that students in all five streams of Community Health – from budding administrators, nutritionists, to family practice physicians – were being exposed to it.

There were other innovative and future-oriented emphases that the federal department was championing and Hastings and Browne were a part of them. A major one was on community health that Browne alluded to. We will explore this further in a subsequent section.

As Chair

Overview

Hastings as departmental chair and subsequently as associate dean guided the department through as profound a period of change as it had ever seen. Many would say this was a result of the dissolution of the School of Hygiene, but actually a process of renewal had started somewhat independent of and prior to this and for different reasons. These reasons revolved around what people like Hastings believed constituted the requisite components of modern health management. The old hospital-centric make-up no longer served, nor did the British-style diploma.

There were a few foci. First was the implementation of the new degree. Some said it was a conversion from a diploma to a master's but it really was much more than that, involving an almost entirely new curriculum and certainly a very different focus. Next was a continuing but stronger emphasis on public health. The department was becoming much more than simply health admin. This probably started under Burns Roth, but Hastings, likely because of his own public health background and interest, reinforced by the history of his family's involvement in public health, took it further.

But there was an additional nuance: Hastings had differentiated himself from his familial public health roots. He was a big proponent of *community* health, and there was a distinction between the two. It had both a programmatic and a managerial focus. Community health involved an integration of health personnel, programs, and consumer involvement. It required very specific managerial skill sets, ones that the DPH and DHA did not emphasize.

Another focus was a much stronger emphasis on research. Next was funding for more staff and the opportunity to hire people with a research inclination. This was likely one of the benefits/incentives as a result of dissolving the School of Hygiene and moving to the Faculty of Medicine. Last was the introduction of a non-professional stream of graduate study and of research degrees at the master's and doctorate levels.

A New Degree, a New Curriculum

A Historical Context

With Hastings in the chair, discussions began in earnest on the type and composition of the professional degree. But these discussions were not new. The Department had not been underway for long before there were discussions on the propriety of the type of degree being awarded, specifically the diploma as opposed to a master's degree.

A master's degree in hospital administration was being discussed as early as 1950. Agnew raised the issue at the Council of the School of Hygiene meeting of May 1950. He noted that accredited schools in the United States providing graduate courses in hospital administration grant a master's degree and that several students who had registered from the United States each year expressed regret that they received a diploma rather than a master's degree. He noted that the university Senate did not want a master's degree awarded unless the candidate had first obtained a bachelor's degree in the area. The Faculty of Social Work was fulfilling this requirement by granting its graduate students a bachelor's degree after their completion of the first year of their graduate course.[36]

A.J. Rhodes discussed the distinction in 1961 in the *CJPH*. Programs of postgraduate instruction in public health in the United States awarded a master's, whereas in Canada they received a diploma. This practice in Canada followed the British custom, which was also adopted in Australia, New Zealand, India, and South Africa.[37] There was also the issue that it was a professional as opposed to an academic qualification.

In his report to the president in 1961 Rhodes noted that a diploma course generally covered a "broad field of study, in contrast to a Toronto Master's programme which is narrower in scope." The diploma in public health was first awarded in 1912 and "is one of the oldest established qualifications in

Public Health in the British Commonwealth." That said, he noted "a need for a higher level course" in some administrative subjects taught in the school and here singled out public health and hospital administration.[38]

Rhodes also chaired a Special Senate Committee on Control of Certificate and Diploma Courses. This information was used by a later committee set up in December 1963 by President Bissell to look into the need for a central School of Graduate Studies. The committee comprised prominent university (and Canadian) intellectuals, including John Cairns, Harry Eastman, Bora Laskin, Northrop Frye, and John Polanyi. It recommended that the DPH, which had international accreditation as the equivalent to an MPH degree, be reformatted as a degree course. The remainder (and these were not just in Hygiene) should be retained as diploma courses.[39]

The Need for New Managerial Skill Sets

Though discussion began on bringing the degree designation more in line with North American practices, other factors had to do with the demands for a much more involved kind of management than had been past practice. This need was presaged by federal reports such as the Hall Commission, but especially provincial reports, of which the Castonguay-Nepveu of Quebec was the most comprehensive. One can see through brief examination what it meant for health-care management. At its centre was the integrated nature of the health-care system.

John Hastings knew Claude Castonguay and Hastings and John Browne interviewed him. Browne notes, "Just as we began the Community Health Centre Project, Claude Castonguay had completed his inquiry into the Quebec system and had become Minister of Health and Social Services, with a mandate to implement his own recommendations. The integrated nature of the Quebec system was an appealing concept, but John realized that the administrative skills required to make it work were not stressed in the DHA program. Other provinces were talking about the usual 'decentralization-regionalization' issues, the solution to which would require cooperative, community-based systems led by skilled administrators."[40]

Cassel noted, "The commission's reforms were more radical than anything attempted elsewhere in Canada. It favoured 'social medicine': an open social model in place of the traditional closed medical model."[41] The Castonguay-Nepveu Report represented three aspects of health care that are important to IHPME. They could be said to be who (government delivered), what (social medicine), and how (an integrated, community-based system).

The report was far reaching in its considerations. It looked at a wide range of factors contributing to health and stressed the need to coordinate the delivery of services: "It is definitely recognized throughout the world and Canada and Quebec in particular, that the State must intervene progressively in the field of public health and health insurance."[42] How it was to do this was crucial and along these lines it noted, "Establishment of a health insurance plan in Quebec offers a unique opportunity to build the field of health into an integrated whole."[43] The "maintenance of good health and recovery demands a complex group of techniques which had long been considered as mutually independent" and it was now "necessary that these techniques be coordinated."[44]

The report stressed prevention as well as treatment. It looked at the connection between sickness and poverty[45] and stressed the role of local and community health centres.[46] One of its major programs was the introduction of *centres local de services communautaires* (CLSCs, local community service centres). Another central feature was regionalization and decentralization.[47] It recommended that "coverage under the plan apply progressively and as conditions and financial resources permit" to areas such as dental care, eye care, drugs, osteopathic care, and chiropody care.[48]

For our purposes, this report is an excellent demonstration of the new needs of the health system. Health was a provincial responsibility, and this report is a clear demonstration of a province taking a comprehensive look at its mandate. It showed how rapidly the health system was transitioning and how complex and interwoven it was becoming. The need for a new type of health manager was clear.

This demonstration of change relates back to the previous section on health system transition. There are several examples in Canadian history, such as the federal Rowell-Sirois Report of 1939, which had its "Red Books," one of which was on health. In Saskatchewan there was with Sigerist Report of 1944, commissioned by Tommy Douglas, that looked at Saskatchewan health care as a system. Douglas's explicit intent was to establish health care as a right, which led him to introduce the first hospital insurance and later medical insurance programs in North America. There was the Dominion-Provincial Conference on Reconstruction of 1945 and its "Green Book" on health; there was a national hospital insurance program made possible by Diefenbaker and his striking of the Hall Commission; and there was the national medical insurance program under Pearson. And Quebec built on this momentum with the Castonguay-Nepveu Report.

What this meant for the department was that there was now a much more complex interrelated health-care system. It required a broadened management focus beyond hospital administration, a more systemic focus on graduating managers able to take their place within the various parts of a health system. There also was the need for a new managerial skill set that could work with multiple stakeholders simultaneously and embraced whole new areas (e.g., community care, prevention). Coterminous with all this was a focus on two activities that are almost inextricably intertwined: graduate education and research.

During this whole process Burns Roth noted that there was a refocusing of the department and, indeed, of the school itself. He said this was evidenced in "the recruitment of a different kind of person who had a more academic approach. When one looks at the changes that have taken place in the last ten years that seems to have been the pattern. The newer people are not as interested in the development of people who can go out and run things but rather in people who can carry out research in why things run as they do."[49]

Development of the New Degree

At the core of the departmental changes was the new degree. Rakow notes that it was not a simple process. There was pressure from graduates and the Society of Graduates in Health Administration.[50] But the university had misgivings about a professional postgraduate degree. The new degree also had to gain the approval of the Ontario Council of Graduate Studies. And there was the issue of a non-professional, graduate degree at the master's and doctoral levels.

As John Browne commented on one of my queries,

> You've got the main point right – U of T saw itself as a strong research university – and there were a lot of moving parts. At that time, SGS as you and I knew it was probably just a decade and a half old and thus very concerned about standards; Sirluck had been invited by Bissell to U of T in the early '60s to strengthen graduate studies and essentially to re-create/re-build SGS (Marty Friedland is quite good on this era). The dust from that debate did not settle for years – almost as bad as the tempest about the creation of the unitary undergraduate departments in 1975![51]

He also noted, "We had spirited discussions about whether to join Div II (Social Sciences) of SGS or Div IV (Health and Medical Sciences). John was adamant that it be Div IV, reasoning that's where Medicine was (our home base), those were the standards we should aspire to meet, and to avoid a growing controversy about a proliferation of new degrees at U of T, then including the MPhil, largely Humanities (Div I), which was labelled by many as the "consolation prize" for a failed/incomplete PhD.[52]

He said,

> Div IV was not "friendly," largely because its paradigms were those of the basic sciences and experimental research. I vividly recall a comment made by a Div IV member when he saw "Introduction the Canadian Health Care System" in the curriculum: "We do *not* teach introductory material in SGS!"; easily dealt with, but you get the idea. We were very fortunate that Jim Ham was Dean of SGS at the time: he was supportive – perhaps because of the PEng degree ? – and helped us move things along, but it was not easy. (Anecdote: after the documentation was ready, but before the MHSc was reviewed by OCGS, Jim chaired a mock "review panel" with some U of T faculty who were experienced OCGS panellists so that we would get a sense of the likely questions: tough going, but excellent preparation).[53]

He observed, "Another element in all this was that the province/OCGS/COU would be creating a new degree designation, the MHSc, so issues like overall need in the province, BIU structures, and sufficient breadth (by which I mean that the designation was broad enough to embrace many fields in order to prevent 'degree designation proliferation') were also in play."[54]

Rakow notes that, prior to becoming acting chair, Hastings had spoken with Mrs Mary Agnew, wife of the late Harvey Agnew, who provided a liaison to Andrew Pattulo of the Kellogg Foundation, which would provide funding for the new degree.[55]

John Browne adds,

> In the early 1970s, JH began a series of conversations with the Kellogg Foundation about a grant to renew the DHA and convert it into a professional masters degree. The grant allowed Robert Baker and me to be hired to staff the "Canadian Health Administrators Study."

> Building on his experience in the Health Centre Study, JH made sure that all types of administrators participated: hospital, long-term care, public health, community boards, etc. The results of the study were published by CPHA and were the foundation on which the new curriculum was built.[56]

There were also other nuances. Browne explains, "We took a particularly Canadian approach to the new degree. Like Harold Innis, we distrusted the American MBA model for a variety of reasons (profit-driven, privately funded system); we also felt that the time had come to abandon the British model as being passé (diplomas). The MHSc was the result; when JH [John Hastings] became head of the Division of Community Health, we exported the model to other departments."[57]

New Staff, New Direction

With Hastings as chair and later as associate dean, a rapid transition of the department began. John Browne was integrally involved. He met with potential new recruits and tried to persuade them to make a move to U of T, negotiated their salaries and support staff, and accompanied Hastings on trips to meet with provincial ministers about possible areas of collaboration. Browne notes that one such trip was to visit Claude Castonguay, as he was implementing the directives of his own report.[58]

Trips like these allowed Hastings and Brown to come into intimate contact with how the Canadian system was transitioning and thereby position the department in the most relevant way possible. Browne's background placed him at the nexus of this transition, having been at the federal Department of Health and Welfare and with a degree of familiarity on Lalonde's and Laframboise's initiatives. It gave him a perspective that complemented that of Hastings in the people and curricula needed for the new/revised department.

WHERE GRADS ENDED UP: V

Meanwhile the program continued to graduate DHAs. Here is another selected list of thesis topics and where grads ended up:

- D. Murray MacKenzie (DHA, 1974) began his career at Mount Sinai and ended it as CEO of North York General. His thesis was "The Administration of Research in the Teaching Hospitals of Toronto." Given the size and prominence today of the research institutes of a number of the teaching hospitals, as well as the fact that some IHPME grads have gone into positions in research administration, it is interesting to see that their management was being thought of as early as 1974.
- Marie Lund (DHA, 1975) was originally from New Brunswick. She received a diploma in nursing from St Mary's Hospital in Montreal and was employed at SickKids as assistant administrator. She was also president of the Home Care Program for Metropolitan Toronto and was an adjunct faculty member of the Department of Health Administration. She was a vice-president of the Canadian College of Health Service Executives Toronto Chapter.
- Murray Martin (DHA, 1975; BAdmin, University of Saskatchewan) was CEO of Hamilton Health Sciences Centre. His thesis was "A Revision of the Quality Review Program at Humber Memorial Hospital."
- Sister Margaret Myatt (DHA, 1975) was CEO of St Joseph's Hospital, Toronto. Her thesis was "Pre-Retirement Counselling Programmes for Hospital Personnel." She received the Robert Wood Johnson Award for 1975.
- Kent Bassett-Spiers (DHA, 1977) was CEO, Ontario Neurotrauma Foundation, and his thesis was "The Detoxification Unit: Origin, Characteristics, Role, Problems, and Opportunities."
- Joseph Mapa (DHA, 1977) spent his entire career at Mount Sinai, ending as CEO. His thesis was "The Problem-Oriented Medical Record: A Description and Analysis if Its Implementation in a Pilot Unit at Mount Sinai Hospital."
- Ron Saddington (DHA, 1977) was CEO of Thunder Bar Regional Health Sciences Centre. His thesis was "The Employee Assistance Program as It Relates to the Chemically Dependent Employee and Sunnybrook Medical Centre." While at Thunder Bay he launched the Thunder Bay Regional Research Institute.

The entry for Sister Myatt points to the fact that a significant number of DHA students were Catholic sisters involved in the administration of their hospitals.[59] This would be the same in the extension course the department helped found that we will look at in the next section. Wall calls them "unlikely entrepreneurs."[60] Their commitment, entrepreneurism and values they brought to health care have been a subject of study in the United States but a number of the findings of this research could apply equally to Canada.

Another Longer Bio

John T. Law came to a graduate degree in health administration from a completely different direction. He already had deep administrative experience. George Beaton noted he was "generally regarded in the hospital field as being a leading 'thinker' in this field."[61] He had been the administrator of one of Canada's premier hospitals and had extensive experience before that. He had been involved in lecturing and administration at the University of Rochester and Yale University. He held administrative positions at Strong Memorial Hospital in Rochester and Grace-New Haven Community Hospital (Yale–New Haven Medical Center), in all some twenty years' experience in American hospitals when he came to SickKids in 1957, which happened to be a period of rapid growth and the transition to hospital insurance.[62]

Notably all his experience was at university-affiliated teaching hospitals while he was also teaching at the university.[63] He was the first professional administrator of SickKids.[64] He left in 1970 to pursue a degree in health admin at U of T but not in the DHA program rather the MSc route. His degree was conferred in 1974.[65]

He returned to the SickKids Board of Trustees in July 1971 with responsibility for long-range planning. He left that position in 1972 to establish and become the first president of the Hospital for Sick Children Foundation. Law understood big hospitals as comparable to big business. It was said he was "a new class of manager for a new era of state health insurance."[66]

Three big challenges he set himself were modernizing the relationship between the hospital and its staff, redefining the role of the board, and fundraising. He strengthened personnel policies, introduced pensions, a forty-hour workweek, better salaries, and a Quarter-Century Club for longtime employees. He redefined the role of the board so that they would be concerned with plans and policies, not day-to-day operations, and looking long- rather than short-term. This included a focus on improving the relationship between the hospital and university and finding ways to evaluate progress in research and treatment. Fundraising had traditionally been to support patient care but in the transition to medicare, raising funds for research was an important new activity.[67] The question was very much how a specialized academic hospital fits into the larger constellation of health care, of university, government, research-funding agencies. But therein was another question: could a board chair in this new world still take a Josephine Kane under his wing?

In another vein, like Wirsig, Law was a strong supporter of a public hospital insurance system, and he would say so publicly, inside the hospital in its newsletter and outside at conferences. His comments and his support were likely important at the time, as Ontario had built up a strong voluntary hospital sector, and there were very real fears it would be eliminated amidst a government takeover. It was a very real fear of administrators and hospital boards, that because the state now provided for everything, people would no longer volunteer. Moreover, this commitment to volunteerism was evident even at the level of the OHA and its setting up of Ontario Blue Cross.

In fact, public hospital insurance strengthened volunteerism, and their interest increased in the era of universal health insurance.[68] Law saw it early on and said so. He became an important early convert. Speaking to a conference of Canadian and American hospital administrators, the American-born Law said he much preferred the Canadian system: Canada now had improved facilities and equipment, greater financial security, more adequate staff, and better salaries for them. A major feature was that the system had built-in accountability. But even more important was that "we are not obligated in our system to pauperize people as a result of large hospital bills."[69]

He noted that Ontario had one of the best-administered plans and probably enjoyed one of the best relationships with hospitals.[70] It was not a hospital insurance system in its classic sense in that services were made "available to all" rather than being equalized to the income from premiums.[71] That said, he did see areas for improvement: there could be more regional planning, better use made of the statistical information made possible by the creation of the commission, and more money put into research on hospital operations and experiments on methods of operating hospitals.[72]

His Thesis

Law's decision to go back to university was an interesting personal choice, the exact opposite of the norm, i.e., after a successful career. His choice of degree was a significant educational choice, going the research rather than the professional route. The professional route probably had little to offer someone with his wealth of experience. In addition, the research route allowed him to gather information and undertake research as the basis for formulating a plan to re-evaluate the role of the board. To go this route was quite apropos, taking an academic path to shed light on an issue of concern to an academic hospital. For an individual with his practical experience to seek out an opportunity to complement it with research knowledge and for the U of T program in health administration to provide that opportunity itself made a statement on the role and value of graduate education.

His thesis topic was the role of hospital boards in Ontario[73] and his supervisor was Burns Roth.[74] It was a very timely topic, for in the implementation of both publicly run hospital and medical insurance programs, the constellation of health care in Canada was changing, and with this were changes in the role of trustees. His choice was current, as it was around this time that the role of the hospital trustee was being debated; it formed part of an interview in *Canadian Hospital* with the head of the Ontario Hospital Service Commission (OHSC).[75]

Another reason for the contemporaneity of his topic was that, as he noted, hospitals had changed drastically since the Second World War. Prior to that they were relatively simple operations. But after the war the range of services they provided, their size and their role in research increased.[76] He noted that prior to the advent of hospital insurance, the primary role of the trustee was financial matters. But hospital insurance changed all that, as with the stroke of a pen hospitals were no longer in a tenuous financial position. Some wondered "whether trustees were really needed now that the financial problems of hospitals were solved."[77] Yet it was soon found that hospital insurance added to rather than subtracted from their responsibilities. One new area was that interrelationships (with other hospitals, other health services, government, universities) became important. Some years before his thesis, Law had voiced the same kind of sentiment: "Trustees have a greater role and a greater responsibility under the present system of government reimbursement than they had in the past."[78] A major reason was that public accountability actually increased.

This was not his original thesis topic. It was to have been on the incentive concept for hospitals as proposed by the OHSC. He had gathered substantial background information and begun to gather data on its degree of use, and reasons for the failure of many institutions to avail themselves of the incentive. But he was forced to abandon this line of research when the OHSC was dissolved and because the imposition of budgetary restrictions by the government "caused a very real distortion in the validity of an incentive plan."[79]

With the introduction of health insurance, a new Ontario Health Insurance Commission was struck, which combined the OHSC, the Ontario Health Services Insurance Plan, and the Health Insurance Registration Board into a new single, integrated entity.[80] The incentive program Law was going to look at had been introduced in 1970 along with global budgeting. The intent of the program was to provide a financial reward to a hospital that had improved on expected results by making its operation more efficient. An OHSC annual report noted there had been considerable interest in the plan and some hospitals had used it, but they did not have data on its viability (they felt it was too early to evaluate the effect its influence may have on future costs).[81] In this way Law's study might have generated some useful data and conclusions of interest to academics, administrators, and the government.

There was also a topic before that one, which was also system-related and submitted as part of his application to the program. It was "A Study Involving Critical Examination of the Organization of Hospital Services Systems (i.e., Federal, Provincial, Local Relations and Influences)."[82]

Comment

Each of his choices of topic was interesting in that each took a systemic focus. This was quite different from the theses of the DHA program, which many times were institution-specific and often concerned with a single issue or department within the institution. Law's thesis not only focused on the system in terms of his topic, it involved surveying and gathering data from other institutions.

His focus was very much in line with where the health-care system was evolving. Prior to the advent of hospital insurance, hospitals were very much a municipal concern and not integrated into any larger whole, so there really was not a system. But with the formation of the OHSC and after the adoption of hospital insurance, this all changed. Hospitals became a provincial responsibility and a hospital system began to emerge. There was concern with how hospitals related with each other in a region. Teaching hospitals emerged as their own entity.

These developments were taken to yet another level when medical insurance was introduced roughly ten years later, which was the time of Law's thesis. Not only were hospitals now funded by the government, so were physicians. Medical insurance meant the whole expanded yet again, and there was now increasing attention to how hospitals integrated into an even larger health system. All of this had implications for hospital trustees.

CHAPTER 13

Moving on Many Fronts: 2

While chair, Hastings continued with themes that had been at the centre of his academic focus. Two were the ideas of a community-focused heath system and the needs of the administrators of the health system.

For Hastings a community-focused health system meant a number of things. One was its ties to the community it served. Another was the health professions coming together as an interdisciplinary group to deliver service. Another was the emphasis on prevention and promotion.

His other area involved educating the people managing the system. Almost immediately he proceeded with the idea of a Canadian health administrators study to gain insight into the issues themselves in the field.[1] Such information formed the basis of the educational program for the department.

TWO IMPORTANT COMMUNITY HEALTH STUDIES

There was substantial activity in the department in the later 1960s and early 1970s. The designation of the degree and the curricula required revision to bring them more in line with contemporary North American standards. There was also the need for a more research-oriented staff and for the department to become more academic rather than practical in its focus. That said, works of its faculty were being cited in selected federal and provincial government reports.

Perhaps most important, there was also much activity in the department in the health care system itself, in two main areas: the evolution of the system (particularly in a need for community care) and assessing the needs of health-care managers. We will look at four examples that cover each of these two areas: the Community Health Centre Project (1971–72), the Sault Ste Marie Group Practice Study (1973), the Ontario Health Administrator Survey (1976), and the Canadian Health Administrators Survey (1981). The results of these activities had a direct bearing on the revisions taking place in the curricula of the professional degree. But the first two of these studies point to the fact that the department was at the cutting edge in looking at alternative methods of health delivery.

The community health centre project kept the department in line with its historical mandate and that of the school, which was to make a difference in the health of the community. It set the stage for the two studies that would follow. For one thing it put the team together that would be involved in the two subsequent studies. For another it identified the need for further information. The study team for the Canadian Health Administrators Survey notes the impetus for the survey originated from the study team's involvement with the Community Health Centre Project. It had proposed a model for the development of the Canadian health-care system. During their research, the dearth of baseline information on Canadian health administrators became glaringly apparent.[2] This coincided with the degree and curricula discussions taking place in the department.

A survey of the Canadian literature turned up a few articles from educators and personnel in the field, and review of the American and British literature revealed some articles and guidelines, but they were based mainly on individual expert opinion rather than any comprehensive body of data. There was also a question about the relevance of each country to the Canadian system. This motivated discussion with the Canadian College of Health Services Executives, which resulted in a proposal to Health and Welfare Canada. While the federal department was considering the proposal, the Ontario Ministry of Health expressed interest in supporting a provincial study. It proved to be a testing ground for the subsequent national study.[3]

Community Health Centre Project (CHCP, 1972)

In 1971 Hastings went on a year's full-time leave to direct a major study of community health centres (CHCs) for the Conference of Health Ministers of Canada. The report was widely praised and solidified his reputation as a leading authority in the field.

This was a visionary document. It sought to move the modality of care away from an emphasis on single, independent physician practitioners to multidisciplinary group models. It also wanted to de-emphasize the use of hospitals.

Background

The project was initiated by the minister of national health and welfare on behalf of the Conference of Health Ministers of Canada for three reasons. The first was accelerating spending on health services. The second was growing belief that a shift from the present emphasis on acute inpatient hospital care to other forms of care such as that provided by community health centres could offer a means to slow the rate of increase. This was based on information on Saskatchewan community clinics and two Ontario group health centre programs. There were also American data on group practice prepayment programs in that country. The third reason was growing belief that community health centres offer an effective response to many health issues other than costs. This included people-centred rather than problem-centred approaches to health care. It singled out the Castonguay-Nepveu Report in that regard.[4]

John Hastings was chair of the committee and project director of the staff that produced the report. John Browne (JB) was head of administration (he was called "head of the secretariat") and assistant to Hastings. The project involved secretariat members visiting every province (some multiple times) and writing every MP "both to see and be seen." Because of the logistics, JB originated a habit he used for the rest of his career. He put up a large, erasable calendar in his office, which displayed six months at a time. He said, "Everything was on that calendar; we worked backwards from deadlines to properly allocate time to each element. For the next three decades, anyone who walked into my office at U of T could see a similar calendar on one of its walls."[5]

Browne notes that the secretariat was given space in the Federal Building at 55 St Clair Avenue East, and the Health Services Branch provided admin support, including accounting, booking travel, and the like, so that secretariat time was spent on the project itself.[6]

And just to show how activities such as these are linked to the fabric of our nation, here is an observation by JB on the effect the CHCP had on him:

> I remember telling the search committee for the Innis Principal that the CHCP made me a Canadian. I had always been a "citizen of Canada," but not really "Canadian": my attitudes were pretty well based in Southern Ontario. I visited and met people from every province (missed

> the Territories; JH took them), spent many hours with each of the committee members individually, and learned that "Toronto" is certainly not "Canada." Not that there is a "Canada" in any unitary sense except as a legal/political entity. We are – and I hope we remain – a conversation in which many voices participate.... The Chief Justice has it so right when she talks about the "living tree."[7]

Progress Reports

A progress report on the work in Hastings's papers references the Hall Commission report that stated an ideal that "the achievement of the highest possible health standards for all our people must become a primary objective of health policy." It goes on to say, "The development of some types of health centre at the community level was essential to provide comprehensive and co-ordinated modern health services to our people."[8] It notes, "The hospital has become the visible sign of community prestige, the symbol of governments in a community," but hospitals "have become the most costly capital and operational entities in the health care system."[9] It then had an interesting section titled "Two New Concepts." They were "the relationship of health care services to social services" and "consumer' 'citizen' or 'community' involvement." In the first, "It has been recognized for some time that many health problems have a socio-economic component and that many socio-economic problems have a health component."[10] This was in line with research emanating from Britain (e.g., the Whitehall Study).

The second stated a premise that "in a democratic society such as ours, health services are essentially an expression of the community's response to the needs perceived collectively by the people comprising it. Individual citizens and groups ... have brought about many developments in our health care system. Hospitals, acceptable education and training levels for health professionals, public health services ... bear eloquent testimony to the dedication and generosity of countless men and women."[11]

Parts of the progress report were quoted in the *Globe and Mail*, which noted that Hastings "said the concept of viewing health care in the context of the total socio-economic, cultural and physical environment is not new," that he quoted a 1920 British report calling for primary health centres, and observed that the Rockefeller Foundation recommended combined centres for health and personal care in the 1920s. It also noted Canadian insurance schemes are based on the sickness insurance and social security concepts of

Europe in the 1930s and 1940s, and that as a result they stress coverage for the treatment of disease, with little emphasis on preventing disease or promoting health.[12]

The project amassed substantial material on the topic. These included 61 commissioned papers, almost exclusively from prominent academics, as well as 127 briefs from organizations, another 77 from individuals (these also included some organizations), and material from a multitude of visits and discussions.[13] One notable commissioned paper was from Dr A.S. Haro of Finland, which spoke of the organization of the Finnish health system. It discussed "polyclinics" and the system's strong community orientation.[14]

The project also had working seminars on issues such as social considerations, existing facilities, medical issues, nurses, allied health personnel, managerial health issues, the relationship of public health departments to CHCs, and the relationship of hospitals to CHCs, among others. The seminars brought a number of experts in the subject area from across Canada to Toronto for one or two days where papers were presented.[15] These different activities point to the fact that running a research project such as this also has an administrative component.

There was also a group of reviewers, prominent people in the health care field,[16] notable for people who had been in the Department of Public Health in Saskatchewan, either during or before the time Hastings spent his two months there. It included people like Fred Mott, Milton Roemer, and Malcolm Taylor. Mel Derrick, who was one of the members of Hastings's project committee, later became a deputy minister to the premier of Saskatchewan and a deputy minister of health in the province. There was also Wendell Macleod, who had been dean of medicine at the University of Saskatchewan while Hastings was there.

The report appeared in three volumes: the report to the ministers, economic aspects of CHCs, and whether they are the health care organization of the future.

A Précis of the Three Volumes

The first volume was in essence the report itself. The other two volumes were more appendices to it. It had three main recommendations:

1 The development by the provinces, in mutual agreement with public and professional groups, of a significant number of community

health centres ... as non-profit corporate bodies in a fully integrated health services system.
2 The immediate and purposeful re-organization and integration of all health services into a health service system ...
3 The immediate initiation by provincial governments of dialogue with the health professions and new and existing health services bodies to plan, budget, implement, co-ordinate and evaluate this system.[17]

It had a number of important principles: a CHC provides initial and continuing care, by a team of professionals that is coordinated with other "social and related services." An important point was that a CHC was both "an organization and service concept." It included an emphasis on quality and on prevention and promotion.[18]

In the second volume its author (Ruderman) set out a number of important observations at the outset, a number of which we would do well to examine today. One, "There is no proof that economies of scale exist and a strong presumption that they do not." And related to the first, "There is no reason for the health authorities to promote bigness as such." Another, that group practices tend of have higher costs of operation than solo practices so that there was no reason for health authorities to promote group practice. However, "There is stronger evidence that group practice of the community-clinic type (as observed in a few localities in Ontario and Saskatchewan) has a lower hospitalization rate than either solo or physician-sponsored group practice."[19]

The third volume was basically a discussion of the possibility of CHCs becoming a significant part of the health-care delivery system.

In regard to the third volume, John Browne, provides context: "Ann [Crichton] was an organizational specialist and she quite rightly pointed out that, whatever finally emerged from the study, the hospital would continue to be 'the engine that drove the system' because of its financial needs, its training programs, and its presence in the mind of the public."[20]

She said as much herself in the third volume: "Hospitals are the status high centres of medical care and the centres of medical education and communication."[21] She recognized that for CHCs to succeed, the financial incentives in the system needed to change: "Presently, it pays consumers of health care to go into hospital and physicians to put their patients into hospital."[22]

Browne also notes, "If you think about it, the emergence of the hospital as the focal point of the Canadian system really only began after WW2 with reconstruction. Burns Roth had a telling anecdote about this: when he was a child and someone said 'my grandmother died,' the response would likely be 'how long did you care for her?'; now, if someone says 'my grandmother died,' the response would be 'how long was she in the hospital?'"[23]

Crichton's volume was also useful in its interpretation of the evolution of the Canadian system since the Hall Commission. This was in terms of federal concerns with rising costs – witness the Task Force on the Cost of Health Services (1969), the Health Manpower Conference (1970), and the Science Council of Canada report on the state of health research.[24] She also noted provincial reports done prior to Hall.[25] Her article provides a very good historical overview of our system for anyone so interested.

She was not sanguine about the challenges, discussing things like the strategy of change, how far and fast it could go, the need for continuous evaluation, issues of consumer involvement and education, and the education of consumers regarding their role, among others.[26]

Comment

The three volumes of the report were interesting documents. There were three different (and very important) perspectives: the report itself, providing an overview of the concept and its application; next, and very important to the ministers and their staffs, the study of the economics of CHCs, including their potential to realize savings in the system; and third a study of CHCs as *the* potential future core component of initial entry to the health system, in essence reorganizing individual medical practice and also examining their relationship to what was then (and still is) a core component: hospitals.

The report was generally well received. The *CMAJ* published the report (the first volume) in its entirety as a supplement to one of its issues.[27] In another issue the CMA president, Dr Gustave Gingras, predicted, "It will rank close to the Hall Commission Report for its impact on health care in Canada" and urged members to read the it. He noted that a "preliminary review indicates several areas where the Association is totally in accord with the policies, positions and opinions."[28]

And, to return to the theme of the impact of department faculty upon health care in Canada, the report itself is an example, and in a number of ways. First was the import of the project itself. It was a major national study placed in the hands of the department to organize, direct, and fulfil. That it could do this is an indicator of the capacity of the department. Department faculty formed the core of the project staff, which oversaw the entire project. The second volume of the report, on the economics of community health centres, was written by a faculty member. Another indication of impact was that a number of department faculty were cited in the second[29] and third volumes of the report.[30] What was also interesting was the Sigerist Report of Saskatchewan was referenced a number of times.[31]

A Thesis Comparing the Hastings Model to the Saskatchewan Model of Community Care

An interesting outgrowth of Hastings's involvement in community health was that it engaged a student who wrote a DPH thesis comparing the community clinic model, which had been developed in Saskatchewan under the Douglas government, with what was called "the Hastings model for community health." It took as its example the Regina Community Clinic, which had been in operation for nearly a decade when the Community Health Centre Project was begun. It was found that the Regina clinic was "essentially meeting the Hastings criteria for a community health centre." There were, however, some differences. The range of services, in terms of the range of medical specialties, was narrower. There was no pharmacy service, because its lease arrangement prohibited one as the result of a privately owned pharmacy in the same leased centre. However, pharmacy services were provided in the Saskatoon and Prince Albert Community Clinics, financed primarily through dispensing fees. At that time Saskatchewan under the Blakeney government insured prescription drugs. It also outlined some other differences.[32]

An interesting finding was that Saskatchewan's community clinics had a lower hospital utilization rate.[33] It concluded that for the Regina centre to truly achieve its goals, the provincial government needed to reaffirm its support of the community health centre concept and pour substantial money into the clinic in order to develop its range of services and those in health education and promotion. It put forward an interesting idea for community health centres to be developed in conjunction with hospitals.[34]

The Sault Study (1973)

Hastings led a study of medical and hospital services of some 3,300 Canadian steelworkers and their families who belonged to a prepaid group practice plan. The study was part of a WHO multi-country comparative study of different organization patterns for the provision of personal health services. It was financed by a Canadian National Health research grant and by WHO.

The data were compared with utilization by the families of fellow members of the same union local whose care was provided by independently practising physicians. It had some rather dramatic findings. For example, it found that, though the group practice had no financial incentive to economize on inpatient care, its rate of hospital utilization was lower by about a quarter.[35]

A second part to the published results was a report on the household survey component of the study. The study populations showed no significant differences in such indices as the incidence of acute illness, the disability due to it, medical attendance in illness, or attitudes to seeking medical care. The differences were in the interactions with the health-care system. For group plan members these were a concentration of services at their health centre, with less use of hospital or other primary care facilities. There were substantially higher surgical rates among the non-group plan participants.[36]

A very interesting piece of information was the sociological aspect of the reaction of different segments of the community to the prepaid group practice plan. John Browne, who worked for Hastings at the time, noted that his "information is received knowledge" from Hastings that

> the doctors in private practice vehemently resisted the clinic: "socialized medicine" and all that (similar language to the doctors' strike in Sask.). The word "communist" was also apparently used (I may have mentioned that the School of Hygiene was known among Toronto physician leaders as "The Little Red School House"). The issue split the community: church choirs broke up, neighbours would no longer speak to one another, but the worst that I recall was JH telling me that children were forbidden from playing with former friends whose parents were members of the Clinic. JH told me about school-yard bullying and name-calling.[37]

HIS PARTICIPATION IN OTHER STUDIES/CONFERENCES

In December 1971 Hastings attended a Canadian conference of deputy ministers of heath and heads of the schools of public health. Chaired by Bernard Bucove of the Toronto School of Hygiene, it looked at the role of health agencies in "tomorrow's world," the roles of schools of public health, and a more specific look at their roles in areas such as health officers, institutional administrators, and health planners, among others.[38]

In December 1972 Hastings attended an international conference sponsored by the Ditchley Foundation of the United Kingdom on the development of health services and medical care in Britain, Canada, and the United States. He was one of six Canadian representatives. Another was Dr Graham Clarkson, then an associate professor of community medicine at the University of Alberta, but also a former deputy minister of public health in Saskatchewan and deputy minister of health in New Brunswick. Another was Dr J.D. Wallace, secretary-general of the Canadian Medical Association and former executive director of Toronto General Hospital.

It had three groups; one looking at medical care, another the structure of health services, and another manpower policies. Dr Hastings was in the second group. Each group produced a report for discussion. The overall objective was to consider the principles on which the health systems of the three countries were based and how adequately they function. Another objective was to look at the health systems of the other two countries to see what elements might be applicable to one's own country.[39]

Still on an international level, he worked for thirty years as a consultant to and an invited participant in conferences, seminars, and studies of the World Health Organization and of the Pan American Health Organization, both of which tried to recruit him during the late 1960s.[40] He also acted as a consultant and expert on many issues relating to community health in Quebec. One of these was Programs in Community Health (1980), and the other was the Commission de l'Enquête sur les Services de Santé (Rochon Commission, 1987).[41]

SCHOOL OF HYGIENE SIXTIETH ANNIVERSARY SYMPOSIUM

In April 1973 the School of Hygiene celebrated its sixtieth anniversary, which it marked with an Anniversary Symposium. The Department of Health Administration was heavily involved. All members of the Planning

Committee (Bucove, Barron, Hastings, and Roth) were from the Department.[42] Ken Clute from the department was the editor of a publication of the addresses. He took his editorial duties very seriously. For example, there is correspondence between him and George Ignatieff clarifying aspects of Dr Ignatieff's address preparatory to its being published.[43]

The symposium had an impressive roster of speakers, who were notable for the range of occupations as well as their seniority. It points to the drawing power of the school. There was the director, Pan American Health Organization; deputy general secretary, Ontario Medical Association; executive director, Canadian Nurses' Association; executive director, Canadian Hospital Association.[44]

Other speakers included Dr Vernon E. Wilson, the immediate past head of Health Services and Mental Health Administration for the US Department of Health, Education, and Welfare (HEW), and James G. Haughton, executive director, Health and Hospitals Governing Commission in Chicago (and who had also been appointed by President Nixon to a HEW task force overseeing Medicaid) as well as those noted below.

The symposium was also notable in the breadth of its topics. It began with Marc Lalonde, minister of national health and welfare, providing the opening address and setting the stage for a changing philosophic context for health. It then had separate speakers on emerging trends on the world scene, United Kingdom, and United States. Then separate speakers on emerging trends in nursing, medical care, and hospitals. There was also a speaker on citizen involvement.

Mr Lalonde's address went on at some length on the work of John Hastings, the Community Health Centre Project, and its importance for the future of Canadian health care. He noted that "the main focus of our time is on first-contact, or primary, ambulatory care services – community health services as we describe them today."[45] He noted how Dr Hastings had been invited by the Conference of Health Ministers of Canada to undertake the CHCP and that its report had generated considerable publicity and discussion.[46]

Sir John Brotherston, chief medical officer of the Scottish Home and Health Department, spoke of an initiative in Scotland to integrate hospitals, the local health authority, and the general practitioner service.[47] He would deliver the 1975 Galton Lecture in the United Kingdom on inequality and its effects on health. George Ignatieff, provost of Trinity College and former ambassador to the UN, spoke of the changing social and political scene, noting the need for "a more rational allocation of economic resources."[48]

Omond Solandt spoke on the impact of science on health. He was an interesting choice not just because of his varied career but also his long history with U of T. He was a graduate of Victoria College (where he got to know another prominent Vic grad, Lester Pearson).[49] He also graduated with other U of T degrees (MA, 1932, Medicine, 1936). He won a scholarship to Cambridge under Alan Drury and was set to teach at Cambridge but with the onset of war became involved in medical and research posts with the British government. He was also a scientific advisor to Lord Louis Mountbatten.

After the war he was founding chair of the Defence Research Board (DRB) in Canada. Ridler notes that Omond's boss at the DRB, Brooke Claxton, minister of national defence, "enjoyed touting the fact that Solandt 'knew more British secrets than the Americans, and more American secrets than the British.'"[50] He was also founding chair of the Science Council of Canada and a former chancellor of U of T. He was the brother of D.Y. Solandt, the second head of Physiology (which had close ties to the school).[51] Both were graduates of Physiological Hygiene (which was part of the school) and both had been mentored by Charles Best. The evolution of Physiology at U of T is not widely known and the distinction between it and Physiological Hygiene can be confusing. The reader is referred to this citation for clarification.[52]

Best's lab was in the Hygiene Building (as the FitzGerald Building was then known).[53] When Solandt was a student, Best was the acting head of the Department of Physiological Hygiene (he later became head), which is listed as one of the departments of the school.[54] He is also listed as an associate director of Connaught (FitzGerald was the director).[55] Omond was at the school from 1931 to 1939, during the time FitzGerald was its head. He spent summers working in Best's lab while he was in medical school.[56] He notes that his goal was a career in clinical research in the hospital.[57] Given that FitzGerald had supported Best's work, and Best's administrative roles in the school and the labs, each of which was directed by FitzGerald, it is likely Omond met FitzGerald. Omond attributed much of his future success to Best's teachings and support.[58] Such mentorship points to another role of U of T. Best acknowledged Omond's contribution in a paper on heparin.[59] Best also co-authored a number of papers with Omond's brother.

Solandt divided his symposium presentation into three parts. The first was the role of research, and he distinguished between basic and clinical research and noted the importance of the latter, which "requires a completely different policy treatment."[60] His clinical research emphasis coincided with an aspect of it that Eugene Vayda, the incoming chair of Health Administration would stress (the area of clinical epidemiology).

Solandt noted that one needed to be careful not to overload the system with more basic research than it can absorb, that new insights cannot be forced.[61] The second influence of science was to improve health delivery systems and this dovetailed with the presentations of Lalonde, Brotherston, and Wilson. Here he noted that the importance of the car to physician productivity (it roughly doubled it) and that things that will improve the health delivery system do not necessarily have anything to do with medical science.[62] He did not think it was possible to have a first-class department that does nothing but teaching, but on the other hand he did not support the view that everyone needs to do research, that "what matters is that there is an enquiring atmosphere pervading the whole institution."[63]

His third area was how the environment affects health, and here he cautioned that one needed to tailor one's thinking to one's immediate environment. He gave the example of air pollution, a problem in Los Angeles but not Manitoba.[64] He concluded his presentation by talking about prevention and suggested "that the public health community should seek a new future role as the focal point for the growth of a broadly conceived science of human ecology" and noted the work of John Ryle in this regard.[65]

He was also a big proponent of government investment in science. He indicated that a country cannot buy technology and effectively use it; "It won't take off and keep going until the knowledge and skills become indigenous and there is continuity."[66] To achieve that, a country must have its own science base.

Bucove provided the concluding remarks and noted he was pleased to hear Solandt and others say that public health is much more than "just the current concern for the delivery of health care services."[67]

CHAPTER 14

Sale of Connaught, Dissolution of the School, Move of the Department

The 1970s proved to be a pivotal era for the department. Its fate was ultimately bound up in two other major events that took place the sale of Connaught Labs and the dissolution of the School of Hygiene.

SALE OF CONNAUGHT LABS (1972)

The sale of Connaught occurred in three stages. Initially it was sold to the Canada Development Corporation (in 1972). Following that there were a series of public share offerings to the Canadian public (1984–86), which saw the CDC completely divest itself of the company. Next, it was purchased by a French multinational corporation, Pasteur Mérieux (1989).[1] In this there was an interesting connection, as Pasteur Mérieux was "at times partly owned by the French government."[2] Allen says, "Sanofi grew out of two government enterprises: Connaught Laboratories ... and Pasteur Mérieux."[3]

The sale had major effects on the university and the school. Both lost a major source of continuing research revenue. While the university received a not insignificant one-time infusion of cash, it lost the source of a continuing revenue. John Hastings said, "I believe that the loss of financial support from Connaught and other endowments was a major factor in the decline of the School of Hygiene."[4]

There had been an almost inextricable symbiotic relationship between the labs and the school, and this was sundered. The labs had been a major source of research ideas and of placement for university graduate students. The sale also placed substantial Canadian intellectual property and expertise into foreign hands.

Ultimately it weakened the school at a crucial time. Hastings said, "There is little question in my mind that as a result of the separation of Connaught and the University of Toronto, the School of Hygiene lost flexibility and also much of its prestige and independence."[5] The reason he said that was that the labs gave the school a financial base that was somewhat independent of the university. He said, "The director of the School had always been able to tap into Connaught money for special activities and functions and initiatives. He had an independence, therefore, from the University of Toronto which was, in some ways, analogous to that of the Medical Faculty."[6]

ROTH RETIRES AS DIRECTOR AND THE PASSING OF BUCOVE (1973)

Roth retired in 1973 and Hastings became interim chair of the department.

Many feel that the premature death of its last director, Bernard Bucove (DPH, 1946), in 1973 may have hastened the school's demise.[7] His faculty position was in the Department of Health Administration.[8] Bucove's credentials in the field of public health were in keeping with the calibre of directors of the school and also representative of the school's many Saskatchewan connections. These, combined with his wide experience, meant the school had a powerful advocate in the overhaul that was underway at the University of Toronto at the time, and particularly during John Evans's presidency, which began in 1972.

Bucove had set up practice in Rockglen, Saskatchewan, in 1939, joined the Royal Canadian Army Medical Corps in 1941, completed the diploma in public health at the School of Hygiene in 1946, and headed back to Saskatchewan to become a regional health officer in the Department of Public Health of Tommy Douglas. He went from there to the state of Washington as a district health officer, rising to positions of greater authority there. In 1968 he left to become health services administrator for New York City and came from there to the School of Hygiene in 1970. While at the school he became chair of the American Association of Public Health (1971).[9]

An interesting aside is that Rhodes had recommend Roth as his successor, but "that did not happen, I'm afraid I don't know why." Rhodes had been under no pressure to resign but he felt that it was time for someone who had more background in health administration, "preferably had got his feet wet," and was not just an academic professor of health administration.[10] It is interesting in that in this he is describing Roth. Also striking is the import he was placing on familiarity with and experience in health administration as a director for the school.

Bucove, who became the fourth director of the school and a professor in the Department of Health Administration, was the first with a primary interest in health administration rather than laboratory medicine.[11] In his first report as director, Bucove paid tribute to FitzGerald, who taught him in public health when he was an undergraduate, and Defries, who was director of the school by the time he obtained his DPH.[12]

One could speculate on what might have been in Bucove's tenure. With his appointment, the Department of Health Administration (and the school) had three of North America's most prominent health administrators (Bucove, Mott, and Roth). Each had been involved in developing and administering leading-edge programs, and each had a strong appreciation of the importance of health administration. When Bucove arrived, he could not focus on strategic planning because his attention was focused on the fate of the school. And then there was his untimely passing. But, had it not been so, with each of these people, with their knowledge, expertise, and ideals, where might the department have gone?

The School of Hygiene was dissolved in 1975.

THE DISSOLUTION OF THE SCHOOL (1975)

Upon assuming his position at the school Bucove was immediately thrust into the vortex of forces pulling for or pushing against the school's demise. One significant factor was that, beginning in the 1960s, public health was losing its profile in North America. Many felt the public health issues of the day, like sanitation, communicable disease, and the like, had been largely solved. Unequal health outcomes due to geography or socio-economic status, already getting substantial attention in the United Kingdom, had yet to be a concern of government or academia in North America. Public health issues like bird flu and SARS had yet to make an appearance. Attention focused even more exclusively on dealing with illness.

And yet Vivek Goel (MSc, Community Health, 1988), as one who was involved in these events as a graduate student at the time and who has been at the senior administrative levels of the university for much of the time since, notes that even as the school was being dissolved, antibiotic-resistant TB was appearing and the first cases of HIV in North America were being seen.[13] This same thought is echoed by Andrew Rhodes, former director of the school, who said in 1985, "It was entirely premature to think that infectious diseases are eradicated; that while smallpox was eradicated with a herculean effort on the part of the world's health organizations, an effort that could hardly ever be repeated, the chance of eradicating other diseases of that nature is very small, and that this whole new disease HIV/AIDS which must have been with us for some time but is only now being recognized and will undoubtedly constitute a very major public health problem. It is already and will be more so in the future."[14]

One could add to that both government officials and academics in Britain were puzzling over the fact that making health care universally available in Britain had hit a ceiling. Initial dramatic improvements in health outcomes had ceased. To be sure, the gains were holding but there was no further improvement. One could not know it at the time, but each of these was calling for a renewed effort on public and population health.

At the time the issues faced by the school in Toronto were also felt in leading US centres such as Johns Hopkins and Harvard. The public health program at the University of Montreal suffered the same fate as Toronto.

Browne notes, "John Evans had just come from McMaster where he reformed, indeed revolutionized, teaching in the medical school. His view – again one of a community/preventive approach – was not in vogue in Toronto ("power medicine" was the description of choice). John E. was of the view that the medical school could only be changed from the inside and the Division of Community Health was, I think, his tool of choice.... [T]he closure of the School was bitterly fought and badly received across the country (except in Quebec) by hospital administrators and medical officers of health."[15]

Roth noted a feeling that there should be closer integration between curative and preventive medicine, that there was a need to cut out the partitioning and barriers to create a "total health system," a holistic approach to health. He felt that many "still think this is a logical development though we haven't succeeded in bringing it off to this point." He was asked by Paul Bator why, and he said, "Because it's too complicated, there are too many different skills, that the scope of knowledge that the practitioners have to have are much too great for them to function across the board. Its just too big a piece of pie to assimilate." He also said we have to look at the enormous expansion in the body of knowledge, as well as its rate of growth and the growth of sub-specializations. He said that they might have been a bit ahead of their time in their focus on a total system.[16]

In another interview Roth noted that it was a fundamental reordering of what the role of the school should be. In his comments, perhaps we see the difference between an individual who throughout his career had been at the front lines in building public health in its broadest sense at the grassroots level, and what was now occurring. This was the emergence of "academic medicine" combined with tertiary-level care. It was resulting in indissoluble relationships between care, teaching, and research, and the emergence of academic health sciences centres in which teaching hospitals and universities were inextricably linked.

The university was breaking new ground, and it was moving public health into this new realm. Whether this new realm necessitated the dissolution of the school is another discussion. Roth noted, "Looking at the Canadian scene in general, it may very well be that the applied instruction of people who are going to have a hands-on approach and effect change out in the community may very well belong in other universities than the University of Toronto, and I can't see anything wrong with that."[17]

He added, "I must confess I did not have the academic approach. I had always been interested in effecting change, not studying whether this kind or that kind of change should be fostered. It all seemed to me to be pretty clear in my philosophy what needed to be done, and the question was to find the best way in which to accomplish it to improve the health status of the people."[18]

What Roth was witnessing was the evolution of a new stratum of health-care delivery, one differentiating itself from what existed, which played a large role at the University of Toronto, likely the result of the size of its medical school. At the time, on the university's southern flank were three large teaching hospitals: Toronto General, the Hospital for Sick Children, and Mount Sinai. Each was a powerful entity; their boards were a virtual who's who of the Canadian corporate elite. Toronto General was the largest hospital in Canada.

And within a short radius of the university were a number of other hospitals involved in clinical teaching; places like Toronto Western, St Michael's, Wellesley, and Women's College Hospitals.

Simultaneously science and medicine were moving to a more academic footing. They were grounded in the pursuit of new knowledge, so research was absolutely essential. It had a point of departure different from what Roth was used to and, indeed, that the school had. In their world, one first had a practical problem and then looked to see how to solve it. That is what FitzGerald did with diseases such as diphtheria. It is what Roth did in the Yukon and Saskatchewan. Each approach also relied on knowledge, and, indeed, the Douglas government's ties to academia were very strong. Further, Roth had had prominent academics in the Department of Public Health – people like Malcolm Taylor and Milton Roemer, each of whom spent his entire career in academia outside of his Saskatchewan sojourn. But this does not mitigate the fact that the FitzGerald, Douglas, and Roth approach was much more applied and much more focused on impact.

And it was a different point of departure. Now academic knowledge had its own momentum. A curiosity-driven research was emerging, constantly pushing at the intellectual frontiers of the discipline, and the discipline itself was generating new theoretical problems to be solved. At this point the application of the knowledge was not clear.

Interestingly enough, today the demarcations between basic and applied research are much more porous, and Roth might find himself much less out of sorts in our present environment. There is a strong push in universities to do something with their basic research, for their research to have a practical application, to go from bench to bedside. Similarly, there are strong links between academia and government on policy development.

Three Reports Before, Four After: Implications for the Department

Reports were prepared on the status of the school or of public health sciences at the university. Three were presented before the dissolution of the school, three after. The three before were the Keats, Peat, Marwick and Co. Report (1968), Presidential Committee of the School of Hygiene (Nikiforuk Report, 1973), and Report of the Hygiene Task Force (Hanley Report, 1974).[19] The ones written after were the Decanal Task Force on Community Health (Hannah Report, 1988), Presidential Commission on the Future of Health Care in Ontario (1990), Presidential Commission on Health Sciences (Leyerle Report, 1993). Then in the 2000s there was a report – not to look at the old school's fate but to establish a new one – the Proposal to Establish a School of Public Health at the University of Toronto (Mustard Report, 2006). The first four reports have been dealt with on another work (see note above), so we will not retrace that information. Rather, as they occur in our chronology we will look at new information in the last two reports, particularly as they involve the department.

In all of this discussion about IHPME, it is important to recall that after 1967 the Department of Health Administration was public health at U of T. So this discussion on whether there should be public health or where it should be had significant implications for department faculty as well as in the focus of a significant part of the department itself.

MOVE OF THE DEPARTMENT TO NEW DIVISION OF COMMUNITY HEALTH IN FACULTY OF MEDICINE

With the dissolution of the School of Hygiene, the Department of Health Administration moved from its position within a stand-alone school (which had the status of a university faculty) to being subsumed as a department in the new Division of Community Health formed within the Faculty of Medicine.

The reasons for the dissolution of the school and the creation of the new division were noted in an article in the *Canadian Journal of Public Health* published some eight months before it was to take effect. The article was written by George Beaton, acting director of the school. It stated, "There have been tremendous strides in the field of public health" and many of the "once major problems of the community are now under control in the Canadian setting."[20] As a result, a new approach was needed. The article also set out what U of T was going to do to make the new division a success.

In the search for an associate dean for the new division, John Hastings was chosen. He was an interesting choice, for Harding le Riche notes he strongly opposed disbandment of the school – so much so that the president, John Evans, commented about it to him at a party at the president's residence; le Riche told Evans that he felt Hastings was "feeling better and will work well in the new organization."[21] John Browne corroborates le Riche's sentiments that Hastings was strongly opposed and adds that Hastings "was convinced that, if the School was abandoned, the University would wind up recreating it, or something very much like it, at some point in the future."[22]

The appointment of Hastings was likely a very good strategic move by the university and it speaks highly about the sophistication of senior administration. His appointment on the one hand would appease those who strongly opposed the decision. On the other hand Hastings's public health credentials were without question, his commitment to public health absolute, so that one could assume with confidence he would work hard to make the division succeed, because in so doing the university would continue in public health education, would continue to contribute to advancing knowledge in the discipline. In sum, public health at the university was preserved.[23]

One might conjecture that in many respects little changed for the department and that on balance the move was positive. Browne notes, "In order to make the division work, John E. gave JH the income from the I'Anson fund for a limited time to help JH build up the research capacity of the Division and to smooth the transition. I have no direct knowledge of what I am about to suggest, but I bet John E. guaranteed that no tenure stream positions would be lost and that more might be added. So – while JH was still chair of HAD (the Health Administration Department) – he would have had the McCracken, Palin, Roth, and perhaps Mott slots he could fill. I personally sounded out Gene V about moving from McMaster, and I negotiated salaries with Maureen Dixon and Raisa Deber. JH used I'Anson funds to launch their research."[24] Palin (DHA, 1953) and McCracken (DHA, 1959) were graduates of the program.[25]

Browne also observes that perhaps the school needed to be broken down in order to be rebuilt properly. Perhaps he has a point. It provided opportunities to the department: it allowed for new faculty, and even more important, for research assistants attached to these faculty. Funding was provided to support the research initiatives of Maureen Dixon and Gene Vayda, and people like Anne Kirkland, Bill Mindel, and Jan Barnsley were brought in as research associates. New space (the McMurrich Building) and the funding for its renovation were found. The entire building was given over to the division, and the department received the whole of the second floor. It is doubtful that any of this would have happened were it not for the relocation of the department.

There was the protection of tenure-stream positions, but even more important, the addition of new positions to hire research-oriented faculty would have been very important to the evolution of the department. Combine that with funds to help launch their research, and one finds that the department was given substantial new resources by which to fundamentally alter its focus from being exclusively practically and professionally oriented to now incorporating an explicit academic and research focus. One could argue that this was exactly what the department needed and was crucial to keeping it relevant, not just to its professional field but to its academic discipline.

Evans did a good deal to ensure that the department would succeed. Funding for new staff and for support for research associates, and the new (refurbished) building were not small measures. Hastings took the ball and ran with it. He found the money to support John Browne with his administrative ability and strategic insight, which, when combined with Hastings's vision and ability to strike a rapport with people, made for a potent combination. Together they refurbished and built what ultimately would be almost a new department, such was the level of change.

With the move of the department, Hastings assumed a new role as associate dean of the new division. He hired a new chair for the department, who would continue actions he had begun for it to refocus itself, revise the curricula of its courses, and the designation of its degree.

Irrespective of one's position on dissolving the school, the attention and resources Evans focused on the new division bore fruit. Bator notes that with the founding of the new division, "while there may be disagreement about its full meaning in terms of future directions, there can be no disagreement about the growth of the Division of Community Health's graduate programs in the professional M.H.Sc. and M.Sc./Ph.D. degrees from the period from 1978 to 1992."[26] He notes that by the end of the period, both streams of graduate work had more than doubled to over 400 students, making Community Health the largest group in Division IV (Life Sciences) at the university. He also notes that these "numbers also established the graduate program in Community Health ... as the largest in Canada, making Community Health the *de facto* national school of Public Health/Community Health in English-speaking Canada."[27]

The Role of David Hewitt

Bator notes, "Much of the credit for the expansion of graduate work in Community Health belongs to Professor David Hewitt."[28] He is a good example of the kind of person the school was attracting: a graduate of Oxford and a member of the MRC Social Medicine Research Unit at Oxford, the first such unit in Britain. The unit had a very strong pedigree, having been headed by people like Jerry Morris and Richard Titmuss.[29] While there, David published with the likes of Roy Acheson, who later became a professor of community medicine at Cambridge.[30] Roy established departments in areas such as epidemiology, public health, and social medicine at universities like Yale, London, and Cambridge. He was also very involved with the Rockefeller Foundation.[31] Roy's younger brother, Donald, served as Britain's chief medical officer of health (1983–91) and author of the Acheson Report on health inequalities.[32]

David was graduate coordinator and later graduate chair of Community Health. He was also the intellectual force behind the development of the core classes that all graduate streams in Community Health took. Bator notes that he "provided a conceptual counterbalance to the increasing specialization in the graduate field of community health."[33] He was a moving force behind the strengthening of the MSc and PhD degree programs during the Hastings and Vayda terms, which saw an increase in student enrolment from 51 in 1982 to 125 in 1988.[34] He played a central role in the development of the new professional degree program.[35]

In 1966 when David was first hired by W.H. le Riche in the Department of Epidemiology and Biometrics, space that was supposed to be renovated by the university for David had not been done and he would not have any good space for his arrival. Dr le Riche was quite exercised about this and wrote directly to the president. The letter illustrates the kind of discourse that can ensue between the likes of people like le Riche and Bissell, with le Riche's imaginative metaphor and Bissell's complete lack of defensiveness.

In his letter he likened the university administration to a "Puffing Billy" locomotive, "a game little engine" producing "quite a lot of smoke," whose "mechanical efficiency is two per cent" and "when the summer comes his wheels fall off." He queried whether "we could not build Billy into a year-round Diesel motor in time for the centennial of 1967." Bissell handwrote on the letter, "J.S. Would you please check into this immediately" and then wrote quite an erudite reply regarding physical facilities and administrative procedures. He noted the "complex urban campus," the number of requests for work, and pleaded "for an element of philosophical resignation ... This University has a long history of administrative self-denial." But what was really interesting was that he said, "I cannot bring this letter to a close without saying how much I admire your Puffing Billy metaphor. I think the estimate of efficiency is too low, but nevertheless the metaphor has an engaging aptness."[36]

FALLOUT FROM THE DECISION

There was substantial fallout from the decision, and though it would become less intense, it did not ever really abate. It remained in the background; questions kept getting raised.

Browne said, "I recall that the debate about closure ran for years: at least two major committees (Ten Cate, Auster) and lots of subcommittees. Five years after the closure, there was a review of the decision – Vivek Goel was a student of mine whom I suggested for the committee. The report confirmed the closure: Vivek was one of a group who submitted a minority dissent. Years later, when he was provost, he proved himself correct by proposing the Dalla Lana School of Public Health. The wheel turns."[37]

COMMENT

Bator earlier made the point of how the school embraced change and had a constant commitment to improvement. A person could extend this point and say the dissolution of the school points to an interesting feature of this action and perhaps a measure of the quality of this university, which is its constant commitment to quality. A number would argue that the dismantling of the school, however misguided, was due to issues regarding its quality.

Such sentiment might be borne out by the subsequent actions of university administrators who sought to provide the proper physical and capital resources to the new division within the Faculty of Medicine. We see that a certain critical mass had already been created with the amalgamation of the Departments of Public Health and Hospital Administration within the school. This was in size of faculty, number of graduate students, and amounts of research being undertaken.

Each was further amplified in the new division. Faculty positions were protected, new positions added, research supported, and new physical facilities provided. An argument could be constructed that what emerged within the division was actually a much stronger Department of Health Administration, one that had a new status within the graduate school of the university, a new curriculum, a new degree designation, a new emphasis on research as well as teaching, and a renewed presence within the university as well as among universities.

One could take this one step further and say that by happy coincidence the leadership of the department proved up to the task and the department went on to successively play to its strengths as well as track to new exigencies emerging in the rapidly evolving field of health care. More specifically, as it turned out, this change for the department proved to be positive. The department not only relocated, it took the opportunity to refocus. It was this change that forced the refocusing and deepening.

The interesting fact is that, unlike what happens many times in the political sphere, the university did not simply dismantle. At the same time attention was simultaneously and very intentionally being focused on how to continue to construct. There was a very clear intent regarding an educational and research mandate and, if one accepts the earlier point made about this being the national school for English-speaking Canada, a clear recognition of another factor – obligation.

John Browne, who was a faculty member at the time, took a view of the closure of the school and relocation of the department that was at variance with the majority. He viewed U of T as a very conservative place. However, every so often the system loosens, and change – even radical change – becomes possible.[38]

All this is true. However, the university did take an entity with a world reputation and dissolve it. This had two effects: it dissolved a momentum and it removed an entity with an international reputation. Many would say the school needed renewal, some would argue it was renewal of a major sort. Nonetheless it was an established entity known among researchers, practitioners, and graduate students. To re-establish such momentum and create a new reputation takes time. It is not automatic.

Having said that, the intent was to rebuild, and the university devoted significant resources – physical, monetary, and organizational – to this end. And it many times revisited the decision. Here one sees the intent of a world-class entity. But should it have kept the organizational edifice, the public face of the school? And, in saying this, did the school itself make a mistake, and seriously weaken itself, when it merged the Department of Public Health into the Department of Health Administration? They were two very distinct entities, each with distinct mandates.

But that said there were two overriding pieces to this transformation. First, the university itself: it gave the reconstituted department the tools it needed to succeed – a physical facility, funds, tenured faculty slots. Second, the new staff of the Department who then ran with it. It moved its professional degree away from a British to a US model and migrated its degree label away from a diploma to a master's designation. This put it much more in line with contemporary North American realities, by far the major market for its graduates. With this went curricular renewal. Research became a major focus and with this obtaining grants and recruiting graduate students.

PART SIX

A Graduate Education Focus: Professional and Academic

CHAPTER 15

A Master's Degree in *Health* Administration

THE DEPARTMENT BEGINS TO DIFFERENTIATE ITSELF

It was not long before the department began to evolve. It began with a focus on hospital administration, and that has remained a piece of its activity. However, in the 1970s this expanded to include management of other aspects of the system, and so the epithet progressed from hospital to health administration as the different types of health organizations grew.

Even before this transformation, it had begun to concern itself increasingly with public health. This could have been the result of its second leader, Burns Roth, who had been the deputy minister of public health in Saskatchewan and who established a solid program in that area in the province. At first this concern of the department took the form of providing academic classes in public health to its students or those of other departments of the School of Hygiene. However, it was not long before forays into research in public health issues began to emerge.

This exploration was greatly amplified and made an explicit focus under its fourth leader, Eugene Vayda. He took on major new challenges; as we mentioned, coincident with his arrival, the degree conferred on students changed from a British-style postgraduate diploma to a professional master's degree. Vayda built on this by adding a new layer of activity: increasing academic focus on graduate education and research.

After Vayda there was the addition of policy and outcomes as areas of activity for teaching and research, and with that its name changed yet again to include these new areas of focus. Some years later there was increasing emphasis on partnerships, particularly between government and the academy, aimed at improving management and outcomes. Along with this was a focus on a new area of activity: innovation. But we get ahead of ourselves. From the chapter headings, the major milestones of the program are apparent.

The field itself was also evolving. While dealing with disease remained a constant theme, prevention became more nuanced. In the late 1950s and early 1960s Britain was beginning to find that initial advances in population health indicators had essentially ground to a halt, and this posed a whole new fertile area for research. The outcome was the identification of areas other than disease that affected health, and this gave rise to the determinants of health in the 1970s. This led to research in health inequalities in the 1980s and links between health outcomes and economic inequalities (related but not the same as health inequalities).

EUGENE VAYDA (1976–83)

The appointment of Gene Vayda was another with a strong public health background. He was acutely aware of FitzGerald's and this university's important role in public health. Indeed, he worked to make possible a written history of this important role (the Bator book).

He was recruited from McMaster University in 1976. He had received his MD from Case Western Reserve Medical School in Cleveland. On graduating he went into private practice and became one of the organizers and first medical director of the first Health Maintenance Organization (HMO) in Cleveland. Through this he maintained a faculty appointment in the Departments of Medicine and Preventive Medicine at Case Western.[1] After completing a fellowship at Yale in 1970, where he met a number of faculty members from the new medical school at McMaster University, he was recruited to McMaster that same year.[2]

John Hastings sent John Browne to McMaster "to talk to Gene to see if he was interested in coming to Toronto and told me to do my best to convince him. If I were to take a guess, I'd say that he thought that Gene would add a medical care dimension to the department since his expertise was in HMO's, an area which would map well on to Canadian developments at the time (health centres, rostering, family practice units, etc.). Jan Barnsley worked with Gene; that was what they both concentrated on."[3] I asked Browne how Hastings knew of Vayda, and Browne said the connection was through Ted Goldberg, who would be the next chair of the department after Vayda.[4]

While head of the department, Vayda oversaw the transition of the professional degree program from a diploma to a master's degree and began to place more emphasis on research. During his term there was a major enhancement of the MSc and PhD programs.[5] Coincident to this was taking the public health focus that had begun with Roth and injecting strong research into it. Also during his term the department moved from the FitzGerald Building to the McMurrich Building, which had been extensively renovated in 1977.[6]

Vayda became the second associate dean of community health in 1983. While in this latter role he changed his mind on the location of teaching and research on public health and advocated a return to an independent school rather than a division within a medical school. Initially he felt that such a school should be located within a medical school, as that had been his experience at Yale, where it worked well. However, U of T had a much more clinically intensive focus in its medical school, and public health did not work as well within that environment.[7]

One important contribution he made to this area was increasing our awareness of the seminal role Canada, indeed this university, had played in the development of public health. It was he who in 1984, after being approached by Bator and Rhodes, searched for and found the funding for the writing of a history of the School of Hygiene – funding that allowed for the hiring of a professional historian (Paul Bator) to do so.[8]

A Professional Master's Degree in Health Administration

Perhaps the most significant program development during Gene Vayda's term was the implementation of a professional master's degree in health administration. It was part of a new master's degree in health sciences, which was meant to replace all of the former diploma degrees. A sub-specialization in health administration was a major component.

One cannot overstate the magnitude of this change. It was not simply a change in degree designation, it was a whole new curriculum, as well as a curriculum with a completely new base of knowledge (a move away from hospital operations and into government policy and academic research).

John Hastings had established a task force in 1975 to look at this, with membership from the Department of Health Administration as well as other departments within the Division of Community Health. It also had external representatives, one of whom was Sidney Liswood, former executive director of Mount Sinai Hospital. In addition to its deliberations, it received written briefs, one of which was from Gerry Turner, executive director of Mount Sinai and chair of the First Year Diploma in Hospital Administration

Task Force. Mr Turner later submitted a separate letter inquiring into the possibility of converting the diploma degree into a master's degree.[9]

The first MHSc class began studies in the fall of 1978. Milton Orris, the program director, arranged for the Ontario government to provide a stipend to these students to help defray the costs.[10]

The Practicum Piece

A number of elements of the diploma program were retained in a different form. The program still extended over a two-year period. There would be eight months of classes (beginning in September), followed by a three-month practicum. In the following September there was another four months of classes, followed by a six-month practicum. This was a change: the practicum piece was shortened from twelve months to nine months, and there were now two practicums. The first practicum was spent in an area that students did not think would be their career focus, while the second was the opposite, spent in an area that would be the career focus. In the second there was also a major paper, which was somewhat analogous to the thesis written during the administrative residency of the diploma program.

The second practicum was somewhat analogous to the residency of the DHA; however, the two practicums taken together gave the student a strong and more varied grounding in the field, given that the first also provided involvement in a whole other area of health administration. This was certainly the case for me, who spent my first practicum under the tutelage of the deputy minister in Alberta. This was at the height of an oil boom, which was ploughing substantial oil royalties into health. This made for substantial activity in the department, the most notable of which was a hospital construction budget of some $760 million.[11] It provided a very stimulating complementary experience to the second practicum, which at that time had already been determined and was going to be in Canada's premiere teaching hospital.[12]

Alberta had a strong heritage in health care. It had experimented with a number of health insurance initiatives beginning in 1930s. It was perhaps because of this that the government took very seriously a commitment to health with a portion of its windfall royalties.

These two new practicums continued a strong practical focus that originated with the diploma program. Agnew and Eugenie Stuart in the diploma program had built a strong residency program. Settings across Canada took the residency very seriously and this continued with the MHSc program.

A Distinctive Element: "The Core Courses"

One unique element of the new degree was the "core courses,"[13] which were compulsory for each of the five streams. There were three courses; in each of three succeeding terms all students in the MHSC program in the Division of Community Health had to take the core classes in common. The class session itself at the time had about 120 students in it, supplemented by tutorials with about 12 students in each. This meant that students in each of the five streams were coming together twice a week and interacting with each other.

The intent was to bring the students from diverse backgrounds and occupations together. The core courses were meant to foster opportunities for meeting and dialogue amongst people from different educational/professional programs. Constructing this opportunity for an intermixture of different professions at the educational level was an ideal that had been in the minds of some in the department for some time.

A number of interdisciplinary personal friendships and professional relationships were formed. But even more important were the perspectives brought to the class and tutorial discussions. Health administrators heard from physicians, nurses, nutritionists, and the like. There was a broadening appreciation of the complexity of the operation and administration of the health-care system. There was a rich element of history to these courses, for many times either the class or the tutorials were housed in the FitzGerald Building (the old School of Hygiene building).

The courses were reminiscent of an observation made by former director Roth some years later. Many, including himself, had felt that there would be a coming together of the health system "into some sort of consistent whole" that would not continue the sometimes quite sharp differentiation between how different sectors of the system were administered (such as hospitals, mental health, public health, etc.). He felt that there would be some sort of universal concern under some type of unified administration. The result was that one thought about what should be done at the educational level and that the sharp separation of the education of various health professionals should be discontinued. This was one reason for the merger of public health and hospital administration.[14]

Roth felt that this thinking was "fifty years ahead of its time" and that had not been borne out in practice. Still, he felt there would come a time when we would attain some "undefinable administrative arrangement that will see a total focus on the health field" and that someday we will "find the mechanism for doing this."[15]

Such thinking was evident in the core courses. In a story recounted in the first session of the very first core class of the new program, the president of a large teaching hospital got into a conversation at a conference with a deputy minister on a topical health issue. During the course of the conversation they found out that they had each been studying in different departments at the School of Hygiene at the same time but had never met each other before. There had never been the opportunity, for example, for physicians in public health to interact with students studying hospital administration and through this to gain an appreciation of the different forms of health-care delivery and of different professional viewpoints.[16]

Browne makes the same point. While doing the Canadian Health Administrator's Study under Hastings he recollected, "We kept running into cases where, while an MOH and a hospital administrator in the same district (in some instances across the street) each graduated from U of T, they had never met each other nor did they have any understanding of what the other really did. This was one factor which led to the Health Administrator's Study and to the MHSc programs."[17]

The three core courses began with the inception of the first MHSc class in 1978. They were Canada's Health Care System (CHL 3001F), Health in Individuals and Communities (CHL 3002S), and Seminars in Community Health Issues (CHL 3003F).[18]

The new curriculum then was to involve two major elements. The first was the course content. The "nut-and-bolts" courses were de-emphasized and in their place was a much more policy-oriented approach. The other element was how the courses were taught and how the new curriculum in each of the departments in the Division of Community Health revolved around the "core courses."

In Health Administration there were, therefore, three levels of courses in the new degree. A compulsory course required for everyone in all five streams (the "core courses"), compulsory courses unique to the stream, and elective courses within the stream.

There was a time (about the mid-1980s) when the department contemplated doing away with the core courses. I was one of those who felt strongly that the substance and the form of the courses should be continued and wrote to David Hewitt, graduate coordinator, strongly endorsing them. I felt that the material gave a solid grounding in current health issues, and the format of the five different streams brought diverse perspectives together.

This was particularly important in learning about differing professional (and latterly cultural) perspectives. Hewitt replied by asking if I was prepared to chair a task force reviewing their status. Ultimately I did not chair the task force, and instead it was Heather Maclean, director of Nutrition Sciences within the Division of Community Health (and later VP, Research at Women's College Hospital), but I was the practitioner member along with faculty representatives from each department within the division. The task force recommended their continuance, which breathed new energy into the courses.

A New Curricular Focus

With the MHSC degree came a very different focus to the classes offered. In the diploma program the classes had been very "nuts and bolts," very oriented toward an operational emphasis of hospitals, i.e., the actual operations of a number of hospital departments. Several of these courses were delivered by actual or former practitioners/administrators.

In the MHSC program full-time academics were delivering the courses, and the focus was much more academic than operational. There was a greater health systems focus, which included looking at its various elements such as community health and health policy at the political level. There was also an examination of organizational design and management theory along with health policy outcomes and evaluation. Research was not yet a culture in the department, but established faculty and new young faculty who were predominately involved in research were delivering a majority of these courses.

Health Admin and Public Health

Gene Vayda pointed to an interesting nuance that had evolved in the department during its latter years in the School of Hygiene, that it had moved far beyond hospital management and providing purely professional education. It had come to include an important public health component and a research function. What Vayda observed was that the Department of Health Administration was public health. What he meant was that the public health program of the School of Hygiene after its dissolution was centred in the Department of Health Administration.[19]

It is hard to pinpoint just when this began. No doubt it was heavily influenced by the merger of the two departments in 1967, but it was likely due in part to the fact that hospitals themselves are an important element of public health. Additionally, people like Burns Roth and Fred Mott had strong public health credentials. And after 1967 its faculty had a strong public heath contingent.

Some recognized the importance of public health and had very worked toward its ideals throughout their previous professional careers outside academia. These were people very much in the mould of the FitzGerald "within reach of everyone" ideal. Roth and Mott had both done important work. Mott had laboured to make health available to everyone with the Farm Security Administration in the United States. Roth had done significant work in true frontier medicine in the Yukon as well as in his public health initiatives in Saskatchewan. Vayda had done important work on prepaid health plans while in Cleveland.

A number of academics also had an interest in the field, including John Hastings, who not only had tirelessly worked toward such principles, but grew up in the milieu of a public health pioneer. Cope Schwenger was a leader with an international reputation in public health gerontology. Also in 1977 he conducted an important study on public health in Toronto. Marion Powell did important work in family planning. Ken Clute wrote a ground-breaking work, *The General Practitioner*, considered the first major attempt to analyze how physicians delivered health care.[20] Robert Langford did work in cigarette smoking and health, health education, and human sexuality. Jim Bell had been medical officer of health for East York. Then, as we noted, there were directors like Hastings, Vayda, and Goldberg, who followed Roth, all of whom had very strong public health credentials.

Vayda himself contributed to the strength in public health with his establishment of Teaching Public Health Units, which was a major contribution to the field. In 1987 he secured funding from the Ontario Ministry of Health to collaborate with some of the health units in the Toronto metropolitan area, first in East York and later in North York. He also initiated discussion for a similar arrangement with the City of Toronto which came into being in 1990. These teaching units opened up the possibility for formal cross-linkages for research and education in public health as well as within the Division of Community Health.[21]

A Push for Research

Vayda was also instrumental in pushing for the development of research while he was chair and later as associate dean, and each succeeding chair continued to build upon his work. It had become an area that was vital to the continued evolution of the department. There comes a time in the development of a discipline when its focus can no longer be solely on practice. It must push at the boundaries of its knowledge. This is important not only to advance the discipline; it also influences the character of its teaching.

As associate dean Vadya worked with the chairs of the department in Community Health (Preventive Medicine, Health Administration, Behavioural Sciences) and the Occupational and Environmental Health Unit to push for more research activity. As a result there was a jump in external funds for research to over $4 million in 1987–88, a figure that was roughly equal to the university budget for the department in the division. By 1991–92 the trend continued to reach roughly double the annual operating costs for the division.[22]

A Clinical Epidemiology Sub-Specialization

Another of Vayda's initiatives, one that would both bolster its research and public health profile, was the development of sub-specialization in clinical epidemiology.

Vayda notes that when he came to U of T one of his goals was to help start a program in clinical epidemiology. To that end he recruited Alan Detsky and Claire Bombardier, who were both physicians and health economists as well as clinical epidemiologists. The U of T program in clinical epidemiology was located in what was then Health Administration because that's where he, Detsky, Bombardier, and Goel were located and where the environment was favourable.[23]

Health Care Research Unit

In 1976 the Ministry of Health in Ontario made funds available for ten research units to conduct research on the health system as well as planning and evaluation in the community. The department's proposal for a Health Care Research Unit (HCRU) received funding and it operated for about ten years. Vayda, with the help of John Hastings, the associate dean, brought in

Jack Williams to head the unit. Dr Williams also taught a course in program evaluation and helped develop the Community Health Appraisal Methods course. HCRU was replaced by the Hospital Management Research Unit as Ministry of Health priorities shifted from pure health services research to health management research.[24]

The HCRU had within its mandate a responsibility to assist community based groups with evaluation and research. It employed four individuals who worked on a wide range of projects. One was a needs assessment for the Ronald McDonald houses, which led to an expansion in the range of services they provided. Another was a needs assessment for a coalition of Chinese service providers, which led to the first nursing/long-term care facility targeted at Chinese seniors.[25]

Work for the Government of Manitoba

Just to point out the profile of people like Vayda, the type of work he became involved in, and how department faculty were seen as a resource by different governments, the following is an example of some interprovincial work. In February 1974 Vayda, along with Graham Clarkson, was appointed by the Department of Health and Social Development in Manitoba to conduct a one-year study of their health sciences centre in Winnipeg. It looked at its future development needs in the context of the overall health facility and program needs of Winnipeg and Manitoba as a whole.

Their study also examined the current facilities and future needs of the health sciences centre and current utilization of health services in Winnipeg, with emphasis on the health sciences centre. It also looked at physician resources and needs and research facility needs, and made recommendations for an orderly and phased development program for the health sciences centre. Their study included particular reference to capital and operating costs of existing and proposed programs and made recommendations in this regard.[26]

A Book on the History of the School of Hygiene

Vayda believed strongly in the need for a history of the School of Hygiene. In 1983 planning began on a School of Hygiene History Project to produce a work for the sixtieth anniversary of the opening of the School of Hygiene

Building in 1987. A planning group of Vayda, Jan Barnsley, John Browne, and Andrew Rhodes was struck. In October of that year Vayda submitted an application to the Hannah Institute for the History of Medicine for funding. Full funding never did materialize, and a combination of small pieces of funding from places like Connaught Labs, Canada Liquid Air, the alumni associations of the school and the division, former and present faculty, Rockefeller Foundation, and Ontario Heritage Foundation allowed the project to proceed in a scaled-down version.[27]

The funding was used to support hiring a full-time researcher in history, Paul Bator, to undertake the project. He also contributed substantial voluntary time. Bator was eminently qualified, having written his dissertation on public health reform in Toronto.[28] The result was the two-volume work, *Within Reach of Everyone*, which has been referenced in this work. Hastings later became a member of the advisory committee for the project and was quite involved in the second volume of the work.

Personnel from the department had their imprint on the project. In addition to Vayda, John Browne, by then principal of Innis College at U of T, provided an office at the college for Bator and Rhodes. Hastings helped secure a publisher for the work.[29]

Contributing to the Debate on Health-Care Delivery

One striking attribute of the leaders of the department/institute has been their willingness to take a stance and wade in on controversial issues. We saw this earlier with people like FitzGerald and Defries on health insurance, and it is evident here with Vayda on the same issue.

Throughout his career Vayda was a tireless proponent of a publicly financed system. Because of his US background, he had seen both. He did not refrain from entering the debate on the Canadian system and what one could describe as an increasing tendency to private initiatives. One example was a review of Vera Ingrid Tarman's *Privatization and Health Care: The Case of Ontario Nursing Homes*, in the CMAJ, which prompted an angry retort from the physician-president of an Ontario nursing home chain and an eloquent response from Vayda.[30]

He wrote an article on the UK system and how, through the Thatcher regime, it was becoming increasingly privatized. One of his more important points was how this transformation was affecting equity. He noted Canada has made concerted efforts to maintain equity, as have countries like Denmark. However, he said that the United Kingdom, "which assumed world leadership in national health care in 1948, is losing ground."[31]

He also gave a speech to the City Club of Cleveland on the universal health insurance system in Canada and whether there were lessons for the United States. Two important points he made for his US audience were that in Canada public funds are used to pay for a private health care system and that "our problems stem from a diminishing economic carrying capacity in the face of strong public and professional pressure to maintain and expand the scope of services."[32]

In speaking and corresponding with Gene, it is evident he started with the premise that universal health insurance was essential. He wrote, "Once I accepted that fact (very early in my medical career) it became clear from looking at all of the Western countries that had universal insurance that the insurance was publicly funded. I saw and still see universal health insurance as a basic human need."[33]

He acted on his belief. He led a physicians' group supporting Medicare in Cleveland in 1962 and helped to start a prepaid health plan in 1964.

He noted, "When I was interviewed for acceptance to Case Western Reserve University Medical School, the director of admissions asked me what I thought of universal health insurance (socialized medicine). I swallowed and told him I was in favour of it. It turned out, although I didn't find out until later, that he was too."[34]

The Import of Vayda's Tenure

It could be strongly argued that Gene represented an important transition for the department, that as strong as the department was in hospital administration – indeed, it was at the very centre of it in Canada – it needed to change. It needed to broaden its focus beyond hospitals, it needed to move from a concentration on secondary care to one that also concerned itself with primary care, and it needed to move from an almost exclusively practical orientation to one combining practice and research. It got all this with its new chair. Gene was the first non-hospital chair, though Burns Roth was both hospitals and public health. Gene also had a deep knowledge of the intricacies of the US system, which the department perhaps did not take advantage of – at that time not embracing a study of comparative health systems.

This all sounds much more simple than it was. Gene came to the department when there were strong and deep feelings over the dissolution of the School of Hygiene. Moreover, its public health role, which had animated it, was in a very ambiguous and amorphous position within the university.

The department needed to preserve its role in its professional degree but it needed to come at this by injecting a strong element of the fruits of research into its professional curriculum. It needed to establish a credible graduate research program.

Gene was able to shepherd the department through these changes.

CHAPTER 16

A Continued Refocusing

CONFERENCE ON EDUCATION FOR HEALTH SERVICES ADMINISTRATION IN CANADA (1977)

The Conference on Education for Health Administration in Canada was held in 1977 and sponsored by the W.K. Kellogg Foundation, an organization long associated with the department. The department was mentioned as being the first program for health administration in Canada by Andrew Pattulo, vice-president of the foundation, in the opening speech.[1] Educators and practitioners from across Canada attended, and the proceedings were published in English and French by the Canadian College of Health Executives.

Several faculty or graduates of the department were involved in presentations. Carl Meilicke (DHA, 1959), who was directing the Alberta program in health services administration, was co-chair and helped organize the conference. He presented a paper on the emerging needs for graduate education in health administration. Jim McNab (DHA, 1951), president of TGH, responded. Maureen Dixon, program director for the department, was the responder to a paper on education content for health administration. Peter Carruthers (DHA, 1959) was the respondent to a paper on financing education and research in health administration.[2] Robert Defries, former head of the school, was one of the presenters. He was also involved in a previous US initiative sponsored by the foundation, the 1974 *Report of the Commission on Education for Health Administration*.[3]

INTERCONNECTIONS BETWEEN FACULTY, GRADUATES, BUSINESS, AND POLITICS

To demonstrate the interconnections from the department and school that extended into the new Division of Community Health, faculty member Harding le Riche knew DHA graduate Harold Livergant, president of Extendicare, and recounts a party he attended at Livergant's house on 25 November 1978. At it he met Premier Alan Blakeney of Saskatchewan. Livergant was originally from Saskatchewan. Also at the party were other Extendicare staff, including Gerald Hiebert (DHA, 1966, class of 1964), a DHA classmate of Livergant's and now at Extendicare in a senior executive capacity. Other former Hygiene faculty were there, such as Lachlan MacPherson, a professor in microbiology and public health. Also attending was Jack Shapiro,[4] who was active in business and health activities (Toronto Board of Health and Cancer Care Ontario) and received the Order of Canada in 2004.

NEW INITIATIVES

Telemedicine

Telemedicine was a continuing health education activity developed initially as a partnership between TGH and the U of T Faculty of Medicine. In the MHSc program there was no thesis associated with the administrative residency, as in the DHA course. However, there was a major paper connected to the practicum that was due when it concluded. As part of this, Jim McNab, TGH president, asked me to consider doing the major paper on telemedicine and specifically to examine the feasibility of telemedicine for diagnosis and/or continuing education.

Mr McNab had been asked to look into the matter by the Ontario deputy minister of health. I did research on current systems and their application. All were in the United States with the exception of a Newfoundland project run by Dr Max House (later lieutenant governor of Newfoundland) who at that time was part of the Faculty of Medicine at Memorial University. I developed a proposal, which concentrated on continuing education only. In addition to serving as the academic requirement for the practicum portion of the program, it was the basis for a policy proposal to the government and hospital. It was another example of how an academic requirement in such a program can also serve as the basis for the practical application of knowledge.

It was presented to the Medical Advisory Committee and then the Board of TGH in 1980, both of which endorsed it. The next step was to organize a provincial conference to gauge the appetite for such an activity. The ministry sent staffers to the conference, which was held in the spring of 1981 with people from across the province attending. Information from the conference and a portion of the material in the proposal were then condensed into a grant proposal submitted to the Ministry of Health and the Donner Canadian Foundation.

It proposed the development of a continuing health education network initially aimed at the northern part of the province to provide health education and dispel professional isolation among the health professions. The decision was made to limit the activity to purely continuing education and not include diagnosis or treatment. In part this was to diminish concern among northern physicians about disrupting existing referral patterns away from Thunder Bay and Sudbury nodes. A proposal was sent to the ministry and the Donner Foundation later that year. The initiative launched in 1982 and the first hospital site was in North Bay. As an aside, the CEO of the Donner Foundation at the time was Don Rickerd, with whom I would teach at Trinity College at U of T some thirty-five years later.[5]

Initially the project consisted of two partnerships. One was between TGH and the Royal College of Physicians and Surgeons to deliver programs aimed at specialist physicians across Canada. House directed the Royal College portion of the project.

The other partnership was between TGH and the five Ontario medical faculties. The Faculty of Medicine at U of T (including the Department of Health Administration) was the most involved. Fred Fallis, former head of Family Practice at U of T and TGH and at the time the assistant dean for continuing education at the Faculty of Medicine, was the physician lead for U of T.

It was initially called Telemedicine for Ontario. The intent was to limit its focus to physicians but, responding to demand, the initiative soon expanded to provide programming to all health disciplines. The presenters initially were almost all from TGH and U of T, but soon other hospitals and Ontario universities were providing presenters as well, and this expanded even further to include other Canadian universities and hospitals.

The programming package for the fall of 1982 had ten weekly programs aimed at physicians, nurses, and allied health professionals.[6] It caught on immediately. A note from Fallis to Dean F. Lowy in 1982 noted that it was not unusual to have twelve to fifteen distant sites participating.[7] In the 1985–86 programming year a newsletter was initiated. As an illustration of its growing credibility, the May 1986 issue noted that a TFO article had been selected for publication by the University of Wisconsin.[8] Also during that programming year an educational TV series *Ontario Medicine Forum* was initiated on Rogers Cable TV.[9] In 1987 the TFO staff published an article in the *CMAJ*.[10]

The telecommunications technology used in the project differed from that used by House at Memorial University. The Toronto project utilized what were referred to as Convener Kits, manufactured by DAROME Inc. in the United States, which were a speaker and microphone set for on-site receiving and transmitting. The TGH headquarters also purchased a twenty-port teleconferencing bridge from DAROME. I later had TGH partner with DAROME on a Canadian teleconferencing initiative that was run in parallel to the continuing health education activities.

At the conclusion of the TFO project three medical schools chose not to continue for lack of commitment among their faculty and potential financial risk. The activity was reorganized as Telemedicine Canada to recognize its now national scope with TGH and the faculties of medicine at U of T and McMaster University as partners. The initiative continued to grow, and by 1990 its size and scope was over 500 sites, including all of Canada and some international locations.[11]

Over the ensuing years the network continued to expand, this time down the eastern seaboard of the United States. A separately incorporated US subsidiary was formed called Telemedicine USA. The combined Canadian and US operations grew to what was believed to be the largest such network in the world, greatly eclipsing the US networks in the field. I served as board chair, and the project remained a part of my directorate through successive promotions at TGH. Gerard Mercer, whom I hired, was president of both the Canadian and US operations.

The Department of Health Administration was very much a part of this enterprise through presentations by faculty and alumni. There were regularly sections on health administration and also hospital finance in the program calendars for Telemedicine Canada. For example, a sample from an old calendar (fall 1997), lists programs in each of these areas with faculty such as Duncan Sinclair, Tina Smith, Raisa Deber, and George Pink involved. Mercer notes that Louise Lemieux-Charles was another regular presenter.[12] Rhonda Cockerill also spoke on evaluation.[13] These programs were an important continuing education activity for hospital management.

IHPME involvement in this type of activity has continued. Matthew Nelson, who at the time of this writing is a PhD candidate in IHPME, is involved in a related activity, the Ontario Telemedicine Network.

A Class on Hospital-Based Ambulatory Care

In 1982 the department launched a class in hospital-based ambulatory care, an example of how the department was always pushing at the frontiers, exploring new modalities of health delivery. At the time this area was an initiative of the Ontario government, which was seeking alternatives to expensive inpatient care. The class was meant to build on an ambulatory care model being implemented at Toronto General Hospital and to provide information for MHSC students on this new mode of delivery.

The ambulatory care model was incorporated into the plans for a new building at TGH, the Eaton Wing. In 1980 it had been completed, purpose-built for combining this activity with inpatient activity. Each patient floor had an inpatient (Eaton South) and ambulatory section (Eaton North) connected by a centre section (Eaton Centre) that housed teaching and seminar rooms. An important and very novel initiative was that staff physicians relocated their clinical offices from offsite to Eaton North. The intent was to combine inpatient, ambulatory care, and teaching for each clinical specialty as an integrated activity on each single floor.

The hospital developed a whole new set of policies and procedures to guide this new area of activity. The majority of this planning was in the office of the vice-president of medical Affairs, under Dr Blenos Pederson. Pederson hired me to help with the policy development and implementation when the practicum portion of the studies in the MHSC program ended. It was hoped that the TGH ambulatory approach would serve as a model for the rest of the province (and indeed the country).

At the time this seemed like a promising way to combine inpatient and outpatient care and clinical education in one location, along with having all the ancillary services (such as diagnostic, rehab, mental health, and others) close at hand.

I taught the hospital-based ambulatory course under Dr Chan Shah's supervision in the Division of Community Health. It included a section on telemedicine. Shah was the director of the Residency Program in Community Medicine.[14] We also co-authored a chapter in a US-based book on the subject.[15]

TWO MORE STUDIES HEADED BY HASTINGS

In a previous chapter we spoke of two important studies on community health led by Hastings. In Vayda's term, Hastings led two studies on administrators.

Ontario Health Administrator Survey (1976)

The Ontario Health Administrator Survey was supported by a grant from the Ontario Ministry of Health and the Kellogg Foundation. It surveyed health administrators throughout Ontario by a mailed questionnaire and received 796 responses. The study reviewed the literature available on the topic as well as that pertaining to Canada. It noted the lack of Canadian research.[16] The findings were that the "day to day management of the health administration field appears to be in very stable, experienced and well qualified hands."[17]

An interesting finding was high turnover at the ministry. It noted that in a government-financed health care system the ministry administrator is "an overseer of the system as a whole" and "holds ultimate responsibility for health care delivery by all the sectors." Also, in a parliamentary democracy, the career civil service is present in a large sense to counterbalance the transience of elected legislatures. Yet in Ontario the evidence did not support this model, as it showed a high turnover of policymakers. It felt that many "of the problems plaguing the health care system" could "be more effectively approached by a continuity of policy." It also discussed the converse, that is, whether high turnover is an essential element in a process of change. It also noted a high proportion of physicians in the ministry and queried "whether it is appropriate to have public policy decisions in provincial health care developed and directed by administrators trained in an institutionally based technical medical model."[18]

Canadian Health Administrator Study (1981)

The Canadian Health Administrator Study, while it was published in 1981, began its gestation almost as soon as Hastings became chair. It was published in a special issue of the *Canadian Journal of Public Health* as a separate supplement to the March/April 1981 issue. It noted the study had also been suggested in 1973 by Dr William Hacon, director-general, Health

Manpower, Health and Welfare Canada.[19] It was undertaken by a study team from the department, three prominent members of which were Bill Mindell, John Browne, and Jan Barnsley. It surveyed over 4,000 practising health administrators across Canada in 1977–78. The purpose of the study was to describe the health administrators: "their opinions about knowledge areas and skills thought necessary for successful job performance, their interests in continuing education, and trends they feel would affect their work in the future."[20]

One important chapter was on issues and trends in Canadian health care. Five themes emerged, the first three of which were the effects of economic uncertainty, the effect of revised federal-provincial cost-sharing arrangements, and the rise of community support programs. The fourth area was new organizational relationships, which involved a number of trends. One was toward multi-unit management, among hospitals and also between hospitals and related facilities such as nursing homes. Another was new interorganizational relationships involving public health agencies relating more closely to other organizations (such as hospitals) in the system. Yet another trend was the strengthening and continued development of regional planning councils. Another was more complex provincial relationships as health began to involve more than one ministry (such as those concerned with occupational health, housing, employment, and income). The fifth area was increased professionalism and the development of continuing education for health administrators, which involved two main needs: sound initial training and the opportunity for continual updating.[21]

An important part of the last chapter was its reflections on the trends and issues emerging. It noted that administrators expected "to be held increasingly accountable for the use of scarce resources" and having "to choose among competing priorities." There were changing emphases, to ambulatory care, long-term care and rehabilitation, prevention, and promotion. In addition there was growing community and government involvement, regionalization, and integration of services.[22] One could also sense in the report an increasing differentiation among institutions in complexity and the sophistication required to manage them. All of these kinds of issues had a very direct bearing on the type of basic and continuing education required.

ALUMNI

Alumni and Other Practitioner Involvement in the Program

The graduates of the program have always formed an important component of its educational mandate. At times this has also included other non-alumni practitioners.

An example of the latter was Sidney Liswood, CEO, Mount Sinai Hospital, 1954–76. He received an MBA from the University of Chicago, School of Business (Hospital Administration in 1942), and an MPH from Harvard, School of Public Health in 1952 and brought a wealth of experience to the program. He served in the Medical Administrative Corps from 1942 to 1946. After the war he served as administrator of the Beth Israel Hospital in Boston. He was responsible for Mount Sinai in 1962 becoming a teaching hospital affiliated with the University of Toronto. He had a faculty appointment in the Department of Health Administration from 1955 to 1981 and delivered a series of introductory lectures in hospital administration for many years.[23] He endowed a professorship in health-care management at his alma mater (Harvard) as well as Ben-Gurion University of the Negev. The next two Mount Sinai CEOs following Liswood – Gerry Turner and Ted Freedman – were graduates of the program and played important roles in the Society of Graduates.

Jim McNab, throughout his tenure as CEO of Toronto General and later North York General, stayed involved in the program, particularly in mentoring students through its practicum. Hume Martin (MHSc, 1981) noted he was fortunate to have had Jim McNab as a mentor prior to his becoming CEO at North York General after McNab. Martin then went on the Bermuda Hospitals Board, Calgary Regional Health Authority, and Rouge Valley Health System.[24]

Another alumnus involved in the program was Gary Chatfield, who received his diploma in 1961. He was an assistant deputy minister in the Ministry of Health in Ontario, a deputy minister of hospitals and medical care in Alberta, and president of Extendicare. To one ambitious and energetic student he said on the very first day of his practicum that he was going to treat him like an assistant deputy minister. He said, "I know this is not fair, but whoever said it's a fair world?" To a young and eager student, words such as these were very stimulating indeed and made for a very stimulating practicum that amplified the motivation of an individual to do well both academically and professionally.[25]

Tom Closson, a U of T grad but not alumnus of the program, has been very supportive and involved over the years. He has had a career as president of Sunnybrook, Capital Health Region (BC), UHN, and the OHA. He has been a regular guest lecturer in HAD 5010 and a guest speaker at education and research events.

Perhaps foremost among the organizations that had a strong involvement were the University Avenue hospitals (TGH, SickKids, and Mount Sinai).

And it wasn't just the alumni who were important mentors. At TGH, for example, a wider group took an active interest in mentorship and were important to practicum students. At the VP level in the 1980s, Bill Anderson, Bill Louth, Wanda Plachta, and Dorothy Wylie were examples, who automatically took on a guiding role and were all larger-than-life. Bill Anderson was a pathologist who was entrusted by William Boyd to update his classic book on surgical pathology.[26] He was also one of the four co-founders of MDS Health Systems, which became Canada's largest commercial medical diagnostics lab. Dorothy Wylie was an important figure in nursing in Canada and recognized as a mentor in that profession as well. Bill Louth had a steel-trap financial mind. Wanda Plachta was very interested in moving people ahead and in a quiet and very unobtrusive way helped build skill sets in those who spent time with her.

I can attest there was much to be learned from each of these four as well as the CEO (who at the time was Jim McNab, a DHA graduate, and later Vick Stoughton, an American, who provided a glimpse of the American system).

The "admin resident," as the person was known, became an important fixture at TGH. And a number stayed on, hired by the hospital after their residency ended. Les Boehm and Liz McCartney (MHSc, 1980) are examples. Vytas Mickevicius (MHSc, 1983) and Sally Brown (MHSc, 1984) were others. Liz subsequently married another graduate, Michael McCartney (MHSc, 1985), who was hired by Toronto Western Hospital.

The Toronto General and Toronto Western Hospitals merged in 1986 and TWH sent administrative staff to the MHSc program. Two examples were Phyllis Matheson (MHSc, 1985) and Sally Martin (MHSc, 1993), who were originally from Toronto Western.

Graduates took their IHPME education and parlayed it into important careers and remained involved. Mary Jo Hadad (MHSc, 1998) is an example. She joined SickKids in 1984 as an assistant manager in the Neonatal

Intensive Care Unit and was appointed president and CEO of SickKids in November 2004.

Society of Graduates in Health Administration

History

Involvement in the program also took place in an organized form through the Society of Graduates in Health Administration. From the inception of the program in the late 1940s they have maintained a strong role in the program, and this involvement was formalized from the 1950s onward when an alumni association was formed. It has been a venue for continuing education and social functions. It lobbied for the program to change from awarding a diploma to a master's degree, and it has supported various capital improvements.

Graduates' involvement was reinforced by the practicum, the supervisor of which invariably was a graduate of the program. For many years a welcoming reception for incoming students was offered by the society at one of the downtown teaching hospitals close to the FitzGerald or, later, the McMurrich Building.

Alumni also participated in major events of the program. For example, in January 1976, as the program deliberated conversion to a master's degree, Gerry Turner, in his capacity as chair of the First Year Diploma in Hospital Administration Task Force, presented a brief to the associate dean, Community Health. Some of the items included the question of whether there should be a personal interview to determine if applicants "are sufficiently well-rounded." It recommended that the program have core and elective courses (each of which was specified). There should be streaming into areas such as hospitals, extended care facilities, community health centres, and public health, among others. There should be a residency program, and there should be "a blend of theoretical and practical knowledge."[27]

Another example is that Gerry Turner, while he was executive director of Mount Sinai Hospital, for many years chaired an External Advisory Committee. His chairmanship and the membership give some idea of the import both the department and the alumni placed on the committee. In addition to Turner, other members included the deputy minister of health, a former deputy minister of health, and the COO of Toronto Western Hospital, a vice-president of the OHA, among others.[28]

The committee met on a roughly quarterly basis, and it is evident from the minutes of a meeting in 1979 that it took an active interest in matters such as curriculum content and how well students were doing in the courses. They were also attentive to the students' perception of the external pieces to their studies, such as the base hospital, Practicum I and Practicum II.[29] The minutes for a meeting of 1975 pertaining to the diploma program showed similar interest. It was chaired by Mr Ron McQueen (DPH, 1956). It also illustrates the attention of alumni and other administrators to the program. The minutes noted it had thirty-nine attendees, of whom nineteen were either CEOs or their deputies.[30]

Comment

A distinguishing feature of the program through its history has been the involvement of its alumni, which began with the program's inception and was born out of practice. Its founders felt that what was needed in the Canada of the interwar period (1930s) was a professional cadre of hospital managers. This led the school to structure a new degree, one that would be along the same lines as the diploma in public health, but this time in hospital administration. The intent was the same, just as the DPH was meant to graduate public health administrators, so too the new diploma did the same with hospital administrators. Its format was a year of class instruction followed by a practicum year with a thesis requirement. It gave the department a very practical character for the first thirty years of its history, as well as a strong link to practitioners.

This has been blurred somewhat as the department, now institute, has become increasingly academic with its emphasis on research. Nonetheless, it is still an important part of the professional degree program.

BURNS ROTH RETIRES AS FACULTY MEMBER

In June 1978 a retirement party was held for Burns Roth at the Faculty Club. The occupation of those at the party spoke to the esteem in which he and perhaps the department as well was held. Some of those attending were Sidney Liswood, former head of Mount Sinai Hospital; Harold Livergant, president of Extendicare; Jim McNab, president of TGH; Boyd Macauley, head of Toronto Western Hospital; Allan Backley, deputy minister of health;

Allan Hay, executive director of the Ontario Hospital Association; Wendell Mcleod former and first dean of medicine at the University of Saskatchewan, and Fred Mott, whom we have already met in these pages, former faculty member and former deputy minister of public health in Saskatchewan.[31] A number of people came from outside Toronto to attend.

RESEARCH AND GRADUATE STUDIES

The addition of research and graduate studies was very timely, adding a new dimension to the teaching of the professional degree in health management. It was significant in that this academic stream of research and graduate students was important as activities in themselves as well as in providing a foundation to give added depth to the teaching of the professional degree program.

The academic field had evolved to such an extent that in order for teaching in the professional degree program to remain current, it could no longer rely solely on an emphasis in practice, as important as that was. It also needed to include some connection to advances in knowledge within the academic realm in order to enhance the management base that was being taught.

THEODORE GOLDBERG (1983–87)

Background

Ted Goldberg's term was cut short by a terminal illness. He was another chair with actual experience in the field of public health, a graduate of the University of Buffalo who had practised social work. He obtained a PhD in political economy from the University of Toronto, where John Hastings was a member of his PhD committee and began his dissertation under Malcolm Taylor while Taylor was at the Department of Political Economy.[32]

After receiving his doctorate he returned to the United States, where he was a medical care consultant for the United Steel Workers and the United Automobile Workers unions. In 1971 he was appointed professor in the Department of Community Health at Wayne State University and in 1976 he became its chair. He returned to Canada to be chair of the Department of Health Administration in 1983. His research centred on the economics of the pharmaceutical industry and generic drug substitution, alternative systems of health-care delivery, collective bargaining in the health-care industry, and health services policy.[33] He also had a background in the practice and teaching of social work.

Goldberg was known for his commitment to accessible and affordable health-care services and to prepaid group practices. He participated in the founding convention of the Group Health Association of America in 1959 and also did some work for the Canadian national offices of the United Steelworkers of America. While there he was instrumental in the development of the Sault Ste Marie and District Group Health Association, the oldest and largest health service organization in Canada, serving on its first Board of Directors. While working for the International Union of United Automobile workers in Detroit he was on the board of directors and for a year was president of the Metropolitan Hospital and Clinic.[34]

In this there was a connection to Fred Mott, as in 1957 Mott had been recruited by Walter Reuther of the United Autoworkers to be executive director of the Community Health Association, a consumer-controlled group prepayment program sponsored by the union for its members and their families in the Detroit metropolitan area.[35] It was under Mott's leadership that the organization bought the Detroit Metropolitan Hospital and built two community clinics.[36]

Goldberg had a keen and wide intellect, and we get a glimpse into his character through published articles that dealt with other than his research interests. One such example illustrates that as a chair of a department undertaking both research and teaching, the importance of the latter was very much a concern for him. In his book review on Derek Bok's *Higher Learning*, we see through the issues he chose to pick out of the former president of Harvard's book just how this concern was crystallized.

He queried why "academics who are so curious about so many things," are "so unready to find out what difference schooling makes in student lives." In an observation that he was sure to encounter when he came to Toronto, he noted the "perennial effort to balance research and teaching functions." This was particularly acute in a department such as his, which was involved in teaching the professions as well as future academics, hence both a teaching and research stream. It is in such a department that teaching takes on a more complex role, for teaching the professions is different from teaching researchers.[37] And, one could argue, teaching the health professions (such as health management) is far different from teaching business management.

He noted Bok's thoughts on the shifting of the centre of gravity from the practical interests of the profession to the more abstract research orientation of the academy. He highlighted a distinction that Bok drew between what Bok termed "the stability in aim and method of curricula in medicine, law and business in contrast to the vacillation and uncertainty that have marked the more 'precarious professions'" of which Goldberg's profession of social work was mentioned as an example. In a world where, rightly, research was becoming so important, he spoke of the "affirmation of the importance of teaching." He highlighted the knowledge explosion where it took Harvard 275 years to collect its first million books and five years to accumulate its most recent million. He singled out Bok's emphasis on ethical issues and social responsibility as well as efforts to develop educational programs to prepare for public service.[38]

Goldberg's thoughts were perhaps implicitly getting at a subtlety of teaching in health at the graduate level. Perhaps in each case (professional and academic) one is teaching leadership. Health administrators are leaders but so are researchers. In the present IHPME a strong argument could be made its research faculty are leaders, and they need to teach the future leaders of research of tomorrow.

During His Term

AUPHA Accreditation

In March 1984 the program underwent an accreditation visit from the Association of University Programs in Health Administration (AUPHA), whose comments were largely positive. Areas noted for improvement included the need for courses in data processing and computer information systems and the physical plant. The open-concept layout of the second floor of the McMurrich Building was not seen to be conducive to a "quiet, confidential setting." Archival correspondence indicates Peggy Leatt as the associate chair was very involved in the preparation for the accreditation visit.[39]

A Continuing Education Program for Physician Administrators

In 1984/85, as a result of a grant received from the Ministry of Health, the department developed programs in management for selected physicians with administrative responsibilities. During that year a ten-day course was developed for psychiatrists, including medical directors of psychiatric hospitals and chiefs of psychiatry of acute general hospitals. It had plans to expand this to medical officers of health for Ontario the next academic year, and chiefs of services in hospitals the year after that. Peggy Leatt was a driving force behind the initiative.[40]

Proposal for an Undergraduate Degree in Health Administration

In 1986 the department, along with Woodsworth College, developed a proposal to start an undergraduate program in health administration, jointly submitted by Goldberg and Dr A. Kruger, principal of Woodsworth College. It noted that the initiative was being undertaken because of the rapid growth of the health-care industry. It observed that while there were opportunities for education for senior managers, it was "becoming clear that many first-line and middle level managers are seeking systematic educational preparation." It suggested that most of the student body would be mature students, people already working in the field. It stated that at that time there was no such undergraduate program in Canada.[41]

The proposal noted that Wordsworth was deemed to be a good partner because it was concerned mainly with meeting the needs of part-time undergraduate students and had experience with working with a variety of faculties toward this end. A task force was formed in July 1985, chaired by Peggy Leatt. Vayda, as associate dean; F.H. Lowy, the dean of medicine; and C. Hollenberg, vice-provost, Health Sciences, were also involved.[42]

Kruger noted that the idea arose out of a discussion with the chief of medical staff at Toronto General Hospital. The chief said to Kruger that capable physicians were promoted to managerial positions and that nothing they learned in medical schools prepared them for the managerial tasks they now faced. He felt that this led to poor decisions and the wasting of large sums of money, and that there needed to be some sort of educational program for people who transited from a purely clinical activity to a clinical/management or a purely management role.[43]

The proposal ultimately foundered in the university's administrative approval process.

Hewitt Facilitates Bator Attending a Rockefeller Conference on Public Health Education

David Hewitt spent a sabbatical year in 1987 with Roy Acheson at Cambridge and told him of Paul Bator's interest in the history of public health education. As a result Acheson invited Bator to a Rockefeller Conference in Italy, which was going to discuss the origins of public health education in the United Kingdom, the United States, and Germany. A number of the discussion questions were very relevant to what was happening at that time in public health education at U of T. One question was, "Has the dogged persistence of the British, of placing responsibility for public health education predominately in the hands of the medical profession been justified?" In Britain many university medical schools were involved in public health education, whereas in the United States it was the opposite – theirs have been for the most part separate schools of public health (though Yale was an exception).[44]

Bator made a presentation whose objective was to inject a Canadian perspective on the themes outlined in a paper by Arthur Viseltear on public health education in the United States. Bator drew connections between the U of T Faculty of Medicine and School of Hygiene and how it was initially influenced by the United Kingdom, then the United States, and Europe. He also noted connections between the school and the Rockefeller Foundation. He noted the Canadian federal system. He mentioned the connection to public health nursing, the Dominion Council of Health, and its being a "staff college" for medical officers of health. One interesting point he made in his paper, which relates directly to IHPME and its role in organization and management, was that FitzGerald's "military health services in wartime" convinced him "that much would be accomplished by a 'unified and coordinated' system of health workers."[45]

An important part of Bator's paper was his elucidation of Fitzgerald's role and Fitzgerald's wrestling with the problem of introducing preventive medicine into the undergraduate medical curriculum. There was also FitzGerald's ideal that public health education included not only physicians but allied health professions as well. In this he strongly asserted it needed to be its own distinct discipline and not part of another field.[46] Bator also emphasized the link between the school and Connaught as "the source of the growth of new scientific expertise.... The concept of a biological laboratory with research and manufacturing activities linked to a school offering public health education programs helped improve general health conditions in Canada."[47]

There are two important distinctive characteristics of the Canadian system that can be gleaned from his paper. One was that the Toronto school could be looked at as a hybrid when compared to the UK and US systems. It was somewhat in the middle, closely connected to a medical school but standing apart. The other was its close relationship to Connaught. Another gleaning was that the school had close links to all three levels of government.

The purpose of the conference was to produce a book on public health education, but Bator's paper was not included.[48] This was an unfortunate omission, as his paper provided a very useful exposé of the emergence of public health education in English Canada and the role of U of T and FitzGerald. Its inclusion would have broadened the compass of the book, as the Canadian achievement was unique.

Some connections of the conference to ground-breaking British work in health inequalities are interesting. One attendee at the conference was Douglas Black, author of the Black Report on that topic, a report the Thatcher government tried to suppress.[49] We noted earlier that Roy's brother Donald later (1998) wrote the sequel to the Black Report. Another connection is that Gene Vayda, who was associate dean at U of T at the time, knew Roy Acheson and Arthur Viseltear, as they were at Yale when he was a fellow in Public Health in their program.[50] The reader will recall that Vayda was financially supporting Bator's work on the history of public health education at U of T.

A REPORT BY DEAN LOWY

In 1987 Dean Lowy produced a report of activities during his term, which included a section on community health. It noted that graduate education had "experienced a steady growth" and that residents in the postgraduate medical program in community health had more than doubled, as had the number of research projects.[51]

Another section called "The Commercialization of Research" was by coincidence almost identical to the title I chose for a graduate course in IHPME some twenty years later.[52]

WHERE GRADS ENDED UP: VI

The following is a selected list of master's grads during the terms of Vayda and Goldberg. The thesis titles are no longer included, as the master's grads did not have to produce a thesis.

Dan Carriere (MHSc, 1980) had a career running hospitals. For a number of years he was president of Southlake Regional Health Centre. He went from there to the private sector and from there to CEO of the Turks and Caicos Islands Hospital.

Camille Orridge (MHSc, 1983) came to Canada from Jamaica and worked as a ward aide at TGH. She was CEO of the Toronto Central Community Care Access Centre and also the Toronto Central LHIN. She was a member of the Advisory Council on the Implementation of National Pharmacare.

Rena Arshinoff (MHSc, 1983), after pursuing a career as an epidemiologist after graduating, embarked on becoming a rabbi, was ordained in 2008, and presently at Baycrest Health Sciences Centre.[53]

Sally Brown (MHSc, 1984), an RN, went from TGH to the Prime Minister's Office, then to the Association of Universities and Colleges Canada, and then to CEO of the Heart and Stroke Foundation of Canada.

Enrique Ruelas, MD (MHSc, 1984), served as secretary of the General Health Council of Mexico, a position that is similar to the US surgeon general. Previously, he was the Mexican vice minister for innovation and quality in the Ministry of Health, where he oversaw the modernization of Mexico's health-care system. He has also been president of the Mexican Hospital Association and dean of the National School of Public Health of Mexico.

John Oliver (MHSc, 1985) was a chartered accountant who became interested in hospitals after doing an audit. He had been an ADM at the Ministry of Health and Long-Term Care and left a position as president and CEO of Halton Healthcare Services to run and be elected a member of Parliament. He was a member of the House of Commons (2015–19) and on its Standing Committee on Health. He decided not to see re-election in 2019.[54]

Sheela Basrur (MD, 1982, MHSc, 1987) was the Toronto medical officer of health who led the city through the SARS crisis of 2003. The *Toronto Star* reported, "In the darkest days of Toronto's fight against SARS, when people were dying and thousands more were quarantined prisoners in their homes, a small, mighty woman took control of the worst public health disaster to grip this city in years."[55] She presented on behalf of Toronto Public Health to the Romanow Commission public hearings held in Toronto on 31 May 2002 (see the section on the commission later in this work). She was subsequently named Ontario chief medical officer. Ontario honoured her legacy by establishing the Sheela Basrur Centre.[56]

CHAPTER 17

Another Transition for the Professional Degree

The tail end of the 1980s saw yet another review of the decision to dissolve the School of Hygiene. It also saw a new chair for the department and an important refocusing of the MHSc degree.

DISCUSSION OF THE DISSOLUTION OF THE SCHOOL CONTINUES (THIRTEEN YEARS AFTER CLOSURE)

Early 1988: Hannah Report

An important internal report was the Decanal Task Force, which was struck in April 1987 and reported in February 1988. It was called the Hannah Report and grew out of a 1980 provostial review of the Faculty of Medicine that raised questions about the future direction of the Division of Community Health. It acknowledged accomplishments of the division, such as the new degree structure and increase of research. It was complimentary of the Hastings and Vayda regimes. Its main concern was transitioning the division to a world-recognized centre for the education of community health experts and an increase in funding to get there. The question was the best structure to achieve this.

There were differing views on this point. Ten of the committee members felt that the best structure was to stay within the Faculty of Medicine but with important conditions, such as support from senior levels, adequate funding, and a good divisional head. Seven members submitted a dissenting view that advocated a return to a distinct and separate institution. The differing proposals on the administrative location for the division appeared as separate and signed appendices (five and six) to the report.

The chair in his letter of transmittal noted that its "recommendation is supported by only a slim majority of the members" and that the "inclusion of these statements has obviated the necessity for a minority report."[1] John

Browne noted, "Walt Hannah was an excellent chair: even-handed, patient, and open-minded. He did us a favour by not voting on the report himself, thereby making the decision seem closer than it actually was."[2] The dissenting members included a number of Health Administration faculty (Browne and Hastings) and Vivek Goel (who at the time was a graduate student in the department representing the Community Health Students Union).[3]

The report noted, "Both groups have the same vision of Community Health, they differ only in their conception of the best Faculty environment to achieve that vision."[4] The dissenters founded their case on the fact that "community health is a discipline, a body of knowledge and its application, in its own right. It is based on a distinct set of assumptions." It then listed what these were: the focus is the community, not the individual; the emphasis is on health, rather than disease; it addresses broader social, economic, environmental, and other factors influencing health. It noted that although medicine shares such assumptions, they are not the primary assumptions.[5]

According to the report, "Community health is fundamentally multidisciplinary, interdisciplinary, multisectoral and intersectoral in its approach." What this meant was that community health "is a distinct end in itself." It should not be limited "conceptually and in application to serving the needs of one discipline." It also noted, "All Canadian universities with faculties of medicine can develop strong Community Medicine Departments if they so choose. Few, if any, are in such an ideal position as the University of Toronto … to develop a separate world-renowned centre for excellence in Community Health research, teaching and practice."[6]

It bears mentioning that one thing demonstrated by the number of these reports was that public health sciences and its positioning within the university occupied university administrators. They did seem to want to get it right, and indeed, as the number of reports suggests, they agonized over the issue.

It also demonstrates that the development of cutting-edge programs is neither automatic nor straightforward. How a program should be configured, the degree of independence it should have within an institution, and where it should sit within an institution are all very important decisions, and as we have seen generated strong and principled stances on the parts of participants.

Late 1988: CJPH *Articles*

The discontent was not just internal to the university. Bator notes that the closing of the School of Hygiene in Toronto along with its counterpart at the Université de Montréal resulted in "the alienation and dissatisfaction of Canadian Public Health professionals," which would "grow over the years."[7]

The issue was also debated in academic journals. John Last, editor of the *Canadian Journal of Public Health*, noted in an editorial in 1988, "The decision more than a decade ago to liquidate the School of Hygiene at the University of Toronto has always seemed to me a short-sighted and unimaginative act.... Those responsible did not behave with a sense of vision about the future health of Canadians. Rather, they seemed to be motivated by a belief that public health training and research could be narrowly based upon a biomedical model."[8]

But it wasn't just the closure itself, it was its implications for the country. Last noted, "Insofar as centres of all-round excellence in public health can be identified in the world, we have none at all in Canada." He called for "at least one centre of genuinely recognizable international stature" that would attract not only the best and brightest of Canadian scholars but also those of other countries. He said without "this degree of intellectual cross-fertilization, public health in Canada will never be anything other than a derivative calling." He added, "Public health is too important to be entrusted to deans of medical schools."[9]

He followed this up with a second editorial some months later where he reiterated that medical schools are an inappropriate setting for teaching and research in public health; that they lack the interdisciplinary nature of public health schools. He added that the "whole thrust of medical education is disease-oriented," whereas public health is "health-oriented" and "population-based rather than focusing on individuals." He called again for "one, preferably more than one, national centre of excellence." He noted that his previous editorial had provoked more letters to the editor, phone calls, and discussion among colleagues than any other editorial topic in the last eight years.[10]

The CJPH reprinted some of the correspondence received, which was notable for its geographical range, with letters coming from different parts of Canada, the United States, and as far away as Israel. The first one printed was from John Hastings, who defended the U of T initiative. Another was from the dean of the Johns Hopkins school, who wrote, "It is most unusual to have a strong public health faculty as a department of a medical school" and added, "I do believe there is a need for a school whose concern is the health of a population rather than the sickness of an individual." Another was from John Evans, who noted the "solutions are not straightforward." Another was from the vice-president, Academic Affairs, York University, who noted that not having a faculty of medicine at the university was in this case an advantage, and they intended to focus on an interdisciplinary approach. Another was from Fraser Mustard, who was dean of medicine at McMaster after Evans, and president of the Canadian Institute for Advanced Research. He directed discussion toward the determinants of health and noted that while this was almost completely absent from medical schools, schools of public health needed to focus more attention on this important topic.[11]

Given opinions such as these and the stellar reputation of the school, one needs to query its dissolution. There is also the issue of moving it and public health from being within an autonomous stand-alone entity within the university to one now nested within a faculty. However, the issues are not straightforward.

There were other matters such as a fear for the cutting-edge, groundbreaking character of the school, which was challenging to the status quo at times. Since its inception, the school was very freethinking, practical, and involved in bettering the health of the ordinary Canadian. It had not only led to discoveries of new vaccines and antitoxins but to their mass availability at an at-cost price that allowed the governments of Ontario and Saskatchewan to make them available to everyone at no cost to the individual. This saved countless lives and countless dollars to provincial treasuries. It had also led to the school being at the forefront of national policy and at every major debate on the possibility of health insurance in Canada.

While on the one hand one could argue for combining the preventive and promotion aspects of health care with the clinical (diagnostic and treatment) aspects, there was a fear for their being subsumed under the vast weight of the illness-care machine that had come to epitomize medicine. That this in many cases was a delicate balance augured for stand-alone schools of public health. And this ignores an entity like IHPME. There is prevention and treatment *and* policy and management and evaluation. This last bit is the hardest to classify and cleanly allocate.[12]

On the one hand, one could also legitimately question whether without such radical surgery the necessary reform and revision within the school and the department could have happened. On the other hand, this was a highly complex issue with a number of very thorny questions, and radical surgery was precisely what was needed. Browne offers that the school was about to break apart anyway, that departments like Microbiology and Parasitology were more properly placed in a science or medical faculty and that the location of preventive medicine was also an open question, given that the Faculty of Medicine had an activity in this area.[13]

There are additional questions such as whether the school could have been reformed internally or incrementally, whether within a highly politicized environment like U of T, Evans would have been able otherwise to direct the funds he did to help support the new division and through this rebuild the department.

We noted earlier that years later John Hastings said he believed "that the loss of financial support from Connaught and other endowments was a major factor in the decline of the School of Hygiene."[14] He said, "As a result of the separation of Connaught and the University of Toronto, the School of Hygiene lost much of its prestige and independence,"[15] because it had been able to tap into Connaught money for initiatives. This gave it a measure of independence from the university, which he said was somewhat analogous to the Faculty of Medicine.[16]

Vivek Goel, who worked a number of years on securing a proper place for public health at the university, reminded me that he was always struck by the phrase on the dissolution of the School of Hygiene written by Friedland in the first edition of his history of U of T (published before the Dalla Lana School was established). At the time Friedland said, "It is likely ... that the University has not heard the last of the question of the proper place of public health in the University of Toronto."[17] The quote also appears on the same page in the second edition of the work, but he also references it in the introduction of the second edition, noting the establishment of the Dalla Lana School, and says, "The issue now appears to have been settled for the foreseeable future."[18]

A CHANGING CONTEXT

When we spoke of the 1962–73 era, we referred to the concentration of hospital care within a short radius of the department. It remains so today. But while the number of hospital beds has stopped growing, the institutions have not. By the 1980s all University Avenue institutions (and some others) had built their own research facilities. This would further broaden the area of health management, as there was now health research management, given that the size of these research institutes rivalled that of small universities. And it continues. We will talk more of this later, but today, on U of T's south-eastern flank, less than a block from the present location of IHPME, we find not only research, but also its application. A biomedical research park, MaRS, spans an entire block. It is located on the original College Street site of Toronto General and has constructed a tower on land once occupied by its Mulock and Larkin Wings on the west and another on where the Burnside Wing was located on the east.

This is research emanating from the "hard" sciences. IHPME soon became interested in this process of discovery. Its predecessor department had already taken an active interest in generating its own research – pioneered by people like Hastings and Vayda, and it really began to take hold in the Leatt era. Then, later, beginning in Louise Lemieux-Charles's era, IHPME went a step further and began to take an interest in the commercial application of research, in the process of taking ideas from the bench to the bedside.

PEGGY LEATT (1988–98)

Peggy Leatt became chair in 1988. She had joined the department in 1980, filling the position vacated by Maureen Dixon, who returned to England and a position with the King's Fund. Leatt had just received her PhD in sociology from the University of Alberta, specializing in complex organizations. During her term as chair the department received strong support from the dean of medicine, not only being protected from budget cuts, but also receiving new faculty positions.[19]

A Modular Format

In 1994 the department began planning to meet the needs of mature applicants working in the field who were looking for the opportunity to pursue further education. It was implemented in the fall of 1994.

Leatt had served as the commissioner of the Accrediting Commission for Education in Health Services Administration and during her tenure had visited twenty-five health administration master's programs across North America. This consolidated her thinking on what was required in the department.[20]

The modular format was one of the biggest changes the department underwent. It involved a complete revamping of class material and how it was delivered. Students did not come for a lecture once per week but rather an intensive series of lectures over a four-day period every three weeks, five times per term. They attended lectures for part of Wednesday, and all day Thursday, Friday, and Saturday. The practicum also changed. It was shortened and had more choices, particularly in the part-time option. Placement opportunities were broadened to include community, policy and planning, and the private sector.

The model chosen was similar to the "On Job – On Campus" model of the University of Michigan. In the new format the fees remained the same. The department did not adopt an executive-type fee structure. This was as the result of work done by the Society of Graduates in Health Administration under the leadership of Barry Monaghan, who was president of the society at the time. He found that the field could not support an executive-type program with a high fee structure similar to that in the university's Executive MBA program.[21]

In a statement to the external reviewers of her department in 1997 Leatt outlined some of the reasons for the switch to the modular format. Managers needed to "have the skills to operate as facilitators, not impediments to change" and the development of skills such as these needed to be "available and accessible by health managers and policy makers in the system as well as those outside the system to be trained for the future."[22]

The new program involved a different kind of learner, an individual who was not a full-time student but rather a full-time worker. A requirement for admission was a minimum of three years' work experience. Students therefore spent much less time on campus. It made for a different kind of commitment. The major commitment of this new cohort was their job as opposed to full-time students for whom it was their studies. It gave the program a different kind of character.

The proportions of this intermixing of practice and theory were altered. The students had a strong practical focus. This practical element was reinforced by practitioner-tutors in two of the program's major classes (HAD 5010 and 5020). Practitioners were also part of the panels used in this class. Yet other academics, other researchers were also part of these panels. And the IHPME faculty involved in teaching were researchers. It made for a very interesting mix.

Vivek Goel noted that today there is substantial emphasis on co-op programs and EMBAs; yet the Institute has been doing this for over twenty years.[23] The modular template Leatt implemented has proven to be enduring, as we will see that it has also been used for the MHI program at IHPME and also for a Master's in Health Administration program at Ryerson University (which was implemented by an IHPME grad).

External Review of the Department

In the fall of 1997 an external review of the department was conducted and its report, submitted in January 1998, was very positive. On its program in health administration the report noted, "Applications to the program have doubled ... and the school has acquired a very positive national and international reputation."[24] On research the report noted that the graduate programs of the department were the largest in Canada.[25] At that time it was receiving $1.5 million per year in research funding – "a good amount even for a university like Toronto where research has a high priority." It noted the establishment of the Hospital Management Research Unit in the Department by the Ministry of Health in 1989, which had been renewed for another five years in 1994.[26]

One item noted in the report was where such departments are situated within a university. It observed that one-third are in each of schools of public health, faculties of management, and other locations (such as faculties of medicine). On the same page it noted that "the Department's MHSc Program is regarded within the academic and professional communities as the leading program in Canada" and that "its activities have earned it a strong leadership position in the country."[27]

A Restructuring of the Department

In April 1998 a restructuring saw increased emphasis on research and graduate education. At this time the Division of Community Health within the Faculty of Medicine was dissolved. In addition the Departments of Preventive Medicine and Biostatistics and Behavioural Sciences merged. The Department of Health Administration became a Graduate Department of Health Administration relating directly to the U of T School of Graduate Studies. At about this time the department received funding for its first research chair (in health management sciences) from Liberty Health.[28]

Hospital Management Research Unit

In 1988 the Ministry of Health in Ontario developed a program for funding research units that were linked to the health system (called System-Linked Research Units). In July 1989 the department was successful in competing for one of nine funded in the province. Peggy Leatt was the principal investigator. Its mandate was to conduct research to improve the organization and management of hospitals. It was also to enhance the hospital system's ability to deliver effective health services. The partner hospital was Sunnybrook Health Sciences Centre, which was where much of the research was conducted. A wide variety of projects were funded over a ten-year period. Additional funding was received from the Hospital Incentive Fund of the Ministry of Health. It was to work jointly with local hospitals in developing and evaluating hospital management innovation.[28] It replaced the Health Care Research Unit.

Core Courses Revised

In 1996 IHPME chose two young faculty at the time, Paul Williams and Raisa Deber, to co-coordinate the core courses. Paul came from Ryerson, where he had set up their health studies program, and Raisa was a Torontonian (and a high school classmate of Tom Closson) who had got a PhD from MIT.[30]

Paul was originally hired on a tenure-track position at Ryerson in 1987 in the School of Politics and Public Administration. But he soon ran into the dean of continuing education, Milton Orris, who was previously program director of the MHSc program in the Department of Health Administration.

Milton bought Paul out of the politics school to create a certificate in long-term care administration and then the undergraduate program in health services management. Peggy Leatt then brought him to U of T to move the policy courses from the old thirteen-week traditional format, into the new modular format, just coming on stream when he was hired in 1993.

Paul always believed in a mix of theory and practice, which was a hallmark of Ryerson's curriculum, and saw the panels and practitioner-tutor seminars as the way of bringing real world experience and insight into the classroom. So academics did what they do best, and tutors and panellists focused on how things play out.[31]

One important characteristic of the core courses was their ability to draw distinguished speakers to present at them. For example, Larry Grossman came while he was minister of health.[32] Raisa Deber arranged for Michael Decter to come while deputy minister of health; Jay Kaufman while deputy minister of treasury board; Margaret Mottershead while senior assistant deputy minister of health (she was later deputy minister).[33]

Under Paul and Raisa the class sessions had a unique structure. It was revised to fit the modular format. They were divided into four sections and took place over a five-hour period. There was a lecture session on a health policy issue. Then a panel of three experts in the area, either academics or practitioners, each of whom made a short presentation, which was followed by questions from the class. Then another lecture on policy and influencers of policy. The last part was a tutorial, which could discuss any of the preceding.

An integral part of the core courses was the tutorials. However, under Paul and Raisa, these changed from being led by faculty to being led by practitioners. They found about a dozen people from diverse aspects of the field to lead them, many of whom would do so for years.[34] The tutorials and the practitioner roles formed an integral part of the course. Tutor packages were prepared for each session, and the tutors were the first line of contact for students and graded all assignments for their group.

The tutorials (and the panels) were another example of continuing practitioner involvement in the institute. They always had more people wanting to be tutorial leaders than were required (a fact that remains to this day). Their eagerness to participate was a sign of the loyalty to the department and the fact that so many wanted to remain in contact.

The assignment format was altered, and instead of essays there was a series of four briefing notes on four different topics (chosen by Paul and Raisa). It was felt this would provide good training for future executives in developing a skill of succinctly summarizing a complex issue into a précis. Each briefing note had to outline a topic (which was usually a health care issue) in five pages according to purpose, background, analysis, and recommendation.

The importance and utility of the briefing notes was underscored in an encounter Paul had with a member of Justin Trudeau's Cabinet. While Paul was at a "Best Brains" conference in Ottawa, he ran into former federal minister of health Jane Philpott (MPH, 2012). She told him she had been in his HAD 5010 class and at the time had worked hard to master the art of writing the four briefing notes. She noted that students had often complained about the amount of effort they spent learning to write them and that now she had a greater appreciation for how important they were, since as a government minister she was constantly having to read them.[35]

INNOVATIVE CLASSES/CONFERENCES

Throughout its history the department/institute has mounted innovative courses aimed either at the student body or as continuing education for professionals. One example is a course "Evaluate Your Programs," which in 1980 was billed as the "21st Annual Refresher Course." It involved topics such as why evaluate, case studies, types of research, cost benefit and effectiveness analysis, and the use of data, among others. Claire Bombardier, John Browne, Raisa Deber, and Jack Williams were the faculty involved.[36] It demonstrates that long before the term *evaluation* was added to the department/institute's title it was looking at issues of evaluation.

HEALTH ADMIN GRADS SECONDED TO THE ONTARIO MINISTRY OF HEALTH

There has always been a close association between the department and the Ontario Ministry of Health, which was reinforced when through the late 1980s and into the 1990s the ministry seconded people from the field to the ministry for roughly twelve- to eighteen -month terms. One intent was to give each segment of the health-care system a better understanding of the other. A number of health admin grads were involved in these secondments to various divisions within the ministry. One example was Les Boehm (MHSc, 1980), who went as a consultant in Institutional Operations. Another was Barry Monahan (DHA, 1974), who was seconded as president of West Park Hospital to the director level in the ministry in Institutional Operations.[37]

Another was Mark Rochon (MHSc, 1980), who went from president of Humber Memorial Hospital to the assistant deputy minister level, where he led the development of policies on the funding and oversight of hospital services in Ontario.

ONTARIO HEALTH SERVICES RESTRUCTURING COMMISSION (HSRC)

An IHPME graduate and an IHPME chair played an important role in this commission. Mark Rochon served as its CEO from April 1996 to August 1998, and Peggy Leatt from September 1998 to April 2000.[38]

The HSRC made binding decisions on the restructuring of hospitals in Ontario and provided policy advice to government on the broader health system. Rochon and Leatt, along with the chair of HSRC, wrote a book on the process.[39]

WHERE GRADS ENDED UP: VII

More information on IHPME grads:

Shirlee Sharkey (MHSc, 1992), is CEO of St Elizabeth Health Care. Her earlier positions have been as a visiting nurse, then in a teaching hospital. She received an honorary doctorate from UOIT in 2017.[40]

Eileen de Villa (MHSc, 1994), Toronto medical officer of health, is also a graduate of U of T medical school (MD, 1998).[41]

Altaf Stationwala (MHSc, 1995; he was in Les Boehm's HAD 5010 tutorial group) was appointed president and CEO of Mackenzie Health in 2010. In June 2015 he established the Mackenzie Innovation Institute (Mi^2).[42] To illustrate the kind of community involvement that Roth referred to, he has spoken a number of times on how the expansion of Mackenzie Health can benefit the community.

Catherine Zahn (MHSc, 1995), is president and CEO, Centre for Addiction and Mental Health. She is also a graduate of U of T medical school with a specialty in neurology.

The academic side was also notable in its grads. Some examples:

Louise Lemieux-Charles (PhD, 1989) was the first PhD graduate of the MSc/PhD program and the first recipient of the Ted Goldberg Award. She has a background in nursing and administration. She was a senior nursing executive at Toronto General and so combined a practical awareness of the needs of the continually evolving and increasingly complex health management system.

Gillian Hawker (MSc, Health Administration, 1993) is Sir John & Lady Eaton Professor and Chair of the Department of Medicine, University of

Toronto. She is a clinical epidemiologist/health services researcher whose research has focused on improving access to and outcomes following care for people with osteoarthritis. She has also been chief of medicine at Women's College Hospital.

PART SEVEN

A Further Broadening of Focus

CHAPTER 18

Adding Policy, Outcomes, and Expanding the Research Mandate

The transformation was important for two reasons: it broadened the research focus, and in doing so it added two new dimensions to the teaching of the professional degree (looking at policy and outcomes).

VIVEK GOEL (1999–2002)

If there is one individual who is central to the revitalization of FitzGerald's ideals of public health at U of T, that person is Vivek Goel. Indeed he is a central figure not just in public health revitalization at U of T but also in Ontario. He was CEO of Public Health Ontario, provost of Health Sciences, then vice-president of Research at U of T. He is also named principal investigator of the Ontario Health Study, launched in 2010 and one of the largest long-term health studies in Canada.

The Program in Clinical Epidemiology Moves to the Department

Vivek Goel was appointed chair of the department in February 1999. Under his leadership the Program in Clinical Epidemiology and the Health Care Research Unit merged with the Department of Health Administration in 2000. He was approached by the dean of medicine, Arnie Aberman, to take the program into the department.

Vivek says that it was a powerful move, for not only did it bring the epidemiologists from the university program into the department, it also brought all the epidemiologists who had a university appointment but were housed in the clinical epidemiology departments of the hospital-based research institutes into the fold. He says it set the department on a trajectory of closer alignment with the clinical sector and gave the department an important new knowledge base for executive and policy development.[1]

Scientist Leadership

A very interesting initiative of Vivek's was what could be interpreted as the beginnings of an exploration of whether research was emerging as a significant new area of activity. And just as the Department of Hospital Administration grew out of a need to provide specialized training for hospital administrators, Vivek began to look at the same for scientist leaders. He notes that around 2000 he and Tina Smith ran a workshop to discuss the creation of a scientist leadership course.[2]

Vivek notes the motivation at the time was the work that was happening with the transformation of MRC to CIHR. He was having regular meetings with leaders of the research institutes at the hospitals, and they were all trying to build their research organizations. That helped flag the need. As well, CIHR was going to have multiple institutes that would need administrative leads. He had also been involved with HEALNet, a national centre of excellence, as scientific program leader and observed the need for preparation of people who could run that type of activity.[3]

Initiatives in Hospital-Based Research

During Goel's time as chair, hospital-based research institutes grew to a size that required their own administrative organizations. As a result some of the IHPME grads started to branch out in what might be called non-traditional areas of health management, i.e., the administration of hospital-based research institutes. In addition to the management of research operations for some, it also involved commercializing health research. It is interesting that this happened during Goel's time as chair, given that he is presently very involved in such activities as vice-president of Research and Innovation at the U of T.

All the large teaching hospitals in downtown Toronto had been involved in research for many years. TGH was involved in insulin research. The pace stepped up after the Second World War. Describing this time, Connor talks of the "inventiveness of these doctors in their workshops" that "pushed the boundaries of medicine in new directions" and research also "became a measure of institutional prestige."[4] It was also unique in that it many times combined basic, applied, and clinical research.

But especially in the 1980s this involvement, in Toronto and elsewhere, began to be formalized within designated large research institutes. By the later 1990s some of them rivalled the size of the research activity of university medical faculties. These institutes were affiliated with faculties of medicine and were involved in teaching graduate students at the respective universities as well as in conducting basic research. The basic research necessarily led to its commercialization.

Over time, these institutes became organizations in their own right, an organization within an organization, a number with budgets well over $100 million and housed in their own dedicated facility. One notable example is the SickKids research institute, the Peter Gilgan Centre for Research and Learning, which at 750,000 square feet, is believed to be the largest children's research tower in the world.[5] It is also an architecturally distinctive building and has been referred to as a "research cathedral."[6] The use of the church metaphor is interesting. The British do the same thing. The *Guardian* has called the building housing the new Francis Crick Institute a "cathedral of science" and an "altar to biomedical science."[7]

SickKids was not alone in building such a facility; the Ontario Cancer Institute, Toronto General, Toronto Western, Mount Sinai, St Michael's Hospital, and Sunnybrook Health Sciences Centre had also built major research facilities. In addition there was MaRS located on TGH land and in its former College Wing. Some of the scientist faculty in these institutes are cross-appointed to IHPME.

As the size of these institutes grew to such levels, it was axiomatic that a new type of manager would be required to run them. Actually two different types of management emerged. The first was in research operations, while the other was in research commercialization. We will look at research commercialization first and research operations in the chapter on Louise Lemieux Charles. The commercialization piece was a spillover into Canada of major new activity that was taking place in the United States in technology transfer as a result of the Bayh-Dole Act.

While at the Sunnybrook Research Institute (SRI) I felt that it needed to become involved in technology transfer and approached Innovations Foundation at U of T to provide this service to SRI. I also hatched the idea of starting a venture-capital research fund and developed the idea of marrying the basic research being conducted at academic institutes with the applied research of big pharma. I worked with Mark Henkelman, vice-president, Research, and Tom Closson, CEO of Sunnybrook Health Sciences Centre on each of these. Each initiative aimed to keep Canadian ideas, activities, and graduates in Canada.

The first initiative was made possible by an innovative program of the Ontario government. It had launched a Community Small Business Investment Fund that provided a tax credit to Labour-Sponsored Venture Capital Corporations that launched such a fund through a university. I approached the Ministry of Finance to see if they would also include hospital-based, university-affiliated research institutes. They agreed and Sunnybrook partnered with Working Ventures Fund to form the first such fund devoted to commercializing medical research, which was noted in the *Report on Business* section of the *Globe and Mail* in January 1999.[8]

Connaught Labs Comes Full Circle

An interesting aspect of the second initiative is that it involved the current incarnation of Connaught Labs. Another was that it brought Connaught Lab activity back to U of T in the sense that it was located at a major U of T affiliate. Yet another was that U of T faculty (Neil Berinstein and Brian Barber) were hired to run the project.

I had canvassed all the major big pharma companies on this idea. As it turned out the denouement put Connaught Labs, which was now a major subsidiary of a French pharmaceutical firm, at the centre of a significant new application of vaccine technology. Pasteur Merieux Connaught Canada (PMCC), which was the company Connaught Labs had been folded into, would strike a partnership with Sunnybrook to locate the world headquarters of their cancer-vaccine project there in 40,000 square feet of purpose-built research space. Also Sunnybrook became a major partner in its Pan-Canadian Cancer Vaccine Network, which meant funding for Sunnybrook scientists involved in cancer vaccine research as well as scientists involved in clinical research. This continued a research thrust initiated all the way back to people like FitzGerald, continued by people like Best, and attracting graduate students like the Solandt brothers.

Technology Partnerships Canada, an agency of Industry Canada, noted that at the time PMC's $350 million investment in this network was the largest single biotechnology investment ever made in Canada.[9] That the whole activity happened in Canada was due to the diligence of the Chrétien government, as Canada was vying with France and Switzerland for the opportunity.

My hope was that having PMCC on site would encourage interaction between scientists involved in the basic research at SRI with those involved in the applied research at PMCC. To encourage such interaction two floors of the Sunnybrook Research Institute were designated as the location for the PMCC activities. Also PMCC and SRI scientists invited each other to their respective seminars. One beneficial result was that a number of U of T graduate students based at SRI were hired by PMCC upon completion of their studies.

As it turned out, the worldwide activities in cancer vaccine were shut down by the French parent company after about ten years. However, now, about ten years after that, it seems the idea has been vindicated, as cancer immunotherapy is one of the hottest areas in immunology, with a substantial portion of immunology conferences devoted to it.[10]

The Connaught Labs connection is still important to the company. PMCC is now known as Sanofi Pasteur. Its website has a history page called "Sanofi Pasteur in Canada," which notes the contribution of J.G. FitzGerald.[11] It also has a separate webpage on FitzGerald called "Our Founder."[12]

The company was also involved in careful restoration of the Barton Avenue Stable, which was originally built in 1913 in William "Billy" Fenton's backyard. Fenton was FitzGerald's assistant at the Ontario Provincial Laboratories. It also had a small lab to prepare diphtheria antitoxin and it was built using funds from FitzGerald's wife's dowry. It was not used for very long and it fell into disrepair, as most of the activity moved to the Antitoxin Laboratories established by the University of Toronto in 1914.

In 1935, to preserve the stable from demolition, it was moved to the rear of the Connaught "Farm" and repaired in the hope of establishing it as a museum. It was moved to another portion of the campus in 1966 where it again fell into disrepair. In 2001 it was moved to its present location at the Heritage Square entrance of the campus. It was carefully restored and a museum created inside in time for the company's ninetieth anniversary in 2004.[13]

Interestingly there is also some awareness in the public mind of FitzGerald. A relatively recent acknowledgement (2004) is a street named after him in north Toronto, almost next to the Connaught campus. Immediately adjacent to the west boundary of the campus is a ravine, and just west of that is Gerry Fitzgerald Drive.[14] In 2014 in downtown Toronto the lane that runs behind Barton Avenue has been named Crestfallen Lane after the name of the first horse he bought to produce the diphtheria antitoxin.[15]

In another example, the chief medical officer of health for Ontario noted FitzGerald's role in combating diphtheria in his 2014 annual report, *Vaccines: The Best Medicine*. In a section of the report, "Ontario Pioneers the

Way," FitzGerald's role in helping make Toronto and Hamilton among the world's first cities to be diphtheria free was noted. His role in Connaught Labs and its role in vaccines was also acknowledged.[16]

Hospital Report Cards

In 1998 and 1999 the Ontario Hospital Association published the first reports on the performance of Ontario's acute care hospital system. The research and data analysis was done by the Department of Health Administration through funds provided by the OHA.[17] The initiative was announced by the OHA at its 1997 Annual Convention. The 1998 (and 1999) report listed Ross Baker as the principal investigator.

The 1998 report noted it "was the first Ontario hospital system report of its kind" and the "most comprehensive report on the performance of hospitals to date in Canada." The hope was that the report "will provide an impetus to move forward in the development of evaluative criteria."[18] It and the 1999 report were examples of the department's move into this important new activity (evaluation) and perhaps a precursor to a change in nomenclature.

The 1999 report listed Ross Baker as first author and had a number of other IHPME faculty such as Adalsteinn Brown (who was completing his PhD studies at Oxford at the time), Geoffrey Anderson, Catherine Montgomery, Michael Murray, and George Pink as co-authors.[19] In addition it involved a number of department staff and graduates in its advisory panels.[20]

The reports were the first provincial multidimensional performance reporting system in Canada, and one of the first balanced scorecard efforts in health care. The report created a foundation for performance measurement and reporting that has since spread across Canada.[21] The report cards were adopted by the WHO and many other countries. One of the people who helped develop their report cards was a colleague of Steini's.[22]

A New Name for the Department

Following the merger, Tina Smith chaired a task force to determine a suitable name for the newly constituted department. A referendum was held among faculty members in February 2001 to decide between "Health Strategies" and "Health Policy, Management and Evaluation," with the latter winning by an overwhelming majority, and the new designation was approved by Governing Council, effective 1 July 2001.[23] It was felt that the initiative to change the moniker would bring it more in line with not only what the department was now doing (also looking at policy) but also to express an objective of its mandate in the contemporary health care scene (looking at and evaluating outcomes).

Building Public Health Capacity

Earlier we mentioned Vivek's work in advocating for more public health education and in establishing a public health agency in Ontario. Each was building public health capacity. Another aspect of his work was the articles he was involved in that disseminated this knowledge, and the amount it was publishing in peer-reviewed journals was coming to be an increasingly important part of the institute. For example in 2004 he was involved in an article that was examining how to make better use of the availability and accessibility of the avalanche of health information and the wish of the public for decisions to be more transparent and explicitly justified.[24]

In another he recounted his experience in building an Ontario public health agency called Public Health Ontario (PHO). He noted that in a short period PHO had grown to be an integral part of the public health system of Ontario and was starting to make a contribution nationally and internationally.[25] He noted that it needed to attain a balance between a number of areas, such as research and service, specialized central capacity and local supports, health protection and health promotion.[26]

LOUISE LEMIEUX-CHARLES (2002–12)

Louise assumed the chair of the renamed department in 2002. A notable initiative of hers was that HPME became an institute (IHPME) in November 2011.

During her term what was called HPME moved into new facilities, the former administrative offices of the Toronto District School Board, now called the Health Sciences Building.

It was actually a bit of an architectural gem, designed for the Toronto Board of Education by the prominent British-Canadian architect Peter Dickinson, while a partner at Page and Steel Architects. The university purchased it in 2003. It had in it a number of murals created by Stefan Fritz and Merton Chambers and an exterior relief by Elizabeth Hahn, which were meant to express the ideals of education. All of these the university preserved, along with a distinctive sixth floor wood-panelled auditorium designed by Dickinson.[27] In addition, wood-panelled conference rooms on the first floor were converted to classrooms, and a wood-panelled mini-auditorium on the same floor was preserved and put into use as a large classroom.

Its official opening was 11 January 2006. Staff and faculty had begun using the building the previous September.[28]

The Department and the Royal Commission on the Future of Health Care in Canada

Staff from the institute were involved in the Romanow Commission on the future of health care. Raisa Deber wrote "Delivering Health Care: Public, Not-for-Profit, or Private?"[29] Greg Marchildon, now a faculty member of IHPME (but not so at the time) was the commission's executive director under Mr Romanow.

One of the strengths of the institute has been its cross-appointed faculty. Linda O'Brien-Pallas from the Bloomberg Faculty of Nursing and cross-appointed to IHPME was co-author of a commission paper on human resource policies.[30] Colleen Flood, also cross-appointed to the institute, co-authored a paper on modernizing the Canada Health Act.[31]

Claus Wirsig, DHA Grad, Presents to the Commission

We noted earlier Claus Wirsig's strong support of public health care. He presented to the Commission on his own behalf. His presentation was aimed at the financial sustainability of Medicare and to this end he advocated for patient participation in decisions about care. What was intriguing about his idea was that he linked it to cost and the patient having some say in the determination of this expense, which is a cost borne by all society. His proposal was for a personal income tax liability, based on a personal tax exemption allotment up front. Only if it was used up would the tax liability be triggered. He felt this would encourage such interaction and at the same time limit costs. He outlined a number of examples of how it works, which elaborated on its benefits.[32]

Romanow evidently had Wirsig's CV at hand in addition to his presentation and complimented him on a "distinguished career" and singled out his Rhodes Scholarship. Romanow queried him further about his idea but said that because of Wirsig's background he was also interested in his views on regionalization and amalgamation, specifically concerning hospitals in Toronto. Wirsig's reply was that he was for rationalization of services but was more for maintaining the independence of facilities. He felt that the more one has regionalization the less attention is paid to individual circumstance.[33]

One comment Wirsig made in response to Romanow's questioning was that "we are getting a lot less healthcare than we are willing to pay for." Another was that "the patients need a mechanism to trigger their involvement in the decision-making." He noted later that there is a basis for a discussion to take place between physician and patient and one not only on health terms but financial ones as well.[34]

Dr Sheela Basrur, IHPME Grad, Presents to the Commission

Dr Basrur presented on behalf of Toronto Public Health, very effectively establishing the importance of public health. She began with an analogy to a river (which was then used throughout her presentation) and noted that we focus very much on the downstream aspect of fishing people out of the river (the analogy being when they are sick) when we should have been involved in preventing them from falling in (or becoming sick) in the first place. She noted that public health focuses on the upstream end. Both aspects are important, and the issue is one of balance.[35]

The hearings of this commission were video recorded so that a person could view the actual presentation as opposed to only reading a transcript (which was the case in the past). In a presentation from someone like Basrur, the viewer can not only hear what she has to say but sees the evident passion of her beliefs and her commitment to public health.

Her presentation was nothing short of excellent. She tied her presentation to that of previous presenters, to an analogy Romanow had made earlier, and used it to buttress her case for more public health resources. She very effectively used one particular quote on public health from the commission's interim report to illustrate the competition for resources between public health and acute care:[36] In a later quote she said, "Some people call for a reinvestment in prevention, I would call for a pre-investment in prevention."[37]

She alluded to a brief they had submitted to the commission in early January and that one of its main points was that "public health must be included as a foundation for our medicare system." She called for far more research into public health interventions.[38] Romanow posed a number of questions to her, including whether she would favour adding another principle to the five in the Canada Health Act (CHA), this one concerned with population health and the determinants of health. She replied that she favoured the mandatory provision of public health services, that it could be the CHA or another statutory mechanism.[39] Interestingly she referred to IHPME grad Wirsig's presentation and illustrated how his idea could also apply to public health and healthy behaviours.[40]

Research as a Distinct Area of Activity

Partnership with UTM in Their Graduate Degree on Innovation

In 2005 the department entered into a partnership with the Department (now Institute) of Management of Innovation at the University of Toronto Mississauga (UTM) to deliver a new graduate program leading to a master's in management of innovation (MMI). This involved working with the Ontario Council of Graduate Studies (OCGS) to get a new graduate degree certified by the provincial government. A major piece of the work was preparation of material for review by a team of three international experts who came to Toronto in May 2006.

It was felt that allowing MMI students the opportunity to learn about issues in health-care delivery would provide an important option in their studies. To this end they were allowed to enrol in a selected range of other HPME courses such as health economics and a class on operations research.

A major piece of the new degree was a new course, HAD 5735, "The Commercialization of Health Research," which grew out of an idea that occurred to me at a Christmas function of the Innovations Foundation (IF) of U of T, which was held at MaRS in 2005. IF was the name of the university's technology transfer arm. I developed an outline for a course that evening and polished it over the next month. At the time I was a tutor in Paul Williams's HAD 5010 course, and in January 2006 I spoke to Williams about my idea. Williams asked for a copy of the proposed course and took it to the HPME program committee. They felt it would be an ideal fit for their partnership with MMI.

My idea was that a class was needed that studied the process of a continuum of health research that culminated in generating a commercial diagnostic or treatment product. This was looking at a different form of innovation as applied to health care. It was not looking at innovation within the delivery system itself but rather the process of taking the fruits of health research out of the lab and to the bedside. This was becoming a major new area of activity. What I wanted to do was study the research process itself. My contention was that health research was becoming an activity that should be studied just like we study health care, that we should study research policy, what works what does not, what we could do better.

The idea was timely, in that the scope of health research at universities was changing. No longer did scientists write only grants and publish papers. There was now developing a third activity and that was doing something with the research, developing a practical application of the research, a product, one that resulted in improvements to patient care.

It was also part of a larger picture that implicitly queried whether health research was becoming a discipline and whether it therefore needed the same academic resources devoted to the analysis of management, policy, and outcomes. In addition, just as the Canada of the 1930s needed to develop a cadre of hospital administrators, and just as the Canada of the 1970s needed to develop health administrators, this was now necessary in the field of research administration. The course that I proposed was reviewed by the OCGS and started in January 2007. In addition to MMI students, HAD 5735 was also open to MHSC students in HPME as well as other U of T graduate students. The MMI partnership continued until the end of the 2015–16 academic year.

Another contribution of HPME was to increase the enrolment level to let MMI students take HAD 5010, "Issues in Health Policy," run by Paul Williams and Raisa Deber. A major part of this course was its tutorials, led by adjunct faculty. I had been leading one of the tutorials since the 1980s (when it was part of the Community Health Division in the Faculty of Medicine). For the partnership two new tutorial sections for MMI students were developed that had an emphasis on innovation, led by faculty with experience in hospital-based research institutes and begun in September 2007. Mark Toone and I led them for a number of years. The intent was to allow for consideration of a research and innovation perspective for MMI students in the tutorials stemming from the health policy issues being discussed in the lecture portion of the course.

National Workshop on Research Leadership and Management

Unbeknownst to me at the time, others shared my ideas on the importance of research management. In 2005 Louise Lemieux-Charles chaired a National Workshop on Research Leadership and Management, in collaboration with

Vivek Goel.[41] However, it was more aimed at research project management, i.e., the training of researchers or researcher/scientist leaders for the management of research projects or teams.[42] The idea I had was more one of research organization management, the fact that research institutes or the research activities in faculties of medicine had grown to such a size that they required professionally trained research administrators.

Involvement in Research Administration

We noted earlier the teaching hospitals forming research institutes as part of their research activity. Perhaps not surprisingly the late 1990s and early 2000s saw IHPME grads branch out into a new area, that of the management of these hospital-based research institutes. Lisa Alcia (MHSc, 1989), Mark Toone (MHSc, 2004), Darryl Yates (MHSc, 2009), and I are examples.[43]

Lisa began her career with the Wellesley Hospital Research Institute and then moved with its VP when he went to University Health Network (UHN). At UHN she oversaw the operations of initially three and later four research Institutes. She is also involved in planning, business development, and risk management for Canada's largest medical research enterprise. Through UHN she provided advice to other research institutes in Canada and the Middle East.

Mark was a scientist working in the United Kingdom when he accepted an administrative position with what is now the Lunenfeld-Tanenbaum Research Institute of Mount Sinai Hospital, where he simultaneously took the MHSc degree (he was in my HAD 5010 tutorial group). Following the health admin program he was appointed director of research operations and among other things took the institutional lead in coordinating the design of research floors as part of a multifunctional building that included the Centre for Phenogenomics, a shared facility operated by Mount Sinai Hospital and the Hospital for Sick Children as a state-of-the-art national research facility. It provides services to users locally, across Canada, and around the world.

I began my career in hospital management but moved over to research admin in the late 1990s at the Sunnybrook Research Institute. My focus was on research operations as well as business development (including tech transfer).

This business development activity in the research institute paralleled a similar focus in some hospitals. In 2005 I met and subsequently collaborated with an Austrian academic, Andreas Eisingerich, who had an interest in business-related activities of hospitals, and as a result he was doing field research in Canada, the United States, and some European countries. He also had an interest in clusters (an interest of mine).[44] What we found was that British hospitals were years ahead of their Canadian counterparts in the renting out of space for commercialization activities. Today it is quite commonplace for Canadian hospitals, particularly academic health sciences centres, to be doing just that. We collaborated on two articles in these areas, one of which was published in the *Harvard Business Review* and another jointly published in the *Wall Street Journal* and MIT *Sloan Management Review*.[45]

Some years later I proposed to Simon Haley at Rogers Media a health research magazine aimed at the general public. The idea was to educate the public more on the benefits and necessity of research as an indirect way to get politicians to become more comfortable providing further funding for it. In my view, knowledge was now a commodity in the new knowledge-based economy, and Canada needed to step up its commitment to the development of new knowledge. *Health Research & Innovation*, with Haley as the editor, launched in the spring of 2012.[46]

There has also been faculty interest in this area. Fiona Miller has a research program that looks at such issues. One example is a very interesting article on the "entrepreneurial hospital." The "entrepreneurial university" has been a catchphrase of late in academic circles, referring to actions to monetize the assets of the academy, especially in trends such as tech transfer. However, there has not been nearly as much attention in the hospital field, and one could add especially in the teaching hospital field, which in so many ways resembles the academy. Her article explores drawing care and research together in new ways.[47]

Another sector of activity is graduate students in the academic (as opposed to professional) program who are doing research in this area.

The Core Courses Evolve into Policy Courses

Over the years the core courses were no longer known as such. The composition of the division changed and the priority placed on bringing together all students within the departments changed as well. Eventually the group of three courses, each with its own distinct theme, and with more than 100 students, shrank to two. And interestingly, though for different reasons, the remaining courses were large ones.

However they were large for a different reason. Rather than a requirement bringing all divisional students together, this course was responding to demand, as a number of other departments or faculties wanted their students to be able to take the course. It is likely that this course became one of the largest graduate classes at U of T. And it could have been larger. The demand kept growing and after a time the decision was taken to limit enrolment.

One practitioner involved as a tutor for many years was Diana Moser (MHSc, 1984), who ended her full-time career as a vice-president, Ambulatory Care and Urban Affairs at Wellesley Hospital. She was chair of the Canadian Society for International Health and served on the boards of Oxfam Canada, the Regent Park Health Centre, and Pathways to Education.

Her husband, Meyer Brownstone, established an award for IHPME students in her name. He was a deputy minister in the Douglas government in Saskatchewan and a member of the Interdepartmental Committee, which in 1959 set out the template for the development of a health insurance program for that province, which later became a template for Canada. He was intimately familiar with the fact that this committee felt that Saskatchewan should not stop with the implementation of physician insurance but should eventually add other benefits (e.g., drugs, dental) as well as build a strong community-based preventive program.[48] He was also involved as a member of a Cabinet group negotiating the government position toward a settlement of the Doctors' Strike of 1962.

He was interviewed on the CBC radio program *Sunday Edition*, which had a program titled "Life-Support: Medicare's Mid-life Crisis" in September 2015, where he was introduced as "one of the architects of medicare" and the last surviving member of the Interdepartmental Committee.[49] He taught in and was chair of the Department of Political Economy at U of T. Each year Rhonda Cockerill brought the winner of the award to meet with Dr Brownstone.

A Research Culture Takes Hold, Influencing MHSC Course Delivery

During Louise's tenure a strong research culture began to take hold in HPME. The number of graduate students was such that they began to form a distinctive element within the department. Faculty had a strong research pedigree. Courses were delivered from their research base and linked to events in the field. It made for a very different intellectual development of administrators.

This had been underway since Gene Vayda's time, but now there was a critical mass in the number of faculty with research as the major focus and the graduate students involved in a research degree. This became even more pronounced during Adelsteinn Brown's term, as we will see.

A New Health Informatics (MHI) Program

HPME began to contemplate health informatics as early as 2001. When he was chair, Vivek Goel co-authored an article in the *CJPH*, the abstract of which said, "Health information infrastructure is being developed across Canada, and health informatics education should be a component of the emerging infrastructure."[50]

Discussions began in the department on a rising need for health informatics professionals: people who could enhance health-care delivery via the collection, analysis, and management of health data, information, and knowledge across multiple points in the health sector. This sparked the program development, which led to a launch in 2008. Julia Zarb, head of the program, notes it was a very complex process to build the curriculum to reflect professional competencies in an arena where there was no professional oversight or central organizing body. There was a significant design, proposal, and implementation process.[51]

The first cohort had five students, which would rise in each succeeding year. It involves IHPME faculty, cross-appointed individuals from the Faculty of Information (iSchool), as well as adjunct faculty drawn from senior health-care leadership.

The initiative once again put IHPME at the leading edge of tackling emerging health issues and meets an educational need, as some feel that Canada has been slow in its development of health informatics programs and then their integration into the curricula of medical and professional courses.[52]

THE RE-ESTABLISHMENT OF A PUBLIC HEALTH SCHOOL AT U OF T

Background

The dissolution of the School of Hygiene in 1975 did not quell the debate on what should be the proper location of the school within the university. Friedland notes that John Hastings and his successor as associate dean of the Community Health division in the Faculty of Medicine, Eugene Vayda, still wanted an independent school of public health like the other two other Rockefeller-funded entities of the 1920s (Harvard and Johns Hopkins) that were regaining strength in the United States. He notes that John Evans and George Connell, both of whom had been involved in the decision to close down Hygiene, later wondered whether the merger had really changed the outlook of the Faculty of Medicine toward either public health or preventive medicine.[53]

FitzGerald himself had been a proponent of a separate school. He viewed preventive medicine as an integral part of public health, and Bator notes he "resisted strongly any move to downgrade preventive medicine from the status of a department of a chair to part of another field."[54]

James FitzGerald notes that the re-establishment of a school of public health was given impetus with the report for the federal government by the dean of medicine, David Naylor, in the wake of the SARS crisis of 2003. Naylor led a team of experts who assessed the country's ability to deal with a major infectious disease outbreak and advocated an overhaul of the public health system, including its educational component.[55]

There was actually a confluence of forces. Naylor's report advocated the establishment of a "Canadian Agency for Public Health" and it, in partnership with provincial and territorial governments, "should directly invest in provincial, territorial, and regional public health science capacity."[56] One could argue that establishing a strong school of public health was a part of this capacity building. At that time an editorial in the *CMAJ* strongly endorsed the report and the establishment of such an agency, saying the National Advisory Committee on SARS and Public Health "issued a thorough, blunt and eminently rational report."[57]

In addition to recommending the establishment of the Public Health Agency of Canada, Naylor pointed to a serious shortfall in public health human resources (specialists in community medicine, public health nurses, infection control specialists, epidemiologists, and the like). He felt that this shortfall could be overcome by re-establishing a school of public health in Toronto. James FitzGerald notes that prior to SARS, the chair of public health sciences at U of T had enlisted a group of colleagues, including Naylor, to champion the idea of a school of public health. After the dissolution of the School of Hygiene, there had been a Department of Public Health within the Faculty of Medicine since 1975. Following the SARS crisis and the release of Naylor's report, the idea of a separate school gained momentum, and U of T developed a plan for a new school.[58]

It began with strengthening the division within the Faculty of Medicine, then progressed to raising money for a new school. This was evident in a U of T publication that appears to have been a fundraising document to solicit funds for such a school. It was titled *Public Health Sciences at the University of Toronto*. In it the dean (and later president) Naylor noted, "As Chair of the National Advisory Committee on SARS and Public Health last year, I had a unique perspective on the role of public health. I quickly learned that our ability to fight outbreaks such as SARS is integrally bound up in the strength of our public health system at all levels."[59]

Another article in the same publication, "The Legacy: Public Health at the U of T," noted, "The University of Toronto was a leader in the public health revolution of the 20th century." The School of Hygiene (and the Department of Public Health) in 1975 had been merged with the Departments of Preventive Medicine and Behavioural Science to form the Division of Community Health in the Faculty of Medicine. It noted in 1997 the Department of Public Health Sciences (PHS) was created "rejuvenating the concept of public health at U of T." The Centre for Health Promotion was integrated into PHS in 1998. It said, "Our vision for a new School of Public Health ... represents the fourth age of public health at U of T.[60]

In this and other articles the history and the link with the School of Hygiene was always front and centre. A message from the chair, Public Health Sciences, noted, "Public health has a long and proud history at the University of Toronto."[61] An article in *UToronto Medicine* about the DLSPH noted, "The just-opened school inherited 81 years of history" and the intent was "to create a school to honour the history of the former School of Hygiene and contribute to Toronto's emergence as one of the top locations worldwide for public health research and education."[62]

Mustard Report (2006)

In 2006 the provost requested that the dean of medicine launch a process to develop the Department of Public Health Sciences into a School of Public Health.[63] The resulting Mustard Report (December 2006) began by noting that in "the brief 100 year period of the 20th century life expectancy increased by more than 30 years." It then noted, "What is not well recognized is that more than 80% of this improvement in life expectancy (25 years) is attributable not to clinical advances in the treatment of illness and disease, but to advances in public health.... Academic public health and public health practice, both in Canada and globally, is in a dramatic period of renewal."[64]

It proposed re-establishing a School of Public Health at the university: "Establishing a School of Public Health at the University of Toronto will build on this tradition of strength in academic public health sciences and provide a dynamic academic centre within the University to align with the renewal of public health in Ontario, in Canada and globally."[65] It also noted, "There is a close collaboration between Public Health Sciences and Health Policy, Management and Evaluation in the pursuit of educational and research missions."[66]

It repeated this sentiment later when it said that HPME "is a central partner in the mission of the School of Public Health." It then went into detail on the strengths HPME would bring. This was interesting in a couple of respects. First, in listing three disciplinary areas that HPME comprises. Second, in differentiating between decision sciences and management sciences and listing the components of each. It said, "This partnership is particularly relevant in the applied field of public health policy and practice, where the disciplinary strengths within HPME in clinical epidemiology, the decision sciences (health economics, program evaluation and system performance measurement) and in the management sciences (human resource planning, health information technology and public health system management) will be crucial partners in the mission of the School of Public Health."[67]

The new school was launched in September 2008. And in the same year, a donation from Paul and Alessandra Dalla Lana gave the school the financial foundation to assemble a teaching staff and build an entity with global aspirations. As a result an independent public health program was re-established that year with the creation of the Dalla Lana School of Public Health (DLSPH).[68] The appointment of Jack Mandel as the founding director to lead the school followed shortly after. He was director until 2010, at which time Louise became interim director until 2012.

The next question was where to situate HPME. For the moment it remained within the Faculty of Medicine; however, the Mustard Report, with its recommendation to include it as part of a new independent school of public health sciences, remained. Unsaid in all this was whether one could have a viable school of public health sciences without a health administration arm. And if the DLSPH proceeded to do this without HPME, was this repeating a duplication that had existed in the School of Hygiene, which had a program of medical care administration within its Department of Public Health. There were also the strengths that HPME would bring. We will see the denouement later in this work.

CHAPTER 19

Once Again Moving on Many Fronts

ADALSTEINN BROWN (2012–2017)

Adalsteinn "Steini" Brown became the director in 2012. He had been appointed to the Dalla Lana chair in Public Health Policy in 2011 and moved from Public Health Sciences to IHPME in 2012 to become director. Past roles included assistant deputy minister (ADM) in the Health System Strategy Division at the Ontario Ministry of Health and Long-term Care, and also ADM in the Science and Research Division at the Ontario Ministry of Research and Innovation. He has had a founding role in consulting, software, and internet companies. In 1996 he co-founded a health-care consulting firm in New York that had offices on Park Avenue. He returned to Ontario in 1998 to be principal investigator for the Ontario Hospital Report Card project, where he led the development of scorecards for acute care, emergency, chronic care, rehabilitation, and mental health for hospitals across Ontario.

He also served as an advisor to the World Health Organization, major hospital networks, health maintenance organizations (HMOs), insurance companies, and investment banks in Canada, the United States, Europe and Asia. He received his bachelor's degree in government from Harvard University and his doctorate from the University of Oxford, where he was a Rhodes Scholar.

At IHPME he pushed further the initiative started under Louise Lemieux-Charles of being at the forefront of making a difference in management, policy formation, and evaluating outcomes. One of his accomplishments was to situate IHPME at a nexus of the complex and interrelated health-care system in order to best serve the system's needs in the three mandate areas of the institute. He developed a strategic plan. Its key areas were partnership, impact, and growth.

The institute began to develop policy papers "to better engage the public in health policy discussions." One set "explored investment in quality improvement capacity-building and patient safety strategies." Another set dealt with health system reconfiguration.[1]

IHPME now offers the largest graduate programs in health services research in English Canada. With over 300 students, 200 core and non-core faculty, and 100 senior health executives in adjunct roles, IHPME has become "a wellspring of opportunity, learning and innovation."[2] It offers three professional programs – a master of health administration, master of health informatics, and an executive master of health informatics. It also offers four research programs at the MSc level and two at the PhD level.[3]

A practice internship has been integral to the program. A twelve-month administrative residency was part of the original curriculum in 1947. Practicum placements remain a cornerstone of IHPME programs. Some programs in each of the professional and research areas offer practicum placements, which bridge the theoretical and applied aspects of learning and allow students to benefit from the institute's rich relationships with the field. In 2016 there were 133 students in practicum placements in four programs (MHI, MHSc, MSc-QIPS, and MSc-SLI).[4] In 2017 this had grown to 152 students in five programs (an Executive MHI program was added).[5]

An interesting piece of his leadership, and one could trace it back to the very beginning of the department in 1947, is the degree to which the chairs were publishing. For example, Brown was involved in an article that looked at transferring knowledge from researchers to users, to evidence-based policy advice to create high-performing systems, and another that asked whether the principles and, more specifically, the tools used in research in the clinical world could apply to civil servants offering advice to politicians.[6]

Brown relinquished his role as chair on 30 June 2017 to become interim dean of Dalla Lana.

THE INSTITUTE REGAINS ITS ROOTS, THE CONTINUING EVOLUTION OF PUBLIC HEALTH AT U OF T

The stature and independence of the school was given further impetus with an application for status as an independent faculty. This coincided with the appointment of its second director, Howard Hu, who arrived in 2012.

The Dalla Lana School became the first new faculty at the University of Toronto in fifteen years in 2013.[7] At that time Hu's status was changed from director to dean. To recognize the divestiture from Medicine, an issue of *U of T Medicine* was devoted to global health. In what it called "Pandemic

3.0" Catherine Whiteside, dean of medicine, noted Medicine's efforts in addressing health, poverty, and inequality and saluted its "newest partner faculty" and listed areas of "collaborative growth."[8]

Howard Hu noted, "Medicine and Public Health will remain forever connected," and "collaborations across the spectrum of clinical and public health sciences will be essential to address the enormous challenges to health of the 21st century." He also noted, "The Faculties of Public Health and Medicine are forging innovative ways to collaborate and blend like never before, rather than work in silos." He noted that a great example is the new Division of Clinical Public Health, which is looking at integrating primary care, preventive medicine, and public health. He said this division is also important in demonstrating a partnership of four entities: the DLSPH, the Department of Family and Community Medicine in the Faculty of Medicine, Public Health Ontario, and other clinical and public health units.[9]

The new entity was very aware of its roots. In 2014 the title of a historical poster series displayed at the DLSPH took the title of the book by Bator and Rhodes, *Within Reach of Everyone*, as its label and in so doing established a connection to the tradition of public health in the School of Hygiene. The poster series was called "Within Reach of Everyone: The Renewal of Public Health at the University of Toronto."[10] We noted earlier this connection was also noted in the "Dean's Message" in its first annual report, which said it was "building on a proud history dating back to the creation of the School of Hygiene in 1927."[11]

And, interestingly, the reconstituted school may well be staking out its own distinguished reputation akin to that of its forerunner, as it was ranked fifth globally among schools of public health in the 2017 Shanghai Rankings.[12]

The (Now) Institute Moves Again

In March 2013 the provost and the president asked the dean of medicine to chair a steering committee to make recommendations to create a stronger and closer collaboration between the DLSPH and IHPME. The committee was to work under several key principles. Chief among them was that the DLSPH, not Medicine, be the lead faculty for IHPME.[13]

The evolution of what began as the Department of Hospital Administration came full circle when on 1 July 2014 it was taken out of the Faculty of Medicine and moved back to within a school of public health (the DLSPH). This move created one of the world's largest public health schools with more than 85 core faculty, 725 partner-based faculty, 596 master's and 233 PhD students, thirty-nine residents and postdocs, and $27.2 million in annual research funding.[14]

Commenting of the synergies of such a union, Adalsteinn Brown said, "Global governments will be looking for assistance in shaping or revising health systems," and "building from IHPME's capacity in policy at all levels, the two academic units will offer a wide range of solutions that extend beyond traditional educational and independent research projects."[15]

IHPME once again became part of a school of public health with international impacts and world-class ambitions. The Steering Committee document noted, "The University of Toronto has committed to creating a leading scholarly centre in public health, health policy, and health services research and administration at the DLSPH."[16] The new dean noted the new school "is expanding its footprint to harness the power of one of the world's leading research, teaching and learning networks." The school used phrases such as "accelerated growth" and "balancing deep local impact with broad global leadership." It hosted events like the "transformative" Global Health Summit of November 2014, the result of two years of planning with more than 750 attendees from around the world and hundreds more remote participants.[17]

PROGRAM ADDITIONS/ENHANCEMENTS

MSc-SLI Degree

In 2016 IHPME launched a new MSc concentration in System Leadership and Innovation (SLI), aimed at undergraduate and postgraduate physicians. Faculty member Geoff Anderson was instrumental in its founding.[18] It focuses on key aspects of physician leadership for system innovation such as leadership and motivation, strategic thinking and planning, research methods for evaluating health system innovation, and policy analysis and techniques for system change. It is offered in two scheduling formats. One is a part-time format so that undergraduate medical students can take it in conjunction with their courses and residents and fellows can pursue it along with their clinical training program. It is also offered in a full-time format.[19]

It graduated its first cohort in November 2018. It is the only one of its kind in Canada. It involves two mandatory practicums, though students can do more. For example, one student did four practicums, one of which was in Jönköping, Sweden, where for seven weeks the student was able to network with quality improvement leaders around the world to see first-hand the Swedish health-care system in operation as well as work as a clinician.[20]

An Executive Stream for the MHI Program

In 2016 an executive steam was added to the MHI degree (EMHI). It is designed for established mid- to senior-career candidates from health care, business, and technology backgrounds. This program option enables students to continue professional employment, sustaining career momentum, while gaining the specialized MHI knowledge. It is a twenty-two-month modular format, which involves an employer-based project. It is for individuals who are already established in health care and health informatics–related roles, and who require a relevant graduate credential to move forward in their careers.[21]

With this new stream there are now two professional informatics degree options. The other is a sixteen-month full-time degree program that combines expertise in health systems with applied knowledge in information and communication technologies. There is also a four-month professional practicum placement that provides experiential learning in government, health-service-provider organizations, and the private sector.

In 2016 the program had thirty-six students, with fifteen in a new 2016 executive stream. So between the two professional streams and the research stream it runs with about ninety students and enrolment is expected to continue to rise as the executive stream evolves.[22]

A Course in Comparative Health-Care Systems

In 2010 IHPME began to offer a comparative health policy course: Comparative Health Care Systems (HAD 5774), which involved a comparative examination of the health systems of the OECD countries. Its focus was on components, processes, and outcomes. These included system principles, structures, financing, and human resources. It also looked at technology, culture, level of centralization, and quality. Particular issues such as equity /inequity at the local, national, and international levels, and the current and future effects of globalization were also examined.

Paul Williams first taught it in 2010 as the third of the policy courses, the others being HAD 5010 and 5020. It was meant to be the capstone. Beginning in 2012 it was a joint course with a university in Mexico. He taught the course online, live, in collaboration with Faculty of Economics and Business, Anahuac University in Mexico City for three years (2012–15). One year they also brought in the University of Central Florida, Department of Health Management and Informatics, although the latter didn't actually enrol students, which left them as junior partners.[23]

Paul noted they found fascinating outlooks on performance measurement and management seen from different national perspectives, with quite different takes on what needs to be done. The Americans and Mexicans preferred organization-centred approaches like Kaiser-Permanente (since both have weak systems but some very strong organizations), while Canadian students preferred system-level approaches borrowed from the United Kingdom.[24]

He also noted they experienced some technical challenges: when the web was slow in Mexico it could be difficult to communicate effectively. When their key faculty partner at Anahuac (who was fluent in English and had lots of international experience) left the university, they couldn't find another faculty partner, so the initiative faded.

FACULTY, ADJUNCT FACULTY, AND SENIOR FELLOWS

A strength of IHPME is its diverse faculty. More than 200 faculty members hold IHPME appointments, representing disciplines that include health policy, organizational management, economics, law, clinical epidemiology, innovation, e-health and technology, sociology and political science.

IHPME has over 130 senior health executives who serve as adjunct faculty, drawn from senior executive levels from across health care to bring their experience and best practices into the learning dialogue in a number of ways. These people serve as guest lecturers, practicum preceptors, and course instructors/tutors, to name a few.

IHPME also has "senior fellows" – individuals who have retired but want to share their experiences with current faculty and students. They are each provided with a small stipend to work with students on joint projects. The institute has had a number of successes with this initiative and is continuing to add new senior fellows to the faculty list.

PARTNERSHIPS

Collaborative Research Centres

IHPME is collaborating with different types of research centres and initiatives. All are collaborations that build bridges between students and faculty at the institute and peers in other national and international centres.[25] Several are very novel. Here is a sampling.

Institute for Circumpolar Health Research

This institute develops research policies that support northern-based research and education. Its aim is to develop a research agenda and research training programs that are specific to the study of circumpolar health systems. It is a partnership between IHPME, the University of Alberta, the Fulbright Arctic Initiative, the Finnmark Hospital Trust in Norway, Ilisimatusarfik at University of Greenland, and a number of northern Canadian First Nations groups.[26] The faculty lead is Adalsteinn Brown.

Other Partnerships

Following is a bit more detail on two different types of partnerships.

Knowledge Transfer

IHPME is active in initiatives to transfer knowledge and spark new dialogue. Emily Seto in MHI is involved in tele-monitoring programs for heart failure patients and chronic kidney disease patients.[27] Ben Chan in Clinical Epidemiology co-led an initiative in Kazakhstan financed by the World Bank to help the government develop a Disease Management Program for chronic diseases such as hypertension and diabetes. As a result of their efforts, patients in polyclinics in two northern cities achieved significant improvements in blood pressure control and in diabetes management.[28] Chan was the inaugural CEO of the Health Quality Council in Saskatchewan.

Karim Keshavjee of MHI is involved in an activity that is very much along the lines of the commercialization of research continuum that Les Boehm's class focuses on. Karim's endeavour demonstrated that it is not only basic science researchers who are involved in such commercialization activity. He was developing an idea, taking this idea to the next stage of a practical application, raising venture capital, and forming a start-up company. Karim used his knowledge of family medicine, combined with knowledge of IT architecture, to develop an algorithm to better manage the data of the electronic medical record. He has formed two start-up companies around these ideas: InfoClin and InfoClin Analytics.[29] He is the CEO of both companies. In addition he has hired three MHI grads.[30]

IHPME Faculty Teaching outside the Institute

In 2014 IHPME entered into another partnership with a suburban campus of U of T, this time the Program of Health Studies at University of Toronto Scarborough Campus (UTSC). It approached IHPME to look into delivering upper-year undergraduate courses for their students. The program was looking to eventually become its own department but at the time was nested in the Department of Anthropology at UTSC. It had medical anthropology as one of its emphases. The program came to IHPME in the fall of 2014, as it was experiencing a large increase in demand for courses in health and wanted to expand its offerings.

The result is two courses developed for UTSC. One is a third-year course developed by Julia Zarb and Emily Seto on an introduction to health information systems. The other is a fourth-year course, an adaptation of my IHPME graduate course on the commercialization of research. It began in the fall of 2015 and proved to be so popular that a summer course was initiated in 2016.

There has also been activity in other U of T federated colleges. In the fall of 2014 I began teaching a health policy course at Trinity College and in the fall of 2015 another in the Trinity One Anne Steacy Health Science and Society Stream. I was subsequently asked to be the faculty coordinator for each of a third- and fourth-year independent study course (also endowed by Anne Steacy). These courses have led to connections at IHPME and the DLSPH, as students have gone on to the MPH and MHI and MHSC programs. I have also referred students to faculty like Mark Dobrow, Greg Marchildon, Raisa Deber, Sara Allin, and Allie Peckham as resource people for their essays. Students have also done practicums at the NAO at IHPME. Raisa has been second reader to some of the sixty-page major papers produced out of the courses. Raisa herself, along with Valerie Rakow, has been teaching an undergraduate course at University College for a number of years.

MAKING A DIFFERENCE

Improving the System

IHPME (and the DLSPH) was involved in a solutions-oriented approach (both nationally and internationally) to address complex health issues.

Walter Wodchis is among the first researchers in Canada to evaluate an entire province's health-care costs. He examined anonymized patient records for nearly 15 million Ontarians over three years and found that 5 per cent of Ontarians account for 65 per cent of provincial health-care costs of individual care. The top 1 per cent accounted for one-third of such costs. His study suggested better community-based care could prevent repeat hospitalization – the most expensive type of care.[31] The study is the largest completed in Canada and was published in the *Canadian Medical Association Journal.*

The CMAJ article notes that in each year a few people have major health events that need to be addressed. The relative rarity and unpredictability of these events underlies the need for health-care insurance. It concluded that improving the sustainability of the health-care system through better management of high-cost users will require a better understanding of the clinical needs of subgroups of this population. It will likely require different tactics for different high-cost populations.[32]

Rob Fowler is collaborating with organizations worldwide to improve the communication and reporting done in outbreaks of novel infections. With a team at the World Health Organization and Oxford University he has developed new reporting that has standardized and improved the quality of data collected. He has found that severe acute respiratory outbreaks leading to high mortality in one in one country may not be cause for panic in another, given the variation in health systems and resources available.[33]

The institute has come a long way since its inception as a department. Each of these studies is an example of how the tools of the academy are being used to solve very practical issues. To be sure, the issues being addressed are immeasurably more complex than those of the 1940s. But the same can be said of the tools being used to address them.

Degree Programs Aimed at Improving the System

IHPME has a number of targeted programs aimed at improving the health system. One is the Health Services Research MSc and PhD degrees. Students receive advanced training in areas such as health services organization and management, health policy, health services outcomes and evaluation, health informatics research, health economics, and health technology assessment.[34]

There is also a MSc in quality improvement and patient safety (MSc-QUIPS). In 2016–17 it was working with its fourth cohort of students, a mix of clinicians and other health professionals.[35] We mentioned earlier the MSc in system leadership and innovation (MSc-SLI). It was been developed with the Undergraduate Medical Education and Postgraduate Medical Education offices in the Faculty of Medicine and allows students to obtain a non-thesis MSc.[36]

Faculty Appearing before US Senate and Canadian House of Commons Committees

Another illustration of faculty making a difference is in their being invited to appear before parliamentary and congressional committees in Canada and the United States.

US Senate Panel

In March 2014 Danielle Martin, a regular panellist in the MHSc course on health policy (HAD 5010), appeared before a US Senate panel, where she spoke about single-payer health models. Her quick wit and intelligent responses, especially with Republican Senator Richard Burr, were widely reported in both US and Canadian media, with the Canadian media reporting on offers for her political candidacy. The senator had hoped to score a few points for high-cost private health care.[37]

He posed a few questions to Dr Martin, each time hoping to advance the cause of his side. Each time his questions were effectively answered. The highlight was his asking, "On average how many Canadian patients on a waiting list die each year? Do you know?" Martin responded, "I don't, sir, but I know that there are 45,000 in America who die waiting because they don't have insurance at all."[38] Martin's responses provoked a flurry of media activity suggesting she run for political office.[39]

The House of Commons Standing Committee on Health

In spring 2016, on two separate occasions, IHPME faculty appeared before the House of Commons Standing Committee on Health to speak about a universal, public drug insurance plan, dubbed pharmacare.

In April 2016 Danielle Martin appeared with Dr Steven Morgan from UBC with whom she'd co-authored a *CMAJ* article on the topic. She noted the issues of an open formulary in giving licence to doctors and other providers to prescribe more expensive medicines when less expensive ones are available that are just as good. She noted that private insurance plans have no incentive to reduce inappropriate prescribing. She also noted that while a number of Canadians were covered through employer-sponsored plans, a significant number had no coverage at all.[40]

In June 2016 Greg Marchildon appeared with former Saskatchewan premier and former chair of the Royal Commission on the Future of Health Care, Roy Romanow. Romanow provided the overview. He spoke about the importance of federal leadership to achieving the goals of a national pharmacare plan and getting us out of our current situation. He said this as a former premier, that the public wants a strong federal role in advancing this much-needed step forward in reform. He queried whether Ottawa will act on this issue, just as Prime Minister Pearson in a minority federal government in the 1960s did, by overcoming opposition to implementing the goals of medicare.[41]

Marchildon spoke of the options for such a program. One was financed in part by the federal government and then administered and financed for the remainder by the provincial and territorial governments. This had analogy to the provision of universal hospital coverage in the 1950s, and then universal medical care coverage in the 1960s. The second option is a national pharmacare program financed and administered entirely by the federal government.[42]

Both sets of presenters, in a spirit reminiscent of the FitzGerald ideal "within reach of everyone," advocated for some form of a public plan.

Collaboration with HOOPP on Health-Care Costs for Retirees

In another example of the breadth of collaboration of IHPME, the Healthcare of Ontario Pension Plan (HOOPP) collaborated with the institute to conduct a study on the impact of out-of-pocket health-care expenses and retirement savings on Canadian retirement security. HOOPP is one of the ten largest pension plans in Canada and to its credit not only invests on behalf of plan members but also conducts research into various aspects of retirement.

This study factored in the wide range of costs associated with long-term care, including publicly funded nursing homes, publicly funded home care, and privately funded assisted living in seniors' residences.

The research found that approximately 323,000 Canadians (41 per cent) who are eighty-five and over have inadequate retirement income once long-term care costs are factored in. This could grow to approximately 815,500 by 2038 if factors remain unchanged. It found the percentage of eighty-five-year-old women with inadequate retirement income rises from 25 to 44 per cent when long-term care costs are considered (the study defines inadequate retirement income as those with less than a 50 per cent net income replacement rate). This kind of retirement insecurity among Canadians has important implications for things like the Guaranteed Income Supplement and Old Age Security, and the health-care system.[43]

The crux of the issue is spending on health-related costs not covered by provincial health-care plans. This affects women in particular. Because they generally live longer, women should expect to pay a lot more in their retirement years for long-term care, home care, and other costs like dental care and drugs not covered by provincial programs. The potential impact is huge. People who start retirement in good shape financially might find themselves with insufficient income if they live long and need long-term care later on. This is of concern to governments, because people strapped for money may neglect their medical needs and put a greater burden on the public health-care system.[44]

These findings point to a crucial aspect of research in general and this research in particular. It points to the foresight that can emanate from research, highlighting emerging issues that will become a significant problem if not dealt with.

CHAPTER 20

Crystallizing the Strengths of a Seventy-Year History

RHONDA COCKERILL (2017–19)

With Steini Brown becoming interim dean of Dalla Lana on 1 July 2017, Rhonda Cockerill became interim director of IHPME.

Rhonda perhaps epitomizes the change that has taken place in IHPME. She was hired by the Department of Health Administration in 1985 as a research associate in the Health Care Research Unit.

She was born and raised in Alberta, with a PhD from Edinburgh. She has teaching responsibilities for program evaluation and quantitative methods. Her research interests focus on the evaluation of community-based programs, and she has been actively involved with the Canadian and American Evaluation Societies. She played a key role in developing and teaching the Critical Skills for Evaluation, a workshop series still being delivered by the Canadian Evaluation Society. She served as program chair for the 1995 International Evaluation Conference. For many years, she was graduate coordinator in IHPME and has supervised/graduated well over twenty doctoral students in her career.

IHPME Facilitates a Syrian Doctor's Education in Public Health

Throughout its history, a distinguishing feature of the School of Hygiene and the Department of Hospital Administration was the international profile of each, one indicator of which was the interest of foreign students in each of their diploma programs. Both this international profile and foreign student interest have continued in the Dalla Lana School and IHPME. A very integral part of this profile is how historically Hygiene and the department and now Dalla Lana and the institute have facilitated the public health training of students from outside Canada.

A recent and unique example was the case of a Syrian physician, Khaled Almilaji, who became a student in the Executive MHI (EMHI) program. He had been enrolled in a master's program in public health at Brown University and had gone to Turkey, which he used as a base to do humanitarian work in Syria. In January 2017 he was preparing to return to the United States and found himself stranded in Turkey after having his visa revoked by the US government. This meant he would not be allowed to continue his studies. He became one of the many targeted by the US administration in its new policy toward foreign nationals from selected predominately Muslim countries. It separated him from his wife, who was also a physician, pregnant, and in the United States.

His interest in public health mirrored some of the School of Hygiene and Connaught Labs initiatives, as he had been involved in a Syrian immunization program against polio. In another similarity to Hygiene, he was involved with WHO in developing an alert program to monitor the spread of communicable diseases in Syria. He had also been involved in providing medical care to injured protesters for which he was arrested, tortured, and put in solitary confinement.[1]

In regard to his predicament at Brown, his dean suggested the Dalla Lana School as an alternative and called Dean Hu. Dean Hu then sent out a note to all program directors in the school and institute, which caught Julia Zarb's interest in Health Informatics, prompting her to converse with Almilaji. This led to a suggestion that the EMHI program might be a good fit, on three levels. His work experience suggested the EMHI might be a better fit than the regular program. There was also his interest in medical data and the fact that its modular format would allow him to continue his humanitarian work in Turkey for people in Syria. Also his work in running the organization in Turkey qualified him for the employment piece of the EMHI program.

Julia notes in a statement that is both credible and modest, that the U of T initiative notwithstanding, something would have happened somewhere eventually. This is quite likely true; however, it does not diminish her accomplishment, nor that of IHPME and U of T. Her own involvement started essentially at the outset, January 2017. After Julia indicated her interest, she noted Dean Hu said, "OK, you're the lead," putting her in charge of the initiative. Time was of the essence, as offers went out to students in the EMHI program in April. They formed a committee and because of the complexity of what was involved, produced a Rasky chart to clarify all the tasks, who was doing them, and the timelines involved.[2]

The IHPME staff came together to make this happen. Steini Brown dealt with university administration, and Rhonda Cockerill began a series of interactions with the School of Graduate Studies to process his application. Rhonda also had to interact with Brown University, as it was impossible to obtain any transcripts from Syria. Julia notes that Rhonda is always so quick to give the credit to everyone else, but "she was like a tiger, brilliant in terms of knowing which levers to push to make things happen." The initial work was to get an admission offer, as that was needed for him to get a Canadian student visa, and one for his wife, as her status depended on his. The student visa allowed admission to Canada.

Julia notes everyone pitched in. Her grad assistant worked on getting them student housing and student health insurance as, given his wife's pregnancy, they were going to need the Canadian health system sooner rather than later.[3] The logistics that needed to be worked out involved more than just the academic piece. What also needed to be secured was funding for his studies and raising the money for this required a major effort.[4]

Almilaji arrived in Toronto on 17 June and was reunited with his wife. The couple moved into U of T family housing and he began his program on full scholarship on 22 June.[5] Julia noted part of the reason she wanted him in the program was because of his positive attitude and his lived experiences and resilience, which she felt would be an important learning occasion for his classmates.[6] She also noted that we tend to be very Canadian-centric in our study of health policy and that to have international students in a program, or one like Almilaji who had been so intimately involved with Syrian health care, provided a whole new perspective for the other students.[7]

David Johnston, while he was governor general, and himself a former university president, made much the same point in a U of T *Varsity* interview, saying, "Students from different parts of Canada and around the world should make up a student body."[8] Yet another perspective was given by two U of T professors in a *Globe and Mail* article that said, given recent events in the United States, Canada should tap into this global talent base.[9]

Comment

Julia's initiative is also important for other reasons. It harkens back to the phrase used to describe FitzGerald's efforts: "within reach of everyone." However, a shortened version, "within reach," might be more evocative. We see a war-torn country like Syria does not have health "within reach" for its people. But, moreover, it also does not have the opportunity for physicians like Almilaji to have a study of public health "within reach." And now in countries like the United States, graduate study of public health is also not "within reach." As Almilaji notes, the US system began to tighten up even before the inauguration, i.e., when Trump had stated his intent as president-elect.[10] Julia has put such education "within reach" of Almilaji, but one could argue she also has set up a chain reaction, facilitating his efforts to put health care "within reach" of at least a portion of the people of his country.

Perhaps it also harkens back to opportunity and futures. IHPME has been in the business of creating them since its inception. Julia has given us a specific example. But one also thinks of the certificate program Agnew had started, or the one started by DHA graduate Meilicke at the University of Saskatchewan, or the master's program he started at the University of Alberta. All have created opportunities and futures.

Julia said, "There was just so much good will to make this happen, I was just so proud of everyone," and added, "It made me so proud to be a part of U of T."[11] Another element is the deep commitment, the profound appreciation for what U of T is, the values it exemplifies, the continuity of these values and the people who live them. It also speaks to the commitment this university feels as a public institution.

The denouement is that Julia met him at the airport when he arrived. She was there when he was reunited with his wife. And the week of 2 October 2017 she had an early Thanksgiving dinner at her home, with her three daughters, Almilaji and his wife, and halal turkey. It all somehow seems just so appropriate – so very U of T, so very Canadian.

In December 2017 Almilaji was awarded the Governor General's Meritorious Service Medal at a ceremony in Ottawa, in recognition for his efforts to provide medical relief and educational training in disaster-stricken areas around the world, particularly Syria.[12]

This is what you get at this institute and this university – a deep commitment to ideals, to people, to the public mission of the place, its history, its links to its past, and its legacy.

New Initiatives

A New Class on Comparative Health Systems

In September 2017 Greg Marchildon launched a new class that was an important complement to his NAO initiative. "Comparative Health Systems and Policy" provided a graduate education opportunity attached to the NAO, which meant that there was a service, education, and research component to the NAO. This is an important tripartite activity and mirrors the three components found in a teaching hospital.

Continued Evolution of the Health Policy Courses

We noted earlier the format of the health policy courses changed. Paul Williams and Raisa Deber continued to be involved for over twenty years. Raisa then relinquished her role when she was asked to co-teach a similar course at Dalla Lana, but Paul continued until his retirement in the summer of 2017. A new young faculty member, Kerry Kuluski, initially took over Raisa's role, and in the fall of 2017 Paul's role.

In HAD 5010 in the early 2000s, students in the health administration stream of IHPME formed the largest group. Next were students from another professional degree within IHPME, the master of health informatics. Next were students from the DLSPH (Family and Community Medicine and the master of public health streams). Finally were students from other faculties such as Education (MEd), Rotman (MBA), Engineering (MASc), Clinical Engineering, from the Institute of Biomaterials and Biomedical Engineering (MHSc), and Public Policy and Governance (MPP).[13] For a number of years (2007–15) there were students from the Institute for Management and Innovation at UTM.

An Advantage of the Modular Program

One advantage of the modular program that HAD 5010 is a part of is the opportunity it affords to health-care professionals in remote parts of the province to access graduate professional education. A student in the 2017–18 MHSc program is a case in point. Karim Suleman works as a physiotherapist in Moose Factory. Moose Factory, with a population of about

2,400 is on Moose Factory Island near the mouth of the Moose River, on the shore of James Bay, 850 kilometres north of Toronto. It is accessible from Moosonee airport by water taxi in the summer, ice road in the winter, and helicopter in the two shoulder seasons (freeze-up and break-up); however, Moosonee is not accessible to the rest of Ontario by road. Moose Factory was established in 1673, the first English-speaking settlement in Ontario and the second Hudson's Bay post established in North America. The term *factory* refers to the jurisdiction of a *factor*, who was an officer of the Hudson's Bay Company.

The advantage the modular program affords in this case is twofold. First, it allows the opportunity for Karim to be in the program while still working. This is an advantage to both him and the people of Moose Factory – the people of a remote northern community who still have his services while he is in the program. Second is the experience both he and his fellow students gain in interacting with each other, as he brings a unique perspective on the issues of the delivery of Canadian health care. The challenges this country faces in health care delivery in what I term its "near north" (provinces bordering on the territories) and its "far north" (the territories) are not generally known.

The Support Staff

No account of the history of IHPME would be complete without mention of its support staff. It is simply not possible to have the calibre of academics, with their range and intensity of activity, in an institute such as this without an equally strong support staff. Not only do these people take care of the myriad details of the everyday running of IHPME, they are in many cases the students' first line of contact and many times a confidant of students. They are a strong advocate for the students.

What is perhaps lesser known is that not only are they committed to education in the sense of the institute's mandate; many of them are pursuing further education themselves. At the time of this writing, one is in the midst of her PhD studies at OISE. Another, Anita Moorehouse, is almost always taking a university course – studying another language or creative writing. Others are taking various university courses.

International Connections

Jerusalem College of Technology

The health informatics program helped launch a certificate in this field at the Jerusalem College of Technology, the first program of its kind in Israel. It launched in 2017 and the Israeli government has given approval for it to evolve into a master's degree.[14]

International Students

Carrying on with the tradition of the School of Hygiene, which always had a substantial contingent of international students, IHPME has a number who are doing very innovative work.

Shandong University Partnership

In 2018 a new two-way educational exchange program was developed between IHPME and Shandong University in China. Master's students from Shandong University are eligible to apply for a master's at IHPME. Upon graduating from that they will return to Shandong University to complete the final year of their master's degree at their home institution. Students from IHPME will be eligible for a travel stipend allowing them to visit Shandong University over the summer term.[15]

A CONTINUING GROWTH OF RESEARCH FOCUS

IHPME seventy years after its founding is a very different entity. Originally started as a department within the School of Hygiene to provide graduate professional education – indeed, one could say it had a large hand in building a new profession – today this activity has been eclipsed by its research enterprise. This research endeavour both undergirds and strengthens its professional component. It brings to the professional teaching the benefit of the latest research in a number of related areas.

While it still has a strong professional degree segment (the MHSc and MHI degrees), this is no longer its exclusive focus and it is very much based on a research foundation. While the professional degree curriculum still utilizes practical input from alumni and other practitioners in teaching and practical settings, the institute has very important research concentrations that underpins these curricula.

What is important in this is that while the research activity complements and influences the graduate professional education, it also exists as its own independent activity.

GRADUATE RESEARCH EDUCATION IS ITS OWN CONSTELLATION

Another piece is the graduate research students, who are an important component of the institute, partly because of their number. There has been a continual, incremental growth in its number of PhD students and postdoctoral positions. Another important piece to this activity is the length of time they are here. For example, in the PhD program many of these students are here for five and six years.

This makes for a certain milieu. The abilities of these PhD students, along with those in the master's programs and the postdoc scholars (not sure that students is the correct term for them), add an important element of energy and creativity to IHPME. Indeed, the interaction of these students with their supervisors forms an important creative or innovation ecosystem – adding new knowledge and insights and advancing our understanding of the discipline and the health-care system itself.

Moreover, the interaction between these students and their supervisors injects a certain creative spark into the institute. It is this interaction itself that can spark creative research insights within both student and faculty. An important source of creative ideas is the graduate students. In the hard sciences these can lead to patentable discoveries. In the soft sciences they can lead to equally important breakthroughs.

In 2017, the seventieth anniversary year, the institute graduated twenty doctoral students,[16] in addition to filling thirteen postdoctoral positions.[17] These numbers were creating a critical mass, for it is not only the research generated by faculty that is important but also that generated by its graduate students. Their own unique potential, their ideas developed in conjunction with their supervisors, independent initiatives such as the student-led co-curricular activities and seminars we spoke of earlier – all of these add an important element of knowledge advancement that did not exist at the founding of the institute seventy years earlier.

The critical mass of graduate activity is also spawning a host of innovative initiatives by IHPME faculty. One of its most distinctive characteristics is its innovations in niche-oriented policy institutes, sustainability and climate change, health economics, physician leadership, and the like. We will deal with some of these later in this work.

Student-Led Co-Curricular Activities

An important new addition to the IHPME intellectual milieu is the amount of student-led co-curricular activities.

An example is an Alumni Mentorship Program started in late 2017. It aimed to connect current MSc and PhD students in the Health Services Research (HSR) stream with HSR alumni. They developed a program outline that presented the vision and purpose of the program as well as an implementation plan, the mentor/student matching process, mentor and mentee responsibilities, and program evaluation.[18]

In addition, an important component of seminars for graduate students and faculty is those run by the IHPME Graduate Students Union (IHPME GSU). Students run an annual Research Day consisting of student posters (with poster awards), expert panel discussion, and a keynote presentation. Research Day was an initiative begun by Vivek Goel when he was chair (likely around the year 2000).[19] The IHPME GSU also organizes a series of Lunch and Learn sessions, Health Policy Rounds, Health Informatics Rounds, a Student Rounds, a peer buddy program, and numerous social events.

WHERE GRADS ENDED UP: VIII

More information on IHPME grads:

Jodeme Goldhar (MHSc, 2001, Arbor Award 2016) has been with the Toronto Central LHIN and the Change Foundation. She also has an MSW from Yeshiva University, New York City, and has been president of the IHPME Society of Graduates.

Lieut. Col. Stephan Plourde (MHSc, 2004) received the Meritorious Service Medal from Governor General David Johnston in 2015 for his work in Afghanistan. He and his team developed and implemented a health services plan for the Afghan National Security Forces. While he was an IHPME student he received the Robert Wood Johnson Award (in 2004).

Ryan Hinds (MHSc, 2018; he was in Les Boehm's HAD 5010 tutorial group) is the lead for community engagement with the Toronto Central LHIN. He played professional football with the CFL and won a Grey Cup with the Edmonton Eskimos. Along with Dean Adalsteinn Brown and Annette Paul, director of advancement, Hinds is co-leading an outreach and access program for youth, with the first pilot at Toronto-area high school, Marc Garneau Collegiate Institute.[20]

The academic side was also notable in its grads. Some examples:

Gustavo Mery (PhD, 2013) in 2017 was an advisor in Health Systems and Services with the Pan American Health Organization/World Health Organization for the Bahamas and Turks and Caicos Islands, and was head of the organization's office in the Bahamas during Hurricane Matthew.

Kadia Petricca (PhD, 2015) came to IHPME having completed a master's in public health at the London School of Hygiene and Tropical Medicine. She went from IHPME to work as a research associate at the Johns Hopkins School of Public Health and is based in Dar es Salaam, Tanzania.

PhD Grad First Director of Ryerson Program in Health Administration

Karen Spalding (PhD, 2005) in 2018 was appointed the first director of the Master of Health Administration – Community Care (MHA-CC) program at Ryerson University. She was a PhD student of Paul Williams and a tutor in his HAD 5010 course in 2016.

Her appointment to the position at Ryerson was an interesting outgrowth of the undergraduate program in health services management Paul started there prior to his coming to IHPME. Each of their cases is another example of IHPME faculty or graduates being involved in seeding other faculties of health administration. Paul is on the Advisory Council for the Health Services Management program and pushed the idea of a focus on community care as the program aimed beyond the undergraduate level. This was the first Canadian graduate degree in this growing sector, which launched in the fall of 2018.

A Different Kind of Diversity

Today the university quite rightly places emphasis on attracting an international student body. However, an article written by an IHPME grad illustrates well that a different type of diversity can bring a richness to IHPME and the university's students and, indeed, to what they bring to their career.

Stephanie Zhou (MSc/MD, 2018) was in the IHPME SLI program and wrote an article in *JAMA* in 2017 that went viral and was reprinted in the *Toronto Star*.[21] She recounted how she grew up in poverty and her background made her feel isolated in school as a child and later in medical school but ultimately helped her empathize with her patients: "To come from this background grants a different, more subtle form of privilege beyond that of wealth and networks. I call it 'empathic privilege,' that allows one to be more cognizant of the social determinants of health that patients often leave unspoken when seeking medical care."[22]

She notes, "The experience has shown me what it feels like to not have choice, to have external factors like money and other people dictate the path of my life. For many patients, it may feel the same – when their bodies and their lives are now in the hands of others."[23]

During her undergraduate career she founded the first chapter of Power Unit Youth Organization to promote youth empowerment and mentorship. It encourages youth to take an interest in local causes and philanthropy.[24]

PART EIGHT

The Influence of J.G. FitzGerald

CHAPTER 21

Connections between FitzGerald and IHPME

NINE CHARACTERISTICS OF THE FITZGERALD APPROACH (AND CONNECTIONS TO IHPME)

One can discern nine characteristics or qualities of the FitzGerald approach (and similarly see each of them in the department that developed within the school). They could also be described as nine innovations FitzGerald initiated. We will briefly describe each of them.

The first involved the tight link between teaching and practice. The curriculum and the faculty in the diploma of public health were very closely connected to public health officers at the municipal, provincial, and national levels. The aim was to produce practitioners for these positions. It would be the same in IHPME: on inception its aim was also to produce practitioners (hospital, later health, administrators).

The second was where he found that organization and management were as important as his public health and clinical laboratory activities. This was a result of his service in the Canadian Army in the First World War.

The third involved his emphasis on research, but here it was a very specific kind of research – practical research, i.e., research toward a defined end or, more specifically, to meet a public need. Defining the need preceded doing the research. For FitzGerald this began with his making antitoxins to combat diphtheria and led to the establishment of Connaught Labs, which was unique for two reasons. First, it was wholly owned by the university. The second involved a very important nuance in his work: he was not interested in making a profit from his discoveries; rather, he wanted to make products available at cost. And not only that. Activities at reducing this cost were as important as those leading to further discovery. The principle guiding him was making health available to all. Today, we would call this the commercialization of research, though his particular application of it would be as unique now as it was then.

The fourth involved an emphasis on health policy. He initiated what is believed to have been the first national committee on public health: the Honorary Advisory Committee of the Connaught Laboratories, which had representation from every province. He also made numerous presentations to parliamentary committees on public health and the need for a government-run health insurance program and how this needed to include public health (prevention), not only treatment.

The fifth was a belief in public assets – assets held in common that had a very strong service component (or mission). In a world that emphasized private commerce, FitzGerald was carving out a role for a public sector.

The sixth was an academia-government interface, and in many ways it grows out of the fourth. FitzGerald had close connections to provincial departments of health as well as is national counterpart. His Honorary Advisory Committee was the precursor to the Dominion Council on Health (which he was a member of).

The seventh was in comparative health systems. FitzGerald was very interested in the health systems of other countries, and he travelled to them to learn more of their activities and what might be gleaned from them and applied back in Canada.

The eighth was the importance of networks (at the national and international levels). In a world that is today characterized by networks, FitzGerald was an early proponent of the phenomenon.

The ninth was history. FitzGerald, like Sigerist at Hopkins, knew health history and how important it was to policy.

We will deal with a number of these in more detail below.

Link between Teaching and Practice

Praxis

We have dealt with much of this throughout this work and will not duplicate it here. FitzGerald was governed by a paramount ideal of impact. What drove his twin ideals of research and education was need. He had to meet a societal need, whether it was in the education of public health officers or developing antitoxins to militate a communicable disease. FitzGerald would not have been a fan of knowledge for the sake of knowledge, or new knowledge not tethered to dealing with a practical need.

He would very much have been a fan of some of the world's best biomedical research organizations, such as the Lister and Pasteur Institutes overseas and the Rockefeller Institute for Medical Research (now Rockefeller University) in New York. Outside of health care he would have been a fan of Bell Labs, the research arm of AT&T and its aim to harness science and technology in the service of a public good, the building a continental telecommunications system.[1]

Solving practical problems for the public good – that would have been what animated him.

Epidemiology

Another connection to future activity in IHPME was FitzGerald's close friend Dr Neil McKinnon, who was a professor of epidemiology and biometrics in the School of Hygiene, established in 1924, making U of T the first university in Canada to have such a department.[2] This was an activity later championed by Gene Vayda, who was recruited to IHPME from the Epidemiology Department at McMaster University.

The Importance of Organization and Management

FitzGerald also had good abilities in organization and management. They were implicit, not something he objectified and wrote about. We see them identified in work he did for the war effort. They were also evident in his management of the school and the labs. One quite simply could not start, grow, and maintain two world-class organizations without such abilities. There had to be capacities in first conceptualizing the organizations that actualized his ideals in public health education and public health products. There also had to be competencies in day-to-day management, in choosing good department and section heads, and in backing good research (most notably Banting and Best).

He embodied sound organizational principles. According to his long-time friend Clarence Farrar, "One of his most felicitous characteristics was his confident facility in delegating responsibility."[3] He could build organizations around an idea. After developing the antitoxin, he could scale up its production, drive down production costs, then convince governments to purchase his products in quantity, thereby ameliorating a disease and strengthening the viability of his entrepreneurial venture.

Canada now had the scientific and production ability to develop its own sources for the biological products indispensable for its public health programs without having to depend on foreign sources.[4] In essence "he created and administered a new industry in Canada" with his antitoxin company.[5] He also created "the first such training center in hygiene and public health in Canada."[6] In view of all this, "it is no wonder that he received the devoted cooperation of the members of his staff and associates."[7]

Principles of Health Management and Public Health Applied to the War Effort

An interesting sidelight in the history of the labs and school (at that time a department of hygiene) is FitzGerald's application of principles of public health and those of health management and organization in the First World War. We saw an earlier notation that supplying serum to servicemen was a priority. It is evident in reviewing FitzGerald's published works for the war period that he applied his knowledge to the health needs of the troops with the same focus and commitment he had directed toward the general population back in Canada. It was really a public health microcosm of the general population (with some special challenges). It presaged the emergence of IHPME in that the tools he used were those of epidemiology and those of the organization and management of services.

For example, in an article he co-authored in 1917 he spoke of the methods necessary to maintain the health of the troops. These were also applied in the military barracks in Canada, which included the need for a "laboratory unit" that did the work of both a public health laboratory and a hospital clinical laboratory.[8] He also noted the need for good preventive health measures and that "In the great wars of the past, plagues have been responsible for more deaths among troops than have any acts of the enemy."[9] His grandson notes, "In past wars, eight soldiers died of disease for every one killed in battle; on the Western front, the Canadians have pulled off a spectacular reversal – only one soldier died of disease for every twenty killed in battle."[10]

Bator and Rhodes note the importance of organization, that Amyot and FitzGerald "helped to organize in the Canadian Army a system to treat and control contagious diseases" and that "the preventive measures adopted by the Canadian Corps in France reversed the trend of more men dying of disease than of wounds."[11] Friedland says the same.[12] Amyot noted that in the Crimean War eight men died of disease for every one who died of wounds and that inoculation was a major factor in this reversal.[13] A significant part of this change was the vaccines supplied by Connaught Labs. There were two significant qualities of the Connaught vaccines; their high quality and the fact that they were roughly a third of the cost of those from foreign suppliers that Canada previously used. Over 250,000 doses of tetanus antitoxin were prepared and sent overseas.[14] Connaught Labs had a strong showing in the First World War, between supplying antitoxins and vaccines and the services of people like Amyot and FitzGerald.

McPhail, in an official history of the medical services of the Canadian forces, notes FitzGerald's contribution in supplying sufficient quantities of the serum to fight tetanus and keep it under control.[15] In his account, he notes that Canadian death rates of the wounded was 11.4 per cent, which is low. However, while he gives a British casualty rate, he does not give a comparable death rate.[16] Shorter notes, "Amid the horrors of the Great War, Canada achieved a significant public relations triumph" by reducing the proportion of soldiers dying from disease to one in twenty from one in eight and that Connaught Laboratories "contributed in no small measure to this reversal, producing one-fifth of the serums used by Britain and her allies."[17]

FitzGerald's organizational capacity and also his ability to choose good people were noted by George Porter, a colleague who also served in the Canadian Medical Corps. Of FitzGerald, he said, "His organizing ability and fine judgment, in choosing promising and capable men for his associates and helpers, were two of his outstanding qualities." He also noted that FitzGerald inspired great loyalty.[18]

FitzGerald himself was explicit in the role of organization. In the Gordon Bell Memorial Lecture in 1928 he referred to the role of organization as an important condition of prevention and public health. And in this he gave the example of "what was accomplished during the Great War as a result of organization."[19]

FitzGerald and Hospital Administration and Public Health Administration

FitzGerald knew of the importance of good management. He practised it, as to scale up his Antitoxin Laboratories as rapidly as he did in 1915 and to produce and ship the volume of sera overseas that he did required no small skill in logistics and management.

He was also not unaware of hospital administration. In his Gordon Bell Lecture he specifically mentioned hospital administration as another area (in addition to medical practice) that could engage physicians.[20]

Because of his close ties to the Faculty of Nursing he would have been aware when the Faculty launched a course in hospital administration in September 1939 (see the section on it in this work).

The School in its diploma of public health program for public health officers recognized the importance of administration. It had classes on public health administration for many years beginning in the 1920s[21] through to the 1930s.[22] One needs to also bear in mind that at the core of FitzGerald's ideas of preventive medicine and public health – in his own words – are "effective administrative procedures."[23]

The contention being made in this work that FitzGerald understood and practised principles of administration is supported in a review article on FitzGerald's biography, *What Disturbs Our Blood*. It offers that the book's contents, and hence FitzGerald's actions, in addition to providing a compelling story in themselves, "may offer a powerful case study for current and future health service management and policy professionals."[24] It notes, "Few books have the makings of both a bestseller and a health administrator's reference."[25] It outlines ten reasons why it could be helpful to health administrators. Among them are descriptions of how research accomplishments occurred, i.e., Canada's "capacity to organize, partner and translate the benefits of research into life- and limb-saving measures as well as better quality of life."[26]

Another is a focus on research institutes, highlighting the importance of not only attending to each research goal but to the environment in which research and innovation can thrive. Another is noting the importance of health care and public health and the importance of integrating the two. Yet another is that the book "describes the histories and origins of many research institutes and academic healthcare organizations in Ontario" and that understanding their stories "enables us to describe the strategies, structures and cultures that yield such successes."[27]

FitzGerald's Emphasis on Management Carried Forward

FitzGerald's emphasis on administration continued under Defries. In the academic year 1940–41 it formed a Sub-Department of Public Health Administration under William Mosley (DPH, 1937),[28] within the Department of Epidemiology and Biometrics. In another example of linkages, many years later Mosley co-authored the report on organized community health services for the Royal Commission on Health Services. The other author was Department of Hospital Administration faculty member J.E.F. Hastings

(DPH, 1954). Defries himself became the head of the sub-department in 1945–46.[29]

Research Application

The research done by the labs, which was closely affiliated to the school, had a similar practical orientation. It was meant to solve health problems; hence it created products such as vaccines and insulin. While in the contemporary vernacular one could say this was the commercialization of research, for what FitzGerald was doing *commercialization* may not be the quite the right term.

Commercialization, as the term is used, is meant to describe the process whereby research generates an economic return. With FitzGerald this was not his primary aim. Rather he wanted to provide a useful product that could help toward the restoration of health. He did not aim to make an economic return and, indeed, he structured the labs to do precisely everything but make an economic return. It paid a royalty to the university (to be reinvested in further research and education) but it did not generate a profit. The aim was the product and making it as widely available as possible.

It is said FitzGerald's vision for Connaught Labs was three-pronged. First was the preparation of a number of low-cost, high-quality preventive medicines available for widespread distribution through provincial health departments at a low enough price that they could make them available at little or no cost. Second was the establishment of a research arm to continue to develop new products to meet the constant threat of infectious diseases prevalent at the time. Third was knowledge-transfer, the provision of undergraduate and graduate education to pass on the knowledge to future generations.[30]

In actuality there were other operative factors as well. To put it in different terms, first was the basic curiosity-driven research in the quest to find antitoxins and vaccines against communicable diseases and, once developed, to conduct further research to continue to drive down price. The discovery piece expanded into funding new areas of research outside that of infectious diseases, such as Banting and Best's research on diabetes. Next was the translation of this research into a practical product that could be made available to the population, which today we would call technology transfer. Finally, was the production of the product itself.

All of these elements can be linked to an area of research and teaching at IHPME, the commercialization of health research in that this involved a continuum of research and product development whose ultimate aim was creating a product that could be put into the marketplace. However, Fitz-Gerald was not concerned with the marketplace per se. From the beginning he had a novel twist to this equation, as he was completely unconcerned with making a profit and equally completely dedicated to making his discoveries available to everyone.

Undergirding such aims were a number of principles. One was making such medicines available at cost. People, especially children, were not to be denied life-saving medicines for want of being able to afford them. Another was that the basic and applied research, the commercialization of this research, the links with public health bodies at the local, provincial, and national levels as a distribution partner, as well as the undergraduate and graduate education that went hand-in-hand with this research activity, forming one vast continuum. The commercialization piece did not necessarily need to be separate, for-profit, and outside of the academic realm and, indeed, in this case was the opposite: publicly owned, non-profit, and within the academy. Finally, the marriage of all these elements could form a virtuous circle, with the proceeds of the sale of the products generating the revenue to sustain research and education.

It generated a kind of mini-innovation ecosystem and anticipated the wider role in the commercialization of research that we see many universities undertaking today. It was a continuum of activity and role that would be illustrated and debated in future classes on the commercialization of health research in the institute, which succeeded the Department of Hospital Administration.

As James FitzGerald would say, "Nearly everyone stands to win – the government, the university, and above all, millions of Canadian citizens, regardless of social class or income."[31] But, as he notes, the druggists and the commercial drug manufacturers are much less enthused, as Gerald's "self-sustaining laboratory devoted to public service" eats into their potential profits.[32]

Another aspect of just how revolutionary (and advanced) FitzGerald's thinking was concerned how he anticipated two things that would become very important in the knowledge-based economy of the twenty-first century. The first was academic-government-business partnerships. This triad generated substantial academic literature, *The Triple Helix* being one example, in which the triple helix was the tripartite partnership.[33] In addition there was a major government report in the United Kingdom, the *Lambert Review of Business-University Collaboration*, which promoted such activity (university-business collaboration).[34] There were also two MIT studies that said discovery cannot be separated from production.[35] All of these were ideas IHPME taught many years later. FitzGerald's action touched on all of them.

This is where JGF was very innovative – his very interesting nuance in the Etzkowitz triad as his third component was not a corporation in a for-profit business, but was instead a corporation wholly owned by the university. It was a powerful combination and a powerful motive. And its particular combination was unique among universities.

Fitzgerald's grandson makes a somewhat similar observation, that the labs and the school after the First World War "are now closely related yet independent units of the university, uniting the functions of teaching, research, manufacturing, and public service."[36] Further, with the establishment of the federal Department of Health (where his colleague John Amyot was its first deputy minister), and the appointment of the Dominion Council of Health (in which FitzGerald had a role), public health is given a new prominence. James FitzGerald notes Connaught is a "modern, state-run bureaucracy, stretching like a gigantic safety net from the Atlantic to the Pacific." He notes as well the labs is "an engine of national influence." All nine provinces freely distribute its products and it has a thriving export market reaching countries as far away as New Zealand, the Caribbean, and China.[37]

By the mid-1930s, with the publication of a classic study of the incidence of diphtheria in 30,000 immunized Ontario schoolchildren and 20,000 unimmunized controls showing a 90 per cent reduction of disease in the immunized group, Connaught had "made history by statistically demonstrating for the first time the value of a non-living vaccine in preventing a specific disease."[38] It also was "acknowledged as the world leader in overcoming the difficulties of producing and distributing on a large scale a safe and effective preventive medicine."[39]

This phrase captures the essence of what Connaught did. It made history. Above all it sought to provide a service – solutions to communicable disease. But it did so in a unique way. It wanted its products to be available to everyone, and this imposed a specific discipline on the company. Also, it sold its products at cost. It had rigorous quality control. It was a unique institution. Perhaps in the end its most significant contribution was what all these characteristics represented. It exemplified that most elusive quality – one difficult to engender and even more difficult to maintain: a culture of innovation and excellence, and equally integral and significant, harnessed in the service of humanity.

James FitzGerald perhaps best encapsulated the contribution of the labs, the school, and their founder (his grandfather) when he said in 2003 that in the wake of AIDS, the water crisis of Walkerton, the re-emergence of virulent drug-resistant diseases "the thrust" of his grandfather's "life's work" in each of these organizations "stands as timeless as ever."[40] This would be further reinforced with the SARS epidemic about a year after his article appeared.

None of this was lost on the university, which, after dissolving it, sought to re-establish a school of public health in the wake of these occurrences, a process in which IHPME faculty was integrally involved.

It is easy to forget just how rare FitzGerald's accomplishment was. Today we have buzzwords such as *technology transfer* and *knowledge translation* to describe two of the processes FitzGerald was driving forward. Yet he was doing this some sixty years before the buzzwords existed.

Vivek Goel, who became chair of IHPME and after that vice-president, Research and Innovation at U of T, noted much the same in a *Globe and Mail* article: "It's been a century since John Gerald FitzGerald combined his passion for medicine, his scientific knowledge and the resources of a major Canadian university to make history.... At the time, there was no road map to guide such a university based endeavour that included teaching, research and manufacturing. There were no tech-transfer offices and no debates on how best to share intellectual property rights or which tax incentives could best support startups. There was a shared desire to put research know-how to work to save lives."[41]

We can continue to find connections between FitzGerald and important medical discoveries of the last century. Henry Mintzberg, in an interview on the CBC *Sunday Edition*, in February 2018 said that the three most important discoveries of the twentieth century came out of non-profit labs: insulin, penicillin, and the polio vaccine.[42] We have seen that FitzGerald, through Connaught Labs, was involved in the funding for insulin. Interestingly, some sixteen years earlier, FitzGerald's grandson notes in a separate article Connaught's involvement in the same three areas. He notes insulin as one of its "major global achievements" and that Connaught "also contributed to the mass production and worldwide distribution of penicillin in the 1940s and the Jonas Salk polio vaccine of the 1950s."[43]

Journalist Linda McQuaig, in a recent book on public enterprise, which deals in part with Connaught Labs, notes that Bator said that, in 1968, Connaught was investing 24 per cent of that in R&D, far more than the private pharmaceutical firms. In fact, with only 2.5 per cent of pharmaceutical sales it was investing 20 per cent of all R&D by the entire industry in Canada.[44] She notes its seminal role in the global eradication of smallpox[45] and penicillin,[46] and its support of medicare.[47]

The Public Mission of the Antitoxin Laboratories

The public mission of the Antitoxin Laboratories began to be apparent shortly after FitzGerald's appointment. The dean of medicine's report to the president for 1914–15 noted, "Some very interesting work was developed in the Antitoxin Laboratory." It went on to note the development of the diphtheria antitoxin, which was being distributed throughout Canada. It noted the lab was also producing tetanus antitoxin for First World War troops. Smallpox vaccine, anti-meningitis serum, typhoid vaccine, and the Pasteur preventive treatment for rabies were other products being produced.[48]

Bator and Rhodes note, "The demands generated by the First World War soon turned FitzGerald's small factory into a wartime industry and thereafter a national institution."[49] FitzGerald's contribution to the war effort was recognized in a Canadian government's official history of the war.[50] The war also stimulated research at the U of T, and FitzGerald's lab was a beneficiary of it.[51]

Life-Saving Medications "Available to All" or "Within Reach of Everyone"

We have noted repeatedly the orientation of the labs to making its products universally available. Batorand Rhodes note that, from its inception, the school had been concerned with providing health to all. As early as 1915, FitzGerald (who founded the Connaught Laboratories in 1914 and later the School of Hygiene in 1927) was working on making a diphtheria antitoxin available to everyone, even the poorest. This included not just availability but also delivering it into the community by establishing "antitoxin depots."[52]

So characteristic was this intent that it formed the title of their book on the history of the school and the labs, *Within Reach of Everyone*. The title came from a phrase in an article on FitzGerald's work that appeared in *Maclean's* magazine in August 1915. The article itself illustrates that FitzGerald's principle was not lost on journalists, as it reveals just how driven by mission some of its early researchers and leaders were, how much they aimed at betterment of the world around them and that their concern was not just improving the lot of a subset of society, but everyone.

It talks about FitzGerald's efforts to combat diphtheria but in particular his efforts to make it available to "the general public practically at cost." It stated that it "is the story of an achievement, an achievement which will mean life and health to many, many Canadian children." It went on to say it "is the tale of how a great life-saving product came to be made by a university." Just how unusual that was at the time was is in its next statement: "An institution whose usual business, as everyone knows, is to develop the youthful mind."[53]

The article noted that FitzGerald was able to set a price that would pay all expenses and "at the same time put the life-saving antitoxin *within reach of everyone* – even the poorest" (my italics). It went on to note that the university was selling the antitoxin for one-fifth to one-tenth the price being asked by private corporations.[54]

FitzGerald himself used much the same phrase. In the Gordon Bell Memorial Lecture of 1928 he queried "whether adequate and satisfactory medical service, preventive and curative, is *within reach of all persons in need* thereof" (my italics).[55] It was an ethic he never lost sight of, as in this phrase he was advocating for health insurance and so was wanting to bring not only the products manufactured by Connaught but health care itself within reach of everyone.

And, interestingly, almost 103 years later, the *Economist* felt the phrase "within reach" very much captured the global intent regarding health care and used it on the cover and in a feature article of its 28 April 2018 issue. It spoke of the need for and advantage of universal health care and captured many of the same ideals FitzGerald had aimed at over a century before.[56]

Principles Established by This Initiative

The *Maclean's* article (perhaps unwittingly) provides early indication of two things. One is a strong Canadian concern for the health of its people. It is easy to see from this how discussions of health insurance took root. Second is a strong public service ethic, the mission of Canadian public institutions, of making a difference, of undertaking research aimed at a practical outcome. What they don't state, but what is implicit in the article, is that actions by people like FitzGerald provide early evidence that visionary leaders and institutions felt strongly that the university was not just a passive transmitter of knowledge, it also had an activist role in the practical application of the fruits of its research, in this case that health needed to be available and to everyone.

What it also states – explicitly this time – is that "there are certain things which must be exploited for the public good," that "those things which have been freely given" should be "open to all," and that no human being "should die for the lack of them."[57] This is an important statement for it (perhaps again) unwittingly illustrates another aspect of this institution: the labs and the School of Hygiene that was to follow were institutions within an institution that provided an important public service – one recognized internationally – and in doing so, in the way that they did this, in the emphases they had, helped define for a young country what it was to be Canadian.

The article concluded by asking, "Why should a university as a corporate body not lead in this education of the public in a new sense? Why should she not reach out to touch the hearts and lives of the people as well as their heads?"[58]

FitzGerald's spirit or values exemplified by the article are nowhere better captured than in a letter he wrote to the president later that year. In December 1915 he convinced the Provincial Health Board of Ontario to agree with the Antitoxin Laboratory to purchase "public health biological products" from the lab and arrange for their distribution "free of charge." He noted, "This makes the Antitoxin Laboratory the official source of public health biological products in Ontario and practically eliminates commercial firms, at present competing, in Ontario." For him this was all part of a plan, as he also noted this "marks the second step in the plan I had in mind when I first undertook this work" (it is not stated what the first step was).[59]

The article and FitzGerald's subsequent letter to the president are important in that they set out his fundamental principles, ones that would guide the labs throughout its existence. The first was to forego personal returns in favour of applying that money to further research.[60] Next, of equal importance to the development of the product was its reduction in price, i.e., producing it at a cost that was affordable to people and to governments.[61] Next, there was a business mission – it needed to be self-sustaining – but there was an equally important public or social mission of the enterprise.

An interesting corollary was that an institute undertaking research in vaccines or antitoxins required a farm. The article notes that the Lister Institute had one (donated by a wealthy peer) and the Pasteur Institute did as well (donated by the French government).[62] This was why the land donated to U of T by Gooderham was so important. There were other unique aspects. The ownership of the enterprise was by a public institution (not private shareholders). A part of its mission was working with governments and/or local health authorities. The enterprise was not only self-sustaining, it was generating revenue for further research activity, intramurally and extramurally.

McQuaig notes it was "focused on health benefits, not on gaining market advantage or pushing up its stock price. While private firms manoeuvered to corner the market on a lucrative drug, Connaught shared its advances with other producers in order to make needed treatments more widely available."[63]

Health Policy: An Abiding Concern for Universal Health Care

In keeping with FitzGerald's objective of having health "available to all," he devoted substantial time to the establishment of universal health care.

There were strong links to later IHPME activities. In the 1960s the Department of Health Administration attracted people with significant health insurance experience (e.g., Burns Roth and Fred Mott), and even more so in the 1970s in the Division of Community Health (e.g., Robin Badgley).[64] But the interest in health insurance long preceded them at the school.

FitzGerald's concern for health policy was carried forward by his protégé, R.D. Defries. Bator and Rhodes note that Defries was a "persuasive lobbyist for national and provincial health policies" and "a pioneer in the establishment of the Canadian health and welfare system."[65]

Links between the War Effort and Attempts at Health Insurance: Connections to IHPME

Bator and Rhodes note that the personal experiences of Amyot and FitzGerald "had an important influence on the development of Canadian public health services," including health insurance, and cite Morton in this regard.[66] Morton felt that military medicine before and after the First World War was an important precursor to universal public health care in Canada. He quotes a major in the Canadian Army Medical Corps who, addressing a US audience, said, "The fact that former sailors, soldiers and their families, are protected against the risks of death, accident and ill-health, will inevitably lead towards the extension of social, health and life insurance to all citizens."[67]

Morton notes that people like Major Todd thought that the military "would be the vanguard of a nation protected by health insurance."[68] Of course it was not to be: "Far from expanding its postwar social responsibilities, the government was eager to cut its commitments and reduce its role."[69] Yet Morton notes, "The war *was* a starting point. It had established a new and inescapable link between the state and medical practice … the First World War was the beginning of Canada's experience with publicly financed medical care."[70]

An almost identical scenario would play out in the US military medical corps, specifically the Surgeon General's Office, involving its head and, of greater interest to us, a deputy who would later become a faculty member in the Department of Hospital Administration. Thomas Parran, the surgeon general, and Fred Mott, a deputy surgeon general, were supporters of both Roosevelt's attempt at health insurance and later Truman's, as well as the Hospital Survey and Construction Act of 1946 (Hill-Burton). Both were experts in rural medicine. Parran spoke to a New York audience and wrote an article in 1936 supporting Roosevelt's legislation.[71] Both individuals ran afoul of the AMA for their support. Parran was not reappointed by Truman as a result, and the atmosphere for Mott deteriorated. This allowed him to be enticed by Tommy Douglas in 1944 to come to Saskatchewan to launch the continent's first hospital insurance program, and Roth later lured Mott to Toronto to teach in IHPME.

A Belief in Public Assets

FitzGerald had an abiding belief in the value of public assets. This was more evident in his actions than in anything he wrote. It involved a public commons, i.e., assets held by the community for the good of the community. In his case examples of these public assets included public health delivery, public health education (through a school of public health), academic health research, universal health coverage and universal access (they are not the same).[72] It would be fair to say that he regarded the U of T as an important public asset.

They also included a drug manufacturing and distribution enterprise, one that had intimate links to research and – unique for his time – a social as well as a business mission. It represented a certain genre of the entrepreneurial spirit. In Canada it was more usual (either federally or provincially) to see Crown corporations (in other countries called state-owned enterprises). Many are profit oriented. In Canada, to a lesser degree there are examples of public institutions (such as hospitals or universities) owning enterprises (where surplus revenues are directed to the mission of the parent enterprise).

A recognition of the particular qualities of the school engendered by FitzGerald, and their link to the notion of the school, indeed the university, as being a public asset, was given by Canon H.J. Cody in December 1927. In an address to the Canadian Club of Toronto he spoke of the University of Toronto as being a public servant. One of his illustrations was the School of Hygiene, whose new building he noted had been opened the previous June. Cody went on to become president of U of T and was a graduate of Trinity College (with a doctorate of divinity conferred in 1914).[73]

Cody said, "There is one particular feature of which I would like to speak because it is so new," and then he went on to single out FitzGerald and the School of Hygiene. He also said that FitzGerald had already "made a name and fame for himself" through the Connaught Laboratories. He noted that representatives of the Rockefeller Foundation visited Toronto "and they saw the excellent work already being done by Dr FitzGerald in the Department of Hygiene," which motivated them to found a school of hygiene and provide the money for its operation and a building to house it.[74]

He said,

> The extraordinary thing about this building is that it is Dr FitzGerald's idea and it is unique as far as I am aware and gave the lead to other universities. It is a curious combination. It combines a certain measure of medical education. It combines a large measure of research and then it adds to those two features of teaching and research the third function of providing a public medical service, for it is a manufacturing establishment and it manufactures there all kinds of serums and vaccines which are distributed through the Dominions and far beyond its bounds. The combination is absolutely unique.[75]

As we have seen, unfortunately FitzGerald's belief in public assets would not endure. McQuaig, in a book that champions Canada's record in this area, and that singles out Connaught's contribution, notes the role in divesture played by John Brent, head of IBM Canada, and, at the time, the head of the Connaught committee of the U of T board of governors.[76]

Academic-Government Interface

FitzGerald was constantly interfacing with the federal, municipal, and provincial governments. With him it was an axiom of his praxis; one could truly be effective only if one was at the coalface, and the coalface was the medical officers of health at the city or provincial level or the deputy ministers provincially or federally.

This is an interface that the present dean maintains. "Steini" Brown has led taskforces such as the Minister's Working Group on Transparency and Open Data, the Minister's Roundtable (other ministers of health from across the country) on Pharmacare, and the Minister's Task Force on Lyme Disease. He is a board member of Ontario Health and a member of the Premier's Council.[77]

We will see later that such an interface was carried to a new level by IHPME faculty member Greg Marchildon and his North American Observatory (NAO), which had direct involvement with the national, provincial, and territorial governments. But the degree of this involvement was taken to a different level, which is the topic of our next FitzGerald link to IHPME.

Comparative Health Systems

FitzGerald's interest in universal health care naturally focused attention on the health systems of other countries, and he made extended trips to gather information on aspects of their systems. It was also important for FitzGerald to bring in researchers from other countries to the School of Hygiene.

The connection between the health systems of other countries and IHPME's NAO is in the sense of comparative health systems, but IHPME has elevated it in three senses. It has taken it to a formal organizational level, it includes sub-national systems (in Canada, the United States, and Mexico), and it has formal links to a European and an Asia-Pacific observatory, thereby covering a large portion of the world.

FitzGerald's interest in public health also had an international flavour. In 1933 he wrote of his involvement in the Health Organization of the League of Nations and its "activities of an international character in the prevention and control of disease."[78] He spoke repeatedly of the development of "international public health." He noted its involvement in bringing about the control of widespread outbreaks of epidemic typhus fever, recurrent fever, and Asiatic cholera that menaced the greater part of Europe and that had they not been brought under control, almost certainly they would have spread to all countries.[79] He also noted its role in adopting international standards for various antitoxins.[80]

A Translocal and Transnational Character

Both the school and IHPME had a national and international character from the outset, on a host of fronts. The school and the department had many transnational or international connections. FitzGerald and Defries after him, in their annual reports to the president, most invariably mentioned guest lecturers or visitors from other countries. Both the school and the Department took applicants from other countries.

Jones says it "would be difficult to find a more emblematic symbol of the Canadian nation state" than medicare. And yet at the same time she sees that it (along with public health) "can be seen as embedded in a transnational network of ideas and people who advocated an expanded role for the state in public health and medical care."[81] She is making two points here: the health of populations and the health of individuals. That public health required government involvement, irrespective of whether that was local, provincial, national, or international level, was a fact FitzGerald well recognized.

But Jones also sees a transnational element to a number of figures on the Canadian scene. These include a number that were in the Tommy Douglas Department of Public Health in Saskatchewan. One of the individuals she mentioned, Fred Mott, was also an IHPME faculty member and so can also serve as an example of a transnational element to IHPME.[82]

National and International Networks

An important part of what FitzGerald did was to establish and plug Canada into national and international networks in public health. His work with the International Health Committee of the Rockefeller Foundation and the Health Committee of the League of Nations were illustrative.

Another piece of national and international networks is the people he associated with. An example is that in 1933–34 he was an officer (second vice-president) of the American Public Health Association, serving alongside Thomas Parran Jr, who was the chair of the Executive Board of the Association, also the US Surgeon General, and a known strong proponent of a national public insurance scheme for the United States. John Amyot, who until the year before had been the first federal deputy minister of health, FitzGerald's former boss at Hygiene at the U of T, and a close associate of FitzGerald's, was a member of the executive board under Parran.[83]

He also served with Parran on the International Health Division of the Rockefeller Foundation, where in 1936 both were on the committee of scientific directors of the division.[84]

At the national level there was FitzGerald's involvement with medical officers of health (local and provincial), deputy ministers of health (provincially and federally), the advisory committee he set up at Connaught of senior health officials from across the nation, and the Dominion Council of Health. Through this he and the school influenced the development of public health in Canada locally, provincially, and nationally.

Agnew did the same for the Department of Hospital Administration, but there were differences. He also had a well-developed national network of hospital administrators and connections to all provincial hospital associations. His international network was largely limited to US contacts, and it was not as extensive as his national network, i.e., it did not reach into every state. He did not have the international connections FitzGerald had.

An Example of FitzGerald's Network: Simon Flexner

There was also FitzGerald's relationship with important public health figures who had extensive international involvement, including Simon Flexner, who was the first director of Rockefeller Institute for Medical Research (now called Rockefeller University), generally recognized as one of the top medical research institutes in the world. A CBC *Ideas* interview with a later president, a Canadian, Dr Marc Tessier-Lavigne, noted if it were a country the Rockefeller Institute would rank as number four in the number of Nobel Prizes received.[85]

FitzGerald and Flexner corresponded throughout the late 1910s and into the 1920s, mainly on mutual medical interests. In a number of instances it was FitzGerald requesting copies of Flexner's papers for the Canadian Army Medical Corps. In one letter FitzGerald arranged for him to speak at Convocation Hall in October 1917,[86] in conjunction with the official opening of the Connaught Laboratories. The lecture title was "War Activities of the Rockefeller Institute."[87]

The *Globe* and the *Varsity* in almost identical articles reported on the talk, given on 25 October. They reported that the governor-general and lieutenant-governor for Ontario attended, that Flexner was introduced by Robert Falconer, university president, and was thanked by Dean Clarke (Medicine) and FitzGerald. They noted that both Falconer and FitzGerald "remarked on the high administrative abilities that marked Dr Flexner." Not much has been written about FitzGerald's concern (or talent) in management, but that he would single out Flexner's ability clearly shows that it was something he gave thought to.[88]

Flexner spoke primarily on dealing with wound treatment, very topical for 1917. As a result of "the highly fertilized state of the soil of northern France and Belgium it was found that the wounds of almost all men quickly became infected." This prompted research at the institute and the discovery of the bacillus of "the dreaded 'gaseous,'" along with the belief they had discovered the antitoxin for the treatment of these wounds. He also noted that each fortnight sixteen surgeons from the American army were given instruction in the use of the new antitoxin.[89]

The *Mail and Empire* reported that the microorganism responsible for the condition had been discovered in 1892 but little further work had been done because from then until 1914 only 200 cases of infection had been reported. The bacilli were carried even in new uniforms and they seemed to be "omni-present."[90] The *Toronto Daily News* noted "so virulent were the bacilli that they clung even to sterilized uniforms." It described Flexner as "one of the best-known American men of science and one who had contributed largely to the principles that had revolutionized society."[91]

Fetcher's talk illustrated the challenges of public health, albeit the health challenges of war. Irrespective, his talk demonstrated how the Rockefeller Institute beat a challenge posed by the environment to which the American troops were exposed. Both his talk and FitzGerald's correspondence with him illustrated the kind of network that FitzGerald was constructing with the top scientists and institutions in the world and plainly shows the league he intended the U of T School of Hygiene to function in.

It also demonstrates another quality of FitzGerald's approach: the degree to which he fostered international connections of the labs and the school. It was evident in the number of international students at each organization as well as in the international experts he brought in for special talks.

It also shows another aspect of his approach: public outreach. A number of media accounts of Flexner's talk noted that he presented his topic in a manner that the layperson could understand. One cannot underestimate the value of public education in talks such as this, an educative function amplified by the number of reports of this talk in Toronto's print media.

The International Influence of the School

A letter to FitzGerald from F.P. Gay of the US National Research Council demonstrates the importance of the school as an international model. Dr Gay noted that he had been entertaining Dr Leon Bernard, professor of hygiene at the University of Paris, who had been instructed by the French government to establish an institute of hygiene. To that end the International Health Board of the Rockefeller Foundation had sent him to the United States to see what they had in the field. He had been to the Rockefeller Institute and the School of Public Health at Johns Hopkins, both of which he viewed as exceptional. But they were also exceptional in the amount of money expended on them – a level of financing that could not be accomplished under ordinary conditions elsewhere. He noted that he considered the best work in instruction and service under ordinary financial conditions as being done at the School of Hygiene in Toronto.[92]

There was a second letter to this effect, this one from Wicliffe Rose of the International Health Board, who passed on a statement made by Bernard on the impressions of his visit to the University of Toronto. It said that Toronto had "the best system existing anywhere in the world." In this he was referring to the city, the university (i.e., FitzGerald's school), social service (by which FitzGerald notes he meant public health nursing), and the hospitals.[93]

CHAPTER 22

The Legacy of FitzGerald

FITZGERALD'S IMPACT

Another important historical component in understanding the chronicle of IHPME is the impact of FitzGerald. He left a huge imprint. He had passed away seven years before the IHPME's predecessor department started, but his figure still loomed large. The School of Hygiene was his creation, in most cases the people running it and its departments picked by him and, indeed, a number trained by him.

In addition, a number of his activities were an almost exact mirror of those that IHPME eventually concerned itself with and, indeed, adopted in its nomenclature (health policy, management, and evaluation). We will describe them briefly.

FitzGerald exerted an important influence on IHPME in two senses. The first was in an institutional sense – he founded two institutions whose activities had links to IHPME. The second sense was in personal activities that had a link to activities that IHPME would pursue.

LINKS BETWEEN IHPME, SCHOOL OF HYGIENE, AND DALLA LANA SCHOOL

Another reason for delving into this historical and organizational context is that it is a legacy that lives on and a history that the present Dalla Lana School feels it is important to remember. It notes the contribution of FitzGerald in several of its reports. In the first annual report for Dalla Lana, Howard Hu, its second director, noted its "proud history" in reference to the school.[1] A thirty-six-page report for potential funders for what became the Dalla Lana School taps into this legacy, as it begins with a chapter on the School of Hygiene. Incidentally, the link to IHPME is also evident, as its second chapter is on IHPME.[2]

In IHPME the director, Adelsteinn Brown, noted FitzGerald's contribution in the 2016 annual highlights of the institute. He also noted "the extent to which our Institute is formed by the contributions of those who came before" and that "our greatest strength is in how we use or own history – our understanding of the research, the teaching and the leaders that have shaped us."[3]

When Brown became interim dean of Dalla Lana, he emphasized the history of the school by a number of initiatives. The main one was creating two history walls. In the main hallway leading to the administrative offices on both sides of the corridor on the sixth floor of the Health Sciences Building are a series of panels depicting a timeline of significant events from the early 1900s to the present. I provided information to the curators on the IHPME piece. This area was featured at U of T Homecoming 2018.

In one of the main reception areas on the same floor are two portrait walls, with FitzGerald's portrait, along with portraits and pictures of other former heads of the school and its departments, along with distinguished faculty and grads. As well in this area there are two of FitzGerald's desks identified by a small gold plaque, and there is a heavy, oak conference table (believed to have come from the conference room for faculty in the building funded by the Rockefeller Foundation) in one of the main meeting rooms. Brown has FitzGerald's bookcase (also identified by a small gold plaque) in the dean's office. There is a section on the Dalla Lana School website on School of Hygiene history.

AN ETHIC OF PUBLIC SERVICE IN TEACHING, RESEARCH, PRODUCT DEVELOPMENT

Bator notes that the labs and the school were part of FitzGerald's master plan to improve general health conditions and that FitzGerald "regarded teaching in conjunction with research and the provision of public service as the essentials of public health work."[4] This triad formed a basis of his approach.[5] One could say he proceeded in stages. The first was establishing an antitoxin and vaccine laboratory in 1914 (later expanded and named Connaught Laboratories) and the second restructuring and increasing the staffing of the Department of Hygiene when it was part of the Faculty of Medicine. The third was further restructuring and expanding into a school of hygiene, which had its own building, functioned as an independent division within the university, and was one of the Rockefeller schools of public health (who financed the building). The Rockefeller support not only provided operational and capital funding, it also plugged the school into an international network. Overriding it all was establishing inextricable links between the labs and the school (through cross-appointed staff, labs funding of university and school research) that created synergies between the two.[6]

Defries notes that FitzGerald "never lost sight of" the "place of research in the development of the School of Hygiene" and that the "unique interrelationship which he evolved" between the school and the labs made possible many research studies "which ordinarily could not have been undertaken" in the various departments of the school.[7] FitzGerald himself gave us some indication of this uniqueness when in his last report he said, "It is frequently possible to ascertain facts of theoretical interest and importance while developing practical means of more effectively controlling certain communicable diseases."[8]

The educational contribution of the labs was evident when he said that since 1927 forty-one Connaught Laboratories fellowships had been granted.[9] Defries noted that the provision of these fellowships, along with those of the Rockefeller Foundation "has been an important factor in making possible this large group of trained medical personnel in Canada" and that without them only a small number could have undertaken this postgraduate work.[10]

The product development component was evident in the mandate of the labs to first develop products to improve the health of the population and second continually drive the price of those products down in order to make them as widely available as possible.

AN ETHIC OF PUBLIC SERVICE IN PRACTICE

School of Hygiene the Staff College for Public Health and Hospital Admin

The School of Hygiene had always had a strong emphasis both on and in public health. As Browne pointed out, most of the senior health administrators in Canada had the DPH: "Most of the MOHs [medical officers of health] in Canada at the time held the DPH. JH [John Hastings] and I did the Community Health Centre Study 70–71 and certainly found this to be the case (except in Quebec, where Laval was preeminent)."[11]

Browne's observation is echoed by Bator and extended to include the DHA: "Just as the School of Hygiene constituted the staff college of Public

Health officers in English-speaking Canada for over forty-five years, the School of Hygiene's Department of Hospital Administration assumed a similar role."[12] Bator adds, "What was noteworthy was the extent to which recipients of the Toronto Diploma in Hospital Administration assumed key positions across the continent. By 1970, the graduates ... occupied senior positions in hospitals in nine Canadian provinces from British Columbia to Nova Scotia, fifteen American states from California to Texas to New York, and at least six countries outside the continent, from Barbados and Ecuador to Indonesia and the Philippines."[13]

Andrew Rhodes makes the same point regarding the school by noting that all full-time members of the Dominion Council of Health were its graduates.[14] Bator and Rhodes note that at the fifty-fourth meeting of the council, all but four of the thirteen members were graduated of the school.[15] Bator makes a similar observation of the hospital admin grads: "Because of their record of accomplishment on the job, the hospital administration grads of the school formed a potent lobby."[16]

The Staff College for Saskatchewan

This role of the DPH and DHA programs was particularly evident in Saskatchewan. There were a number of connections of each to the Department of Public Health. Fred Mott was at the Surgeon General's Office and was plucked by Tommy Douglas to implement Saskatchewan's hospital insurance program. An interview with Douglas was instrumental in inspiring a student of the DHA program, Burns Roth, to cut his administrative residency short to come to Saskatchewan to work in the provincial Department of Public Health. The deputy minister in that department just prior to Roth's arrival, Dr C.F.W. Hames, was a DPH grad (1931).[17] Roth would rose to become deputy minister and then returned to Toronto to be the second director of the DHA program, whereupon he convinced Mott to return to Canada to teach in both the hospital administration and public health administration programs. Other DPH grads in the Department of Public Health were F.C. Middleton (DPH, 1925), deputy minister, 1929–34, and M.S. Acker (DPH, 1946), assistant to the deputy minister when Roth was deputy minister.

There was also V.L. Matthews, who received his DPH in 1947. He was born in Saskatchewan, and on his return after graduation he took a position with the Regional Health Service Branch of the Saskatchewan Department of Public Health, while Tommy Douglas was minister. The following year

Matthews became the medical health officer, Swift Current Health Region. While there the first universal hospital and medicare insurance and comprehensive children's dental programs were pioneered and the first regional hospital council formed. Matthews later played a significant role in the development of medicare as a member of the Planning Committee on Medicare and as acting deputy minister of public health after Roth left and when medicare was introduced in July 1962.

Matthews joined the faculty of the College of Medicine at the University of Saskatchewan as professor and head of the Department of Social and Preventive Medicine.[18] This had been an idea of the provincial Department of Public Health (while Douglas was premier and Roth the deputy minister) as well as Dean Wendell Macleod. The new department was intended to forge a vital link between the university and the health problems of the community and would stress the roles of epidemiology and sociology.

Comment

Matthews's career is an almost textbook example of the types of career of certain graduates of the School of Hygiene. We have noted their position in offices of leadership. In Matthews's case it was also in positions at the vanguard of thinking in both population health and curative medicine. The Swift Current Health Region was leading in public health and was actively supported by the Douglas government as a test case for comprehensive, universal health insurance.

CRYSTALLIZING THE FITZGERALD CONTRIBUTION

Throughout his career FitzGerald crossed new frontiers and scaled new heights. He took this university's somewhat tentative and nascent foray into public health and put it squarely at the centre of this activity in Canada and onto the world stage. He took the university into a commercial endeavour, but one with a very distinct quality. It would commercialize medical research and use the proceeds to support further research at the basic and applied levels. Its main aim was not to generate a profit from these activities, it was availability. It would provide these products as close as possible to cost and it would constantly seek to drive down that cost.

Not content with what was taking place in his country, Fitzgerald had a custom of travelling to other countries to seek out and observe first-hand the information he needed, whether this was in methods of dealing with diphtheria or in the application of health insurance. His keen interest in other countries extended to bringing in people from other countries to the school or labs. Today we take this international interchange for granted. However, in the 1920s it was novel and travel was not as developed as it is today. It was an early example of today's global networks in science.

One can discern common elements to his activities: an ethic of public service, the importance of research, of public health, health insurance, prevention, and interestingly, the public's involvement in their health. And within this the emergence of multiple roles of a university – as a centre of teaching, research, entrepreneurship, and public service.

A lot of these values were congruent with FitzGerald's own. They came to permeate both the school and the labs. They included elements such as hiring on the basis of merit, an ethic of service, i.e., a focus on something other than the self, making a difference in people's lives. Research was important, but research aimed at impact. He had a strong belief in public institutions and a public mission – institutions like a U of T, or Canadian hospitals, or departments of public health. A corporation could be a public institution, it could be more than profit-seeking, to the extent to which its mission could be a wholly social mission, and its business wholly aimed toward that mission. And, as a result, its revenues could be ploughed back into the public mission of the university of which it was a part (in his case, research and clinical education).

His grandson noted he "conceived an overarching vision of public health that not only laid the foundations for provincial and federal programs across Canada but also influenced medical research and teaching on an international scale."[19] Further, "As a result in large part of his foresight, within a single generation between the world wars, Canada leaped from colonial backwater to recognized world leader in preventive medicine."[20]

Another important aspect of FitzGerald was his ability to pick people of great ability, dedication, and loyalty to an ideal: people like Defries and McKinnon, and many others.

Robert Defries, the first student in the public health program at U of T and the individual who took over the directorship of the school and the labs on FitzGerald's death, summed up the contribution of his mentor and colleague. FitzGerald had set himself to create "within this university, a non-commercial scientific institute" to fulfil two functions "in the interests of medical public service": research in preventive medicine and development of biological products that "might be supplied throughout Canada" and "would ensure their being of high quality and low price." This was made possible by the "promotion of intimate relationships and integration among teaching, research and public service."[21]

In Defries we see that the quality of leadership witnessed in FitzGerald carried forward. Defries was recognized for it. In 1954 he become the first Canadian to receive the prestigious Lasker Award. Former U.S. President Harry Truman took it upon himself to attend the ceremony to personally thank him for his work in mitigating the incidence of polio.[22]

We spoke at the outset of this work of recent academic literature that links health to nation-building. FitzGerald's actions in areas such as communicable disease, public health, the Dominion Council of Health, School of Hygiene, and Connaught Labs were definitely nation-building. Add to that his idea of combining research, education, and the production of vaccines and serums in a single facility, as well as his concept of producing a range of high-quality preventive medicines manufactured at costs low enough to make them universally available.

He was also playing into the strong hand of what I will refer to as Canada's "health heritage," a label that one could attach to Canada's historic concern with both public health and health care. In this case we are concerned with public health and the strong leadership of J.W.S. McCullough and Charles Hastings regarding the provincial and Toronto boards of health respectively. In fact, this is an under-examined area – the degree to which the health reforms being undertaken by McCullough and Hastings were complemented by the initiatives of FitzGerald at the university.

Bator's dissertation was on what was taking place at the city of Toronto with reference as well to the province. However, he does not deal with what was taking place at U of T.[23] There is a question about the complementarity of what was taking place at the boards of health and what was taking place in public health at the university.

Bator notes, "Even before Toronto became noteworthy as the home of the inventor of insulin, it received international acclaim for the operation of its health department."[24] Moreover doctors and nurses from Toronto's Department of Health were very much oriented toward "improved life for the ordinary man, woman and child."[25] There was the province supplying FitzGerald's diphtheria toxoid for free. In this way these departments were consistent with the theme associated with FitzGerald of bringing health "within reach of everyone."

Perhaps as a portent of things to come in the importance of administration and hence for the school to start a formal program in administration is how administration was emphasized when speaking of Toronto's public health achievements. Bator stated that "Toronto's Department of Public Health was a model of public health administration.[26] Or, a related statement, that a "cornerstone" of the department and "Hastings's greatest achievement" was "a competent administration."[27]

There is a nuance, however, that the reader needs to bear in mind when the school started its Department of Hospital Administration: with this new department, the school was adding a new dimension, moving into the realm of acute-care health delivery in addition to public health delivery and health-care administration in addition to public health administration.

What we are also witnessing with FitzGerald's actions is a progressive involvement in the areas we identified in these linkage areas. All are a portent of the formation of IHPME.

FitzGerald and Agnew

FitzGerald and G. Harvey Agnew, the first director of the Department of Hospital Administration, knew each other. Both were active in the Canadian Medical Association and they served on its committees together, one of which was the Special Committee of Hospital Service.[28] FitzGerald was on the CMA's executive committee when Agnew was active in its Department of Hospital Service.[29]

SUCH GENIUS IS A DELICATE BALANCE

Much that has been written on FitzGerald's passing focuses on his mental health, and increasing the awareness of this important issue and the empathy for it is a good thing. However, another aspect to his untimely passing has to do with the genius of the man, and his type of genius is a delicate balance.

There are his intuitive abilities regarding his research and that of others, his ability to pick people of singular dedication, and to create a culture of excellence in two world-class organizations. There is his intellectual and organizational genius. His establishing two complementary organizations, each gaining an international reputation, were phenomenal. Similarly, his writings on diphtheria and preventive medicine were noteworthy. His concern with medical education, the role of public health and particularly the role of nurses were ahead of his time.[30]

His close colleague Don Fraser eulogized him in the proceedings of the Royal Society of Canada: "Too few are given the qualities of executive ability, singleness of purpose, imagination and vision, combined with gentleness, modesty, and charm of character in such large measure as Dr FitzGerald possessed."[31] Of note is his reference to FitzGerald's executive ability.

Michael Bliss says he "was a towering figure, perhaps the single most important public health entrepreneur Canada has yet produced.... In the first third of the 20th century, he was everywhere on Canadian and international medical stages, knew everyone in the worlds of psychiatry, public health, pharmaceuticals (he and Connaught were at the centre of the production of insulin), academic medicine, and was widely respected for his industry, character, and good judgment. His seemed a career of almost Oslerian dimensions."[32] He says FitzGerald was associated "with some of Canada's greatest 20th-century medical achievements."[33]

However, it goes beyond this. There are his views on the marriage of theory and practice, and similarly of basic and applied research, and the strong applied orientation of the school he founded. There was the strong interrelationship between the school and labs, each energizing the other, described as "two halves of one whole."[34] He was at least one full generation, arguably two, ahead of his time.

That has to be a lonely quest. A person at the frontiers – of knowledge or its application – is out there alone, pushing back present and establishing future intellectual borders. There are both benign (the inertia of conventional wisdom) and more malevolent (the envy of the lesser mortals) forces to contend with – a constant drag. In FitzGerald there were also the constant demands on him, especially as his reputation grew, and being able to deal with them while at the same moment finding time for the continued development of his own intellectual creativity – another part of the balance.

This is "the stress of a crowded life."[35] Some details on FitzGerald's crowded life are "racing back and forth from country to country," meetings in Manhattan for the International Health Division of the Rockefeller Foundation, then Geneva and the Health Organization of the League of Nations, then Ottawa for the Dominion Council of Health's three-day meetings.[36] And this is on top of his work, directing the two organizations he founded and his own research.

The delicate balance is mediating all this – the forces of his own personality, the almost insatiable demands on his time, and the need for quietude that one needs in order to recharge. It was not an easy task, for him or the others of his ilk. Bliss notes, "A very large number of FitzGerald relatives, friends, and professional associates including such giants of Canadian medicine as Banting and Best, were also mentally ill, unstable, and/or addicted to alcohol or drugs."[37]

Bliss may be onto something here, for what is the cost of being at the frontier alone? How do you sustain the aloneness of that part of your life and yet remain a part of the social fabric in all others? Most important, how do you reconcile the two? And this may not be only the province of exceptional people like FitzGerald. Social isolation is perceptual as well as actual. Most anyone can feel alone. FitzGerald's situation poses the eternal question, if it persists, how can it be mitigated?

Another aspect to this is not necessarily the sole province of genius but more of ambition: what one reaches for. Here Bliss also has a comment: FitzGerald was part of "a medical generation brought up to aspire to more than their temperaments could sustain."[38] A corollary is that there is a toll exacted for high aspiration, of driving oneself to that degree almost constantly.

Another toll (and here we are in the province of IHPME) is the one exacted for administering organizations distinguished by their size, complexity, and international stature – organizations like a faculty of medicine, a school of hygiene, or a major enterprise like the labs. FitzGerald, remarkably, at one point in his life was doing all three, as well as his major extra involvements like the Rockefeller Foundation and the Health Committee of the League of Nations. But running such organizations exacts a price. One sees the same in individuals who run the major academic health sciences centres, places of almost unimaginable complexity, places like a UHN or a SickKids.

In all of these there is an almost byzantine complexity, which begins with the ambitions of the organizations themselves. A school of hygiene, a U of T, TGH, or SickKids aspires to be world-class; it wants to lead internationally. Its ambitions are high, and the people who work in them of similar ambition. The aim and maintaining their place takes tremendous energy. All of this exacts a price for senior administrators or senior medical staff – and on myriad levels – one's health, marriage, children.

FitzGerald was subject to three huge stresses, one the stress of his genius, of articulating the ideals of his vision of public health in Canada. The second was the stress of running the two large and complex organizations he founded. The third was coping with his own fame, for fame itself can be a huge stress, particularly in maintaining one's sense of self amidst the persona. And this coupled with the demands arising from the fame to consult or be various committees, many outside Toronto (or even Canada).

So we can discuss FitzGerald's mental health, and even what might have been his fatal flaws, but one needs to couch it within the almost impossible demands that arose from his accomplishments, and those he placed on himself. And in doing this one needs to acknowledge the essential heroism of the man – and through FitzGerald recognize this in many others, even if not many can match the true scope of his efforts.

Other elements have to do with the milieu of the time. Today, his ideals – his strong emphasis on practice, on impact, to harness academia to solve real-life issues, the quest to bridge the gap between academia and society – these are common currency; then, not so much so. Add another novel twist, the marriage of an academic teaching and research enterprise and a manufacturing enterprise.

Another strong lesson from his passing is how we forge a culture of excellence, the establishment of a meritocracy, the fostering of a culture that incubates and supports the genius among us. But perhaps the most important question is how we forge a culture that can catch us as we fall, that can act as a kind of balm for the troubled soul.

One can liken the time leading to FitzGerald's passing to that of a falling leaf. Often the leaf can be caught as it gently falls to the ground. We can liken this to opportunities for intervention and, indeed, in FitzGerald's case, these were tried. But the corollary is to have a society of sophistication, quality, and community in which there is something to reach for, a new ledge from which to continue the ascent.

PART NINE

Outcomes of the IHPME Approach

CHAPTER 23

Range of Activity

Today research has greatly eclipsed professional education in the IHPME. This is not to diminish the importance of the latter, but rather to point out the degree of new activity that has been undertaken by the institute. Research faculty are also involved in delivering substantial course content of the professional curriculum. They often utilize and refer to the work of other research faculty in their lectures and readings.

Current experimentation could not take place with policy institutes at IHPME if it did not have a very strong research capacity. And research is more than the papers being cranked out, it is the capacity of IHPME to use its research tools for research questions posed by stakeholders like the Ministry of Health and Long-Term Care (MOHLTC) or OMA. Further it is networks, particularly ones that are international (such as on integrated care or comparative systems).

SOME PROMINENT RESEARCH ACTIVITY

IHPME has undertaken initiatives that are future-oriented and could be significant additions to its mandate as well as make significant contributions to the future of health policy in Canada.

High-Performing Systems

Faculty member Ross Baker has been in involved in researching high-performing systems. He has a number of publications analyzing such systems.

Alaska and the "Customer-Owner" Model

One study supported by the Canadian Health Services Research Foundation looks at three systems (in Alaska, Utah, and Sweden).[1] The intent is to discern which elements of their success could be exported to Canada. Much of Baker's research is intriguing, and the Alaska model on the Nuka System of Care and their customer-owner model has caught the attention of the Ministry of Health and Long-Term Care in Ontario.

While the Nuka System is aimed at Indigenous peoples, the deputy minister of health and long-term care, in an address sponsored by IHPME graduate students, noted that Ontario would like to examine how it might be applied here for the whole population.[2] It is an intriguing idea: he noted one could say in a public system like Ontario's the people are "customer owners."

The deputy minister's talk was another example of how high-ranking Ontario civil servants take the time to speak to IHPME students. Students invariably find such talks interesting and motivating.

Another study, sponsored by the OHA, also looked at high-performing systems and was notable for an appendix that listed a number of studies that have been done on such systems.[3] This was a reanalysis of the High Performing Health Care systems work that was initially funded through the Ministry of Health and Long-Term Care. There was also a patient engagement element to it. There was also a larger patient project funded by the Ontario Foundation for Health Innovation (which was founded by the OHA).[4]

It bears mentioning that IHPME has long had a relationship with the OHA. Given that it is Ontario's hospital association, it will not be surprising to learn this started with the very inception of the program. It has included IHPME grads who have served on OHA committees as well as its board.

Patient Engagement: IHPME and SPOR

There is increasing democratization in health care, specifically patient engagement in their care and also in research, and there has been substantial activity in this area in Europe and the United Kingdom.

Along this line IHPME has also been involved in an innovative project of the CIHR. It is in their Strategy for Patient-Oriented Research (SPOR) program, which aims for a continuum of research that engages patients as partners. It aspires to apply research knowledge to improve health-care systems and practices, and its goal is to foster evidence-informed health care by bringing innovative diagnostic and therapeutic approaches to the point of care. It is a partnership between the CIHR and provincial and territorial ministries.

Alison Paprica at IHPME led the development of the business plan for the Ontario SPOR SUPPORT Unit (OSSU), a $100-million, five-year, joint federal/provincial funded platform to support and enhance patient-oriented research.[5] Fiona Miller directs a series of patient-oriented health research seminars sponsored by OSSU.[6]

One part of this platform was a series of seminars conducted through the academic year put together by Fiona Miller. They brought in prominent academics to speak of their experiences in involving patients in research and/or care. One example was Deborah Marshall from the University of Calgary, who spoke of the Patient and Community Engagement Research program she runs in Calgary. One of the interesting aspects about this program was that patients bring their experience of diagnosis, treatment, support, and self-management to improving the health-care system. They also can become involved in patient-led research after participating in a year of course work and a year of practical research experience under an established academic researcher.

Another example is Dr Stephen Peckham (who had a cross-appointment with IHPME), who spoke of his experience in researching different types of patient involvement in health-care policy in the United Kingdom. He is at the Centre for Health Services Studies at the University of Kent. He presented a historical overview of initiatives the UK government has developed since the 1960s to encourage patient participation. He also reviewed barriers they face to more or effective participation. The centre has a specific initiative aimed at public engagement, which connects research activities to the general public through public talks and exhibitions, press and social media activities.

What is interesting about the U of T seminars is that not only faculty attended but also patients and the public, so they became a way of building greater awareness in the public.

Another piece was that the institute was contracted to do three White Papers for OSSU on research relevance and public/patient/community engagement in health research, with a focus on engagement as an issue for health research systems.[7]

Research Management

In 2016, Louise Lemieux-Charles and Alison Paprica planned a research leadership day, in collaboration with Vivek Goel and U of T researchers, to discern what type of need might exist to cultivate leadership and management skills amongst scientists and researchers. As a result, Vivek, through his Office of the Vice-President, Research and Innovation partnered with the School of Continuing Studies and worked with Alison to develop a research project management course offered through the school. The first session was held in the fall of 2017.

The reader will recall that scientist/researcher leadership was Vivek's initiative when he was institute chair. He says it fell off his radar when he moved to other roles – but now that he is back in research he sees that it remains an unmet need. He adds that he now also sees a major need for training for people involved in research governance – that researchers wind up on boards with very little understanding or preparation for their role.[8]

Community-Based Services

There is a certain continuity in this area. The work of Robert Defries and William Mosley and the East York Health Unit (1940s), that of Hastings and Mosley for the Hall Commission (1960s), and Hastings and the Community Health Centre Project (1970s) has seen a renewed interest. Professor Emeritus Paul Williams focused on community-based services while at IHPME. He, along with Janet Lum at Ryerson, started the Canadian Research Network for Care in the Community.[9] It is aimed to promote knowledge generation and knowledge translation in home and community care. They have organized many international symposia and presented at many international symposia organized by others on cutting-edge best practices in home and community care from around the world. They have visited and worked with leading community agencies in Ontario and internationally in countries like Japan, China, England, and the Netherlands.[10]

Another perspective on community-based, cooperative medicine is offered by Greg Marchildon, who was involved in updating an important work on the history of community clinics in Saskatchewan. His introduction demonstrates important perspectives that IHPME faculty are offering on critiquing the Douglas model of medicare, which served as the national template. He notes that Alan Blakeney, who was a Cabinet minister in the Douglas government, noted that the Saskatoon Agreement, which ended the Doctors' Strike, involved a major concession, in that the government agreed not to radically change how medical care was delivered by physicians. This was very much against the ideals of Stan Rands, a founder of the community clinic movement in Saskatchewan, who wanted a policy that would transform the delivery of health care, not merely the funding mechanism.[11]

To do this Rands wanted a particular type of co-operative group practice: the community clinic, which would be controlled by the consumer of health services and would redress the traditional inequality between doctor and patient. He saw an inherent contradiction in the Douglas medicare plan. On the one hand, as a funding mechanism, it established health care as a right. On the other, in terms of delivery, the fee-for-service method of payment and the private, for-profit, small business organizational framework had physicians treating health care as a commodity. This framework also inhibited the establishment of preventive care.[12]

Community clinics embodied a number of specific principles: they were collaborative, community-based group practices, they were interdisciplinary, and they involved other health professions. Their governance was community-based (boards of clinic members).

Marchildon's introduction in the revised edition of the book by Rands (cited above) provides a description of a community health-care movement that survives to this day in Saskatchewan. It is also an important historical descriptor of a comprehensive alternative to health-care delivery at the primary level. As such it broadens the dialogue in this area. The collaborative work of Williams at IHPME and Lum at Ryerson provided an important source of academic expertise that was an important resource for strengthening the community health movement at the local, national, and international levels.

There are important activities underway here. Paul and Janet are involved in building capacity – in the community health movement to be sure, but also in the Canadian system. Marchildon is building awareness, providing a historical and analytical framework that gets at some of the subtle (and not so subtle) nuances of medicare.

His discussion of linkages between the Saskatoon Agreement and primary care sets up a more sophisticated understanding of some of the foundations of Canadian medicare. It is an example of how IHPME faculty are developing conceptual models that complement the capacity-building of Williams and Lum. His explication of the tensions that surround the Saskatoon Agreement – but even more important in how it set in train a certain path of health-care delivery – is important to an understanding of some of the limitations of our present system. His analysis sets out the importance of history in Canadian health care. He points out that "the reform of primary care remains one of the most intractable pieces of the health care reform puzzle, and the potential for reform remains constrained by the Saskatoon Agreement."[13]

AN OUTWARD FOCUS

A Nexus

As the reader has no doubt gleaned by now, the institute/department has been at a nexus throughout its history. We have seen faculty involved in government studies, commissions, and standing committees of Parliament. But we may be seeing an intensification of such activity that shows no signs of abetting.

Perhaps the mission of the university is expanding. Increasingly it is seen as housing centres of expertise, which can be manifested in various ways. They can bring people together by mounting seminars or conferences in certain subject areas. Ideally these attract not just faculty or students from academia but also members of the public, journalists, civil servants, businesspeople, and politicians.

A number of activities of IHPME reinforce a vital role of the university. The university of the twenty-first century has an expanded role in our society for many reasons, not least of which is the knowledge-based economy, which characterizes this era and is the currency of the university. Here the university becomes a nexus, a focal point bringing diverse groups of people together.

This position becomes important on many levels. One is bringing diverse faculty students, and the public together. It points to the fact that the university of the twenty-first century has an outreach function; it needs to engage with the society at large.

Another reason for its importance is the stimulation of bringing diverse faculty together to dialogue on common issues. This nexus becomes a vibrant part and result of the university, a vital part of our global village, and an integral part to forging a strong societal fabric.

Throughout its history IHPME has been a nexus on many levels. In its beginning was its strong relationship with hospital administrators across the country. Also during this time it was in connections to a progressive, activist government in Saskatchewan, which saw this department, indeed the school it was associated with, as a recruiting ground and educational resource for further education for that government's best and brightest.

IHPME is a nexus between academia (including faculty and students), hospitals, and government. In the 1970s this expanded to include other health organizations. Later it added research, in addition to professional education.

One could argue that with the NAO and ACE the nexus between governments (national or sub-national) is deepening and, importantly broadening, in that graduate students are involved in these activities.

But IHPME has been a nexus for student-practitioner interactions. We had this originally with the strong relationships between students and hospital preceptors. People like Jim McNab, Gerry Turner, Ron McQueen, or Ted Freedman did not just graduate and go their way. They remained actively involved with the program as guest lecturers and actively involved with admin resident students at their hospital.

When the department became part of the new Division of Community Health the core courses were a nexus. In the more recent past, the way HAD 5010 was organized when it became part of the modular program in the 1990s created a nexus. This included its "expert panels," bringing in faculty from other universities or practitioners from different facets of health care. This was important not just in bringing practitioners into the classes. It was important in a much more subtle way, in the student-to-practitioner interaction that took place during the class break.

At these classes one invariably saw students in earnest conversation with presenters, no doubt about an issue in the student's mind sparked by the presentation. Such discussions invariably continued in the tutorials afterward. The importance of these informal discussions and of the opportunity for this interaction (nexus) cannot be overstressed.

Another aspect was the involvement of practitioners as tutors. This provided another type of nexus. It allowed practitioners to retain an academic involvement and students to gain a practical-world perspective.

A case in point was in HAD 5020 in 2018. Paul Williams had its last class on pharmacare, which was very topical at that time. It had been an issue in the 2015 federal election, Ontario had announced a plan for people twenty-four and under in its 2017 budget (called OHIP+), and it was an issue in the Ontario 2018 election, which was underway at the time. Paul brought in three experts from three different areas (a physician, academic, and journalist) for the panel part of the class. The physician, Danyall Raza, was chair of Canadian Doctors for Medicare and had a degree from Harvard. The academic, Katherine Boothe, a McMaster professor, had written a book on the subject comparing Canada, Australia, and the United States. The freelance journalist, Vanessa Milne, had written for many of Canada's leading publications.[14] Their perspectives shed important light on a complex topic and this, combined with the substance of Paul's lecture, set the stage for a lively tutorial discussion.

Another part of this nexus is the seminars organized by graduate students. Once again the intellectual thought of IHPME is being fertilized by bringing in outside perspectives.

One can also take this notion of nexus and put it on a larger canvas, the university as nexus. We spoke at the outset of this university's sense of place. There is another aspect to this sense of place. The historian Fernand Braudel says that certain phenomena in life are world-oriented in their character. There are countries that have "world economies" and "world cities," and these economies and cities look outward to their counterparts in other parts of the world as much as they do inward to the country within which they are located.[15]

One could say that Toronto, with its degree of cultural and ethnic diversity, is such a city for Canada. One could also argue, though Braudel does not say this, that there is yet another world category, such a thing as "world universities." They, like the city within which they are located, look outward. A number of qualities that make them so. They have a larger proportion of foreign students, their faculty are involved in research projects that are either international in their orientation or include international networks. Their students have more opportunity to do a part of their studies or summer projects in foreign countries. Discussions in the halls more often focus on global issues.

One could also say that another distinguishing factor in such universities is that they carry with them not just the hopes and aspirations of those in the city in which they are located, but the hopes and aspirations of a province and of a nation as well. Their institutional interactions and the interactions of their faculty are on a global stage. They have a global imprint. Such universities are at a nexus. They bridge interactions and mediate the interface between the global and local.

An Intersection

A very interesting function for IHPME is its role at an intersection of stakeholders, including academia, government, NGOs, industry (business), and the public in the development and evaluation of policy and health-care delivery. Within the institute are striking initiatives coming at this from centres of expertise within the institute and with different emphases. It points to the myriad ways that IHPME links itself to practice and involves its alumni and other practitioners in its activities.

We spoke of this at the beginning of the work. One example is health insurance, where the School of Hygiene, School of Nursing, and Department of Hospital Administration were involved. With the School of Hygiene (FitzGerald, Defries) and School of Nursing (Gunn) we see different people focusing on it, and for differing reasons. With the department it was a concern of Agnew's. For FitzGerald and Defries it was part of their objective of health available for all, as it was for Gunn, but it was also part of extending the goal of public health nursing delivery and recognition of the role of nurses as its own distinct activity.

The interconnectedness of all this is evident when we see the (primarily physician) public health training of the School of Hygiene linked to public health nursing at the university level, which is linked to a major hospital nursing school under Gunn, because even though it was separate from the mission of her (hospital) nursing school, she felt it was a very important area of nursing training.

Added to this was the School of Hygiene's connection to local and provincial officers of health and the Dominion Council of Health.

An Emphasis on Practice

There are two aspects to this emphasis. The first concerns the priority in the hospital administration diploma program, which was almost exclusively the nuts-and-bolts of hospital operation. Unlike today, it was not built upon an academic foundation of a body of research in policy, outcomes, or management. Nor did it take into account new or emerging areas such as integrated care, sustainability, or agency.

The second concerns the broader area of the tension between an emphasis on practical as opposed to theoretical knowledge. A lot of the practical orientation originated from FitzGerald's intent to have maximal impact on the health of the population. Throughout his tenure this led to the school's tight relationship with the city and province, indeed with other provinces and the federal government as well. This kept the school closely focused on the practical needs for good public health training. We noted earlier the Ontario Department of Health approaching FitzGerald with its intent to have mandatory minimum requirements for public health officers and for the school's to help to mount programs to achieve this goal.

An integral part of the emphasis on practice was practicums, the inception of which can be traced back to the DPH degree. It had a three-month term of public health practice in a health department in the summer between the two academic years.[16] The DHA had a twelve-month practicum, the MHSc at inception two practicums (four- and six-month terms), and one with the modular program. The Dalla Lana School has a required practicum (sixteen weeks) in its MPH degree, with the option for a second (twelve weeks).

All this emphasis on practice, through practicums or a curricular emphasis, is in line with a recent emphasis of the Ontario government on experiential learning, which is occurring at all levels of education, from primary through to tertiary. Both the Ministry of Education and the Ministry of Advanced Education and Skills Development have made experiential learning a priority.

In June 2016 the Premier's Highly Skilled Workforce Expert Panel released a report on how experiential learning is a vital component to building the workforce of tomorrow.[17] Later that year the Ministry of Education released *Community-Connected Experiential Learning*,[18] which was followed by the Career Ready Fund in September 2017 to support experiential learning at Ontario's universities and colleges.[19] In that same month U of T solicited applications for funding from undergraduate divisions wanting to support experiential learning.[20] One only needs to search "experiential learning" to find a host of Ontario and Canadian universities as well as the Council of Ontario Universities emphasizing it.[21]

It is worth noting IHPME has been incorporating experiential learning through its practicums since its inception seventy years ago. And it has broadened its application. It was a core of the diploma and still forms a core of the MHSc degree, but it is now also included in the MHI, EMHI, and MSc-SLI degrees.

Academia and Board Memberships

A number of IHPME faculty are involved in governance, which spans the range of organizations from NGOs to hospitals to policy institutes to start-ups.

Current and past directors typically serve on important boards. Vivek Goel is on the board of the Canadian Institute for Health Information (CIHI) and Louise Lemieux-Charles on the board of North York General. Adalsteinn Brown is on the Canadian Association for Health Services and Policy Research and a series of incubator and business accelerator boards.

Faculty members are also active in this area. To give just a few examples, Ross Baker has been on the Saskatchewan Health Quality Council since 2007. Saskatchewan was the first province in Canada to set up a quality council. He was appointed to the board of University Health Network in 2017 as well as chair of their Safety and Quality Committee. Greg Marchildon is on the boards of the Champlain Society and Broadbent Institute and was chair of the Saskatchewan Health Research Foundation.

A Strong National and International Orientation

We have seen how the school and the department were considered as national schools in their respective areas. We have also seen how people like FitzGerald and Defries were part not only of entities like the Dominion Council of Health but also international organizations like the Health Committee of the League of Nations and the World Health Organization.

We have also seen that international students were part of both the school and the department. This continued with the institute. And in particular we have seen how the institute took this one step further to facilitate enrolment of at least one individual who was interested in public health from a war-torn country, indeed, an individual who actualized this interest by pursuing humanitarian activities while in the Executive MHI program.

We have also seen internationally focused entities such as the North American Observatory and Institute for Circumpolar Research. This international stance was complemented by graduate courses with an international orientation such as HAD 7001, "Comparative Health Systems and Policy."

A very distinct characteristic of the school, the institute, and the university is the degree to which they all are outward facing, i.e., looking to the world as a whole and with interactions in many different parts of it, in essence a bridge between Canada and the world. This can involve faculty interacting with faculty in other parts of the world, students from other countries coming to the school or institute, or activities of the institute (like the NAO) using the world as their backdrop.

The Power of Example

Another important role played by faculty, adjunct faculty, and alumni is that of example. The Eugenie Stuart Award seeks to recognize this by having awards in categories such as best mentor, best thesis supervisor, best instructor, best director, and best course preparation. The role played by tutors in HAD 5010 is another example. Similar is the power of mentorship, especially among external administrative officers in practicum settings within the MHSc and MHI degree programs. Supplementing this was the initiative of the IHPME Graduate Students Union developed for HSR students in the MSc and PhD programs.

In this work we have seen instances of the mentorship role played by executives at Toronto General, and the importance of mentorship is widely recognized. David Johnston, while he was governor general, and himself a former academic, recounted the influence George Wald, a Nobel Laureate at Harvard, on him: one lecture he attended led to a "moment of epiphany." He said that an interdisciplinary approach allows one "to triangulate and look at problems from a different angle."[22]

And to further illustrate the power of example and the impact of an interdisciplinary approach, Lewis Auerbach, a classmate of Johnston's, in an introduction to Wald's Massey Lectures, noted the *Harvard Crimson* reported that Wald's course "'turned more scientists into poets, and more poets into scientists, than any course ever taught on this campus.'"[23] The emphasis on an interdisciplinary approach is one IHPME has emphasized since its inception.

Academic Entrepreneurism

Some of the activities in IHPME could be called academic entrepreneurism – not in the sense of building profitable enterprises but in building enterprises with an academic and public purpose. These include Greg Marchildon's work on the NAO, Steini Brown and Mark Dobrow on C3, Mark Dobrow on ACE, Audrey Laporte on the Canadian Centre for Health Economics, and Paul Williams on community-based workshops and seminars. For each of them – conceiving the idea, developing a proposal and building a business around it, obtaining funds, hiring staff, and just generally dealing with all the operational issues around making each organization self-sustaining – falls into this realm.

A similar argument but with a different nuance could be made for the tight relationship of FitzGerald's activity in research and its application, and the virtuous circle of each reinforcing the other in the founding of the School of Hygiene. Or, in a different but related case, his developing products to meet a public need, in always driving down the price of those products, in forming a company to take them from the bench to the bedside – this is a kind of entrepreneurism where an academic or social mission is as important as a business one. The business in this sense is not in building for-profit activity but a viable pursuit.

An IHPME webpage lists nine such initiatives, ranging from health economics, evidence-based policy development, health system performance, and driving excellence in the health system, to public health strategies.[24] One could argue that their existence is evidence of IHPME encouraging such entrepreneurial initiatives among its faculty. Greg Marchildon notes they also bring in additional students and resources that would not otherwise be available to IHPME.[25]

All the individuals mentioned really function as CEOs – with all the operational issues and responsibilities that this entails in what one could call academic-business ventures. Even though these initiatives are not businesses per se, they nonetheless have certain elements of business ventures.

One could also include developing new programs like MHI, SLI, or IDEAS. Here one is not creating a business per se but trying to develop a self-sustaining pursuit. These IHPME activities do not have the same corporate emphasis as FitzGerald's, but they are still building businesses in the sense of viable organizational entities. The main difference here is that the social (educational, service, societal) mission as opposed to business (profit) is predominant.

Yet another aspect involves a class like HAD 5010, which under Paul Williams's direction grew to include students from several faculties, an external panel of three experts, and a dozen or so external tutors. This is also a form of entrepreneurism, of always expanding its reach, involving a greater variety of experts in order to deliver the richest content and provide the fullest opportunities for interaction.

We are seeing entrepreneurism in two important respects. One is the creative function of starting and operating a new activity that provides a product and employs people. The other is furthering public institutions, which it does in a number of respects. It furthers the activities of this university, but it also furthers other public physical institutions such as government, hospitals, and other health-care organizations as well as non-physical institutions such as health insurance.

Most often when one speaks of entrepreneurism one is speaking of business activity, and when this occurs in the university one is referring to patents and start-ups. But there is a very important entrepreneurial component in public institutions that IHPME is supporting. A nurse developing a new process in patient care as a result of an IDEAS seminar would be another example.

Fundraising

An important activity in IHPME and Dalla Lana is fundraising. Because of the long history of Dalla Lana and IHPME there already are a number of student awards that represent powerful examples of the generosity of faculty, business, and alumni. For the year 2018, Steini Brown, while interim dean of Dalla Lana, offered to match donations by current and former faculty.

As well Dalla Lana created an office of advancement to spearhead fundraising. An important piece of their activity is not only the fundraising itself but also the events that bring faculty, alumni, and the public together.

Interfaces

A major distinguishing feature of the institute (and the school) throughout their history could be what one might label as interfaces. We noted earlier that the Etzkowitz and the Lambert Report talked about business-academic-government partnerships, and this has become an important theme in many countries.

The institute (and the school), and the department before it, were pursuing interfaces long before such a collaboration became a concept or a trend. We see it in the school's longstanding involvement with the Rockefeller Foundation and the department with the Kellogg Foundation.

Connaught Labs was a business-academic interface, but what was most fascinating about it is that it was one initiated by the school. And it had unique features in that Connaught was wholly owned by the university and was more service than profit oriented. Nonetheless, it paid royalties to the school, which were a major source of research funding. Many years later, Telemedicine Canada was quite similar. Its initial two owners were U of T and TGH, and it was more service than profit oriented.

An example of an academic-government interface is the Centre for Evidence and Health in All Policies (CEHIAP). Another is Ross Baker's work on high-performing systems. The NAO is another example, and while it is not a formal example, it is a nascent policy institute indicative of a comment we will quote in detail later of Martel's on policy institutes being at the intersection of ideas, institutions, and interests. The NAO takes this interface one step further in its studies of comparative systems.

What we have seen is a successive expansion of interface building. Initially it was academic-government/field. The school and the department had very close connections to the field. With the school this was with the municipal offices of public health and provincial ministries of health (particularly those of Ontario and Saskatchewan, though one could add the federal department to the mix). With the department it was with hospital CEOs across the nation. The practicum portion of the diploma curriculum strongly reinforced this. Saskatchewan almost immediately added a nuance, as in 1947 it had launched its hospital insurance program, which started a new division within its Department of Public Health, and Burns Roth from the university department cut his studies short to be its head. More recently the modular approach in the MHSC and MHI streams geared to full-time workers is another example of an academic-field interface.

Another type of interface is the tight relationship between the school (basic research), the labs (applied research), and health sciences centres such as TGH and SickKids (clinical research). The department/institute had its own variant on at least two aspects, with its emphasis on clinical epidemiology.

From this one moved to academic-government/field-business (with Connaught Labs) and from this to academic-government/field-business-public with the close ties of the school and the labs to meeting the public's needs in amelioration of communicable disease. Today there is an additional nuance to this fourth component in that the institute intentionally reaches out to the public in inviting them to seminar presentations. It expands the role of the university. It moves beyond the education of students, the continuing education of professionals, to a public outreach role, i.e., building awareness in the public on health, in a strengthening of democratic decision-making.

Linkages

Another commonality between the two was the number and intricacy of their linkages. FitzGerald was very involved with the top people in his field, such as Flexner, Parran, and the like. IHPME is much the same.

CHAPTER 24

Institution-Building

SETTING CONTEXT

A very important question is the degree to which the School of Hygiene and IHPME have historically been a part of institution-building. For example, how responsible have they been in founding and maintaining public health in Canada, establishing hospitals as centres of care, supporting health insurance, or helping to develop a professional public service in municipal, provincial, and federal health departments?

This institution-building takes place on multiple levels. On the one hand there is the building of organizational institutions like those mentioned above. One the other there is the building of less tangible institutions such as a research mentality, and along with this, capability – in other words, capacity-building. The question here is the degree to which an institute like IHPME is necessary for and an essential part of a nation's capacity to build and maintain hospitals, a universal health insurance system, public health, or new areas like patient involvement in research or the patient as agent.

And if we fold the Dalla Lana School into the mix, how necessary are such institutions to build a nation's capacity to deal with health inequalities, economic inequalities as they apply to health, the determinants of health, pandemics, and the like?

Recent literature from the Health Foundation in Britain regards their National Health Service as an anchor institution. This means many things, one of the primary ones its role as an essential national institution. But it also means its importance in supporting local economies and providing a focal point for communities.[1] The applicability to us is whether IHPME and Dalla Lana are an important support to health care as an anchor institution in Canada.

There is also the establishment of processes, ways of doing things, a certain discipline of action. There is the building of human and social capital.

One can point to the Department of Public Health in Saskatchewan during the Douglas era, which sent a number of people to the school or the DOHA for training in public health or hospital administration. The same was true for Ontario and other provinces.

Bator notes that the school "was the primary public health education centre in the country for decades" and that it "trained most of the health officers who established the municipal, federal and provincial public health services in Canada."[2] We have seen the same is said of the what was then the department and hospital administrators. In addition, the "bridging of the gap between medical research in the laboratory and the saving of human lives" animated the school and its staff "for almost fifty years."[3]

IHPME has been intimately involved in building Canadian public institutions. It all began with an ideal, "health for all," to construct a phrase, or as *Maclean's* magazine expressed it in 1915, "within reach of everyone." It began in FitzGerald's lab and led to the founding of Connaught Labs. One could argue that the DOHA grew out of the school's recognition that in the post–Second World War era an old institution (the hospital) was emerging in a new and powerful guise as a centrepiece of curative medicine. The ideal predated the school and even the DOHA but it would frame each of them. People like Agnew or Roth spent a good part of their lives trying to actualize this ideal regarding hospital care. And each was contained in helping to build another public institution, one of society's oldest institutions, the university.

What the preceding indicates is that the labs, school, and department were institution building in the sense of fostering other Canadian institutions. They themselves were also being built as institutions. The establishment of the labs in 1913 grew out of an urgent need by the provincial medical officer of health in Ontario, who faced many urgent public health problems. Diphtheria was the scourge of the day, but there were others. The death rate from TB was triple what it would be in the 1950s, typhoid fever was prevalent, and infant mortality two and a half times the 1950s rate.[4]

In 1924 the school was made possible by the Rockefeller Foundation grant and the decision to fund a school in Canada was influenced by the fact that the city of Toronto had an outstanding Department of Health. Also, by that time the labs provided an activity that was essential to the successful development of postgraduate teaching: research.[5]

We noted the department was formed as a new public institution (the hospital) was becoming much more predominant, and it grew as this new public institution grew. It was the pre-eminent educational facility for training in hospital administration in Canada. In fact it contributed to the emerging strength and quality of hospitals. Faculty in both the school and the department became involved in other new institutions: hospital, later medical, insurance; community care centres, primary care – the list goes on. The practicum aspect of the curriculum cemented practitioner involvement in teaching that continues to this day.

The importance of what the school and institute do is because societal health is not automatic. Nor is it necessarily tied to a certain level of economic development or prosperity, as is commonly believed. Szreter notes the importance of this institution building when he says, "Wealth and health ideally should go together, but history shows that any polity needs a rich endowment of institutional and civic resources for its citizens to achieve this ideal."[6]

He goes on to say, "It is still commonly assumed as a primary lesson of history that the process of economic growth automatically brings with it improvements in population health.... But the human record in fact shows no *necessary*, direct relationship between economic advance and population health, but rather a more ambivalent and contingent relationship.... Indeed, in almost every historical case, the first and most direct effect of rapid economic growth has been a negative impact on population health."[7]

He says it has been the "extensive 'welfare states' that have primarily provided the crucial mechanism" enabling countries to experience rapid rates of economic growth while minimizing the disruptive impact on people's health."[8] The School of Hygiene, IHPME, and the DLSPH, for Canada, have helped shape the Canadian version of the welfare state, and have helped mitigate the untoward effects of rapid economic growth.

Thoughts such as these raise important questions not only about the importance of places like the School of Hygiene, IHPME, and the DLSPH, and their role in building institutions, it also raises how important each is as an institution itself. And further how important are they not just as teaching and research tools but as repositories of knowledge? How important is it that an institution like U of T or IHPME has 189 and 70 years respectively of accumulated knowledge and history? Is knowledge aggregative, and does an institutional memory of knowledge matter?

The Importance of Location

In the early twenty-first century, health care has evolved into a very complex interdisciplinary matrix. U of T and its affiliated academic health sciences centres epitomize its fundamental characteristics. Toronto has what must be one of the world's pre-eminent medical clusters, one that is distinctively at the city's urban heart.

First are the university's health sciences faculties – Medicine, Public Health, Nursing, Pharmacy – all clustered at the southeast corner of its St George campus. Just across from this point are four large teaching hospitals: Toronto General, SickKids, Princess Margaret, and Mount Sinai, along with two specialized facilities, Women's College and Toronto Rehab. Princess Margaret actually began life as the Ontario Institute of Radiotherapy at TGH.[9] All of these hospitals have research institutes affiliated with the university. Also across the street is MaRS, a biomedical research park. This cluster covers the entire spectrum of health care from teaching, research (basic, applied, and clinical), patient care (primary to tertiary), to health entrepreneurship.

One wonders if there has been some intentionality to this placement, as the university moved its faculties of Nursing and Pharmacy to this corner of the campus. And the ministry relocated Princess Margaret Hospital to this location in the 1990s.

And in another distinctive aspect to this cluster, it is adjacent to the government seat of power and within blocks of the nation's corporate and financial centre. Links can be found between IHPME and all of these components.

A CHRYSALIS?

An important fact in this history is that for a time what was then the Department of Health Administration was an organizational container, a vessel that embodied and kept alive the values of the School of Hygiene. It encapsulated these values, and as such represented a kind of continuity and transmission agent between the original school and the Dalla Lana School that would later emerge. Bear in mind that in the original school the Department of Hospital Administration had merged with the Department of Public Health during Roth's tenure, so that after the School of Hygiene's dissolution this combined department kept alive academic activity in public health.

It was a department that survived intact in the intervening period between the two schools and always had a significant role of its own because of its mission in professional education. It also had its own independent reputation (in health administration circles) and a strong alumni in its Society of Graduates, many of whom were in prominent positions at leading Canadian institutions – places like Mount Sinai, Toronto General, and Sick Children's Hospitals.

This heritage is important to the Dalla Lana School, whose history section on its website details and pays homage to FitzGerald and the former school.[10] The DLSPH commissioned a professional historian to create this website history section, which goes into substantial detail on some of the significant players such as J. Amyot, D. Fraser, and R. Defries, to name only a few.

This history mentions people from IHPME like John Hastings, Louise Lemieux-Charles, and Vivek Goel who were very involved in both health administration and public health. They were also active in getting a new school established. And they as well as others such as Gene Vayda and Steini Brown played crucial roles in the evolution of the department/institute as it went through its roles in Hygiene, Medicine, and Dalla Lana. Also these individuals were important supporters of a public health school. Yet another connection is David Naylor (also a faculty member) and his role in establishing the DLSPH. This is to say that while there were many U of T faculty over the years who pushed for a new school, an important continuing focus came from IHPME.

The website states that with the IHPME transfer from Medicine to Dalla Lana, the latter became the largest school of public health in Canada and one of the largest in the world.[11]

CUTTING EDGE

The department was and is always at the cutting edge. Either the School of Hygiene or the department (now institute) was advancing the frontiers of knowledge.

The institute remains at the forefront with initiatives like the NAO, which looks at systems comparatively, not only among nations but within subnational entities as well. Or CEHIAP, providing policy advice to government, which could prove synergistic for both organizations; that academic-government partnerships yield better policy; that the research and analysis that the academy can provide – this aggregate knowledge is very important to policy development in the knowledge society.

Steini Brown pushed this further with his emphasis on partnerships and collaboration. An important part of IHPME has been its multidisciplinary nature. Rhonda Cockerill notes this and identifies that this means that its "impact becomes much wider."[12]

The institute has been constantly pushing at the edges. It, and the school before it, began with a very practical focus. It worked, as the graduates of each became leaders in their field. As Goel noted, the department had incorporated an internship piece to its curriculum that, along with its later move to modular study, presaged the co-op programs that are popular today. The debate on moving to a professional graduate degree pushed a university with a research-intensive agenda to consider another form of graduate study, and this in turn pushed the department to move into research and academic degrees, which gave new depth to its professional studies.

A PROVINCIAL/NATIONAL RESOURCE

As one of the larger health management and policy institutes, IHPME continued to be at the centre of health care in Ontario. But it had grown in its sophistication, which had paced that of the health care system itself. It was at the centre of a much more holistic, inextricable entity, one immeasurably more complex and almost byzantine in its interconnectedness to all facets of individual and social well-being. And it continued to be situated within a world-class school of public health.

The institute has had a fascinating evolution. It began with an exclusively practical focus. Archival records show a very nuts-and-bolts collection of classes on the practicalities of running a hospital, which included topics like medical staff organization, hospital bylaws, the governing board, unions, personnel management, and public relations, to name a few.[13] This characteristic was buttressed by the topics of the theses written in the second year of the diploma program. It is almost the polar opposite of the focus today.

In addition the academic and research role has eclipsed the professional role of the institute. And today what is deemed necessary for professional education is a much more nuanced approach to management. It needs to include an education on issues such as health policy, intervention outcomes, service quality, the importance of innovation – an approach that is geared toward leadership as much as management.

Perhaps some of the reasons are that health-care professionals and organizations are more than just that in many communities. They are integral parts of the community fabric. And to take it one step further, when one gets into levels such as the CEOs of large teaching hospitals or senior civil servants at the director, ADM or DM level, decisions are being made for organizations whose budgets extend into the hundreds of millions, even billions of dollars. Or to take another perspective, decisions are being made that affect entire health systems. The people making those decisions need to be schooled in particular skill sets. The institute has kept and needs to keep pace with the level of complexity and sophistication involved.

We have seen in these pages the institute has always been able to attract individuals of top calibre. At the faculty level this has been evident in the contributions these people have made. At the student level it has been evident in the positions of leadership these people have attained.

The leadership of faculty and chairs are equally fascinating. They have not been just strong academically. They have been requested to share their insights at provincial legislatures, the federal Parliament, and the US Congress. The public record of such appearances is fascinating to read. Some of these appearances have resulted in national press coverage that has not only focused on the quality of information presented, but also debating skills that have bested the grandstanding of politicians.

It raises a series of questions. Is there another role for institutes like IHPME? Health is the biggest single line item in our provincial budgets. In countries (unlike ours), that do not have regional legislatures, many times it is their largest national budget item. Bator notes that what was then a department served as our national school of public health and also the staff college of public health officers and hospital administrators.[14] So it serves a very useful role. But is it more than this? Is there an additional role? And do we get a glimpse of it through initiatives like CEHIAP and the Mowat Centre? Is there a need for government, indeed, not just government but a province or a country, to have a *capability* such as an IHPME?

Does an institute like IHPME, or a Mowat Centre, or a Munk School of Global Affairs serve as a resource (provincial or national) that governments can draw upon, in these cases in health, public policy, and international affairs respectively? And is this a competence that is essential for governments to be able to access? Should governments be able to draw upon such expertise, and do they, and is the net effect of having done so in many cases better decisions? Has IHPME evolved into much more than teaching? Is it at one and the same time a centre of expertise to be consulted, a node in an international network in its various specialty areas? Is this now the new multifaceted role of IHPME?

A primary characteristic of the School of Hygiene, its departments, and above all its people, is competence. But in rare instances you've had something more, you've had the extraordinary, and not just the extraordinary in science as important as that is, but the extraordinary in character, in caring, in asserting the dignity, indeed the right, of everyone to have access to health care. And then to have it delivered in the best manner possible. This is the legacy of the school and the department. The University of Toronto has always had some of the best medical minds. It has fallen to the department, now institute, to graduate the professionals who can envisage the best way to get it to the people and then manage an organization that can bring it all to fruition.

This idea could be extended to U of T itself. Is it a provincial and national resource? Arguments can certainly be made along such lines. Also institutions such as the Robarts Library were originally conceived as a resource for all universities in the province. President Cody once remarked to the Canadian Club of Toronto that U of T had the alternate title of University of Ontario and that the lieutenant-governor-in-council had the legal power to make such a change under certain conditions of ratification from the U of T Senate and Board of Governors.[15]

U of T also used this term in advertisements for university programs. A full-page ad listing its programs in the *University of Toronto Monthly* begins with the header "The University of Toronto" and then in parentheses "The Provincial University of Ontario." This ad appears in the issue just before the opening of the School of Hygiene and it has a section that begins, "Attention is drawn to a new feature." The next few sentences are about the school, its departments, and Connaught Labs. It notes, "Teaching, research, and public service are the functions of this School and of the Connaught Laboratories."[16]

AND TO COMPLETE THE CIRCLE: INTEGRATING THIS INTO PUBLIC HEALTH

Throughout this work we noted links between the department/institute to public health at U of T. In some important ways it added to the traditional concept of public health. For example, the school had a very successful assessment and action ability in public health. Through its contacts it had an excellent grasp of what was needed, and it developed a very good educational program to develop in its students an assessment and action function. DPH people were doers, very good at determining what needed to be done and then doing it.

Shortly after the Department of Hospital Administration merged with that of Public Health, it added a third function, which resulted in assessment-action-evaluation.[17] An important step toward this was during Vayda's time when an ability in clinical epidemiology was begun. Today this has grown to a faculty including more than eighty leading epidemiology researchers, spanning multiple departments, disciplines, and institutions. It is enhanced by collaborations with University of Toronto clinical departments and affiliated teaching hospitals. It has an international reputation for excellence in clinical, health database, and decision sciences research. The program is very competitive, with one in five applicants gaining acceptance. More than 80 per cent of students are awarded peer-reviewed research fellowships and have a high rate of successful grant applications and publications in academic journals.[18] The director of the program is Dr Rob Fowler.

The role in developing physician leadership that the school established has been continued by the institute and augmented by the addition of this evaluation component evidenced in its programs in clinical epidemiology and SLI.

Through this evolving history the Faculty of Medicine saw its Division of Community Health fill the function of a school of public health. In 1990 Dean John Dirks referred to it as "'the unique equivalent of a School of Public Health in English-speaking Canada.'"[19] The Faculty of Medicine's Academic Plan for 2000–4 noted that programs in clinical epidemiology and health-care research moved into the graduate department of health administration "'significantly strengthened what constitutes Canada's only "school" of public health.'"[20]

SHOULD RESEARCH EMERGE AS ITS OWN DISCIPLINE?

We have noted earlier the need for research to emerge as a separate and distinct discipline – that its import to the knowledge-based economy is such that it should be studied as an subject in its own right. There is a nuance here in that research is usually regarded as an activity and here it is being suggested it should also be a subject, i.e., its own field of study. There should be an emphasis on studying research policy, metrics, and outcomes. A graduate professional degree should be developed to train research administrators, just as one was developed by this very department in 1947 to train hospital administrators. There should be a distinction between research project management (i.e., middle management) and research enterprise management (i.e., executive management). There should be courses for research/scientist-leaders just as there are for physician-leaders.

Then as a separate but related activity, and one that will undergird the professional degree, there should be an academic degree: the opportunity for academic graduate work in research on research at the master's and PhD level. The academic degree should be built on full-time academic staff in sub-specialty areas such as innovation, technology transfer, comparative research systems, and the like.

All of this recognizes that the research enterprise is now one of scope and scale. A number of Canadian research institutes rival faculties of medicine in the amount of research funding they attract. This makes for very specialized organizational enterprises with specialized needs in administration, financial management (especially grant accounting), human resources, public relations, technology transfer, and the like.

The fruits of research, both through new products or new companies formed around them, are becoming important new sources of jobs and tax revenues for countries. Its import to a national economy means there are aspects like national innovation systems or, in a decentralized federation like Canada, the United States, or Australia, subnational systems like regional (or provincial) innovation systems. There is the balance between basic, applied, and clinical research. In health there is the relation between research, patient care, and teaching (and this at both the clinical and scientific, graduate and undergraduate level). All of this points to the need for a specialized study of this subject.

A question is whether we are seeing what might evolve into the emergence of this possible new area of study through initiatives such as Vivek Goel and Tina Smith ran in 2000, the National Workshop on Research Leadership and Management in 2005 that Louise Lemieux-Charles chaired, and the new course in 2017 in the School of Continuing Studies.

One could question whether this emphasis on research administration is the same beginning that we saw in 1947 with the emphasis on hospital administration, i.e., an emphasis on professional management that later evolved into the academic study of a system. In the former case it was a health system (emerging in the twentieth century) and perhaps in our prospective case it is a research system (emerging in the twenty-first century).

PART TEN

IHPME and the University's Role in the Twenty-First Century

IHPME and the DLSPH have placed themselves at the centre of the evolving role of the university. It is my contention that the university has an expanded role in society in this twenty-first century knowledge-based economy. Because universities generate knowledge, they are important generators of new economic activity through their discoveries, which lead to patents and new company formation. In this, and the fact that they are large employers, they are economic engines.

However, they are also essential in another very important sense as well. They can help to solve pressing issues of our time by being a resource in areas such as policy development and building better public awareness of such issues. Though it is more recent that our economy has moved to a knowledge-based footing, i.e., that knowledge has become the product as well as the means, knowledge has always been a very important factor in health care.

While research into health policy and health outcomes does not have the same direct economic benefit to society in the sense of job creation or additional tax revenues, it does have a very real benefit in cost reduction and better health outcomes. Because of the importance that society places on health, anything that IHPME or the DLSPH can do to help improve our delivery system, develop new policy, or to foster a more involved public can aid in the overall strengthening of our Canadian system.

IHPME and the DLSPH are very much participants in this expanding role of the university. They are originating new and significant initiatives that arise from the creativity of the faculty within the institute and the school. We will look at some of these in this section. These include four new focus areas for universities: university-based policy institutes, public engagement, communication, and impact. While we will regard them separately, they are interrelated.

CHAPTER 25

University-Based Policy Institutes

The first new focus area for universities is the development of university-based policy institutes. For our purposes we will call them such; however, one could get into a discussion on whether these initiatives are all policy institutes or whether some might be more appropriately called research centres. For the sake of simplicity we will use a single term. Policy institutes are themselves not a new thing. Two of the most pre-eminent, the Royal Institute of International Affairs (RIIA) in the United Kingdom and the Council on Foreign Relations (CFR) in the United States, were formed by a group of academics after the First World War to help prevent the next war. They were quite an innovative idea, as what these academics sought to do was provide the perspective of history and its disciplines (tools) to help in the analysis of events in international relations. In essence they were focused research.

Though not academically based, they had very close ties to academia and became an important resource for academics. But perhaps more important, they also became a very important resource for governments (both politicians and civil servants) and journalists. Also one of their objectives was to build public awareness.

A very exciting new area of IHPME is work some of its faculty are doing developing policy institutes. However, unlike the RIIA and the CFR, IHPME's policy institutes are university-based, which is a very interesting Canadian variant. What these represent for IHPME and the DLSPH is a very interesting focus of its disciplinary and its research skills.

One of these is an initiative Steini Brown began while director of IHPME and he has continued as dean of the DLSPH. It is a concept that has been germinating for some time but with the last few years is beginning to see greater definition in the development of separate initiatives led by different faculty emphasizing different areas of expertise. Some very important inaugural events took place in 2017 and 2018. In 2017 the NAO was launched and in 2018 C3 had its first symposium featuring international speakers and discussing issues regarding policy institutes such as their impact.

Academic research is the foundation, but within these institutes it is focused research. The definition and form are still evolving, but one can discern some common elements: a common aim (improving the health system), involving graduate students, and crossovers between the institutes, i.e., a sharing of people, utilizing a diversity of expertise.

OF ACADEMIA AND POLICY

Academia and policy is another way a university's expertise can be utilized, i.e., in interested stakeholders seeking out faculty for independent, expert advice. This can have a spillover affect when faculty involve graduate and/or postgraduate students in such projects. IHPME is very much at the centre of this approach.

Converge3

A very innovative initiative of IHPME and the Ontario government was creating Converge3 (C3),[1] originally called the Centre for Evidence and Health in All Policies (CEHIAP).

It is funded by the Ministry of Health and Long-Term Care and was created in 2016. It was felt there was a need to better understand the ongoing and potential impact of existing and new programs and policies. This was in order to identify the most effective ways of promoting higher overall health, a more equitable distribution of health, and to realize a more sustainable system.[2]

The intent was to build capacity to estimate the costs and benefits of different options and to assess options using an equity lens, and to root this on evidence-based assessments. It felt this enhanced capacity would help to identify which programs/options were likely to work or not work and would help assess the potential benefits of alternative programs and approaches.

The ministry's program description noted that jurisdictions in the United States and United Kingdom were using such measures to assess return on investment, how initiatives (such as better housing for certain population groups) or health equity audits could have an impact on health inequalities.

It felt Ontario already had expertise and data infrastructure at the university, hospital, and government levels. The issue was to harness and focus it. The intent of C3 was to be a trusted and useful source of advice by creating a network of experts and establishing a partnership among Ontario's current areas of expertise. These included the Institute for Clinical Evaluative Sciences, the Ottawa Hospital Research Institute, Health Quality Ontario, Public Health Ontario, the Li Ka Shing Knowledge Institute of St Michael's Hospital, McMaster University, and the University of Toronto.

C3 is developing questions for analysis, doing the analysis, and communicating the results. In essence it is an independent public policy think tank devoted to health. IHPME is one of its nodes and its administrative home.

C3 is also sponsoring lectures on cutting-edge issues in health. An example was its June 2018 inaugural afternoon symposium on enhancing evidence infrastructure to inform policy. Mark Dobrow notes it was designed "to bring together senior health system decision-makers and policy-makers, researchers, and patient/public representatives to discuss contemporary thinking and approaches for strengthening evidence infrastructure to inform policy."[3] The symposium's featured speakers were the heads of the Government Outcomes Lab (GO-Lab) at Oxford University, the Jameel Poverty Action Lab (J-PAL) at MIT, and the Washington State Institute for Public Policy. An important part of bringing these heads together was that C3 staff met with them during the morning prior to the afternoon symposium. The importance of this sharing of ideas and best practices among the four organizations cannot be overemphasized.

The genesis of C3 was that during time spent in senior government positions, Jonathan Weisstub and Adalsteinn Brown identified a gap between the evidence needed to budget effectively in government and the evidence that was routinely available to decision-makers. Following a long consultation across several ministries, Cabinet office, and the Office of the Premier of Ontario, they developed a proposal for a new approach to evidence generation that would focus on producing reports and analysis that could be used to evaluate the efficiency, effectiveness, and equity of current and upcoming spending decisions.

Key to realizing this vision was seed funding from the Rossy Family Foundation that supported the preliminary work and allowed Weisstub and Brown to engage with decision-makers and experts as they developed and refined the proposal to maximize the benefit for the province. To speed the development and implementation of the work and leverage the outstanding research across the province, they created a network built on the strongest scholarly institutions across Ontario and an advisory committee of political and public service leaders.

It produced its first reports on the effectiveness of workfare-based health benefits in 2018. Its first executive director (Mark Dobrow) and scientific director (Ahmed Bayoumi) joined in 2017, along with the co-chairs of the Advisory Committee (Jonathan Weisstub and Hugh Segal).[4]

North American Observatory on Health Systems and Policies

The North American Observatory on Health Systems and Policies (NAO) is a collaborative partnership of researchers, research organizations, governments, and health organizations promoting evidence-informed health-system policy decision-making. Because of the high degree of health system decentralization in the United States and Canada, the NAO is committed to focusing attention not only on national systems but on sub-national systems as well, i.e., state and provincial health systems. It also seeks to create a basis for more systematic health system and policy comparisons among sub-national political entities.[5]

The official launch of the NAO took place on 6 February 2017. Dr Bob Bell, the deputy minister, Ministry of Health and Long-Term Care for Ontario, spoke, as did Roy Romanow, former premier of Saskatchewan and former chair of the Royal Commission on the Future of Health Care. Romanow's address was important in that he was able to offer insight into the potential of the observatory based on his previous experience as premier and royal commissioner.

Romanow noted the NAO's independence from government and interest groups. In addition, "As Royal Commissioner it became abundantly clear to me that Canada depends upon the academic community to suggest and research ways and governance structures that can lead to timely and responsive research and advice to our citizens and governments." He noted that "academic research and thought produces powerful, positive results in the formulation of public policy." He said this "was confirmed when the Royal Commission engaged some of the top minds in health care policy to produce original research on a wide range of important topics," including IHPME faculty. He noted we need such an observatory "capable of rigorously comparing and evaluating the impact of innovations" and that "the road that evidence may lead us can be very uncomfortable – even threatening – to the governors, managers, and users of health care." But that should not lead us to "deny the power of evidence and rigorous analysis and evaluation,"[6] or to learn from the policy experiments.

Gregory Marchildon is the IHPME faculty lead and founding director of NAO. He is also the Canadian representative on the Health Systems and Policy Monitor network of the European Observatory on Health Systems and Policies.[7] The idea for the NAO grew out of his involvement with the European Observatory, and that work grew out of his involvement with Romanow's royal commission. We mentioned earlier he had been executive director of the commission. He has had extensive government experience and has written widely in the area of health policy. He has also been secretary to the Cabinet and deputy minister to the premier in the Romanow government and had advised Cabinet on the establishment of the Fyke Commission (which was struck to review medicare in Saskatchewan).[8]

Romanow noted Marchildon's other experience, that in government together they had dealt with issues of national unity, the Quebec Referendum of 1995, major trade conflicts with the United States, modernization of government institutions, and development of new policies and reforms across social and economic sectors to meet the needs of the time.[9] One delicate issue was the consolidation of hospitals in the cities and closure of a number of small hospitals in villages and towns in Saskatchewan.

The NAO reports on policy reforms and innovations as well as health system performance. A large part of its mandate is comparative analyses. Its ambition is to be the North American counterpart to the European Observatory on Health Systems and Policies (EO) and the Asia-Pacific Observatory (APO). Although the sub-state focus of the NAO differentiates it from the EO and APO, it is understood that that the more extensive study of systems and policies at this level in constitutional federations will provide a foundation for better national-level studies, which in turn will permit more useful comparison studies between North American countries and those in Europe and Asia.[10]

A significant strength of the NAO will be its ties to the EO and APO and their extensive studies on the health systems of the various countries. This will be important, not just in the NAO's work with outside organizations but also as a source for graduate students in IHPME doing work on comparative systems.

Its first academic hub is at IHPME, but it expects to establish an academic hub in the United States and also Mexico. It will also develop a network of academics from other North American centres. It is expected that government and health organization NAO members will call upon it to provide an analysis on an existing or emerging policy issue or problem. This could also include a "rapid response." The working paper version of such studies will be posted on the NAO website for public use. NAO members will include federal and provincial/state governments as well as publicly financed health agencies and organizations.[11]

The NAO is important in three respects. In the first, it draws attention to an emerging area, comparative studies, which is becoming important across a host of disciplines. Second, it moves into a relatively unexplored area of discourse – comparative health systems, one that could be called health in a global context. And in doing so a distinction gets drawn between this and the more generally studied area of global health. Second, in looking at this new context, the NAO not only examines national actors but subnational entities as well. While this is important for its area of geographic concentration (North America), it is a methodology that focuses attention on and could also be applied to other areas of the world where there are large nations and/or similarly decentralized systems with subnational political entities.

Another nuance to this concentration on sub-national entities is the national network of expertise that the NAO is building. As part of this concentration in 2018 the NAO began a series of provincial and territorial health system profiles. As Greg Marchildon, the series editor, notes, "There is not, and never has been, a single Canadian health system. As subnational jurisdictions in one of the most decentralized federations in the world, provincial and territorial governments are the principle stewards for publicly financed health services and coverage in Canada."[12]

In Canada the provinces have substantial autonomy in health. It is precisely this degree of latitude that allowed an energetic and creative provincial premier who knew full well the constraints – and opportunities – that this afforded to launch a North American first. It allowed his province to break out of the US-like health trajectory that had been Canada's lot and prove to the rest of the country in 1947 that a government-run hospital insurance system was not only possible, it was highly efficient. Ten years later, through a prime minister's initiative (incidentally a prime minister [Diefenbaker] from Saskatchewan) the nation itself broke out of this US mould.

The first instalment in the NAO series is a health system profile of Nova Scotia.[13] This book, and the series itself, will be an important research and teaching tool for academics. It will address an area in which there was a paucity of information. In Canada we tend to look at and study medicare as a national phenomenon. And yet in this highly decentralized federation, and given that constitutionally health is a provincial responsibility, each of the provinces has grappled with health issues throughout its history. It is very much an understudied area, and Canadians need to become more fully aware of just how deep our health roots go and how innovative we have been in each of our provinces.

Saskatchewan pioneered in health insurance. And yet BC in the 1920s and again in the 1930s was an important player here, as was Quebec with the Castonguay-Nepvue Report.[14] Paul Williams brought to my attention that there is a more recent Quebec innovation:[15] Hébert's Autonomy Insurance Act of 2013,[16] which aimed to provide second-tier health insurance for seniors. It was based on a White Paper, *Autonomy for All*[17] but was not passed, as the PQ government was defeated in a snap election after its introduction. Indeed, as the NAO's provincial profiles will demonstrate, each province has its own story to tell and the NAO is proving to be important in ushering in comparative health systems scholarship, not only among national systems but in sub-national ones as well. Hébert, a geriatrician, was health minister in Quebec at the time and is a faculty member in IHPME's Quebec analogue, now called the Département de gestion, d'évaluation et de politique de santé at Université de Montréal. We noted earlier it had been started by a DHA grad. Greg has a Quebec academic at work on a health system profile for Quebec.

A strong argument could be made that robust policymaking in a nation is enhanced by looking at the best practices of one's peers. In addition, in nations with highly decentralized health systems (such as Canada and the United States) this is further enhanced when not just the policies of national entities are studied but sub-national entities as well. It points to the fact that IHPME is about two things. It is about building "national competency," which in other terms could be called a national capacity in management and policymaking. But it is also about "global fluency." When regarding a country's health system, discourse should not be just a closed loop, i.e., always internally focused within the nation. A country should also be looking at what others are doing. It should also lend its own expertise when possible.

The activities of the NAO are important not only for works such as these but also for the experts in each province that Greg is assembling in what will undoubtedly become a national network. In this there are links to

FitzGerald's intent of developing a national network with his Honorary Advisory Committee.

The NAO is also important for how it is helping to build capacity. It focuses on four areas: research into health systems, its rapid reviews, its Canadian profile series, and the NAO Lecture Series. The rapid reviews are "environmental scans or quick literature reviews on policy issues identified as urgent" by clients.[18] The Lecture Series "brings leading scholars and great thinkers from around the world ... to present their applied research on comparative health systems and policies."[19] It is also closely allied to graduate education in comparative health systems.

At the time of writing it has two important projects underway. One is a study of health policy in federal systems. In the Americas it is looking at Canada, the United States, Mexico, and Brazil. It is also examining European systems like Germany, Austria, and Switzerland. This is some very important work in comparative systems and is yielding very important new knowledge on the challenges and opportunities such systems present to health policy. A second study is for the OMA on patients' perceptions of the health system. The OMA wants to use this information to determine how they should help influence health policy in Ontario.

Undergraduate and Graduate Education

The NAO is also proving to be an important source for undergraduate and graduate education in comparative health systems, and more specifically an important vehicle for high-ability students at the undergraduate and graduate levels. At a research-intensive university like U of T it is important to provide early opportunities for a specific cohort of student, one that has an almost insatiable curiosity and drive.

I have funnelled both undergraduates and graduates to NAO activities though health policy courses I teach at Trinity College. I arranged for a former Trinity College graduate, now doing a graduate degree at McMaster, to do a practicum at the NAO in the spring-summer of 2019.

Another instance was a NAO Lecture in February 2019.[20] I had a fourth-year undergrad, Grace Harn, who had come to me to do a paper on the National Health Insurance (NHI) system of Taiwan. When I learned of the NAO Lecture on the NHI, I contacted Grace. When she saw the name of the presenter, she mentioned that she had used a couple of the papers of Dr Tsung-

Mei Cheng in her essay and would be very excited to hear the lecture. Though the seminar was aimed mainly at graduate students and faculty, I knew Greg Marchildon and Sara Allin well and it wasn't a problem to have her attend.

She asked if it might be possible that she meet Cheng and I put this request to Greg and Sara. They went one better and invited her to a lunch with Cheng. On the way to the lunch she phoned her father in Taiwan. Her family has a great depth in health care. Her father had been a director of the Department of Health in Kaohsiung, Taiwan's second city, and knew the vice-president of Taiwan as well as the health minister whom Cheng had visited.

There were other connections: Grace's mother is a pharmacist, and her maternal grandfather was a physician who had started and operated a hospital in rural Taiwan and worked with a former president of the country.[21] Her parents continue to run this hospital. The story of her grandfather's concern for the people resonates well with FitzGerald and our own health-care history.[22] Needless to say, the student was deeply grateful for the opportunity that Greg and Sara made possible.

Grace's parents subsequently visited Canada for her graduation, and, along with her older sister, we all had a long visit and discussed both public health and illness care in Taiwan in depth, on the basis of her father's wide experience in each area. I gave them a tour of the Dalla Lana School of Public Health, which was especially relevant given her father's background. Her father noted that he became the director of health for the city of Kaohsiung when they were dealing with an outbreak of dengue fever and two months later with SARS.[23]

It could be argued that the opportunity that Greg and Sara afforded this student is crucial for this university in being able to engage the curiosity and energy of a certain cohort of its undergrads. A certain group of high-ability undergrads have a curiosity, intellectual range, and depth that needs to be engaged beyond what regular classes can provide. This needs to be done throughout the undergraduate experience but is especially relevant for a fourth-year student contemplating her options.

In this case it led to a conversation about the public health programs at U of T and Princeton. It also led to a discussion of a new MHSc program (in physiology) being started for September 2019, her application to it, and the possibility of her doing a practicum with either the NAO or C3 in IHPME. It also led to a discussion of a Canadian-style health insurance system that was adopted in another country – a country that has taken the Canadian model much further than the Canadians themselves, in the range of benefits and their use of an IT backbone for an electronic health record for providers and citizens.

The subsequent meeting with Grace's family was especially fruitful, as there is no comparison to talking with someone who has both the education and range of experience of her father. It is especially edifying for me to get into an in-depth discussion of the links between public health and health systems with that of government policy in different eras, such as when the country was a Japanese colony, the Chiang Kai-shek administration, and the present administration. These are the types of discussions that should be taking place at a world university such as U of T, and internationally recognized programs like IHPME and the DLSPH.

Exporting Our Knowledge

This lecture also points to an important example of how Canada is exporting its knowledge and how IHPME is becoming part of international networks. In this case Greg Marchildon has done work on the Canadian model and the NHI in Taiwan with Tsung-Mei Cheng and Uwe Reinhardt (another Princeton academic). When they were considering universal health insurance, Uwe had recommended to the Taiwan government that they adopt the Canadian single-payer model. He had been a student at the University of Saskatchewan in 1962 when that province implemented the template on which the Canadian system is based.[24] He had also been a classmate of future premier Roy Romanow.[25]

In 2005, in Taipei at the tenth-year anniversary of the NHI, Greg, along with four other international experts (including Uwe Reinhardt), was asked to speak on health reform in their respective countries. The formal title was "International Symposium: Toward an Equitable, Efficient and High Quality National Health Insurance."[26]

What Greg is doing with the NAO, and with students at this university, is continuing the tradition established by FitzGerald at the inception of the School of Hygiene. For FitzGerald, international connections with other health systems were important. Equally important was attracting international students.

Accessing Centre for Expertise (ACE)

ACE was an idea of Mark Dobrow's, based on the premise that IHPME represents a critically important breadth and depth of expertise that allows an informed multidisciplinary perspective on a wide range of issues facing health system stakeholders.

ACE takes this as a base and uses it to provide a consultation service to representatives of health system organizations to discuss their systems' needs with a member of the ACE team. The consultant can provide preliminary guidance, including identifying which IHPME experts could provide further expertise to inform the issue at hand.

ACE can also coordinate research services to help an organization make more evidence-informed decisions. This can include preparing different types of reports to address an organization's needs.

An interesting aspect of ACE is its student involvement in various projects. It also collaborates with other IHPME policy institutes such as the NAO.[27]

Others

IHPME has other policy institutes that, like the NAO and C3, are niche oriented. Greg Marchildon prefers to call them "research centres," and that may be a more apt term.[28] These (with their faculty lead) include the Canadian Centre for Health Economics (Audrey Laporte), which aims to be a centre for health economics research in Canada. It sponsors a weekly Health Economics Series during the academic year involving visiting Canadian and international speakers. There is also the Strategy Design and Evaluation Initiative (Rob Schwartz), which is concerned with whether, how, when, and why public health strategies deployed to alleviate complex problems realize greater and lesser degrees of success.

There is the Health System Performance Research Network (Walter Wodchis), which has a focus on performance measurement and improvement, and the Centre for Sustainable Health Systems (Fiona Miller), which looks at local, national, and international efforts to improve the environmental and social sustainability of health systems. The DLSPH also has its own set of such activities.

THE TOOLS OF POLICY ANALYSIS

The tools of health policy institutes – and indeed of health policy formulation and analysis – go beyond those of the discipline of health policy. They include those of other disciplines such as economics, history, and political science. And indeed Greg Marchildon in IHPME is one example of a faculty member who includes perspectives of history and political science in his writing, the former due to a lifelong interest, the latter because of his government experience. There is academic literature to support such an approach.[29]

IHPME AND TIES TO OTHER POLICY INSTITUTES

The IHPME connection to policy institutes is a continuation of a long-standing practice and has clear links to other Canadian policy institutes. We are concerned with interactions with other policy institutes and analogies to yet others. The latter first. The NAO and its internationalist orientation – that is looking at health systems other than our own – continues an inclination (spoken of earlier) of J.G. FitzGerald.

There is a connection to a larger, Canadian impulse, specifically an internationalist focus. In this it reaches back to one of the earliest Canadian policy institutes, the Canadian Institute of International Affairs, which also had an internationalist focus, and an organization that we previously noted had strong representation from this university.

There is, however, a differentiation in purpose. The IHPME institutes are aimed much more at being useful to policy. I asked Greg Marchildon, who we noted is the founder of three such institutes, what motivated him to do this. Likely as a result of his senior government experience, he said it was to provide a linkage between the applied policy scholars in the academy with government. He noted that government lacked the ability of deep policy research necessary for groundbreaking policy. On the day-to-day operational matters they were very good but not the deep policy areas.[30]

It is evident in speaking with him that there has been a certain progression in his thought. He differentiated between the Saskatchewan Institute of Public Policy (SIPP), the Johnson-Shoyama School, and the NAO. Put simply, SIPP was a Saskatchewan game, Johnson-Shoyama a Canadian game, while the NAO is global. This difference is manifest in two main ways: the students it attracts and the research it does. In research, the question the NAO asks itself is where it sits in relation to other global centres in its projects and publications.[31]

This NAO activity is also linked to the parent university. We spoke earlier about the Braudelian concept of world economies and world cities, and now we extend this to a new concept: world universities. In another section we also noted making universities more outward facing. The NAO is very much an extension of the outreach function of a university, moving IHPME toward the world stage. In so doing it is helping position U of T on the world stage, which is very much a role this university should be pursuing.

Greg was involved with the EO before starting the NAO; it began when he went back to university life after the Royal Commission on Health Services in January 2003. He was asked by the EO to present to a group of social democratic health ministers from Europe at a meeting in Stockholm that month. He then went to Spain, where he was part of the EO team presenting to the president and health minister as they considered a major reform package involving the autonomous communities. He continued his work with the EO over the years, including preparing the Health System in Transition (HiT) studies[32] for them for Canada and working on rapid responses, and presenting to governments (e.g., South Korea and Taiwan).[33]

This impetus of applied policy scholarship is somewhat the same as the mandate of the RIIA (Chatham House). Parmar notes, "It was to be an active, working institution for the scientific, non-political and non-ideological study of foreign affairs; an expert organization dedicated to educating the public, and furnishing policymakers with the factual basis upon which to make 'sound' policy and 'sound' public opinion."[34]

This was different from the object of the CIIA, which was "to promote through study, discussion, lectures, and public addresses ... an understanding of international questions."[35] An integral component of the CIIA was the establishment of branch units in major Canadian cities.[36]

Another tie is that, through Steini Brown, and previously in Gene Vayda's era, IHPME has had strong connections to the King's Fund. From 1974 through 1985, John Hastings coordinated study visits and participated in some programs in London. Also, he and his family lived at the King's Fund College during several visits in London.[37] In the 1980s the Department of Health Administration has sent MHSC grads to the United Kingdom for a three-week intensive with the fund in London with reciprocal visits arranged by the King's Fund to Toronto. A former faculty member (Maureen Dixon) from the United Kingdom lectured at the King's Fund (and in 1986 became director of the Institute for Health Services Management).

IHPME faculty have been involved in King's Fund major events. For example, an international seminar held in London and sponsored by the fund on the role of health service administrators saw DHA alum Peter Carruthers and adjunct faculty member J. Boyd McAulay present papers. The Canadians were very much a part of the discussions and were cited in the book that was published on the proceedings.[38] Former faculty member John Browne has been a part of the planning committee for a King's Fund event.[39]

While Steini was director of IHPME and as Dean of Dalla Lana he has maintained strong ties with King's Fund, particularly its former CEO, Chris Ham, whom he has had to Canada on two extended visits.

A TECHNOLOGY OF KNOWLEDGE

At IHPME is there almost a "technology of knowledge" at work? The question implies using knowledge itself and the methodology of research as a tool or technique. Through its policy institutes, IHPME is developing a particular skill that allows it apply its expertise in health disciplines, combined with its research prowess, in new ways. And it is simultaneously expanding its scope of activity, now no longer working only with other academics but also with practitioners, individually or organizationally (in governments and NGOs).[40]

It is creating its own new organizations to focus on these applications of knowledge. It is forming project-oriented teams from within IHPME and DLSPH for its assignments. It is utilizing expertise from inside and outside the school and institute. It is involving PhDs and postdocs. It is not only task-oriented; to use Steini and Rhonda's phrase, it is pushing the research out through its client activity and seminars.

The reason one speaks of a technology of knowledge is because not only is the knowledge itself important, so too is how this knowledge is applied – again to use Steini and Rhonda's phrase, how it is pushed out. This is where this technique or technology comes into play. Crafting this knowledge for the public, politicians, civil servants, and journalists is all very different. Communicating knowledge is itself a discipline. The Certificate in Health Impact gets at this.

There is the issue of developing the tools so that university-based policy institutes can be a resource for government. Another issue is using the knowledge to encourage dialogue, bringing diverse people together to dialogue and increase their awareness of common issues.

COMMENT

Through IHPME's policy institutes we are seeing a difference in degree and depth. Degree is in the interface between academia and outside organizations, a big one of which is government. Before it was sporadic, people were sought out for intense bursts of activity related to a government need. Now it is more or less continuous.

Depth is on three levels. In the first, IHPME now has a somewhat different faculty. They have not only academic and research experience but also practical experience. For example Mark Dobrow worked at Cancer Care Ontario and in senior management at the Health Council of Canada. Greg Marchildon worked in the Romanow government in Saskatchewan at the deputy minister level and then on the Romanow Commission. Steini Brown was in start-ups and at the ADM level in the Ontario government. The second involves the depth of education of individuals such as these. Mark did a postdoc at the London School of Hygiene and Tropical Medicine. Greg got his PhD from the London School of Economics. Steini has degrees from Harvard and Oxford.

The third is in a depth of experience with policy institutes. For example, with Greg Marchildon the NAO was not the first policy institute he was instrumental in founding. He played a similar role in the Saskatchewan Institute of Public Policy (SIPP), founded by the Romanow government, and a similar role in the Johnson-Shoyama School of Public Policy at the University of Regina.[41] Mark parlayed his experience with the Health Council of Canada into ACE and C3. Steini had his role as ADM of two government ministries and in his role as a cofounder with C3 was involved in an environmental scan that looked at similar organizations across North America.

This depth of experience, particularly the government involvement each of these three individuals have had, gives them a keen appreciation for the needs of government and other organizations in order for academia to be a valuable input. It also maintains the tight link to practice and making a difference that has existed ever since FitzGerald and the founding of the School of Hygiene.

We are seeing that the ability to gather, analyse, and interpret information is important. Public policy formulation is complex. In our present knowledge-based society, policy development has become a highly sophisticated activity in recognition of the complexities involved. This is particularly so in health, with its complex subject matter, strong feelings of the public, and powerful interest groups. Governments and others need access to the expertise, critical insight, and the dispassionate analysis of academia. And academia is more than just the sum of its information-gathering and processing capabilities. These in themselves are a discipline, a process. It is the process as much as the product that governments require.

In this way these initiatives represent unique and creative partnerships. They give government and others access to research and give academia the opportunity to see its research have an application and make a difference in policy and programs.

The NAO recognizes another important component of this process – its comparative and global context. Governments look more frequently to other governments for best practices when developing policy. There is also growing public awareness of what is taking place in other countries. It makes increasing sense that governments take these factors into account. But the NAO takes this expanded view one step further. Its ties to the European and Asia-Pacific Observatories are an extension of its transnational perspective and will give it a truly global reach.

Questions, therefore, are whether university-based policy institutes such as C3 (the former CEHIAP), ACE, and the NAO will become an increasingly important activity, and even more significant, whether they will be a capability or capacity nations need to have. Or whether governments will increasingly seed them in academic settings, and whether they will become a new area of activity for universities. There is also the question of whether they will be a nexus, a convergence point, bringing together politicians, civil servants, journalists, businesspeople, professors, students, and the public.

This has proven to be the case for the RIIA. Martel notes, "The most interesting thing about the Royal Institute of International Affairs is its central location at the intersection of ideas, institutions and interests of twentieth-century Britain."[42] The same could be said of IHPME in health in Canada.

Similarly the same could be said of the School of Hygiene and DLSPH. And one could argue C3 and the NAO are moving into this realm.

Another analogy to the RIIA is its comparative focus, which is very similar to that of the NAO and C3. For the RIIA this comparative focus was pioneered in current affairs and foreign relations in the 1920s by its first research director, Arnold J. Toynbee, who began an annual *Survey of International Affairs*. He later (the 1930s) applied the same comparative thinking to history in a multivolume theoretical *Study of History*.[43] He, like FitzGerald at roughly the same time, was combining research, practice, and impact. IHPME and the DLSPH are making the comparative study that Toynbee applied in history to be focused on health systems and an important part of their academic activity through the NAO. The NAO is also giving this comparative approach a new application through its director, Greg Marchildon, who is very interestingly applying the comparative lens to the sub-national as well as the national realm.

This comparative approach could be applied in other disciplinary areas. One wonders what new truths would be uncovered if we studied comparative tax systems in our management schools, or comparative economic systems in departments of economics, or comparative analyses of welfare states in schools of public policy. These types of knowledge could be very useful when looking at comparative health systems.

There is also a precedent for a think tank or policy institute in health. We noted earlier the King's Fund of the United Kingdom, founded in 1897 as a charity to support London's voluntary hospitals but transformed itself into an educational centre and policy institute after the founding of the NHS. An article in *Lancet* notes a statement by a former UK minister of health: "As Enoch Powell once remarked, recalling Voltaire's view of God: 'If the King's Fund had not existed, it would have been necessary to invent it.'"[44] Perhaps the same might be said some day of C3 and the NAO.

What is incontrovertible is that policy institutes have proliferated and become increasingly central to decision-making. They are at the leading edge of trying to make sense of the complexity of the development of modern public policy. They seek to apply the intellectual frameworks, the mental discipline of academia, one could perhaps say a kind of scientific method to the study of their area.[45]

They could well be a portent of the future. McGann suggests they constitute a fifth estate and refers to a Duke University academic who says they address the public interest from a wider perspective than any of the first three estates and in greater depth than the fourth.[46]

One could ask whether IHPME (and U of T) is onto something here. Are policy institutes a new and necessary institution in the knowledge-based society? Can a strong argument be made for locating them on university campuses? With Converge3, ACE, and the NAO, IHPME is moving into this important new application of intellectual knowledge, joining other U of T–based policy institutes such as the Mowat Centre (at the former School of Public Policy & Governance) and the Munk School of Global Affairs. It is an area that is also proliferating in Canada.[47] It also poses the question of whether there is a need to study research itself and very closely allied to this, innovation, in more depth in a similar such institute.

Activities such as the NAO and C3 begin to move IHPME into the realm of activities of policy institutes. However, one needs to be careful with the nomenclature as, while there are similarities, the IHPME – and indeed the Mowat and Munk – initiatives differ in a number of important respects. Perhaps the most important is that, unlike many other examples of policy institutes, they do not have an advocacy function, they are nested in a university, and they involve graduate education. One wonders whether this university is evolving a new form – perhaps a distinctly Canadian form – of such policy institutes.

This is new territory for the IHPME. It is a very important point of departure and it recognizes a need within the health-care system. History may prove that it is also moving IHPME into a very important activity that will become increasingly important.

One purpose of policy institutes has been to respond to a need in society, particularly in government, to be able to deal with the increasingly complex events happening around them. There is the need to be able to unpack and sort through this complexity and to bring information, past and present, to bear. To do this they need people with a certain analytical tools, who think within certain mental frameworks. They need to be at a certain remove from government. Research is integral.

Two of the original and most powerful policy institutes were (and are) the Royal Institute for International Affairs (UK) and the Council on Foreign Relations (US). Canada was an early leader in this area with the establishment of the Canadian Institute of International Affairs (CIIA). It had significant ties to this university, and a number of its academics were integrally involved in the CIIA.[48] A former head of the CIIA and university faculty member at Trinity College, John Holmes, captured some of the significant qualities of such a research institute when he talked about growing "intellectually in the company of the country's brightest and best" and in the CIIA providing an outlet "about the better reordering of the world."[49] It is a sentiment that could be applied to ACE, C3, and the NAO.

Since these early beginnings, think tanks have proliferated in number and areas of study. They are vehicles of increasing public awareness. But importantly they also constitute "the shadowy outlines of a global public space."[50] And they are beginning to focus attention on global public policy. Within this there is a clear need for a concentration on health as well.

If anything, the need for policy institutes has grown. Though they began for the most part in international affairs, there is a clear need for them in health, itself increasingly an international affair. Health is complex, idiosyncratic, rooted in a nation, or, in the case of a geographically large, highly decentralized federation like Canada, one of continental scale, and it can be rooted both nationally and sub-nationally. Health has very powerful and influential professions. Issues such as health insurance, the determinants of health, and health inequalities touch on a number of government departments. There is a need to build public awareness and involvement. It is timely that IHPME undertakes its initiatives in policy institutes. It is a natural offshoot of two areas (health systems and public health) that have a rich history at this university.

And one of the good qualities of these IHPME initiatives is the number of seminars that enterprises such as the NAO and Converge3 are sponsoring that bring together faculty, students, and the public. Each has an important seminar series in its respective domain. This is important both in creating dialogue as well as in building public awareness. The NAO brings in speakers each year from other health-care systems. C3 sponsors symposia in specific topics that bring in speakers from other countries. One example was its symposium in June 2018, noted earlier, that discussed enhancing evidence infrastructure to inform policy and brought in international experts from such organizations to discuss their experience. Not only was it good in its subject matter but also in the linkages that IHPME through C3 is establishing with other research institutes in other parts of the world.

Along the same vein, the evolutionary aspect of such initiatives is attracting the attention of donors and through them the establishment of related activities. Through an endowment and the leadership of Steini Brown in Dalla Lana an important DLSPH lecture series has been fine-tuned. It has been reordered into a threefold format of keynote speaker, panel, and audience questions. Further, in this reordering, Steini involved the deputy minister of health in choosing the areas of emphasis. The deputy minister also agreed to moderate the panel discussions. In Steini's words the lectures are meant to be transformative in their impact.[51]

Another related activity is a student award established in IHPME that provides a prize for the cutting-edge issues being addressed through looking at comparative health systems. Rhonda Cockerill and Greg Marchildon were instrumental in working with the donor on establishing this award.

Another aspect is the linkages with like-minded organizations and academic centres that are arising out of the NAO and C3. The sharing of information, seminars, and symposia are proving to be an important learning experience for their staffs as well as the health community generally.

All of this points to the present sophistication of the research activity. Organizations like the NAO, C3, ACE, GO-Labs, and J-PAL are very focused, directed research activities. They not only do research in specific areas, they are nested in or have important links to academia, and not only influence government policy but engage in activities such as testing important policy questions with randomized evaluations. They build an evidence base out of which emerge interventions that can improve the efficiency and effectiveness of health care delivery and point to new directions. They are a long way beyond the traditional paradigm of writing grants and publishing papers.

Moreover the people running such organizations are not only research scholars in their own right but engage in the research management of multifaceted organizations dealing with a complex array of subjects, stakeholders, and mandates. For example though they stress evidence-based decision-making, they are at pains to point out that other factors are given weight, such as powerful interest groups, the politicians' perception of the art of the possible, and the feelings of the public on health-care issues.

A question for consideration is whether the NAO, C3, and ACE are a continuation of the School of Hygiene (now the DLSPH) and IHPME is part of the larger picture, i.e., constantly moving at the edges of policy development, bringing information and analysis to decision-makers. Another question is whether they are an extension of FitzGerald and his Honorary Advisory Committee, a twenty-first-century version of the intent of FitzGerald's committee.

A further question is whether the location of these institutes – in this city, university, and institute – demonstrates that each is moving onto the world stage. This is demonstrated particularly in the case of the NAO. Three levels of location noted above are at play here. Toronto is a world city, U of T a world university, and IHPME an institute with international connections. Was the international stature of each a component of Marchildon's success in bringing the NAO here?

An interesting aspect of each of the NAO, C3, and ACE is just how tightly each of them has been interwoven into the educational mission of IHPME. Each has been involving faculty and interestingly graduate students and postdocs in its projects. Mark is involving PhD students in C3. Greg is having his postdoc work on two chapters of the Ontario book, which is part of an NAO series on provincial health systems. The NAO and ACE are continuing the strong involvement the DLSPH and IHPME have had in practicums. Each has taken on students in internships and practicums for students from this and other universities (Queen's and Ottawa).[52]

They have also involved students in special activities. Students have commented on how tremendously motivating this is. Allie Peckham, Greg's postdoc at the time, noted the "privilege" of being able to attend a reception for Bernie Sanders at the president's residence and meeting Roy Romanow at the NAO launch.[53] The import of this is that these are tomorrow's scientists, doctors, and administrators, and this interweaving of education, research, practice, and theory is a powerful learning tool.

There is also a question of whether IHPME is moving us back toward or continuing a tradition that Canada has carved out in policy institutes. To examine this possibility we turn to reflections made on what was one of Canada's oldest policy institutes. In a draft of a speech we noted earlier, John Holmes got at some of the other important facets of a policy institute, particularly a Canadian one when he said, "The CIIA was a product of the conviction, or rather the hope, that war might be exorcised if policy-making were more widely shared, if the public was better educated in international politics, and diplomacy was open."[54] Such a comment can be applied to health. Here, too, if policymaking were more widely shared, if the public were better educated in health policy, if discussions were more open, might we get more accountable, sophisticated, and leading-edge health policy?

Holmes continued, "There was in this belief some of the romantic Wilsonian heresy that a sweet peaceful populace was always being led into war by scheming and, as we would now say, power hungry politicians and envoys extraordinaire. There were those, however, who more soundly realized that the public itself had to be tamed of its nationalist passions by a wider understanding of their consequences."[55] Here too we have applicability to health. The public is led by governments and powerful interests. But, particularly in health, there are strong feelings of the public itself, which definitely need to be taken into account by politicians and policymaking civil servants, and if not tamed at least attenuated by policy institutes.

Holmes also said, "I am convinced, nevertheless, that there would have been more errors and illusions had it not been for the books, the articles, the pamphlets, the speeches, for which we had been responsible and for the voices trained in CIIA seminars speaking out."[56] Does this speak to the importance of the publications and the public seminars that the NAO and DLSPH are sponsoring?

It all points to the fact that IHPME and the DLSPH, with their emphasis on policy institutes, are taking us to the leading edge of academic research. They are pushing the boundaries, taking research out of academe, using their expertise to work with government and non-government organizations toward furthering the latter's objectives through the former's abilities.

Canada has a long history in policy institutes. The CIIA, which we talked about earlier, was founded in 1928. In September 1968 Prime Minister Pierre Trudeau used the occasion of his first Speech from the Throne to call for the creation of an independent policy institute, noting, "It would be useful to have available to all governments an institute where long-term research and thinking can be carried out into governmental matters of all kinds."[57]

This led to the Ritchie Report of 1969 and the creation of the Institute for Research on Public Policy in 1972.[58] Ronald Ritchie had been a VP at Imperial Oil and executive director of the Glassco Commission on Government Organization. One of the people he consulted when writing the report was A.W. Johnson, who is well known to Marchildon. An aim of the report was to outline the need for "a form of research oriented to the making of public policy – research aimed – specifically at illuminating the choices to be made by public policy makers" — in other words "the need for organized research and analysis for public policy questions."[59]

Ritchie's statement points to the success of the RIIA and at one point could have been applied to its Canadian counterpart, the CIIA. They become a nexus for all sorts of activity. One only need look at the kind of people who pass through its doors to attend events or give addresses – presidents, prime ministers, senior ministers. Almost anyone who is anyone does not pass through London without making a stop at the RIIA.

It is not different at Munk. Often a black Suburban is parked outside the entrance, signalling that someone of import is inside. Former director Janice Stein confirmed that Munk provides such unofficial consultations.[60] And, regarding the CIIA, one can comb through the personal correspondence of John Holmes at the Trinity Archives to find letters with a veritable who's who of Canada, with governors general, prime ministers, premiers, ministers, journalists, and academics, including the likes of Lester Pearson, Vincent Massey, John Kenneth Galbraith, to name only a few.[61] It points to a fact that they, and the people involved in them, become a nexus.

A POSSIBLE FUTURE POLICY INSTITUTE

All of this presents the question of whether IHPME or the DLSPH needs another policy institute – one with a different mandate. Roughly ten years ago Chatham House began to look at health issues and today it is very focused on universal health coverage. The King's Fund is constantly looking at the NHS and emerging issues in health care. The Health Foundation has been important in leading-edge activities, such as looking at the NHS as an anchor institution and "health in all policies" initiatives from around the world. Each organization is looking at overarching questions and with a broad mandate. The question for Canada and the DLSPH is whether we need to do the same.

There are many reasons for this possibility. One is to add to our policymaking capacity. Another is to educate the Canadian public. Yet another is to plug Canada into an international network of institutes that are dealing with such questions, places like Chatham House, the King's Fund, the Health Foundation, and others.

Another huge one is to discern emerging trends and influence the dialogue. We noted earlier the dramatic illustration in the Chatham House conference in the fall of 1941 that noted the entire structure of medical services after the war might be on a basis completely different from the one before the war.[62] Given what transpired in Britain fifteen months later with the Beveridge Report, four years later with the landslide election of the Atlee government, and a short while later with the NHS, the statement was predictive. It points to how such policy institutes can discern emerging trends.

Another outgrowth of a top-tier policy institute is the interchanges it sets up between academia, the institute, and government. Most of Chatham House was moved to Oxford University and absorbed into the British

Foreign Office during the war. Arnold Toynbee, Chatham's director of research (who also had an appointment with the University of London) headed up the staff.[63] He developed papers for wartime committees of the British government on what post-war Britain might look like, and social policies figured into his calculations.[64] If IHPME and DLSPH were to develop such a policy institute might it evolve into a similar nexus?

Another crucial question is whether such an institute is necessary in order that it can interact with its other international counterparts because health systems (health-care delivery and universal health coverage) and public health are increasingly becoming international concerns. The need would seem evident, as in each of these areas the issues transcend national boundaries. With health systems the UN passage of a special resolution on universal health coverage in December 2012,[65] as well as in public health issues of vaccination, disease outbreaks, and epidemics[66] would seem to indicate need for an organization that can take its place within such an international network.

The question in all of this is what the model might be for such an institute. I would contend that there are important elements in each of the RIIA, CIIA, King's Fund, and Health Foundation. Each should be studied to discern elements that might be germane to forming a distinctly Canadian entity.

The primary issue is that Canada does not have an institute in the league of the British institutes – one sufficiently endowed to have staying power, with the independence to tackle difficult issues, the emphasis on communication, and the ability to bring our different communities together (in Chatham House Rule discussions) that each of these has. This includes being able to have a permanent staff that can be constantly scanning the horizon for the cutting-edge issues and can be interacting with other institutes doing the same.

CHAPTER 26

Communication, Impact, Public Engagement

COMMUNICATION

Steini Brown emphasized the importance of communication, and Rhonda continued to do so. This is important on a number of levels. Because it is a public institution, one can argue that a university should inform the public on what it is doing. Or for fund-raising one needs to be able to tell potential donors the same thing.

Perhaps the most crucial of these levels is the university emphasizing the importance of transmitting its academic knowledge in a form that the public can access. This is not as simple as it sounds. Being able to talk to or write for a public audience is very different from doing the same for an academic one. Not everyone is good at both.

Here, again linked to the knowledge-based society, one can question whether research has reached its full potential if it is seen only by an academic audience. This type of argument has been made on the determinants of health – one reasons that governments have been unable to devote more resources to this area is that most of the public is unaware of them. There have been vast volumes of literature written on the area, but it has been for about 1 per cent of the public, i.e., an academic audience.

Steini Brown notes that the King's Fund in the United Kingdom has as many people in its communication department as in its policy and research department, and that they use social media and public engagement as a key channel to influence stakeholders.[1] It has a webpage called "Health and Care Explained," which reveals a separate page of videos, articles, and seminar announcements.[2]

Steini also began a communications activity within IHPME when he was director. A major part of this fell under Rhonda while she was deputy director; however she continued the emphasis when she became interim director.

At first this involved using existing staff and contracting out specialized activities but eventually a dedicated communications officer was hired.

A result was establishment of a monthly newsletter, *IHPME Connect*. Another result was an electronic presence for IHPME with a continuing emphasis on its webpages. Rhonda notes that for both Steini and her it was important to "push the research out," i.e., to get it out into the public weal. This was especially important for IHPME, given its multidisciplinary nature, its large number of adjunct faculty, and its emphasis on applied research.[3]

This emphasis on communications extends to IHPME programs. The NAO has created a broad web presence, with links to the other North American hubs (US and Mexico) as well as to the European and Asia-Pacific Observatories. It also posts its health systems profiles, comparative data on national and sub-national systems, research, lecture series, and events, among others. It has its own YouTube channel, which has recordings of the lectures.[4]

Within IHPME, Health System Performance Research Network (HSPRN) and C3 also have a broad web presence. HSPRN, for example, has online links to current and past projects, reports, publications, applied health research questions, hospital performance results, and others.

This emphasis on the communication of complex knowledge to a lay audience has a long history. Donald T. Fraser, who was hired by J.G. FitzGerald, had such a talent. In 1925, with George Porter, he produced a health book for children, the *Canadian Health Book*.[5] It was also printed as the *Ontario Public School Health Book*.[6]

The book began with the story of how the Duke of Normandy, the eldest son of William the Conqueror, wounded in the siege of Jerusalem in the First Crusade, went to Salerno, Italy, home of the most skilful physicians in Europe. Before he departed, the physicians of the college wrote a book for him, *The Regimen of Health*, which was handwritten, since printing had not yet been invented. It became one of the most famous books on health in the early centuries and was read for hundreds of years.[7]

Fraser also wrote articles on topics like immunization, one of which appeared in the *Canadian Forum*.[8] Another example of his work was a broadcast on CKCL on the prevention of diphtheria and scarlet fever.[9]

A Pilot Project in Health Impact Communication

In communication, in July 2018 the DLSPH embarked on a Certificate in Health Impact pilot program, whose major aim was to increase the impact of what the DLSPH (and IHPME) does. The certificate focuses on journalism disciplines and partners with the Fellowship in Global Journalism (FGJ) program at the Munk School of Global Affairs and Public Policy.

It is very cutting-edge, basically building on DLSPH and IHPME research strengths and moving it into building skill sets to be able to demonstrate research impact, which is increasingly becoming a part of the rubric for grant proposals. But even more important it is seeking to build a skill set so that graduates and faculty can précis highly complex issues in order to advocate to politicians, journalists, and the public.

The aims of the program are to teach people how to influence public discussion by exposing important issues, get editors and politicians excited by nuanced ideas, and maximize public impact through solid reporting and communications.[10]

A DLSPH webpage on the certificate notes that journalism disciplines will help participants maximize public impact by exposing important, underreported issues, compete for research funding as public impact becomes a key granting criterion, and meet professional competencies in public health and medicine including communications, advocacy, leadership, and knowledge translation in scholarship.[11]

It notes that journalism disciplines will help "lead fraught, politically charged public issues to equitable, evidence-based outcomes." It has as mentors people like the former managing editor of the *Globe and Mail*, the former foreign editor of the *Los Angeles Times*, and the former foreign correspondent of the *Wall Street Journal*.[12] An aim of the pilot is to gather research data on how best to teach this material to health professionals and scholars in the future.[13]

The pilot is funded by the Office of the Vice-President, Research and Innovation, whose incumbent is Vivek Goel (who, you will recall, is an IHPME grad). It began as a Munk-DLSPH initiative and is now solely a DLSPH initiative open to its faculty, students, and alumni (which includes IHPME) and to the Faculty of Medicine (senior residents and faculty), as well as other U of T health faculties.

A major reason behind the certificate idea was that the Munk Fellowship in Global Journalism was finding that nearly 30 per cent of participants in their Fellows program have been health researchers and professionals, far more than from any other field. One of them, Rebecca Fortin, is listed as an MHSc grad from Dalla Lana.[14] These health specialists have, in turn, generated a disproportionate degree of the program's success in published stories.[15]

Alumni have gone on to significant positions. They have become staff or regular contributors to the *Dallas Morning News* (health correspondent), CNN (health contributor), *Chatelaine* magazine (health columnist), CBC News (health contributor), and the *Montreal Gazette* (health contributor). Others are with *VICE* (senior reporter), the *National Post* (deputy comments editor), the *Financial Times* (New York bureau), the *Wall Street Journal* (London bureau), the *Economist*, and *Foreign Policy*.[16]

The certificate proposal notes major research foundations now include public impact as a key research criterion. This includes the investigator helping to "shape a sustained public discussion" in the field of their research. It aims to help build competencies in health advocacy, leadership, collaboration, and communication. It's an emerging dimension of scholarship.[17]

The fellowship from which the Certificate program is drawn has "gained international attention as the only program in the world designed specifically to recruit highly qualified professionals and scholars internationally and mentor their work as independent journalists." Its alumni have earned major recognition, including a Pulitzer finalist, Emmy Award winner, Emmy finalist, and two Chawkers Fellows, among others. The fellowship has attracted attention from leading academic programs outside U of T. For example, in the past the Rhodes Trust has invited the FGJ director to teach workshops at Oxford and now has asked him to develop a "Bearing Witness" workshop for all first-year Rhodes Scholars.[18]

This emphasis on communication is not new for IHPME. When I shared the announcement of the Certificate of Health Impact program with former IHPME faculty member and Innis College principal John Browne, he noted that when John Hastings finished the work on the Community Health Center project for the Conference of Health Ministers of Canada, Hastings volunteered members of the team to go to any province or meet with any group to explain what they did, how they did it, and why it mattered. Browne noted that Hastings felt that those who made statements about public policy had an obligation to explain why they made them and what their effect might be.[19]

Communication with Whom?

There are some interesting connections between what the DLSPH and Munk School is doing and what many would regard as one of the premiere policy institutes in the world. It is instructive that one of the original documents setting out the premises of one of the world's pre-eminent policy institutes, the RIIA, more popularly known as Chatham House, expressed some of the same ideals as are contained in this pilot. It noted, "Public opinion is and should be to an increasing extent the determining factor in the sphere of foreign no less than that of domestic affairs."[20]

It noted, and here watch for the distinction, "Public opinion in questions of foreign policy is guided by a comparatively small number of experts, to a far greater extent than in social questions, of which a larger proportion of the electorates have personal experience." So "the first object of the Institute was to enable those who influence public opinion on international questions to write or speak with a better knowledge of the subjects they handle."[21]

What the RIIA was therefore trying to build was greater public awareness in order to influence better policy and, ultimately, build a stronger democracy. Through all of this the quality of the knowledge base was crucial.

How Does It All Link Together?

This latest initiative of the DLSPH is part of a wider canvas, one that IHPME is an integral part of. First is the world-class school of public health and its foundation of basic and applied research and graduate education. Next are the university-based policy institutes (or research centres, as Marchildon would call them), which at once are two things: focused research and meeting places. They utilize the research skills and knowledge of IHPME toward applied ends. These can be for governments, health-care organizations, or other interested parties.

Through the seminars they offer, such as the former Leadership Series within the DLSPH and both the Symposia of C3 and the NAO Lecture Series in IHPME, they are meeting places bringing people together in dialogue. The DLSPH and the NAO post these seminars on the web so that the public can also access them. Through their project work they foster interactions between academics (both faculty and graduate students) with government or

NGO staff. Through things like *IHPME Connect* or the *DLSPH Newsletter* they push the research out – to varied audiences.

But then we get much more intent and focused on this – the communication piece. The traditional part is academics writing for other academics in peer-reviewed journals or grant applications, or academics presenting at academic conferences. But an increasingly important part is academics writing or speaking to non-academics. This non-academic piece can take the form of academics needing to communicate via either the written or spoken word to advocate for an evidence-based position. It can be by academics pitching stories to media who can spread the word further and enhance public awareness, it can also be academics writing to decision-makers such as politicians or influential businesspeople, or it can be academics writing for newspapers or appearing on radio or television and in this way reaching the public at large.

The communication piece is both an outcome and a process. The outcome is where there is a "story" in it. The process is its conveyance – the basis for getting others interested. But it's also a way of framing, formatting the information. These are the journalist disciplines. It all has to do with "scholarship for impact" – complex, nuanced ideas (expressed well and in brief) to senior decision-makers, senior editors of various media.

The import of what Brown and Steiner are doing was emphasized at the National Health Conference in the United States in 1938. It was by invitation with representatives from a broad range of stakeholders concerned with health, including a few journalists. One was Fulton Oursler, editor-in-chief of *Liberty*. He noted a woman who had been commissioned by the US government to look into the affairs of the Indigenous people. She wrote a notable report and nothing happened. But afterward she wrote a novel that used the information contained in the report. The novel was *Ramona*, its author Helen Hunt Jackson, and it chronicled such tragedies that an avalanche of public opinion formed and forced reforms.[22]

But Oursler also noted that public opinion "is a tricky thing, and it needs expert handling." He gave a second example of Upton Sinclair who, in *The Jungle*, was wanting "to excite American sympathy" for stockyard workers. Yet what the public read into his novel was the need for better food laws and that, not better working conditions, was the outcome.[23]

Another skill set of journalists was demonstrated at this meeting by Myron Weiss, associate editor of *Time*. The substance of his remarks highlighted their ability to know their own stance on a situation (in this case health insurance) and yet equally value the other side of an issue and present both sides to the public clearly and objectively.[24]

So the importance of the communication piece cannot be overstated. The knowledge value is greatly diminished if its distribution is narrow. But the message is equally important.

Comment

These initiatives in communication within IHPME build on a foundation in the academic literature on the importance of scientific communication. They have an important precedent, particularly in the United Kingdom. The Bodmer Report by the Royal Society noted that "a better understanding of science can be a major element in promoting national prosperity, in raising the quality of public and private decision-making and in enriching the life of the individual."[25] Various bodies representing UK science were sufficiently enthusiastic about the report to fund schemes to encourage scientists to improve the communication of science to the public. Also the Imperial College in London established a professorship on the Public Understanding of Science.[26]

The third report of the House of Lords Select Committee on Science and Technology, *Science and Society*, was evidence of the acceptance by the UK government of the need for science communication to be framed in the public's terms. It recognized that to be of real value in a public policy context, scientific knowledge needed to be reframed to engage audiences on their terms, i.e., specific to their understanding and background and not in the terms of those of the scientific community.[27] The UK government also established a Government Office for Science (GO-Science) to support evidence-based decision-making.

Through its own communications activity and initiatives such as C3, the NAO, and ACE, IHPME is communicating the results of its research as well as supporting governments in evidence-based decisions. This is particularly important in health, where the effect of better public awareness is intimately connected to better policy and better quality of life.

One could contend that such initiatives within IHPME were taking the FitzGerald motif "within reach" – or ours, "available to all" – into a new realm. What was being made available in these instances was not (as in

FitzGerald's time) a physical product (such as a vaccine) but rather an ethereal one (knowledge). Knowledge itself was now the product. It had moved from being a means toward an end to the end itself.

It also places IHPME in a new realm in that IHPME can be sourced not only for the specialized knowledge it is generating but also for the methods it employs to get that knowledge out to multiple audiences.

Between DLSPH and IHPME, it is also evidence of movement on a wide of variety of fronts, developing a broad skill set of building and running policy institutes and reaching media editors and decision-makers.

One can point to an analogy between what DLSPH and IHPME are doing and what the RIIA and the CFR were doing in the 1920s. The crux of the challenge is unpacking complex issues in an evidence-based manner. In the 1920s the issue was international relations. The emergence of the nation state as the predominant political form and the globalizing world had made for a radical increase in scale and complexity. The same is true today in individual health and health insurance or population health and health determinants.

Common elements are knowledge to be communicated and used for active participation in the process, to create a climate of opinion that will nurture more measured debate, to promote an awakening public interest, encouraging academic research in their respective areas (health and international affairs respectively), and to provide leading forums for experts and policymakers from several walks of institutional life.

The emphasis on communicating for impact is an apt segue into impact in broader terms.

IHPME AND DLSPH IMPACT

What much of the preceding is aiming at in the university-based policy institutes and the communication piece is impact. Throughout its history the DLSPH, including the School of Hygiene, has had its eye on making a difference, the outcome of which was impact. Much the same can be said of IHPME. J.G. FitzGerald, Harvey Agnew, Gene Vayda, really all the directors and a disproportionate number of the faculty; these people wanted to make a difference; more on this in the next chapter.

Impact is another important focus of the university of the twenty-first century. It is taking the academy out of the academy, linking it to a broader public. As Rhonda and Steini say, it is "pushing the research out."

Former IHPME director and present DLSPH dean Brown is focusing on impact by encouraging the university-based policy institutes, lectures like Bernie Sanders, the Dean's Leadership Series, the Boehm Lectures, and the NAO lectures.

All of these are bridging the divide between academia and society at large. The policy institutes do it by focusing the knowledge and the skill sets of the researcher on practical needs, particularly of governments, but other interested organizations as well. The lectures bring our communities together, people together in dialogue – either faculty and students of different disciplines or these in addition to the public.

The DLSPH's website headline on its certificate pilot implicitly notes the power of communication and an emphasis on impact: "Improve health outcomes by using journalism skills to shape a smarter public discussion on health."[28] By setting up the pilot the DLSPH is taking account not only the tremendous importance of the power of communication but also its skill set and how it can make IHPME graduates more effective.

It was the same when Dean Brown, at the time IHPME's director, became involved in the CIHR Health Systems Impact Fellowships. His intent in co-leading the CIHR-sponsored Training Modernization Working Group was to develop new competencies for PhD students in health services and policy research. Recall he noted to me that these were necessary to have greater impact on health policy and practice and accelerate the transition to a learning health system.[29]

Health Systems Impact Fellowships

In 2015 Adalsteinn Brown (with Stephen Bornstein at Memorial University) led the CIHR-sponsored Training Modernization Working Group. This group developed a list of new competencies necessary for PhD students in Health Services and Policy Research to have greater impact on health policy and practice and accelerate the transition to a learning health system.[30]

Within eighteen months the new competencies and a set of tools (including curriculum elements) had been developed, and CIHR had launched the first competition for Health System Impact Fellows where PhDs in health services and policy research were matched with employers ranging from ministries of health to charities to private sector companies.[31]

By 2018 the cadre of these fellows had grown to nearly 100 across the country, and they met annually with their mentors (including deputy ministers and CEOs of health-care providers) and health system leaders to review progress and refine the program. Program support continued to be administered out of IHPME and the doctoral fellowship launched in 2018.

Comment

Steini is not alone in his focus on impact. Other countries focus on links between research, innovation, and impact. For example the UK Research and Innovation has a mandate is to work "in partnership with universities, research organisations, businesses, charities, and government to create the best possible environment for research and innovation to flourish."[32] Universities like Oxford and Cambridge have a webpage on impact,[33] as do many other UK universities. The MRC has a section on its website "Investing for Impact."[34]

The British government also has a chief scientific advisor, and its departments have their own scientific advisors.[35] It also has a Government Office for Science, whose mandate is "to ensure that government policies and decisions are informed by the best scientific evidence and strategic long-term thinking."[36]

In the United States the National Science Foundation has the "Broader Impact Review Criterion," which includes elements such as "dissemination to enhance scientific and technological understanding" and "benefits to society."[37]

Given this increasing focus on impact by other universities and granting agencies, Steini, through the certificate pilot, is ensuring that the DLSPH (and IHPME) can build a skill set in this area.

PUBLIC ENGAGEMENT

Another very important area is public engagement, which can take three forms: public lectures delivered specifically for a public audience, and specialized academic lectures whose audience is academicians or graduate students but which the public is free to attend.

The Boehm Lectures

The Boehm Lectures are a DLSPH lecture series to engage health system and government leaders. When Steini Brown became interim dean there was a series of lectures called the Dean's Leadership Series. Steini wanted to reconstitute them and make them "transformative" by bringing in external experts to provide their insights on pressing issues. He considered several options such as rebranding the existing series, but after he was confirmed as the new dean and partly as a result of a donor, who believed strongly in this area and expressed interest in funding them, he decided on developing a new series.

He refocused on transforming public health and health care, supported by the Dean's Office and run jointly by a DLSPH and an IHPME faculty member. The intent was to bring in global leaders in fields covered by the DLSPH and IHPME. What was very interesting was that he involved Helen Angus, the Ontario deputy minister of health and long-term care in developing the parameters of the series.

The series is intended to centre on three themes: leading-edge options to integrate care, improved access to care using new models, and building new models of public health and health care into the health system. There are two to three panel-style lectures a year on these themes with a mix of local and international speakers on each. The deputy minister agreed to be part of an additional lecture on what it takes to be a leader in the health-care system and moderated the first panel. There will also be a lecture focusing on leadership in public health.[38] What was noteworthy in this was Steini's focus on public health and health care, as well as his involvement of a senior government official.

His objective was to create an opportunity to engage the health system and public leaders in discussion about critical and pressing issues in public health and health systems.[39] He worked with the donor to create a forum for academic-government discussion somewhat along the lines of Chatham House and the King's Fund in the United Kingdom. Steini and the donor were of similar minds on a constellation of initiatives that were needed for communication, impact, and public engagement. Both knew of the King's Fund and Chatham House. The donor had a graduate degree from IHPME as well as a graduate degree in history and had provided Steini with material on Chatham House. His thesis had been on the work of Arnold J. Toynbee who, in addition to his theoretical work in history, had also been research director for Chatham House.

Steini outlined his idea for the lecture series in correspondence to Annette Paul (director of advancement, DLSPH) and the donor that sought to capture the tenor of the discussions between him and the donor. He wrote a preamble for the donor document. His précis was a wonderful reconnoitre of past, present, and anticipated future cutting-edge leadership that at once captured the deep history of the school and pointed to its ambitious aims. It also indicated how he saw the lectures integrating into the mission of the school.

Because it captures the essence of the DLSPH as well as the School of Hygiene, it deserves to be quoted in its entirety:

> The Dalla Lana School of Public health is building on a century's worth of leadership and achievement. The dominant themes of impact and partnership that shaped the early years of the School of Hygiene still shape our School today. The production of toxoid here made Toronto and Hamilton the first Diphtheria-free cities.
>
> We see the same impact today in our faculty's work on high users of health care, the opioid crisis, Ebola, Assisted Death, and big data. We can continue to build on this tradition and culture by creating the global model of engaged public health and health systems research. This model could help meet the most pressing needs in Canada and serve as a beacon of innovation and excellence, much like McMaster did with Problem-based Learning in Medicine in the 1970s.
>
> However, such a model depends on strong communication and outreach to expert, elite and general public audiences about pressing public health and health systems issues and ways to solve or even prevent these issues. To this end, the [donor's name] gift will provide funding for a series of lectures every year that put a spotlight on major public health and health systems issues.
>
> The lectures will match global leaders with expertise at the DLSPH and will be open to the faculty, staff, students and alumni of the School as well as to the general public. They will also create the opportunity for associated events like Chatham House Rule sessions that can bring together leaders in a way to help solve these issues.[40]

At the inaugural lecture Steini captured his intent and that of the donor. He said their purpose was to "create opportunities to engage all of our communities and engage all of our communities in discussions about the health and healthcare system that we want and I think that we feel that we deserve."[41]

"The Warmth of the Shadow"

Planning for this new series also illustrated the erudition of IHPME and DLSPH staff. The reader will recall support staff involved in continuing education and degree courses. It is illustrative that in a meeting discussing the objectives of the new lecture series, Annette Paul voiced a thought – a phrase – that expressed a deep ideal for her. She wasn't sure whether she had thought it up on her own or had seen it somewhere. The phrase was "the warmth of the shadow," and it was evident that, irrespective of its origin, she had given it her own meaning.[42] To her it had to do with the atmosphere or aura created by the ideal leader: you wanted to be in their shadow.[43] One might also add that you sought to emulate them, that they produced a sense of dedication and commitment among staff.

One could build on her thought and also say it involved the warmth, inclusion, the ambiance cast – an aura born not only of competence but more importantly of character. There is a certain character amongst the leadership and faculty of IHPME. There is "the warmth of the shadow" of the intensity of their commitment to graduate education and in making a health system better. There is "the warmth of the shadow" that intuits and actualizes the best of potentials of colleagues and students.

It is a wonderfully evocative phrase that one could extend and say also applied to the "warmth of the shadow" cast by the School of Hygiene, the DLSPH, or IHPME. In the case of Hygiene it would certainly be an apt phrase for the families who no longer had to face the heart-wrenching occasion of watching their child die of diphtheria. All of these organizations cast a large shadow, not just among the people they graduated but also within their respective fields of endeavour. This was due in no small measure to their relationships with practitioners.

At IHPME and its predecessor departments it is the same with people like Eugenie Stuart. Or FitzGerald and Defries at Hygiene. They were people who not only cast a large shadow but also someone to whom others gravitated, people in whose presence others wanted to be.

Public Lecture: Speech by Bernie Sanders Sponsored by DLSPH and the NAO

A very powerful example of public engagement was the institute's participation in special events. One such event was a talk by US Senator Bernie Sanders, at the time a candidate to be the 2016 Democratic nominee for president and an outspoken advocate in the United States for a public health insurance system. His talk, "What the US Can Learn from Canadian Health Care," was sponsored by the Dalla Lana School and the NAO at IHPME. The NAO director and IHPME faculty member was integrally involved. It also included a discussion of his widely publicized plan "Medicare for All." He was joined in his discussion by Danielle Martin, adjunct faculty member of IHPME.

The event was free to people on a first-come, first-served basis. He came to speak at Convocation Hall, the university's largest assembly hall, on 29 October 2017. Tickets became available at 10:00 a.m. on 20 October and a Toronto radio station reported were fully subscribed "within seconds."[44] This meant the level of interest was such that the entire capacity of Convocation Hall, of over 1,700 people, was filled in moments. The event was also live-streamed. The premier of Ontario introduced Mr Sanders.

His speech touched on many themes: the breadth of health insurance benefits, social determinants of health, increasing economic inequality (and its effects on health), and powerful entrenched interests that do not want a public system.[45] It was widely reported in the media. Martin asked Sanders what we could do to help, and the *Globe and Mail* noted his response: "I know Canadians are well known throughout the world as kind and gentle people. Be a little louder. Stand up and fight for what you have achieved."[46] The *Globe* added that while Canada looks good when compared to the US system, a Commonwealth Fund report ranked it ninth out of ten countries.

The report of the *Toronto Star* emphasized the points Sanders made on how extreme right-wing movements are capturing the political agenda, which is resulting in "a shrinking middle class and extreme inequality" and that this is threatening health and democracies. It also noted his comment that "Canadians make more noise about the benefits of universal access."[47]

The *New York Times* also reported on his visit, suggesting he learned five lessons from his weekend in Canada. Greg Marchildon was mentioned in the article and its quote of him formed the subject line of one of the lessons (that he's a "rock star"). It also noted the enthusiasm of the student crowd, that Convocation Hall was full, that "he received repeated and sustained standing ovations," and that "college students waited for hours" to be admitted and hear him speak.[48] The *Varsity* noted, "Convocation Hall buzzed with energy."[49] I was in the audience and there was a palpable sense of energy, excitement and expectation.

Sanders's appearance implicitly pointed to how important it was to make the event free, open to all, and to bring such a prominent person to the university to speak of such a topical area in health-care delivery.

Another important outcome was the discussion it generated amongst students and faculty. I was personally involved in discussions on Sanders's talk in classes at IHPME, UTSC, and Trinity College. Some of the students had managed to get tickets for the talk, while others listened to the live stream.

Former NDP national leader Ed Broadbent in thanking Sanders called him "North America's leading social democrat."[50]

This is one example of public outreach at the NAO. Another is its sponsorship of individuals from different health-care systems from around the world to present seminars on the significant characteristics of their systems.

Shortly after the Sanders lecture, I suggested to Marchildon to get the Harvard political philosopher Michael J. Sandel for a future talk. Sandel is famous for his "Justice" course, which has been taken by over 15,000 students at Harvard,[51] and tens of millions around the world have viewed it online.[52] Sandel delivered the prestigious Reith Lectures for the BBC. Steini Brown took his course while an undergraduate at Harvard.[53]

NAO Lectures

The 2017–18 academic year was the first year for the NAO lectures, and they were an important new addition for IHPME. Greg Marchildon is bringing people in from around the world. Here are some examples of people, places, and topics: Miguel González-Block, Anahuac University, on universal health coverage in Mexico; James Gillespie, University of Sydney, on private insurance in Australia and Canada; Martin McKee, London School of Hygiene and Tropical Medicine, on comparing the performance of health systems worldwide; Bruce Rosen, Smokler Center for Health Policy Research, Israel, on dual public-private physician practice in Israel and Canada.

I attended a number of these sessions. The types of information being provided on the national systems of these countries and then the comparisons the listener could make to the Canadian system was very useful.

Disseminating Academic Knowledge

IHPME has been a part of a transformation at the university. Many have said that universities need to move beyond their teaching and research mandate to active participation in dissemination of that knowledge. Beginning in the 1980s and the passage of the Bayh-Dole Act in the United States, this took the form of emphasis on the application of this knowledge and the emergence of a new area of activity: technology transfer. The objective was to use knowledge as more than a means to an end, to become the end itself, i.e., a marketable product. In health this meant universities would become active participants in the development of new drugs and diagnostics. The IHPME class on the commercialization of research (mentioned earlier) looked at this process.

We will see further in this section that during this period the United Kingdom began to bridge the divide between the academic and the public. In the twenty-first century this is taking place on a much wider scale in the United Kingdom with a host of activities, which include the MRC initiative on public engagement[54] and reports on access to information,[55] as well as specialized activities such as the Foresight Programme and the Government Office for Science (GO-Science), to name just a few.[56]

In this century this knowledge dissemination takes on a new dimension with emphasis on public outreach. This means that the university must transmit its knowledge not just to students and other academics but also to the public. The public needs to have a greater awareness of issues in areas such as health, international relations, and the economy, and the university has an integral role in this. At U of T, the Munk School of Global Affairs and Public Policy posts a number of its seminars on its website and opens their attendance to the public. IHPME (and the DLSPH) has done the same, with seminars, semi-annual symposia, and White Papers that highlight important areas of policy for the public.

The SPOR seminar series run by Fiona Miller on citizen participation in care and citizen participation in research is another example of this public outreach, but it also takes public participation a step further in that each is related to a concept of the patient as agent, that is, the patient as more than a passive recipient.

Public engagement is another area in which the United Kingdom is active. The MRC devotes a page on its website to public engagement.[57] The Wellcome Trust does the same, along with a Public Engagement Fund.[58] The UK

National Coordinating Centre for Public Engagement has a publication called *The Engaged University*.[59] Universities such as Oxford and Cambridge (and many other UK universities) have public engagement sites.

COMMENT

One wonders if when one takes together the four elements of university-based policy institutes, communication, public engagement, and impact, it points to an increasing responsibility passing to universities to maintain things like a health system and whether this binds the university more tightly to its society.

PART ELEVEN

Final Thoughts

CHAPTER 27

Outcomes

CROSS-CUTTING THEMES BETWEEN THE SCHOOL OF HYGIENE AND IHPME

In commenting on the first draft of this manuscript Adalsteinn Brown concluded that six key themes illustrate the close connection between IHPME and the School of Hygiene, which intertwine through the history of the two.[1] They are the following.

A Focus on Impact

We just spoke of a focus on impact in the preceding chapter. However, impact at IHPME and the DLSPH has deep historical roots, which reach back to FitzGerald and his staff. Their focus was concentrated on application. These people wanted to make a difference. It was not enough for them to engage solely in theoretical exploration; knowledge for knowledge's sake was not enough. This focus has prevailed.

It is evident in the School of Hygiene's major influence on public health where so many of the positions of significance were filled by DPH grads or that almost all deputy ministers on the Dominion Council of Health were DPH grads. There is FitzGerald's research on diphtheria and his founding of Connaught Labs. And, since Connaught had an intimate relation with the school, it could be any of its many products – the diphtheria antitoxin, funding Banting and Best's research on diabetes, or the polio vaccine, to name only a few.

IHPME had its health administrator study, Hastings's work on community health, and the involvement of faculty in two royal commissions. More recent are its policy institutes like C3 and the NAO.

Tight Connections to the Local Community

Tight connections to the local community can be the connections of the department/institute to hospital administrators and in turn the administrators' connections to the community, connections of the school to local and provincial medical officers of health, or, to broaden the radius of community, connections to provincial and federal departments of health.

And there is a nuance to the term *community*, for IHPME serves multiple communities. *Local* is an apt term. But in a global world, what is local? Is it the teaching hospitals at IHPME's doorstep? Is it Toronto and the health-care organizations within its environs? Is it Ontario, other provinces, Canada? Or, and we see this with some of the scholarship of the faculty, or the observatory on health systems (NAO), is it – to use the term of another Canadian – the "global village"?

Some of these global connections were evident early on, such as FitzGerald's travels in the 1920s to view the social policies of Scandinavia, or in the1930s to survey the teaching of preventive medicine in other countries.

Reliance on People Inside and Outside the Academy

Reliance on people inside and outside the academy is linked to the first two and connotes the school's emphasis on a close working relationship with medical officers of health on solving health issues. Two examples would be FitzGerald's relation with the medical officers of health in Saskatchewan and Ontario regarding the distribution of antitoxins. In IHPME it involves its relationship with hospital CEOs in the practicum portion of the DPH or MHSC.

A Constant Deepening of the Scholarship and Growth in Programming

IHPME and the school were intimately tied to the evolution of the Canadian health-care scene. IHPME began with a singular focus on hospital management. But by the 1960s it was impossible to ignore the intrusion of other aspects of the health system such as health delivery through community health mechanisms, or in the 1970s emerging issues such as clinical epidemiology, geriatrics, and health law, or in the 1980s health economics. It was also becoming harder to separate institutional health delivery (such as hospitals) from the wider area of public health, which was perhaps evident in the merger of the Departments of Hospital Administration and Public Health in 1967.

Brown notes that over the period of transitioning into the faculty of medicine and back out (and across different graduate units) the quality of scholarship seems to have deepened at every turn.[2] And the transitions seem to have energized as opposed to debilitated the department/institute. Coincident with a deepening of scholarship was expansion of teaching activity at the professional and academic levels as well as an expansion of the breadth of academic interest.

Related to this is that the department/institute was very able to hold its own in an environment in which the bar was set very high. For many years it was part of a school with an international reputation. Yet within that, and within a few years of its inception, it established a very solid national reputation. Just as the school was responsible for most prominent medical officers of health, the same could be said of the department graduates and hospital CEOs.

Continual Diversification

Continual diversification is in line with faculty's increasingly nuanced understanding of how complex health is, on perhaps two levels. One is in the continual broadening of academic focus of IHPME in systemic areas noted above, or moving into other areas like health informatics, high-performing systems, comparative systems, or physician leadership. Or the School of Hygiene and its pushing into areas such as nutrition, or the reconstituted Dalla Lana School and its areas of global health and Indigenous health.

The other level is a movement into completely new areas, one of which is the research activity itself, which is a twofold activity. It is not just to broaden a knowledge base. It is also to look toward the practical application of the knowledge.

One example is the application of research and scientific principles to government decision-making; another is the commercialization of medical sciences basic research. An example of the former is the IHPME Graduate Students Union hosting John Preece to talk about the Government Office for Science in the United Kingdom and their push for evidence-based decision-making at all levels.[3] An example of the latter was IHPME's partnership with the Institute of Management of Innovation at UTM and Boehm's graduate course, which looked at the whole area of the commercialization of health research. Another is IHPME's agreement with the Health Sciences Program at UTSC and the adaptation of his graduate course to fourth-year undergrads at UTSC.

Some of IHPME's grad students have become interested in exploring aspects of the commercialization of health research. Many are interfacing with an organization a block away from IHPME – MaRS – which is pushing the envelope on taking science from bench to bedside. It is an organization that is at once major research park, innovation hub, and entrepreneurial incubator; one at a nexus, bridging divides, with links to basic research, technology transfer, venture capital, government, and business.

The example of MaRS and its focus has connections to faculty member Naylor. While president of U of T he was very concerned with government support for research and also in the university doing something with this research. Under his successor, U of T has an equity stake in MaRS. As mentioned earlier, while not a major focus of IHPME, commercialization is an interest area in both teaching and research.

Another aspect is a constant pushing of the envelope, teasing out new ideas. The institute has constantly pushed into new areas of policy and management. At present it is venturing into very innovative areas, such as the institute's forays into patient engagement in research and patient engagement in care and its partnership with OSSU. Another is the exploration of high-cost users and how attention to the determinants of health could mitigate these costs. The NAO is another, as is the commercialization of health research.

Lots of In and Out: People Moving Seamlessly between Academia and the Field

Naylor is a good example of movement between academia and the field. Rhodes Scholar, former dean of medicine, and president of this university, at various stages he has been student, clinician, epidemiologist, founder and first CEO of ICES, and now a member of faculty and sponsor of one of the institute's awards.

We have the present dean of DLSPH, former head of IHPME, also a Rhodes Scholar, company founder in Manhattan, ADM in two government ministries, and now back in academia.

We have the head of the NAO, a former deputy minister of two Saskatchewan departments, executive director of a royal commission, and now an academic.

In addition to the movement in and out of academia, these roles embody the sophistication and complexity of management at high levels, of pushing policy to its limits, and tackling large risks in doing so, and all with the aim to ensure that Canada has a place in a rapidly evolving global knowledge-based arena of which health is very much an integral part.

Tom Closson and Mark Rochon are other examples, graduates of this university and IHPME respectively, former CEOs, and now involved with IHPME – "practidemics," as Greg Marchildon calls them.

The other issue in all this is whether this is a tradition that senior administrators in the civil service or tertiary hospitals should aspire to. There is a precedent. British historian Arnold J. Toynbee noted that in the Late Victorian era a British civil servant was appointed not only on the basis of proficiency in office but also in scholarship. And such individuals were also expected, and indeed often encouraged, to keep up such scholarship thereafter alongside their official work.[4]

IHPME AND THE UNIVERSITY AVENUE URBAN MEDICAL CLUSTER

Also near the inception of IHPME there was another new major activity underway. We noted earlier that during the 1950s, almost right next door to IHPME, there were the beginnings of the University Avenue cluster of hospitals. TGH, already at this location, expanded on its site. SickKids and Mount Sinai relocated to a University Avenue address. All were hospitals whose administrative teams a number of IHPME grads would join.[5] And a number of these same individuals remained involved with IHPME as guest lecturers, seminar leaders, and the like.

There were other relocations to University Avenue. In 1978 Queen Elizabeth Hospital opened in the location of the former New Mount Sinai Hospital (which had been relocated in a new building next door).[6] It became the Toronto Rehabilitation Institute in 1997 with merger of the Queen Elizabeth and Hillcrest Hospitals. Another IHPME grad, Mark Rochon, was its CEO for a number of years.

In the 1990s SickKids built out to Elizabeth Street, a long block east of University Avenue. TGH had long ago built out to this location. In the mid-1990s

Princess Margaret Hospital and its research institute, the Ontario Cancer Institute, relocated to University Avenue.[7] As we have seen, this combination of a research institute affiliated with a teaching hospital was characteristic of the University Avenue hospitals. And IHPME grads were involved, with a number becoming involved in the new area of research administration, as these research institutes reached a critical mass of operations.

Also at around this time UHN and Mount Sinai began leasing space in the Ontario Hydro building at the corner of University Avenue and College Street, so that by the 2010s they were leasing about a third of its office space.[8] In 2005 Phase I of MaRS opened on a portion of TGH property, including its original College Street building. Its website calls it the "the world's largest innovation hub" with a title that encapsulates the theme of the section, "Place Matters."[9] MaRS serves a number of purposes. It is an office/laboratory location for spin-off and related service companies and is also a conference centre.

In the 2010s Women's College Hospital built a new facility at the north head of Elizabeth Street (which dead-ended at the Women's College property).

The U of T Role in the Medical Cluster

The U of T is also an integral part of this urban medical cluster. It has a number of related facilities "clustered" at the northwest end of the cluster, the southeast end of the campus. These include existing buildings such as the Faculty of Medicine, Donnelly Centre for Cellular and Biomolecular Research, McMurrich Building, FitzGerald Building, David C. Naylor Building, and the Banting and Best Centre for Innovation and Entrepreneurship.

In the 2000s in this area a number of other buildings were constructed or purchased. The Toronto District School Board headquarters became the Health Sciences Building; a half-block from MaRS, it brought together IHPME, the Dalla Lana School of Public Health, and the Bloomberg School of Nursing. The Faculty of Pharmacy moved into new facilities at the corner of College and University Avenue. Both Pharmacy and Nursing moved from buildings further away from this cluster.

The U of T has built on the physical aspects of this cluster by adding organizational entities to help facilitate commercial outcomes from research. It added incubators and commercialization support services located in this cluster area. There is the Health Innovation Hub almost next door to IHPME (on McCaul Street), and across the street from MaRS (and about a block from IHPME), U of T Entrepreneurship and the Impact Centre: Science to Society are housed in the Banting and Best Centre for Innovation and Entrepreneurship. Essentially next door to the Banting and Best Centre is University of Toronto Early Stage Technology (UTEST) Program, which provides companies with start-up funding, mentoring, and space in the centre to new companies.[10]

A webpage on U of T Entrepreneurship points toward a history of innovation and discovery at U of T, noting that Banting and Best were "U of T's first and most successful entrepreneurs."[11] One might amend this by saying they were *among* the first, as there was also J.G. FitzGerald and his founding of Connaught Labs, which took place a number of years before their insulin discovery and funded their research.

These U of T initiatives are becoming part of a larger canvas. Both Toronto and U of T are becoming recognized for innovation and start-ups. The *Globe and Mail* noted, "The U of T is among the leaders in North America for research-based startups."[12] And Reuters rates U of T Canada's most innovative university and one of the top thirty institutions worldwide.[13] Toronto is being called Silicon Valley North[14] and the New Silicon Valley, the latter a term used by *Toronto Life* as the cover story for its October 2017 edition.[15]

A not insignificant part of all this is this urban medical cluster of teaching hospitals, their associated research institutes, the collection of university health sciences faculties, a biomedical research park, and a university innovation hub that is "a launch pad for start-ups, a platform for researchers and a home to innovators."[16] Equally important are global linkages as scientists and academics in this urban medical cluster take their place as a part of international networks in their respective areas.

Another advantage to this urban location is its proximity to related facilities. It is within a few blocks of Ryerson University and their health sciences activities. IHPME staff are involved in teaching there. Also the medical cluster is within blocks of Canada's financial centre.

The Boundaries of the Cluster Expand: A Toronto Urban Medical Cluster

We noted that facilities are concentrated at or immediately adjacent to University Avenue, but one needs only broaden the radius to include other facilities, such as Toronto Western Hospital, St Michael's Hospital, and the

Centre for Addiction and Mental Health (CAMH), each of which has its own research institute. Further to the north is the Sunnybrook Health Sciences Centre, again with its own research institute.

A recent example of the growth and vitality of this cluster is CAMH receiving a $100-million donation from an anonymous donor for mental health research. The *Globe and Mail* noted, "It is a powerful endorsement of the Canadian research enterprise and young researchers in particular" and went on to say, "At a time when public investment in health research is stagnant, it's the kind of bold, innovative gesture we should be seeing from the federal government, not just from private donors."[17]

A *Toronto Star* article reported, "The donation is by far the largest ever given to a mental health centre in Canada and one of only a handful of that magnitude bestowed on any health organization in the country."[18] It noted that this latest donation was one of a growing number of major donations and it listed a number of them to Toronto and GTA health-care facilities, including a $100 million additional donation by Peter Munk to UHN for the cardiac centre that bears his name and a $130 million donation by the Rogers family to establish the Ted Rogers Centre for Heart Research.[19] This list shows just how important hospital-based research and the public system is, and that, as we have seen, involvement of some of the most prominent people in Canada in our hospitals is a tradition that reaches far back in our history.

IHPME and the Knowledge-Based Economy

And these donations point to just how important research is becoming. IHPME is a part of it. The VP of research and innovation at U of T is an alum and former chair of IHPME. It is attracting people from start-ups to its MHSc and MHI programs. Also we previously noted faculty member Karim Keshavjee and his start-up (which has hired MHI grads), which is housed in space at Ryerson University.

In other examples of IHPME involvement, earlier we noted MHSc grads involved in research administration, and Ross Baker and his research on high-performing systems and Fiona Miller and her work on tech transfer. There was also the partnership with IMI at UTM and the research commercialization class IHPME taught for UTM and UTSC students.

A Nuance in IHPME's Involvement in the Innovative Economy

IHPME is also connected to changes in society at large. What IHPME is all about – knowledge – is assuming an increasing role in society, so much so that many say that the world is transitioning from a resource- and manufacturing-based economy to a knowledge-based economy. Research is an integral part of this transformation and is a major part of IHPME in that IHPME, with its own initiatives, is in the midst of knowledge-related programs and activities.

But IHPME's involvement in research and the utility and aim of its research is different from what has come to be considered the norm for universities and we have outlined thus far in this section. The primary aim of initiatives like MaRS or the university incubators, indeed, society at large, is the commercialization of research, i.e., research aimed toward business ends, in other words the development of a marketable product.

However, with IHPME, although it studies and teaches in research commercialization, its ends are more geared toward what could be called non-commercializable research. Its research is aimed not at private profit-making ends but toward more public-oriented ends, such as at making a public health-care system better. This will not result in increased profits but in a more efficient use of public money and better quality of care. When allied to DLSPH research in public health, this expands to better health generally for the population at large.

One could point to any number of IHPME faculty and their research. A case in point is Emily Musing (MHSc, 2003, Arbor Award, 2011) and her involvement in the Caring Safely program at UHN. It will result in better patient outcomes and a reduction in preventable hospital errors, which cost almost $400 million per year.[20] Another is Ross Baker, who does research in patient outcomes as well as in high-performing systems.

In essence IHPME is emphasizing an equally important part of the knowledge-based economy, which is research aimed at the common good, which is very much in line with the goals of J.G. FitzGerald when he founded the School of Hygiene and Connaught Labs before it. In our own time with health care forming the largest single budget line in provincial budgets, this aim of IHPME to use knowledge and research to make a public system better, to improve population health, focuses attention on an area of research and innovation that is under-represented in the academic literature and in the public mind.

When governments write reports on and people think of the knowledge-based economy, innovation, and entrepreneurship, it is toward commercializing research, forming a start-up company, and the like. Academics studying the area write and look almost exclusively at studies aimed at improving research and innovative activity toward business ends. There is a large and growing literature in this area, an area that a number of U of T faculty are involved in.[21]

A typical example is the chapter in a recent book by one of Canada's most successful entrepreneurs and venture capitalists. It talks of discovery research and suggests that basic research is aimed at discovery, not commercialization.[22] And yet almost anyone involved in research commercialization will say that basic and discovery research is the fertile field from which commercialization grows. Put another way, it fuels the commercialization pipeline, so there is a very real connection.

Yet within this research environment there is a subtle nuance. An equally important part of research and innovation is improving the public commons – areas that improve the public good – areas in health care such as public health, global health, determinants of health, health inequalities, and health systems, among others. Outside of health this includes climate change or ecology. These are areas that have only the remotest hope of yielding a commercial product while at the same time can make real and meaningful difference in people's lives and overall health.

IHPME shines a light on such areas. When we advocate for governments to increase research funding and to promote initiatives that encourage innovation it should not just be in the so-called hard sciences, IT, and engineering, but also in areas that help build the public commons. We should also advocate the crucial importance of non-commercializable research in areas highlighted above, and, indeed, research that brings the two cultures together, as famously advocated over sixty years ago by C.P. Snow.[23]

IHPME is moving on a number of fronts, highlighting the importance of research to governments and of informing the public on research, and emphasizing the importance of research to strengthening a public health system.

The Importance of IHPME's Location

IHPME has always had a very favourable location near the southeast corner of the campus, which placed in in close proximity to the Ontario Legislature, the Ministry of Health, and a number of Toronto's, indeed Canada's, larger hospitals, such as Toronto General, Toronto Western, SickKids, Mount Sinai, Queen Elizabeth, St Michael's, Wellesley, Women's College, Orthopaedic and Arthritic, and Central.

Proximity to these major facilities mattered. It gave students a unique access, and the fact that IHPME and the Department of Hospital Administration before it was in the midst of these facilities had an influence. If my thoughts while a student are any indication, students walked past them and wondered about their future roles and actions. I recall walking past various buildings of the TGH campus, the historic College Wing with its dome, or tall, thin Norman Urquhart Wing as symbols of Canada's leading hospital. These centres were looked upon as leaders in Canadian health care. Their proximity meant that they were always in the mind of faculty and students. Faculty referred to them in classes.

When I was a student, the school was located in the McMurrich Building, which was essentially across the street from the legislature, and on occasion I would walk across to listen to Question Period or watch the House in session. This involved watching people like William Davis and Stephen Lewis in debate, or people like Davis and his ministers responding to questions.

If anything, the intensity of this location is amplified today as MaRS, the Faculties of Nursing and Pharmacy, and the Dalla Lana School of Public Health have been added to this mix. The recently announced Schwartz Reisman Innovation Centre will further enhance this mix.

IHPME's Role in Producing Leaders for the Toronto Urban Medical Cluster

This discussion points to the role of IHPME in this constellation. In the past, IHPME has produced this nation's hospital leaders, and they have been at all hospital levels, from primary through to quaternary. These levels point to a complexity of care. What we now have is a complexity of role.

The academic health sciences centres that form the Toronto medical cluster have been based on the tripartite role of patient care, teaching, and research. However, this last role has expanded such that the research institutes of these facilities are rivalling the size of some medical faculties, indeed, some universities. Further, with their emphasis on research commercialization, they are becoming economic engines in themselves. In their work on non-commercializable research they are generating important new insight in health outcomes. In this area their interactions with each other, with health sciences faculties at the university, with research parks like MaRS, and with the venture capital community all point to an exponential increase of complexity.

And this raises the question of who will run these organizations and what is the IHPME role in this, especially given that it is such a small subset of the total hospital management milieu. Yet the small numbers of IHPME graduates belies their influence. And we are not talking of only CEOs, there are also the VP-, AVP-, and director-level positions. It points to the fact that while the majority of people being graduated go to community hospitals or community-oriented organizations, people are still needed who can run the large health science centres and their university-affiliated research institutes.

Charles Hollenberg, former physician-in-chief at TGH and former vice-provost of the university addressed the issue when he said, "The kind of administrator that we need as the chief operating officer of a large teaching hospital has to be very different from what we've had in the past," and we cannot "assume that an individual who has done a reasonable job as an executive director of a community hospital has the basic capability to be executive director of a teaching hospital." Such individuals need to understand the complexities of dealing with how faculties of medicine operate, the medical education process, medical research, and the regionalization of medical services. They need to understand the rapid scale-up of research activities in both commercial and non-commercial areas. He added, "We should be looking to train a new variety of hospital administrator" who has these skills.[24]

He raises a very important question – not just about the complexity of interrelationships, but also how to understand the milieu, gain a feel for the tenor and the pulse of these super-large organizations. This includes how to effect change, within them and within the system, the evolving landscape (e.g., transition to a knowledge economy) they are part of, and what this means to things like their research mandate. They are entities unto themselves.

TIES BETWEEN IHPME AND HEALTH SYSTEM GROWTH

We spoke at the beginning of this work of a possible link between IHPME and the Canadian health system writ large. Let's crystalize some of what we have outlined here. Two major new areas can be outlined. The first involves governments initiating a major new public program, which results in health ministries becoming the largest single line item in provincial budgets. The second is a very twenty-first-century concept, that of clusters, and a very distinctive application of that concept.

IHPME and Government

What occurred almost immediately, basically coincident with IHPMES inception, was that governments began building new capabilities. In Saskatchewan this involved the administration of a major new hospital (insurance) program. In all provinces health ministries began administering activities resulting from the federal hospital construction grants, which were sometimes supplemented by their own grants. Saskatchewan created a whole new division in its Department of Public Health to deal with this and outgrowths of its hospital insurance program. Burns Roth went from the IHPME program to be its head. We saw Ed Wahn had preceded Roth to Saskatchewan and convinced Roth to come.

In the 1950s Paul Martin Sr at the federal level built a capability in health insurance – in a move very reminiscent of FitzGerald – with his surveys of insurance programs in other countries. In the latter 1950s and early 1960s health ministries of all provinces became involved in administering hospital insurance programs as a result of Diefenbaker's amendments to the Hospital Insurance and Diagnostic Services Act.

Next came Saskatchewan in the early 1960s undertaking a further expansion in its ministry with its implementation of medical insurance. Burns Roth had begun this process and left Saskatchewan to head up IHPME just as it went into full gear. By the latter 1960s and early 1970s all provincial governments followed suit as a result of Pearson's National Medical Care Insurance Act (passed 1966, implemented 1968). And this begat a whole new concern of governments, that of a health system. And isn't it interesting that IHPME would change its name (and its focus) in the latter 1960s to a Department of *Health* Administration.

What one had in effect was the beginning of the largest government activity in Canada and a whole new emphasis on public services. Health ministries grew to be the largest government departments. It began with Saskatchewan staffing-up its Department of Public Health when Tommy Douglas in 1944 took on being its minister as well as premier. The earliest IHPME grads were among these new staff. He then created a Hospital Services Plan in 1947 to manage his hospital insurance program.

Other provinces followed suit. Ontario created the Hospital Services Commission in 1957. Taylor gives a sense of the outcomes across the country when he notes that the Catonguary-Nepvue report in Quebec "set a new standard for all government departments in Quebec and for many health commissions and departments in Canada." He noted a "new bureaucracy had been created."[25] Claude Castonguay resigned from the commission to become minister of health for Quebec. John Hastings knew him well.

IHPME and the Intensification of Scale and Scope

What we see here is an intensification of scale. We spoke earlier about how the department/institute kept pace with the evolving complexity of the health-care system. However, in addition to a systemic evolution we spoke of was an evolving complexity of hospitals and the system itself. This was in addition to what we saw at the outset of this book – that at the time of the department's inception hospitals were rapidly expanding in numbers in both Canada and the United States. It was also in addition to the fact that they had and still have a place in the public imagination.

As an organization they evolved. This was at its most concentrated at the apex, the tertiary hospitals. It is unclear exactly when this happened. Certain hospitals began to differentiate themselves very early. Almost as soon as there were medical schools, hospitals like a TGH became involved in clinical teaching, initially for physicians but soon enough for the allied medical faculties as well.

Not so long after this they also became a kind of workshop for certain physicians who couldn't help but tackle the seemingly intractable problems of patient care. And so within certain hospitals a research activity began to take hold. But this was a research borne not so much out of theory as out of practice, and so it had much more of what today is called applied research and clinical research.

We noted earlier hospitals' evolution to health sciences centres. There was a continued intensification of scale; they continued to scale-up. We noted the size of major Ontario hospitals in the 1960s. They became not only larger but also more diverse. We noted earlier in reference to TGH in the 1980s the tertiary centres began an emphasis on ambulatory care, which became an activity equal in emphasis to inpatient care. In the 1990s health-care restructuring in Ontario resulted in fewer but larger hospitals.

Hospitals reinforced another trend. The multiplicity of specializations led to dedicated demographic or disease facilities such as children's hospitals, mental health hospitals, cancer hospitals, and rehabilitation and chronic care hospitals. In many instances these agglomerations became like small cities in themselves.

IHPME and the Integral Nature of Health Care

Recent indications amplify the idea of how integral health carc is – initiatives that are positioning health care increasingly at the centre of communities/societies.

The Health Foundation and the King's Find are looking at the NHS as an anchor institution for local communities[26] – an idea that could be applied to medicare and hospitals in Canada. On the one hand we have a very decentralized federation that presents challenges the NHS does not have. On the other this is not an adequate reason to not look at how provincial health insurance plans and hospitals could strengthen local communities.

There is also the idea of "health in all policies," which says that health considerations need to move beyond the borders of health ministries.[27] It recognizes that to adequately deal with the social determinants of health requires that we de-silo health; we need to factor health into *all* government policies.

Related to an all-policy approach is another initiative of the Health Foundation: "healthy lives." Its basic premise is that the health of populations is one of a nation's greatest assets, and it needs to be looked at and invested in as asset-building.[28] The objectives are economic prosperity and a flourishing society. And importantly this is not only a role for the public sector. The private sector also needs to be involved; they need to recognize that strong communities and families are fundamental to their business model and to the nation they are a part of.[29] It is a more positive and broader approach to health. It moves beyond the individual and illness to the population as a whole and promoting health and well-being within that population.

One could add to this universal health coverage (UHC) and the emphasis it is given worldwide, but particularly at Chatham House in the United Kingdom.[30] What this means for Canada and the opportunity it presents is that its variant of UHC is exportable.

The issue for IHPME and the DLSPH is that if we are seeing health become even more central and even more pervasive to societies, what are the curriculum implications? The issue for Canada is whether we are innovating at the level of a United Kingdom. We have presented three very innovative, new directions of the United Kingdom; do we have something comparable? And, in the fourth area the same question is whether Canada with its own variant of UHC is continuing to innovate and update what is an exportable commodity.

And, to come back to IHPME and the DLSPH, what is their role in helping Canada innovate in each of these four areas? What is their part in keeping Canada at the vanguard? Is this where they need an academically based policy institute that punches at the level of a Chatham House, King's Fund, and Health Foundation?

The Multiplicity of Roles of IHPME MHSc Grads

Many people would regard it as incontrovertible that a strength of Canadian health care is its public institutions. This had manifested itself in a number of ways. We noted earlier in this work the deputy minister's comments on Ontario hospital voluntary boards being the best in the world. We have seen historical examples of Canadian philanthropy such as that of David Fasken and Toronto Western.

A significant strength of the Canadian public hospital system is the involvement of the Canadian community in hospital volunteer activities, at the board level, or in donations. And there are multiple communities in this regard, which range from local communities surrounding Canada's community hospitals to the community of Canada's financial titans who seek to fund cutting-edge research at Canada's most prominent academic health sciences centres. It is at the apex of the system, its leading edge, where institutions have an almost insatiable appetite for financial resources to push the boundaries of clinical care and health research.

The donation to CAMH is a case in point. Its CEO is IHPME alum Catherine Zahn, and the donation points to just how complex being CEO of a tertiary centre has become. It, and others like it, points to how big the research enterprise of these hospitals – aptly called health sciences centres – is becoming.

The constituency of such hospitals is broad, including patients, students, universities, government, voluntary boards, and donors. It also harkens back to what began as the original role of IHPME, that of hospital management. It underscores a role of IHPME in graduating people with the tools to take on these highly complex institutions.

Providing Leadership in Other Related Public Sector Organizations

IHPME faculty and grads have also provided leadership in other related public sector organizations. Two notable ones are the Hospitals of Ontario Pension Plan (HOOPP) and the Change Foundation.

OHA

We saw earlier the close relationship of Harvey Agnew and the OHA, and the involvement of Eugenie Stuart in OHA conventions. This was supplemented by the involvement of graduates in a number of OHA activities, such as presentations at OHA conventions and serving on the OHA Board of Directors, including serving as chair. Some of the grads who did so include P.R. Carruthers, J.H. Carter, G.P. Turner, G. Pierce (DHA, 1967), D.M. MacKenzie, L. Steven, T. Dagnone, and M. Rochon.[31] A. Stationwala is the present chair.

The chairs took an active role in OHA activities. Under P. Carruthers four new committees emerged, in trustees, research and development, government relations and communications, and priorities and planning.[32] L. Steven was involved in Safeguarding Patient Care while chair.[33] The OHA launched strategic planning under the leadership of T. Dagnone and Warren Chant (DHA, 1977).[34]

Mark Rochon urged the government of the day to appreciate that improving the health system required multiple strategies. For example, the government wished to reduce wait times in ERs but didn't appreciate that out-of-hospital care (home and long-term care, for example) needed to be addressed to improve health system performance. This was important because he felt the OHA was shifting from a focus on advocacy for hospitals to advocacy for the health system. It led, for example, to promoting more funding for home care, even if that meant less funding for hospitals.[35]

There were other collaborations. In January 1963 the OHA contributed to the production of several educational filmstrips developed by the Department of Hospital Administration.[36]

HOOPP

Al Whiting made a comment earlier in this work on the value of HOOPP to retirees. IHPME grads have been a part of the governance of HOOPP, and it was a role that many took quite seriously as it affected their pension and that of their staffs. I recall that William Louth, the executive vice-president at Toronto General, who was himself a chartered accountant, took a keen interest in HOOPP operations and talked many times to HOOPP staff and board members about pension policy. At the time he was working for DHA grad Jim McNab.

Mark Rochon (MHSc, 1980) was involved with something called HOOPP Settlers as part of his OHA Board role. When he was OHA Board chair he pushed a policy to ensure that the OHA nominees to the board had appropriate competencies.[37]

HOOPP has become one of the world's strongest defined-benefit pension plans. In a World Bank report it was ranked first (along with the Ontario Teachers' Pension Plan) for investment performance by its global peers.[38] The report also noted that what they termed a "Canadian model" of public pensions was garnering international attention.[39] The report noted that publications such as the *Economist, Fortune*, and the *Financial Times* "have highlighted the unique approach and success of these growing public pension institutions" in Canada.[40]

The Change Foundation

The Change Foundation was formed in 1997 with proceeds from the sale of Blue Cross. It is an independent health policy think tank, modelled after the King's Fund in the United Kingdom, that works to inform positive change in Ontario's health system.[41] IHPME faculty/grads have received grants as well as being involved in its administration. Vivek Goel and Louise Lemieux Charles have served on its board,[42] and Shirlee Sharkey has been the board chair.[43] Jodeme Goldhar has been very involved in Change Foundation activities.

INTERSECTIONS

A Practice, Education, Research Tripartite Activity

The school and the institute were focused on practice (or performing a service), graduate education, and research that mutually reinforced and synergized each other. The practice component was in a tight connection to the community being served, whether it was in public health, patient care, a profession, the government, or other areas. It was also in the practitioner involvement in the program, which has been a strength of IHPME ever since it was founded in 1947.

The graduate education piece began with professional degree offerings in public health and hospital administration and expanded into academic degrees at the master's and doctorate levels. Research was always present but received an increasing emphasis. It also broadened to include basic, applied, and clinical research.

FitzGerald had a variant of this. We saw earlier that he was a bit more specific in his practice component, as his triad was teaching, research, and public service. In fact he noted this triad in his very first *Report to the President* in 1914.[44]

A Second Tripartite Activity: Academia, Government, and Public Enterprise

Another aspect of this triad is the close connections between the academy (and here we include the university, school, department, and institute), the government, and the field (which in our case can be either public institutions like hospitals or publicly administered health insurance plans).

We spoke earlier about Etzkowitz's "triple helix" (academia, government, and business) and the Lambert Report by the UK government, which dealt with business-university partnerships. In each there has been substantial attention given to focusing the fruits of publicly supported research on commercialization by the private sector. The importance for us is that both the institute and the school have been practising this for decades, each since its inception, long before Etzkowitz coined the term.

We noted a nuance in the school and labs, since the business component was owned by the university so that in essence it was a business component for the public good in three respects: its products priced at cost, the revenue it generated through a royalty stream that was ploughed back into research, and the jobs it created.

A key aspect of this triad was that the old manufacturing- and resource-based economy mainly involved a government-business interface. The new knowledge-based economy added a third component, universities, signalling their importance as economic engines. The School of Hygiene had come at this in a different way in that its application of the triad was for the public good, even though the economic aspects (increased government revenues and jobs) were also fully in place.

With the institute the business component was replaced with public institutions (e.g., hospitals community health centres, and health insurance commissions) it interacted with.

This points to a potential new triad of research and policy emphasis. We note that the focus of Etzkowitz's book and the Lambert Report is on strengthening the academic-business interface, with government as an important facilitator (hence the triad). But what about a similar paradigm aimed at strengthening the academic-public sector interface? What about research that is aimed at building strong public institutions?

This is not to disparage nor redirect attention away from the academic-business interface. But it is to recognize that a significant strength of any society is to have a strong and viable set of public institutions. The NHS in Britain is an example. Our universities, hospitals, and provincial health insurance plans in Canada are another, as are our Crown corporations. Publicly owned businesses in which this university was involved, like the former Connaught Labs or Telemedicine Canada, are another. Our pooled pension plans like HOOPP, Teachers, and OMERS for public institutions in Ontario are another, as are our sovereign wealth funds like the Alberta Heritage Savings Trust Fund and Northwest Territories Heritage Fund.

In fact Canada has a strong tradition of public enterprise, arguably a distinct characteristic of our national identity. Outstanding examples include Tommy Douglas and his hospital insurance plan of 1947 as well as his Crown corporations, which succeeded where private enterprise could not.[45] He then dipped into this university and IHPME's predecessor department for administrators to staff his hospitals and health insurance commission. But Douglas was not alone. There are numerous other examples of public enterprise in Canada.[46] Earlier we noted earlier IHPME initiatives like the NAO, C3.

One could say IHPME and its predecessor incarnations have been strengthening our health system institutions implicitly (through their professional education programs). But what about a broader and more explicit focus? This looks toward research that carves out the public sector as a topic of study and looks at how we strengthen our academic health sciences centres, our community hospitals, community health agencies, and public health offices. It looks toward research that puts our provincial health insurance plans under the same microscope under which the King's Fund and Health Foundation in Britain put the NHS. It looks at focusing attention so that we have studies like the Lambert Report but aimed at the public, not private, sector. The question for IHPME and the DLSPH is whether they have a role in fostering this. One could then ask whether other faculties in this university have a role in a similar focus on strengthening public enterprise in Canada.

What we advocate here amounts to strengthening Canadian sovereignty, to building Canadian capacity in areas noted above, and in fostering public institutions that are recognized as global leaders.

A Didactic University-Government Activity

The School of Hygiene and now the Dalla Lana School as well as IHPME have also been exhibiting a didactic university-government activity. But this is toward an end different from that of the tripartite university, government, business activity of Etzkowitz, which was aimed at an economic outcome. This one is a purpose-oriented activity to be a resource to governments. An example is the NAO, which provides research and consultation to national and sub-national governments.

It is an example of governments tapping into the expertise of academia, which has a long tradition. The United Kingdom did this in the First World War with the establishment of the Political Intelligence Department, which seconded Oxford historians. The Rowell-Sirois Commission did it in Canada in the late 1930s and the Hall Commission in the 1960s. But now we have purpose-driven units within academia set up specifically for that purpose.

Historically one had this in the close relationship that the School of Hygiene had to municipal and provincial public health officials, which began with FitzGerald and continued with subsequent directors.

THE IDEA OF NATION-BUILDING REVISITED

At the outset we said that recent literature suggests that health and health care can be looked at from the perspective of nation-building.

One could certainly make a strong case that the School of Hygiene, Departments of Hospital and Health Administration, and now the Dalla Lana School are very much a part of it. We had FitzGerald and his work to eradicate the scourge of diphtheria, not just in developing the antitoxin but in constantly driving its price down, and in working with local and provincial departments of public health to make it available to their citizens. We had his work in establishing a school of public health at this university, which in essence was a national school devoted in large measure to public health administration. We had his involvement in public health at the local, provincial, national, and international levels.

Similarly, Harvey Agnew, in IHPME's predecessor, the Department of Hospital Administration within this school, had the same concern about the administration of a public institution and development of a program to support it, but this time aimed at hospitals. It had the same national scope but this time with hospitals. There was also his concern, not just for management, but also for hospital construction and for funds for running them, this fostering of community spirit (in addition to providing a needed service), that this was nation-building.

Agnew's successor, Burns Roth, in delivering medical care in northern BC and running a hospital in Whitehorse, Yukon, was nation-building. The same can be said of his work with the Department of Public Health in Saskatchewan, simultaneously emphasizing universal health care as well as preventive care and public health. This vast experience was brought to the Toronto DHA program, where he also found time to be very involved in the Home Care Program for Metropolitan Toronto.

One could easily argue that the series of provincial and territorial health system profiles that Greg Marchildon is coordinating – this building of public awareness – is nation-building. Similarly, one could argue that the work of Hastings with the Conference of Health Ministers of Canada on community health centres was another example, and there is Steini Brown's work on C3.

We could give any number of additional examples of how the actions of faculty or graduates in Hygiene, Departments of Hospital and Health Administration, IHPME, and the DLSPH can be seen as nation-building.

HOSPITAL TRUSTEESHIP

In this work we have noted the involvement of a DHA graduate Sid Parsons and a hospital trustee Ted Hughes on an issue of hospital closure and of the involvement of Judge Hughes on the Saskatchewan and Canadian hospital associations as well as his work on the role of trustees. We noted MSc (Health Administration) student John Law's thesis topic on the role of hospital boards while Burns Roth was chair of the DOHA. There have also been articles by DPH and MHSC grads in *Leadership in Health Services*.[47] Prior to that the CHA had a journal titled *Hospital Trustee*. But it points to an area that neither the DOHA or IHPME has been involved in educationally.

This could be a continuing education opportunity for IHPME. The reader will recall that a deputy minister of health, Bob Bell, speaking at IHPME, noted that Ontario's volunteer hospital boards were "the best in the world."[48] Many in Ontario would agree with him. But a corollary is that it points to an opportunity. Hospitals and their role are becoming ever more complex. An ever increasing quality of trusteeship strengthens the role of the administrator, that of the hospital in its community, and of its relationship with government.

This has traditionally been a role for hospital associations in Canada and the United States. Both the Canadian and American hospital associations had a journal for hospital trustees. In addition, *Canadian Hospital* periodically had articles on hospital trusteeship.[49]

However, an argument could be made for the role of an academic centre to supplement the hospital association involvement or to be done in conjunction with it. One could make this argument in general terms – it would be beneficial to have such academically based continuing education for the trustees of all hospital boards, particularly so for the trustees of tertiary and quaternary health sciences centres, which themselves have such a large academic orientation.

IHPME is ideally positioned to play an effective role with its emphasis on management, quality, evaluation, and policy. Unlike hospital associations, it brings the mindset or mental discipline of the researcher to the equation. The aim is to build the quality of trusteeship, knowing that in doing so one is improving the system itself. It should be noted that the Rotman School at U of T has a program for corporate directors that it conducts with an association, the Institute of Corporate Directors.[50]

CHAPTER 28

Conclusion

DEPTH

Depth has three levels. First, the bench strength of the faculty. Faculty had extensive government, i.e., policy involvement. This included people like Roth and Marchildon who had deputy minister (DM) positions. Or Brown at the assistant deputy minister (ADM) level. Or graduates: Chatfield at the ADM and DM levels, or Rochon as ADM.

Faculty continued to play to their strengths. For example, Marchildon was approached by the Myanmar government twice (2014 and 2018) to help broker a peace for the central government. Health was only a small part of their need; their greater interest was in utilizing his knowledge of decentralized federations and his experience as deputy minister for the Premier's Office.[1]

Second, changing the intellectual landscape: Marchildon persuaded Johnson to recast and publish his Harvard dissertation on the Douglas government. Or his work coordinating individual studies of the evolution of provincial health systems. And Baker worked on high-performing systems.

Third, accomplishments: royal commission involvement: Hastings (Hall Commission), Marchildon (Romanow Commission); policy involvement: Hastings, his work with the Council of Ministers. Or one could point to business involvement: Livergant (Extendicare), McQueen (Agnew-Peckham). Or teaching hospital involvement: McNab (TGH), Turner, Freedman, Mapa (Mount Sinai); Hunt, Hadad (HSC); Dagnone (RUH, UH), Steven (Sunnybrook).

In addition, the department/institute constantly reinvented itself. We see under each successive director important new initiatives undertaken that broadened its activity and also contributed meaningfully to the continued evolution of the Canadian health-care system. This was due to the quality of faculty recruited at each step along the way.

IN CLOSING

The Program

An intriguing characteristic of the original department was the speed with which it assumed national leadership in its field, no doubt due to the prominence and connections of its first director. It is probably also the result of its placement within a school that also had a national as well as international footprint and its absorbing some of the elements of that culture. Evidence of its success is in the large number of applicants it received and in the leadership position attained by its graduates, not only in hospitals across the country, but also in those of world-class standing such as TGH and SickKids. The same could be said of graduates rising to the rank of deputy minister.

It is unclear that selling the labs, thereby severing the link between the labs and the school, then dissolving the school and putting some of its constituent parts within the Faculty of Medicine met expectations. The university (and Canada) lost momentum in public health; it also lost momentum in discovery research and a synergistic relationship between the two. Canada lost a company, its expertise and intellectual property to a foreign multinational.

What became IHPME ultimately flourished, but a very relevant question is whether this was somewhat inevitable, given the progressive leadership of the institute with its groundbreaking initiatives and recruitment of outstanding faculty. The answer is complex, as IHPME appears to have been energized by its relocations. The DLSPH could well serve as a yet another springboard to enhance what is taking place in IHPME.

The institute is a very different entity from its predecessor. It still has a strong practical focus, which has been strengthened by the introduction of the modular programs in health administration and health informatics, each of which focuses its intake on practitioners, people already working in the field. They bring their own unique perspectives based on their experience.

But this is no longer the sine qua non of the institute. Undergirding this practical focus, and the professional degree programs, is now a strong research faculty and a bright cadre of graduate students in master's, PhD, and postdoctoral programs. In this the institute has not only staked out an important new activity but also provided what could be the foundation to an important new climate for teaching in professional degree programs, one that uses research to inform practice.

Health Informatics has done just that. It has two streams in its MHI program, one that is modular and another that takes newly minted undergraduates in a regular full-time program. It makes for a rich student mixture with students in the modular stream, in a regular full-time professional stream, and in academic MSc and PhD programs.

And the decision to reconstitute a school of public health has borne substantial fruit, as we noted earlier with its number five position in the Shanghai rankings. But it is even more remarkable that this position of the DLSPH is part of a larger picture where U of T placed in the top ten in seven subject areas.[2] Importantly, as we have seen in this work, IHPME is both benefiter from and contributor to this position.

The People

One cannot come away from rooting through the archives and listening to hours upon hours of tapes on the history of the school and its departments by former directors without getting a sense of who these people were. Their reflections based on a lifetime of experience, the depth of their insight, their intense commitment – to their discipline, to graduate education, to building the health-care system of their country, give one a clear sense of the high calibre of these people.

One also gained a sense of these people as being at an intellectual frontier. They headed a school or one its departments that had leadership positions. Yet they continually questioned and re-evaluated their direction. For example, a large debate in the school in its final years was one between an applied, i.e., a practical, and a theoretical focus. Along with this was a debate on research and to what degree it should be emphasized, indeed, whether it should be applied or theoretical in its focus. That IHPME has been able to successfully pursue both is no small achievement.

One cannot but be in awe and somewhat humbled listening to these people, people who were a product of their experience, the scope and range of their thoughts. There were people like Mott who put in place the first hospital insurance program in North America, and who, along with Roth, built a provincial department of public health that earned an international reputation. Or Roth in his university role, along with Rhodes and Beaton, ruminating on the direction science and research were taking, sensing a tension within this university between using them to further theory or practice. For, given the high bar the U of T set for itself, at that time it was felt that a choice needed to be made, that it was very difficult to do both. These were individuals who had no rancour or resentment with a road taken they themselves would not have taken, such was their admiration and commitment to the university, its departments, and its disciplines.

It is challenging to convey the proper sense of these leaders, and those of the faculty who stand out, and their contribution to the knowledge of their discipline, but especially their strong desire to make a difference in the health care of this country. Given the sense of Canadians and how they hold health care as a public commons, what these people did is nation-building. Canada has pushed at many physical and geographic frontiers. Here, it pushed at intellectual and social frontiers no less formidable.

The people themselves put it most eloquently. Recently Ahmed Bayoumi, who has been a part of IHPME as both student and professor (in Clinical Epidemiology and Health Services Research), said, "IHPME students graduate with knowledge and skills on par with the very best programs internationally.... The large number of our graduates who have gone on to be global leaders in health research and health systems is a testament to the commitment of our faculty and our students to work at the very top of their fields."[3]

He then went on to make a statement that will dovetail perfectly with that of another IHPME faculty member. It points to the kind of creative, synergistic relationship that can be set up between faculty and student, teaching and research, where each energizes the other. He said, "That level of education also means that education is bidirectional – faculty teach but also learn from students."[4] Wendy Ungar, who has led the MSc in health technology assessment management, said, "A lot of my work is inspired by IHPME students' interests. Their passion to understand and assess emerging technologies is endlessly motivating. They are using cutting edge research methods and I am constantly learning from them."[5]

Rhonda Cockerill emphasized the talent of the students: "I never cease to be amazed at the depth and experience and talent in our student body. Over the past five years, we have added a number of new programs in recognition of emerging trends in healthcare. These have added great depth to our educational offerings, but what has not changed is the amazing talent found in every cohort."[6]

Its Contribution

These areas are getting at three results of the present IHPME. Bayoumi speaks of the synergies created from combining research and teaching. Ungar speaks to the synergies created between faculty and students and the importance of the student denominator. Rhonda speaks to the depth of student talent, to which could be added that of faculty. All of them speak to what we could call building capability and capacity. What IHPME is doing is giving Canada a capability and capacity in its "PME" areas. This is crucial. A country's good policy and management does not just happen. It takes the talent of first-class faculty and the synergy that arises between such faculty and equally talented students, tomorrow's leaders.

What governments need are institutes like IHPME that they can turn to as a resource. IHPME has deep expertise here with faculty that have been involved in government (Steini Brown, Greg Marchildon, and Mark Dobrow) and others seen as a resource to government (Ross Baker and Walter Wodchis).

Next, the potential; it is fashionable to talk about clusters. One could argue the University Avenue hospitals, their research institutes, the University of Toronto Faculty of Medicine, and the Dalla Lana School (of which IHPME is a part) form one of the world's great medical clusters, with their threefold concentration of patient care, teaching, and research. To this one could add a fourth component, application, recognizing that research lends itself to a kind of academic entrepreneurism, which can take place in either the private or public sectors.

And one could go further and argue that the responsibility of Ontario, indeed Canada, is to resource this world-class cluster. It's a tall order and one that in some ways goes against the Canadian grain. Canada likes to spread its support for its public institutions, and there are many good arguments for doing so. However, there are equally good arguments to differentiate and appropriately resource its world-class institutions and the personnel within them. The question for IHPME concerns its role in this potential.

Finally, through a study such as this, and many others that Canadian academics have made of the Canadian system, one quality of our system becomes apparent. We say that Canadian medicare is part of our identity. This statement could be broadened to Canadian health care generally. Canada has evolved a very distinctive health-care system. It has done so on the shoulders of many giants of the field – diverse people like a J.G. FitzGerald (an academic) or Tommy Douglas (a politician) and so many others. It is a public system, and its evolution has been on the foundation of public institutions such as health insurance, hospitals, IHPME, and the School of Hygiene, which form a kind of bedrock of the system. It is very much a heritage that should be treasured. It is also one that should be recognized as an essential characteristic of the Canadian identity.

This account, of necessity, has had to choose from the contributions of many, many individuals over the years. In having done so, it must be stressed that this is not to diminish in any way the great contribution of all of the people who have passed through these doors – people who have given unwaveringly throughout their careers, people who have influenced the lives of future practitioners and graduate students. This institute has contributed much to our Canadian health system. Its contribution rests on the shoulders of *all* of these people. They have travelled the length and breadth of this nation accumulating data for research or to administer complex facilities. They applied what they learned in professional roles or disseminated their knowledge through countless journal articles. They have prepared lectures without number to pass it on – to educate the next generation. This work stands as a testimony to their dedication.

This institute had its beginnings in a school that used research toward very practical ends. In the beginning the department that grew into the institute was almost exclusively practically oriented – the unprecedented and rapid growth of hospitals necessitated professional management. The institute was at the centre of establishing a new profession in this regard. And the heights that these graduates attained speaks to how well it discharged this activity. And it points to another piece of the Canadian identity, that it is characterized by an inclination of competence and earnestness.

But having said this, it wasn't long before this exclusive practical orientation gave way to an increasingly academic one, as some faculty began exploring new areas. It now pushes at the boundaries of its discipline in so many ways: high-performing systems, high-cost users, patient involvement in research, public and patient involvement in policy. It is increasingly being seen as a resource for government and NGOs.

We have unique characteristics in this school its departments and institutes. One is prompted to ask, Is this what makes this University – and this nation – strong? Though U of T is an Ontario-based university, is its national scope a source of strength? We see it in FitzGerald in the School of Hygiene and its connections to public health activities and people across the country.

Similarly we see it in Agnew in the Department of Hospital Administration in its hospital residency program that spanned the country and its graduates that came from and ended up across the country. We saw it in Hastings and Browne and their travels across the country. We see it in the more recent Brown and his work on circumpolar health.

Moreover, is the relationship of Saskatchewan, as a provincial example, with the school and the department another sign of the strength of this university and nation? Canada on the one hand is a highly decentralized federation. It can be prone to provincial parochialism. And yet, this fact notwithstanding, it is a nation where one province did not hesitate to forge links with a university in another province, links of an interprovincial or federal-provincial nature to solve health issues, educate health-care managers, or in order to build a stronger health system.

Moreover does this Saskatchewan–U of T connection illustrate how two entities at the cutting edge are just naturally drawn to each other? Saskatchewan's pioneering in public health under Maurice Seymour established important connections to the school during FitzGerald's time. Subsequent hospital and public health initiatives of the Douglas and Lloyd administrations established important connections to the Agnew and Roth eras in the Departments of Hospital Administration and Health Administration. Roth went from being a deputy minister in Saskatchewan to director of Hospital Administration at this university. Swanson had gone from a faculty position in Hospital Administration to executive director of the University Hospital in Saskatoon. We have previously noted these and other in-and-out people moving from the University Department of Hospital Administration to the Department of Public Health in Saskatchewan or Saskatchewan hospitals and back again.

There is also the interest of faculty had in Saskatchewan. Gene Vayda notes that while he was at McMaster University (in the early 1970s) he got funding for a conference for a second look at the Doctors' Strike, which drew a crowd from all over Canada.[7]

It may be linked to a comment our recent governor general made in a recent book on Canadian innovation in which he asks, "What is it about Saskatchewan? The province seems to be the birthplace of a disproportionately large number of advances in the delivery of health care."[8] It's a comment made not only from the perspective of his vice-regal office but also as a former academic and university president. Malcolm Taylor makes a similar comment regarding Saskatchewan's prominence in hospital and later health insurance. He queries why the Saskatchewan contribution to the process was so important and hints that it might have been its leadership.[9] Given Saskatchewan's cutting-edge activity in health, it is perhaps not hard to see its affinity and connection with a major academic department in the discipline doing the same.

This school and this department/institute have been at the forefront of the building of the Canadian system. The school, and Connaught Labs that was so intimately connected to it, mitigated the worst effects of a number of communicable diseases. It did this through discovery, the development of marketable products, and constantly driving down their price to make them widely available. But it also quickly found that organization and management were central to this success. In this way the genesis of IHPME in 1947 was somewhat inevitable.

The school and the department/institute were also at the centre of the evolution of this system. We tend to look at a select number of dramatic events, such as medical insurance, as being defining moments, and, indeed, they were. However, very early on, Canada began to set the tone of its health system, to differentiate itself from its southern neighbour. Canadians looked to government at the federal, provincial, and municipal levels to solve the ravages of diseases such as diphtheria, and people like FitzGerald in its public institutions rose to the challenge.

These public institutions included the three levels of government. They also included institutions like U of T, which, through its School of Hygiene, was involved at a variety of levels, from local and provincial boards of health, to the Dominion Council of Health. It funded research aimed at applied outcomes and played a significant role in addressing diseases such as diphtheria, diabetes, and polio. It had a significant involvement in both world wars.

It came as no surprise that this involvement extended to another public institution that was growing throughout Canada, one that was becoming an important new modality of care, as well as the proud symbol of communities' commitment to health care. They elicited untold hours of voluntarism at a host of levels in support of their mission. The school responded to a need for a new breed of manager to operate these new facilities, which had a level of complexity quite unlike anything else in society.

There was another aspect to this contribution, and here the school anticipated what would become an established act of universities. This had to do not only with their educational role or their research role, but an added economic role. Vivek Goel, former chair of IHPME and now vice-president, Research and Innovation at the U of T, noted in a *Globe and Mail* article, "One hundred years ago, Dr FitzGerald was moved to action as he witnessed diphtheria claim the lives of children. He saw a need and mobilized his scientific knowledge and university resources to make it right. He did so not to make money or create jobs, but in focusing on what was right, he achieved both of those in spades. That's the model that we need to emulate – combining passion, knowledge, and institutional support in new ways to make a difference that benefits us all."[10] And one is reminded of his overriding aim that it be "within reach," "available to all."

Canadians expected state support to deal with diseases like these and others like tuberculosis, cancer, and polio. FitzGerald and his successors rose to this challenge as well. Canadians expected state support for the building and operations of hospitals. They evolved a unique mechanism of a private corporation that was publicly administered and funded. In fact what we see in the evolution of the Canadian health system is a successive layering over time of responses to challenges from which a unique character of its health system emerges.

It raises the issue of the impact that an institute such as IHPME has had – on students and on the health-care scene. It began with hospital management, but as the system grew and continued to evolve, new and important other areas began to emerge and IHPME was at the forefront of addressing them, hence its nomenclature that highlights its commitment to policy and outcomes. And if we to look at present areas of concentration in IHPME we see it is the same today, with it at the vanguard of areas such as integrated care, public engagement, and the learning health system.

And in terms of impact it all comes back to people – the faculty of IHPME and how they have helped grow a system and the professionals who work within it. It is hard to know how many young minds and characters have been shaped by their time at this institute and this university.

One recalls an earlier statement by Farley that the International Health Division of the Rockefeller Foundation had a pattern of judging a program by the calibre of the personnel involved. This institute, the two schools of public health, the faculties of medicine and nursing, the university itself, have seen people of unrivalled ability walk their halls – people who have had international impact, people whose intelligence and dedication is almost palpable. It is easy in their shadow to lose sight of the countless others with high ability and equal dedication who have made their contribution. We need to celebrate all these people.

This is a great institute and a great university. U of T does well in international metrics, and this is an objective measure. There is also a subjective component, one based on objective evidence but moving beyond that as a sole measure of the quality of the institution. An aspect of this measure is how seriously U of T takes its public mandate. An example is J.G. FitzGerald starting not one, but two world-class organizations within the university, each dedicated to a public purpose.

When the Rockefeller Foundation picked three places in the world in the 1920s that it would seed as schools of public health, it picked Harvard, Johns Hopkins, and U of T. We see not only groundbreaking discoveries such as insulin that FitzGerald helped to fund, we also see an unwavering commitment to making health care available to all, "within reach of everyone."

And similarly, when the Kellogg Foundation was going to fund four places in hospital administration, it looked to U of T. And the university and the school rose to the challenge. We saw how quickly the institute ramped up a hospital management program of national stature. We saw the types of people it attracted, people like Burns Roth who was a deputy minister in one of the best departments of public health in the world. We see Fred Mott, recruited by Roth, a foremost authority in health insurance and rural health, and another former Saskatchewan deputy minister. We see the institute constantly pushing at the boundaries, consistently reinventing itself, not just to evolve with the evolving health system but to lead it.

Its roots lay in what we had in the early 1900s, a group of dedicated physicians at this university who had an overriding concern for public health. There was a very specific nuance to that concern, one that was in complete sync with the evolution of the Canadian health scene: it needed to truly benefit everyone with its results. But these same individuals quickly found that in articulating this concern, one was necessarily and successively involved in organization and management, in systems, in policy, and in assessing outcomes – the very activities IHPME practises today.

But it is not only what IHPME practises, it is how. It is not only competence, but also character. That IHPME is the former is without question, and all the traditional measures such as publications, citations, and impact-factors provide objective measures. But the latter really sets it apart, though this may be part of a larger picture in that it may be a part of what sets U of T apart and what puts IHPME squarely at the centre of what U of T is.

It was noted that IHPME stepped up to the plate for a young Syrian doctor who was denied re-entry into the United States to continue graduate studies. But it says so much more than the stepping up for one person, as important as that was. It is the values that this action embodies. This institute, this university is about so much more than simply imparting knowledge. As complex as this is, it is the simple part.

The more so are the values of humanity it imparts, that it lives. J.G. FitzGerald was going to make his antitoxins and vaccines, "within reach" – available to everyone. With the insulin discovery they took out a patent not to make the IP proprietary but to do the exact opposite. The School of Hygiene was turning out a phalanx of public health administrators to bring population health to everyone. This institute began with hospitals because they rapidly emerged as centres of care. And in Canada they were also rooted in a public as opposed to a private (for-profit) mission. They were (and are) a public trust. In this vast country the public's commitment to their local hospital stands as a common thread across this nation.

But in the twenty-first century the mission of this institute in these values is expanding. Its orbit is increasing. It now not only puts this education "within reach" of Canadians, including a young physiotherapist from Moose Factory, it defends a Syrian's right to have such education "within reach." It not only examines health policy in Ontario, but also in other provinces, and federally. Through the NAO it looks at it in the context of other national and sub-national entities, which is very appropriate for a North American continent with three large federated countries. It not only looks at the challenges of health in the north – and here we need to separate Canada into the near north and the far north – in terms of the far north it looks at circumpolar health care, i.e., the common challenges among countries in health care in the far north.

The common denominator of all this is people. One needs only talk to the faculty involved to get a clear sense of their deep commitment to education, but ultimately to people. These faculty, students, and alumni make a difference. This work stands as a testament to all of these people. Their caring deepens our humanity. It is enriching to know them.

ITS LINKS TO OUR HISTORY

And through all this we have IHPME, intentionally or not, moving in lockstep with the evolution of the system writ large. At each successive stage of the evolution of the Canadian system one can see an evolution in IHPME. At its founding in 1947 there was substantial hospital activity taking place around it, in Canada and the United States, particularly in Saskatchewan, which began rapid expansion of hospitals with the implementation that year of hospital insurance. And one of IHPME's very first students went to that province to join the Tommy Douglas team. Hospital activity across the country was given an impetus with the passage of the health grants legislation in 1948.

The original Department of Hospital Administration program merged with public health and renamed itself as *health* administration in 1967. On 1 July 1968 Canadian medicare, which focused on a Canadian health system, became a reality. Then in the 1970s the Council of Ministers and the department (under John Hastings) explored community health options. And so it goes.

System complexity continues apace, in everything from the development of public policy, health, from primary care to community health centres, to patient as agent. Graduating managers who take their place in everything from hospitals in myriad cities and towns across Canada – places where the administrator is looked upon not only as a manager but as a prominent person in the community. Or managers delivering health in Canada's frontiers – its near north (Moose Factory) or far north (its territories).

Or at the apex, academic health science centres of almost unimaginable complexity, institutions that are small communities in themselves, with more than 10,000 employees and $1 billion in annual expenditures. Institutions that combine patient care with the education of the future providers of that care. Institutions with research institutes that are establishments in themselves, organizations that rival the size of some universities, but with a wider variety of research, a greater emphasis on applied and clinical research. And IHPME is placing managers in all these institutions.

But this is not the end of the story. IHPME's research has eclipsed its professional management. And its professional management curriculum is in many ways built upon a research foundation. This research emphasis is exactly what is needed to deal with system complexity. Further, maintaining and improving the quality of the system is built upon academic evaluation. This ability is also a resource for governments and other organizations for project-related work.

IHPME has evolved through all this – from a concentration on *hospital* administration at a very applied level, to *health* administration, to combining research with management instruction, to moving beyond institutional management to a focus on policy and evaluation, then from a teaching and research centre to a policy institute.

IHPME has endeavoured to provide managers for this system. It had attempted to conduct research on and for the system and educate other researchers who will critically appraise the system.

Faculty were successively involved in teaching, first in hospital operations, later community health, health policy, program evaluation, health epidemiology, health informatics, technology transfer, the list goes on – a successive layering of new academic activity. And their grads were involved in aspects of institutional operations.

Faculty like J.G. FitzGerald, H. Agnew, and B. Roth were bound up in our national history. It is the same with institutions in the Toronto cluster (e.g., TGH, TWH, PMH, SickKids, and others). The same could be said of institutions across Canada. Building these institutions were stretch goals for Canada. And now the new frontier is building research institutes, which represent similar stretch goals. One cannot separate the history of IHPME (or that of U of T) from this larger history. And this larger history might also be that the fact that these are all public institutions, a piece of the Canadian identity – the value it places in its public institutions.

Recall that Charles Dickens wrote the GOSH into the public's heart. This gets at it precisely. Canadian medicare, the NHS, GOSH, the School of Hygiene, Connaught Labs, our hospitals – these reside in the public's heart. And they have been written there by people like Barrie, Dickens, and Braithwaite. They have also been written there by the countless people who have worked in these institutions. Graduates of IHPME, but also everyone who has worked in such institutions and formed a bond with them or identified with public health insurance. One need only talk to some of these individuals to see how such sentiments are written into their hearts. This has become a public trust that IHPME has been charged with.

And this public trust is complex, for IHPME is furthering not only what medicare is but what medicare symbolizes. And the latter is equally important and just as complex as the first. Danny Boyle gets at it with his choreography of the NHS and GOSH at the London 2012 Olympics. Dickens and Braithwaite get at it in their writing of their respective country's pre-eminent children's hospitals. All of these institutions – children's hospitals, community general hospitals, a school of hygiene, a department of hospital administration – they embody and they capture an essence of the human spirit. We see in this work people like FitzGerald, Defries, Eugenie Stuart, Elizabeth McMaster, Edith Kathleen Russell, and Jean Gunn – people of a singular dedication and ability. There are countless others. One does not pore through all the archival materials without getting to know these people and their singular dedication to their work, to an ideal, to the students, all of which come together to building health care in Canada.

And speaking of students or graduates, the contribution of neither can be ignored. Students in the professional programs bring a particular combination of practicality and academic curiosity. There are now a large number of students in the research programs and they much add to the research climate of the institute.

Then there are the graduates. For about the first fifty years of the program they were predominately in health administration. As the result of space considerations, in these pages we have seen brief vignettes of all too few of them. They give but a glimpse of their cumulative contributions. We have noted that hospitals are prominent institutions in Canada. In many communities they are *the* prominent institution, and hospital administrators are looked upon not only for their role in the hospital but also as community leaders.

We Canadians tend to be a deferential lot. But these graduates made Canada proud. Canada took an approach to health administration slightly different from that of the United Kingdom and the United States. But these graduates put Canada on the map internationally. We may be deferential, but we are also earnest. We have seen in our too few vignettes how these MHSC graduates distinguished themselves, leading in their community and their profession.

There is a certain current of history in this. FitzGerald was a graduate of this university. Roth almost was but didn't quite graduate from IHPME's predecessor department, such was the urgency he felt to become part of the Tommy Douglas experiment in health.

At all times IHPME has been a part of and ahead of this current, this wave. It initially concentrated on hospitals, then moved to a concern with the administration of other organizations, and from this to policy, and then outcomes. Given all this, throughout its seventy-year history, throughout the commitment of its faculty, students, and alumni, throughout its place in this great university, it has had a fascinating evolution. It has moved from a purely practical orientation to now one of a major research focus, and this has come full circle. Even today, through its research, IHPME seeks to make a practical difference, to have impact, which is what FitzGerald so clearly emphasized.

We see how interlinked it all is. Public health, public health nursing, public health administration, hospital administration, nurses involved in hospital administration, prevention, and more.

We spoke of wonder. Now it is at a different level. There is a sense of wonder at the ability of FitzGerald and the good he did for the health-care scene in Canada, in everything from public health, medicines at cost, medical education, to health promotion; and this is by no means an exhaustive list. There are people like Burns Roth, Robert Defries, Eugenie Stuart – earnest people of exceptional ability.

Throughout the history of IHPME or the DLSPH, there has been a building of capacity. In the 1920s Canada needed to be doing so in public health, in the 1940s it needed to be doing so in hospital administration, in the 1960s in health administration, in the 1990s in policy and evaluation, and in the 2010s in comparative systems (and in Canada especially in comparative sub-national systems), evidence-based analysis, informatics, and the like. In fact, is our health-care system ever really truly ours if we cannot take it to this higher intellectual level?

IHPME has had a successive layering of new activity upon old and with this continually evolved to areas of greater complexity. It has pursued each of its areas with great sophistication. For example, at its inception and through the 1950s it was involved solely in teaching hospital administration. But even then it had some of the characteristics we have identified – an outward focus. The program was immediately of national scope. It was also immediately part of the national dialogue in its area, in response to the school's choice of director, Harvey Agnew, and his connections across Canada and his role in *Canadian Hospital*. The department was not only graduating new administrators, it was expanding the dialogue in its field.

In the 1960s its subject area expanded; it was now *health* administration. The 1970s saw new attention to research in addition to teaching; the 1980s a move into graduate education to supplement that in professional education; the 1990s moving into policy and evaluation; the 2000s into research administration; and the 2010s into comparative systems.

The study of comparative systems is really resurrecting something with which FitzGerald was concerned throughout his international initiatives – its international focus. It is linked with Toronto being identified as a world city. U of T is becoming a world university, with its large proportion of foreign students, the Munk School of Global Affairs, and IHPME's Shandong University partnership, and IHPME with the NAO is furthering this mission.

And within this continual expansion one has the complexity of the mission. On the one hand there is academic research, all very dispassionate.

And yet the subject matter is anything but. The subject that IHPME and Dalla Lana deal with encompasses our most cherished institutions. We have seen how the British feel very strongly about the NHS and their hospitals, so much so that they showcased it at the 2012 London Olympics opening ceremony. We have seen how an author like J.M. Barrie was moved to support a children's hospital through an assignment of rights of one of the world's most popular children's tales – an act that somehow makes the story itself just that much more heart-warming. We have seen Canadians are no different in medicare or their hospitals.

We have noted the allusions to health-care and nation-building by both academics and politicians. In the former we note our own heavyweights in this arena, people like J.G. FitzGerald, and the people he hired, heavyweights in their own right, like Defries and Fraser. Regarding the latter, Tommy Douglas stands out, charting a new course for his province and his nation.

Douglas's actions necessitated a new type of sophistication in government, and with one of our early alums he set about building a Department of Public Health and a civil service that was without equal. Douglas took health personally; a health mission was written into his heart. This is why he took it as his ministerial portfolio in his first term. This played right into the hands of IHPME's predecessor department. Douglas hired some of its earliest grads and over the years hired others and sent others to Toronto to the program, one of which was Burns Roth, who grew up around hospitals, was one of the earliest students of this program, but one who early on saw that they were part of a larger picture. As Douglas's deputy minister of public health he built one of the outstanding departments in its field, one that almost immediately combined public health with health care. The same thing happened when he came to run IHPME's predecessor department, the school combined the same two entities under him.

To jump to the present, we see IHPME and Dalla Lana faculty pushing the envelope in their own right, through their teaching, their research, and what we have called their academic entrepreneurism, their setting up new organizational entities to bring knowledge to bear, to have impact.

With Steini Browne we have the same kind of insight, this same pushing of the envelope. He did it with IHPME and he does it now with Dalla Lana. Through him we see the university extending its mandate, emphasizing communication and impact, engaging with government and public. We see him working with a donor on a lecture series to bring distinguished speakers, faculty, practitioners, and the public together in dialogue. We see actions such as these and the contemplation of a health policy institute as actions to further build the health heritage of this nation.

It is easy to miss the magnitude of the accomplishment of launching this program in 1947, placing it within a school of public health and almost immediately making it into a pre-eminent program in the world. Its location within a public health school was a particularly important decision for, in Canada (unlike the United States), the values of public health are much more akin to health management than are those of business.

Then in the same year Douglas launched his hospital insurance initiative, which ultimately drew Burns Roth to Saskatchewan. Unbeknownst at the time, Canada was differentiating itself from the United States in health care and building a unique part of its identity. This started with hospital insurance in 1947, particularly with medical insurance in Saskatchewan in 1962. And here there are connections to the school, for Robin Badgley ended up here after he left the Saskatchewan experiment in preventive and community medicine.

The DOHA folded in public health in 1967 and then pushed into research in the 1970s. Now its research is every bit as important as its professional degrees. It is even more remarkable how it is using its research expertise to launch of new activities that move this research into an applied activity. IHPME has actually become very entrepreneurial in its research applications. It is easy to miss the magnitude of these outcomes, and Canadians are prone to such an oversight.

There is another very subtle factor in this history easily overlooked: whether IHPME and the DLSPH have been integral participants in one of the twentieth century's greatest achievements. Many would argue that the post–Second World War notion of universal, comprehensive health-care coverage pursued in conjunction with public health has been important, not just in improving health generally but in promoting human solidarity and community.

We see that in granting an equal right to health without distinction, people are joined to one another in a unique way. That is why a Danny Boyle singles it out in an Olympic opening broadcast around the world. That is why the UN comes together to pass a special resolution to have UHC as a world objective. That is why the people of the United Kingdom and Canada rank their national health systems as their most cherished institution in repeated polls.

All this points to yet another subtlety: whether IHPME, the DLSPH, and their faculty and graduates are vouchsafing one of humanity's more significant accomplishments. In the grand sweep of history UHC is very young, but it is gaining momentum. And other universal programs are being contemplated. Add to this the global concern for public health. Where this will all lead is anyone's guess. But the question it raises is whether health is the ultimate unifier of humanity.

We can be sure of the necessity of IHPME and its parent the DLSPH. As noted earlier in this work, universal health programs are amongst the largest peacetime initiatives ever undertaken. They go hand-in-hand with public health, which has a longer history. But knowledge never stands still. The research base of the IHPME and the DLSPH is absolutely fundamental, not only to its graduate professional education but also as a resource for governments and civil services. This type of capacity, to generate the managers and researchers, to have the research expertise available for external clients, is a national resource.

It is a chain of continual beginnings. Today IHPME, with its breadth and depth of research expertise, its connection to health-care institutions, to different levels of government, its cadre of bright young graduate students and postdocs, is at a threshold. It is a formidable combination.

Stay tuned.

Notes

ACKNOWLEDGMENTS

1 Nancy Williams and Marie Scott-Baron, eds, *Reflections of a Neighbourhood: Huron-Sussex from UTS to Stop Spadina* (Toronto: Words Indeed Publishing, 2013), 218, 220. Harold Averill was instrumental in getting this book published. It won a North America–wide Independent Book Publisher Award. The University of Toronto is a part of this neighbourhood.

ABBREVIATIONS

1 The journal was renamed in 1943. It had been known as the *Canadian Public Health Journal*. It was felt that the rearrangement of the words in the title better centred attention on "public health." See Editorial Section, "The Canadian Journal of Public Health," *Canadian Journal of Public Health* 34, no. 1 (January 1943): 39.

CHAPTER ONE

1 See United Nations, General Assembly, "Global Health and Foreign Policy," Resolution 67/81, 12 December 2012, https://www.un.org/en/ga/search/view_doc.asp?symbol=A/RES/67/81.
2 The caption on the cover is "Within Reach, Universal Health Care Worldwide," *Economist*, 28 April 2018.
3 See Oxfam, *Public Good or Private Wealth*, 2019, https://oxfamilibrary.openrepository.com/bitstream/handle/10546/620599/bp-public-good-or-private-wealth-210119-en.pdf.
4 See General Assembly of the United Nations, "Moving Together to Build a Healthier World."
5 See Chatham House, "Universal Health Cover Forum," https://www.chathamhouse.org/about/structure/global-health-security/universal-health-coverage-policy-forum-project.
6 See Robert Yates, "Universal Health Coverage Is a Potent Vote Winner," 9 December 2016, Chatham House, Royal Institute of International Affairs, https://www.chathamhouse.org/expert/comment/universal-health-coverage-potent-vote-winner.
7 L. Boehm and Mark Dobrow, with Robert Yates, personal conversation (via Skype), 3 July 2019.
8 Department of Health Administration, *The Program in Hospital Administration: Past, Present and Future*, June 1961, 1, A1998-0023/002, University of Toronto Archives and Records Management Services (UTARMS).
9 See Nicholas Timmins, *The Five Giants: A Biography of the Welfare State*

(London: HarperCollins, 1995) – the entire book is interesting, but especially chaps 1–3 on Beveridge and related events and chaps 6–7 on the NHS; Charles Webster, *The National Health Service: A Political History* (Oxford: Oxford University Press, 1998). In each case the original editions are cited, as they are deemed to be the best version.

10 See Eric Manheimer, *Twelve Patients: Life and Death at Bellevue Hospital* (New York: Grand Central Publishing, 2012); see 339–40 for the genesis of the book. See also *Newsweek*, "World's Best Hospitals 2019," 2019, https://www.newsweek.com/best-hospitals-2019.

11 Fernand Braudel, *Afterthoughts on Material Civilization and Capitalism*, trans. Patricia M. Ranum (Baltimore, MD: Johns Hopkins University Press, 1977), 9. This book is the published version of a lecture series delivered at Johns Hopkins in 1974.

12 Braudel, *Afterthoughts on Material Civilization and Capitalism*, 10.

13 Braudel, *Afterthoughts on Material Civilization and Capitalism*, 10.

14 Braudel, *Afterthoughts on Material Civilization and Capitalism*, 10.

15 Antoine Prost, "Public and Private Spheres in France," in *A History of Private Life*, vol. 5, *Riddles of Identity in Modern Times*, ed. Antoine Prost and Gérard Vincent, trans. Arthur Goldhammer (Cambridge, MA: Belnap of Harvard University Press, 1991), 98.

16 This is a select list that especially gets at a description of the times and the magnitude of what was accomplished: Correlli Barnett, *The Audit of War: The Illusion and Reality of Britain as a Great Nation* (London: Macmillan, 1986), chap. 1, "The Dream of New Jerusalem," esp. 14–32. See also the books listed in note 9 above.

17 Barnett, *Audit of War*, 19.

18 Saskatchewan, Legislative Assembly, "Budget Debate," *Debates*, 18 March 1947, http://docs.legassembly.sk.ca/legdocs/Legislative%20Assembly/Hansard/10L4S/470318Debates.pdf.

19 Malcolm G. Taylor, *Health Insurance and Canadian Public Policy: The Seven Decisions That Created the Canadian Health Insurance System and Their Outcomes*, 3rd ed. (Montreal and Kingston: McGill-Queen's University Press, 2009), 111.

20 Great Britain, House of Commons, *Parliamentary Debates*, 5th ser., vol. 26, 1911 (London: His Majesty's Stationery Office, 1911), 25 May 1911, coll. 509.

21 Dorothy Porter, *Health, Civilization and the State: A History of Public Health from Ancient to Modern Times* (London: Routledge, 1999), 216.

22 Porter, *Health, Civilization and the State*, 215.

23 Porter, *Health, Civilization and the State*, 217.

24 Saskatchewan, Health Services Planning Commission, *Report on Operations of the Saskatchewan Hospital Services Plan, Covering the Organization Period in 1946 and the Calendar Year 1947* (Regina: Thos. H. McConica, King's Printer, 1948), 9, 13.

25 For the scope of the BC service, see British Columbia, *Fifth Annual Report B.C. Hospital Insurance Service, January 1st to December 31st 1953* (Victoria: Don McDiarmid, Queen's Printer, 1954), 9–16.

26 See interview with Burns Roth, audiocassette #1/6, School of Hygiene History Project, B89-0009, UTARMS. See also F.B. Roth, "Division of Hospital Administration and Standards," in Saskatchewan, *Annual Report of the Department of Public Health, 1950–51* (Regina: Thos. H. McConica, Queen's Printer,

1952), 80. Roth became director of the Division of Hospital Administration and Standards in 1950.

27 See "People," *Canadian Hospital* 47, no. 9 (September 1970): 21.

28 "People," 21.

29 The Whitehall I study. The archives are housed at the London School of Hygiene and Tropical Medicine, https://www.lshtm.ac.uk/research/library-archives-service/archives/whitehall-study-archive-collection.

30 Marc Lalonde, *A New Perspective on the Health of Canadians* (Ottawa: Minister of Supply and Services Canada, 1974).

31 Great Britain, House of Commons, *Debates*, vol. 447, Mr Bevan, 9 February 1948 (London: HMSO, 1948), coll. 50.

32 Timmins, *Five Giants*, 4–5.

33 Meeting between Chris Ham and me, 12 November 2019.

34 Great Britain, House of Commons, *Debates*, vol. 447, Mr Bevan.

35 Here is a select list. On the school, the best source is Bator's *Within Reach of Everyone*, which is cited numerous times in this work. On the labs there are two by its former director, the person who followed and was the protégé of FitzGerald, Robert Defries. They are *The Connaught Medical Research Laboratories, 1914–1949* ([Toronto: University of Toronto, 1950]), and *The First Forty Years, 1914–1955, Connaught Medical Research Laboratories, University of Toronto* (Toronto: University of Toronto Press, 1968).

36 University of Toronto, *A First Look*, 1, n.d., UTARMS. The publication is bound U of T calendar material for 1978–79.

37 University of Toronto, *First Look*, 2.

38 University of Toronto, *First Look*, 6.

39 University of Toronto, *Register of the University of Toronto for the Year 1920*, 44.

40 University of Toronto, *First Look*, 6. See also Martin L. Friedland, *The University of Toronto: A History* (Toronto: University of Toronto Press, 2002), 158–61, 164–6, 168.

41 Correspondence with John Browne, 19 May 2018.

42 School of Hygiene, *Twenty-Third Annual Report, 1947–1948*, 3, file "School of Hygiene Annual Report, 1941–1955," S013.002, UTARMS.

43 "Draft Speaking Points, Bernie Sanders Convocation Hall Event," 1, author's personal records. I was also in the audience for this event.

44 "Draft Speaking Points." The three sections in quotations occur on 2, 3, and 1 respectively.

45 Frederick D. Mott, "Some Aspects of the Case for State Medicine," *McGill Medical Undergraduate Journal* 1 (January 1932): 6.

46 See Noah Miller, "The Ten Best Hospitals in the World," *Newsweek*, 20 March 2019, https://www.newsweek.com/2019/04/05/10-best-hospitals-world-1368512.html.

47 See, for example, *For the Common Good, Superintendent's Report, Toronto General Hospital, 1923*.

48 *For the Common Good*, 1.

49 The hospital's war scars are still evident. The ruin of the former Rudolf Virchow Lecture Hall, host to some of the top minds in the world, was destroyed by bombing toward the end of the Second World War. It was restored, but not fully, in the 1990s and is used for scientific conferences, press conferences, formal events, and concerts.

50 David Oshinsky, *Bellevue: Three Centuries of Medicine and Mayhem at America's Most Storied Hospital* (New York: Doubleday, 2016), 318.
51 Virginia Berridge, *Public Health: A Very Short Introduction* (Oxford: Oxford University Press, 2016), 23.
52 Martin L. Friedland, *The University of Toronto: A History*, 2nd ed. (Toronto: University of Toronto Press, 2013), 669.
53 John Farley, *To Cast Out Disease: A History of the International Health Division of the Rockefeller Foundation, 1913–1951* (New York: Oxford University Press, 2004), 221.
54 "Interview with Dr Burns Roth, Reel #1," 16 July 1985, 2, transcript, School of Hygiene History Project, B89-0009, UTARMS. Note, this item comes in four different media: a written transcript (which is an abridgement), the original reel-to-reel, an audiocassette, and a digitized form done in 2017 (which vastly improved the sound quality by eliminating almost all of the interference). The last version became available only late in the development of the manuscript, so the other forms were also used.
55 "Interview with G.H. Beaton," 20 August 1985, 41:39, digitized audio recording, School of Hygiene History Project, B1989-0009_05S, UTARMS.

CHAPTER TWO

1 See Glen O'Hara and George Campbell Gosling, "Healthcare as Nation-Building in the Twentieth Century: The Case of the British National Health Service," in *Healthcare in Private and Public from the Early Modern Period to 2000*, ed. Paul Weindling (London: Routledge, 2015), 123. See also Lutz Lessering, "Introduction to the Book Series 'German Social Policy,'" in Michael Stolleis, *Origins of the German Welfare State: Social Policy in Germany to 1945*, trans. Thomas Dunlap (Heidelberg: Springer, 2013), 1.
2 O'Hara and Gosling, "Healthcare as Nation-Building," 127.
3 Tom Parkin, "What Canada Needs Now Is Another Tommy Douglas," *Maclean's*, 2 May 2018, https://www.macleans.ca/opinion/what-canada-needs-now-is-another-tommy-douglas/.
4 See Lutz Lessering, "Nation State and Welfare State: An Intellectual and Political History," *Journal of European Social Policy* 13, no. 2 (May 2003): 175.
5 O'Hara and Gosling, "Healthcare as Nation-Building," 123.
6 Webster, *National Health Service*, 8. There is a second edition of this work, but the first edition is the better one. Another good history by the same author is *The Health Services since the War*, 2 vols (London: HMSO, 1988).
7 Webster, *National Health Service*, 132.
8 Thomas H. Marshall, *Citizenship.Social Class and Other Essays* (Cambridge: Cambridge University Press, 1950), 56.
9 Ilona Kickbusch and Christian Franz, "Conceptualizing the Health Economy," in *The Road to Universal Health Coverage: Innovation, Equity, and the New Health Economy*, ed. Jeffrey L. Sturchio, Ilona Kickbusch, and Louis Galambos (Baltimore, MD: Johns Hopkins University Press, 2018), 19.
10 Kickbusch and Franz, "Conceptualizing the Health Economy," 18.
11 Pascal Zurn, Jim Campbell, Jeremy Lauer, Ibadat Dhillon, Tana Wuliji, and Jean-Louis Arcand, "The Relationship between Health Employment and Economic Growth," in Sturchio, Kickbusch, and Galambos, *Road to Universal Health Coverage*, 45.

12 Kickbusch and Franz, "Conceptualizing the Health Economy," 19.
13 Kickbusch and Franz, "Conceptualizing the Health Economy," 25.
14 Sarah Reed, Anya Göpfert, Suzanne Wood, Dominique Allwood, and Will Warburton, *Building Healthier Communities: The Role of the NHS as an Anchor Institution* (London: Health Foundation, August 2019).
15 See Porter, *Health, Civilization and the State*, 232–4.
16 O'Hara and Gosling, "Healthcare as Nation-Building," 129.
17 Royal Institute of International Affairs, "Memorandum on Important Changes in the Labour Situation and Social Conditions in Great Britain since the Outbreak of War," document no. 17, Conference on North Atlantic Relations, 4–9 September 1941, 17.
18 Correspondence with Chatham House staff (19 August 2019) indicates that the conference was convened by the American Committee for International Studies and held at Proul's Neck, Maine.
19 Richard M. Titmuss, *Problems of Social Policy* (London: His Majesty's Stationery Office, 1950), 504.
20 Webster, *National Health Service*, 2.
21 Webster, *National Health Service*, 2.
22 Great Britain, *Parliamentary Debates*, 5th ser., vol. 487, session 1950–51, 23 April 1951 (London: His Majesty's Stationery Office, 1951), coll. 38.
23 Great Britain, *Parliamentary Debates*, 5th ser., vol. 487, session 1950–51, 23 April 1951, colls 38–9.
24 Great Britain, *Parliamentary Debates*, 5th ser., vol. 487, session 1950–51, 23 April 1951, coll. 42.
25 Nigel Lawson, *The View from No. 11: Memoirs of a Tory Radical* (London: Bantam, 1992), 613. He notes on this page it was also the third-largest employer and bureaucracy in the world (after the Indian railway system and the Red Army).
26 Charles Webster, "Introduction," in *Aneurin Bevan on the National Health Service*, ed. Charles Webster (Oxford: University of Oxford, Wellcome Unit for the History of Medicine, 1991), 1.
27 Peter Baldwin, *The Politics of Social Solidarity: Class Bases of the European Welfare State, 1875–1975* (Cambridge: Cambridge University Press, 1990), 1.
28 Baldwin, *Politics of Social Solidarity*, 1.
29 Baldwin, *Politics of Social Solidarity*, 1.
30 For an excerpt of the 29 November 2004 broadcast, see CBC, "And the Greatest Canadian of All Time Is …," https://www.cbc.ca/archives/entry/and-the-greatest-canadian-of-all-time-is. See also Guy Dixon, "The Greatest Canadian," *Globe and Mail*, 30 November 2004, https://www.theglobeandmail.com/arts/the-greatest-canadian/article1144309/.
31 Thomas Piketty, *Capital in the Twenty-First Century* (Cambridge, MA: Belknap of Harvard University Press, 2014), 629n12.
32 Webster, *National Health Service*, 29.
33 Ipsos MORI, *State of the Nation 2013: Where Is Bittersweet Britain Heading?* (London: British Future, 2013) 26; see also 16–17. See also Mark Britnell, *In Search of the Perfect Health System* (London: Palgrave, 2015), 3.
34 See Anna Quigley, "Maintaining Pride in the NHS: The Challenge for the New NHS Chief Exec," Ipsos MORI, 8 May 2014, https://www.ipsos.com/ipsos-mori/en-uk/maintaining-pride-nhs-challenge-new-nhs-chief-exec.
35 Webster, "Introduction," 1.

36 Samuel Osborne, "Danny Boyle Claims Tories Tried to Axe NHS Celebration in London 2012 Olympics Opening Ceremony," *Independent*, 10 July 2016, http://www.independent.co.uk/news/uk/politics/danny-boyle-nhs-celebration-tories-london-2012-olympics-opening-ceremony-a7129186.html.
37 *Telegraph*, "The NHS Is Our World Champion," 5 August 2012, http://www.telegraph.co.uk/news/health/9453653/The-NHS-is-our-world-champion.html.
38 Gordon Rayner, "London 2012: Breathtaking, Brash and Bonkers … an Utterly British Olympic Opening Ceremony," *Telegraph*, 27 July 2012.
39 Britnell, *In Search of the Perfect Health System*, 3.
40 See Bruce Cheadle, "Universal Health Care Much Loved among Canadians, Monarchy Less So," *Globe and Mail*, 25 November 2012, https://www.theglobeandmail.com/news/national/universal-health-care-much-loved-among-canadians-monarchy-less-important-poll/article5640454.
41 André Picard, "Why Health Care Is a Lose-Lose Issue for Politicians," *Globe and Mail*, 16 September 2015, http://www.theglobeandmail.com/opinion/why-no-one-talks-about-health-care-on-the-hustings/article26374042/.
42 Picard, "Why Health Care Is a Lose-Lose Issue."
43 Alan Sleator and Denise Winn, *Great Ormond Street: Behind the Scenes of the World's Most Famous Children's Hospital* (London: Ebury, 1996).
44 See "History," Great Ormand Street Hospital, https://www.gosh.org/about-us/peter-pan/history; and Library.IT Services, "The Most Generous Gift: Peter Pan, J.M. Barrie, and Great Ormond Street Hospital," UCL, 1 December 2015, https://blogs.ucl.ac.uk/library-news/2015/12/the-most-generous-gift/#.W6ELfa2ZMXo.
45 Jules Kosky and Raymond J. Lunnon, *Great Ormond Street and the Story of Medicine* (London: Hospitals for Sick Children in association with Granta Editions, 1991), 37. See "J.M. Barrie and Peter Pan," 36–7, for background to the Barrie gift. See also 53 for the expiration of the rights in 1987 and the House of Lords moving an amendment to the new copyright bill in 1988 giving GOSH the right to receive royalties from Peter Pan in perpetuity. Note, the book is introduced by a letter from Diana, Princess of Wales, who served as president from 1989 until her death.
46 Jules Kosky, *Mutual Friends: Charles Dickens and Great Ormond Street Children's Hospital* (London: Weidenfeld and Nicolson, 1989), 1. See also Nick Baldwin, "Charles Dickens: A Most Unusual Celebrity Endorsement for GOSH," *Independent*, 19 December 2015, http://www.independent.co.uk/voices/campaigns/give-to-gosh/charles-dickens-a-most-unusual-celebrity-endorsement-for-gosh-a6780096.html.
47 Charles Dickens, "Drooping Buds," *Household Words*, no. 106, 3 April 1852, 45–8.
48 Kosky, *Mutual Friends*, 4–5.
49 Joseph deBettencourt, "A Hospital for Sick Children," *Hektoen International* 9, no. 4 (Fall 2017), http://hekint.org/2017/12/22/hospital-sick-children/#.
50 *An Appeal to the Public in Behalf of a Hospital for Sick Children* (London, 1850), 3. Note that although the book does not list an author, Kosky and Lunnon attribute it to the founder of GOSH, Dr Charles West; see Kosky and Lunnon, *Great Ormond Street*, 1.
51 *Appeal to the Public*, 4–5.
52 *Appeal to the Public*, 7.
53 *Appeal to the Public*, 7–8.

54 *Appeal to the Public*, 8.
55 David Wright, *SickKids: The History of the Hospital for Sick Children* (Toronto: University of Toronto Press, 2016), 301.
56 Max Braithwaite, *Sick Kids: The Story of the Hospital for Sick Children in Toronto* (Toronto: McClelland and Stewart, 1974).
57 Judith Young, “A Divine Mission: Elizabeth McMaster and the Hospital for Sick Children, 1875–92,” *Canadian Bulletin of Medical History* 11 (1994): 72.
58 Braithwaite, *Sick Kids*, 73.
59 Wright, *SickKids*, 68.
60 Braithwaite, *Sick Kids*, 202. Carl Hunt received his DHA in 1961.
61 Braithwaite, *Sick Kids*, 29.
62 Josephine Kane, *The History of the Hospital for Sick Children, College Street, Toronto, Ont., Canada, and the Lakeside Home for Little Children, Summer Branch of the Hospital, Toronto Island* (Toronto: [s.n., 1918?]), 68.
63 L. McMaster, *Christmas in the Hospital for Sick Children, Toronto; A Letter to the Well Children of Canada, Who Helped to Make Christmas a Happy Time for Their Little Sick Friends* (Toronto: Hart, 1888), 8.
64 Young, “Divine Mission,” 72.
65 *The Report of the Loyal and Patriotic Society of Upper Canada, with an Appendix and a List of Subscribers and Benefactors* (Montreal: William Gray, 1817), 60.
66 C.K. Clarke, *A History of the Toronto General Hospital, Including an Account of the Medal of the Loyal and Patriotic Society* (Toronto: William Briggs, 1913), 12.
67 Natalie Riegler, *Jean I. Gunn: Nursing Leader* (Markham, ON: Associated Medical Services / Hannah Institute for the History of Medicine, and Fitzhenry and Whiteside, 1997), 210.
68 Riegler, *Jean I. Gunn*, 213.
69 Harvey Agnew and Burns Roth would be two examples.

CHAPTER THREE

1 See Hazel I. Miller, “The Hospital in the Public Health Plan,” *Canadian Journal of Public Health* 45, no. 12 (December 1954): 519–23. Ms Miller at the time was director of nursing at Reddy Memorial Hospital.
2 See James FitzGerald, *What Disturbs Our Blood: A Son’s Quest to Redeem the Past* (Toronto: Random House Canada, 2010). Note, this book won the 2010 Writers’ Trust Non-Fiction Prize. See also R.D. Defries, “Obituaries: Dr John Gerald FitzGerald,” CMAJ 43, no. 2 (August 1940): 190–2.
3 FitzGerald, *What Disturbs Our Blood*, 2.
4 FitzGerald, *What Disturbs Our Blood*, 144.
5 FitzGerald, *What Disturbs Our Blood*, 160.
6 FitzGerald, *What Disturbs Our Blood*, 161.
7 FitzGerald, *What Disturbs Our Blood*, 229.
8 W.G. Cosbie, *The Toronto General Hospital, 1819–1965: A Chronicle* (Toronto: Macmillan of Canada, 1975), 11.
9 FitzGerald, *What Disturbs Our Blood*, 162, 232.
10 Cosbie, *Toronto General Hospital*, 216.
11 Cosbie, *Toronto General Hospital*, 216–17.
12 FitzGerald, *What Disturbs Our Blood*, 276.
13 FitzGerald, *What Disturbs Our Blood*, 239.

14 "The Fiftieth Anniversary of the Sheppard and Enoch Pratt Hospital," in *The Fiftieth Anniversary of the Sheppard and Enoch Pratt Hospital, 1891–1941, November 29, 1941*, 25, Clarence B. Farrar fonds, B1999-0011/022(20), UTARMS.
15 This was a branch of the Canadian Social Hygiene Council. In 1935 its Canadian parent became the Health League of Canada.
16 J.G. FitzGerald, "The Future of Public Health," *Public Health Journal* 19, no. 4 (April 192): 154. Note, this was also published as a reprint in *Studies from the Connaught Laboratories, University of Toronto*, 3:254–7.
17 FitzGerald, "Future of Public Health," 154.
18 FitzGerald, "Future of Public Health," 155.
19 FitzGerald, "Future of Public Health," 155.
20 FitzGerald, "Future of Public Health," 155.
21 FitzGerald, "Future of Public Health," 155.
22 Farley, *To Cast Out Disease*, 223. See also 222, 167n39. See 321 for other references to the School of Hygiene.
23 Farley, *To Cast Out Disease*, 216.
24 J.G. FitzGerald, "Report of the Director of the Connaught and Antitoxin Laboratories," in *President's Report, for the Year Ending June 30, 1918*, 26.
25 Sandra Frances McRae, "The 'Scientific Spirit' in Medicine at the University of Toronto, 1880–1910" (PhD diss., University of Toronto, 1987), 315.
26 McRae, "'Scientific Spirit,'" 318.
27 McRae, "'Scientific Spirit,'" 20–1.
28 Michael Bliss, "The Aetiology of the Discovery of Insulin," in *Health, Disease and Medicine: Essays in Canadian History*, ed. Charles G. Roland (Toronto: Clarke, Irwin, 1984, published for the Hannah Institute for the History of Medicine), 338; quoted in McRae, "'Scientific Spirit,'" 7.
29 Marianne P. Fedunkiw, *Rockefeller Foundation Funding and Medical Education in Toronto, Montreal, and Halifax* (Montreal and Kingston: McGill-Queen's University Press, 2005), 77, 83.
30 They were: FitzGerald (MD, 1903), Frederick Banting (MD, 1922), Best (BA, 1921; MD, 1925). Sylvia Lassam at the Trinity College Archives notes Collip was a student at Trinity (BA, 1912); personal correspondence between the author and Lassam, 27 September 2017.
31 Fedunkiw, *Rockefeller Foundation Funding and Medical Education*, 51, 69.
32 J.G. FitzGerald, "Report of the Director of the Antitoxin Laboratory," in *President's Report, for the Year Ending June 30, 1914*, 25.
33 Fedunkiw, *Rockefeller Foundation Funding and Medical Education*, 82–3.
34 Ontario, Legislative Assembly, *Report of the Special Committee Appointed by the Legislature to Inquire into the Organization and Administration of the University of Toronto* (Toronto: Clarkson W. James, King's Printer, 1923), 17.
35 *John Robert Evans, Finding Aid*, "Biographical Sketch by Harold Averill," 2, B2006-0027, UTARMS.
36 My perception is reinforced by Bator's statement in a report to the dean where he spoke of "FitzGerald's master plan for the School of teaching, researching and public service." See *University of Toronto School of Hygiene History Project: A Report to the Dean, Faculty of Medicine, University of Toronto, with an Application for Further Funding*, 8 March 1987, 11, Paul Adolphus Bator fonds, B90-0035/002(10), UTARMS.

37 Edward Shorter, *Partnership for Excellence: Medicine at the University of Toronto and Academic Hospitals* (Toronto: University of Toronto Press, 2013), 59. See also James FitzGerald, "Sins of the Fathers," *Toronto Life* 36, no. 2 (February 2002): 69–70. Note, this article won a National Magazine Award and sparked *What Disturbs Our Blood.*

38 Shorter, *Partnership for Excellence*, 59.

39 Clippings file "FitzGerald, John Gerald," A1973-0026/103(66), UTARMS; *Globe and Mail*, "Laboratory in Stable Grows to World Fame," 2 December 1946.

40 "The Antitoxin Laboratory of the University of Toronto," editorial, *CMAJ* 7, no. 3 (March 1917): 255–6.

41 J.G. FitzGerald to Edmund Osler, 31 March 1914, "Correspondence: FitzGerald, John Gerald, March–May 1914," /028(085), A67-0007, UTARMS.

42 J.G. FitzGerald to President Falconer, 3 May 1915, "Correspondence: FitzGerald, John Gerald, December 1914–June 1915," /034(015), A67-0007, UTARMS.

43 J.G. FitzGerald, "The Work of the Antitoxin Laboratory," *University of Toronto Monthly* 47, no. 3 (December 1916): 95–9. Note, from November 1907 to November 1918 it was known as *University Monthly.*

44 FitzGerald, "Work of the Antitoxin Laboratory," 99.

45 Trinity Medical School was a precursor to the U of T Faculty of Medicine, into which it merged when Trinity College became a federated college of the University of Toronto in 1904. It had various names. It started out as the Faculty of Medicine at Trinity College, 1850–57. The faculty all resigned when the college (Strachan) insisted that all students be Anglicans! Then it started again in 1870 as the Trinity Medical School. Around 1880 it was upgraded to the Trinity Medical College, and this was the name until it was incorporated into the Faculty of Medicine at U of T in 1904 (personal correspondence with Sylvia Lassam, Trinity College archivist, 5 May 2017).

46 *Register of the University of Toronto for the Year 1920*, 267, P1978-0166(07), UTARMS.

47 "The Organizing Committee of the Canadian Public Health Association, 1910: Maurice Macdonald Seymour, 1857–1929," *Canadian Journal of Public Health* 50, no. 7 (July 1959): 297.

48 C. Stuart Huston, "Saskatchewan's Municipal Doctors a Forerunner of the Medicare System That Developed 50 Years Later," *CMAJ* 151, no. 11 (1 December 1994): 1642.

49 "Seymour, Maurice Macdonald," alumni card, Department of Alumni and Development, A2003-0005, UTARMS. See also *Register of the University of Toronto for the Year 1920*, 267.

50 *Register of the University of Toronto for the Year 1920*, 267.

51 Sylvia Lassam, Trinity College archivist, 23 May 2017, personal correspondence.

52 See, for example, *Studies, from the Research Division, Connaught Antitoxin Laboratories, University of Toronto*, vol. 1, *1919–1922* (Toronto: University of Toronto Press, 1922).

53 *Mail and Empire*, "Splendid Gift to University," 26 October 1917, 4.

54 *Mail and Empire*, "Splendid Gift to University," 4.

55 *Toronto Daily News*, "New Laboratories Opened by Duke," 26 October 1917, 3.

56 *Toronto Daily Star*, "Duke Departs after Busy Day, Opens New College Farm, and Attends Banquet and University Lecture," 26 October 1917, 5.

57 Mariana Mazzucato, *The Entrepreneurial State: Debunking Public vs Private Sector Myths*, rev. ed. (New York: Public Affairs, 2015), 1–5.

58 Christopher J. Rutty, "Personality, Politics, and Canadian Public Health: The Origins of Connaught Medical Research Laboratories, University of Toronto, 1888–1917," in *Essays in Honour of Michael Bliss*, ed. E.A. Heaman, Alison Li, and Shelley McKellar (Toronto: University of Toronto Press, 2008), 273. Another work on Connaught Laboratories (but only to 1955) is Robert D. Defries, *The First Forty Years, 1914–1955, Connaught Medical Research Laboratories, University of Toronto* (Toronto: University of Toronto Press, 1968).

59 Christopher J. Rutty, "'Do Something! ... Do Anything!' Poliomyelitis in Canada, 1927–1962" (PhD diss., University of Toronto, 1995), 4.

60 Rutty, "Personality, Politics, and Canadian Public Health," 273.

61 Connaught Medical Research Laboratories, University of Toronto, *Forty-First Annual Report, 1953–54*, 5.

62 For a list of articles and books on the Labs, see Rutty, "Personality, Politics, and Canadian Public Health," 297–8nn2, 3.

63 "Treatment of Diphtheria with Anti-Toxine," editorial, *Canada Lancet* 27 (February 1895): 189–90.

64 "The Value of Diphtheria Antitoxin," editorial, *Canada Lancet* 38, no. 9 (May 1905): 836–7.

65 "Discovery and Commercialism," editorial, *Canada Lancet* 39, no. 5 (January 1906): 463–4.

66 J.G. FitzGerald to Falconer, 10 September 1917, "Correspondence: FitzGerald, John Gerald, July 1917–March 1918," /047a(038), A67-0007, UTARMS.

67 FitzGerald to Falconer, 10 September 1917.

68 Office of the President (Falconer), A67-0007, UTARMS; see FitzGerald to Falconer, 3 December 1917; also "Proposed Outline of Letter to Premier of Each Province Inviting a Nomination of a Representative to Act on the Honorary Advisory Committee of the Connaught and Antitoxin Laboratories, University of Toronto"; and "Further Material for Letter to Provincial Premiers, in Reference to the Appointment of Honorary Advisory Committee, Antitoxin Laboratory." The latter two are in the same file folder but have no date.

69 J.G. FitzGerald, "Report of the Director of the Connaught and Antitoxin Laboratories," in *President's Report, for the Year Ending June 30, 1918*, 27. (It also named seven members and whom they represented.) See also Defries, *First Forty Years*, 34–5 (he has a list of nine members). Defries's list has additional names to those given in the *President's Report*. Names familiar to the reader would be J.W.S. McCullough (Ontario) and M.M. Seymour (Saskatchewan). See also Rutty, "'Do Something!,'" 6.

70 J.G. FitzGerald, "Report of the Director of the Connaught and Antitoxin Laboratories," in *President's Report, for the Year Ending June 30, 1920*, 26. Note, FitzGerald's reports are collected in a bound volume of annual reports from 1914 to 1934 at the Sanofi Pasteur Connaught Archives (SP-C Archives, acc. 83-005-03).

71 J.G. FitzGerald, "Report of the Director of the Connaught Antitoxin Laboratories," in *President's Report, for the Year Ending June 30, 1919*, 24. It is interesting in these president's reports to see how the nomenclature of the Labs changes. In the footnotes above we saw it as the Connaught and Antitoxin

Laboratories, here it is the Connaught Antitoxin Laboratories, and with the discovery of insulin in the 1920s it will change yet again to the Connaught Laboratories.

72 James FitzGerald, "The Troubled Healer," *U of T Magazine, Souvenir Edition* 29, no. 3 (Spring 2002): 91.

73 Defries, *First Forty Years*, 34–5.

74 See vol. 9 of *Public Health Journal*, e.g., "The Proposed Ministry of Health," "Editorial: A Federal Department of Public Health" (January 1918): 40; "Editorial: A Federal Department" (February 1918): 92; "Editorial: A Federal Department of Health" (March 1918): 144; "Editorial: A Federal Department of Health" (April 1918): 198; "Editorial: A Federal Department of Health" (July 1918): 345; "A Ministry of Health" (December 1918): 573–9.

75 Paul Adolphus Bator and Andrew James Rhodes, *Within Reach of Everyone: A History of the University of Toronto School of Hygiene and the Connaught Laboratories* (Ottawa: Canadian Public Health Association, 1990), 1:25.

76 Bator and Rhodes, *Within Reach of Everyone*, 1:134.

77 Bator and Rhodes, *Within Reach of Everyone*, 1:25.

78 File 1, Dominion Council of Health, Meetings 1–6, 1919–22, coll. R-1367, acc. R-88-40, Saskatchewan Archives Board (SAB).

79 "Some of the Work of the Department of Hygiene at the University of Toronto," *Canadian Journal of Medicine and Surgery* 42, no. 4 (October 1917): 93.

80 "Some of the Work," *Canadian Journal of Medicine and Surgery*, 95.

81 Frederick Edwards, "A Peacetime Munitions Plant," *Maclean's* 41, no. 2 (15 January 1928): 4.

82 Edwards, "Peacetime Munitions Plant," 4.

83 Edwards, "Peacetime Munitions Plant," 63.

84 J.G.F., "Opening of the Connaught Laboratories at the University Farm," *University of Toronto Monthly* 48, no. 2 (November 1917): 78–9.

85 "Connaught Laboratories to Publish Research Papers," *University of Toronto Monthly* 22, no. 8 (May 1922): 352.

86 FitzGerald, *What Disturbs Our Blood*, 239. See also Dalla Lana, "Within Reach of Everyone," 1 May 2014, http://www.dlsph.utoronto.ca/2014/05/within-reach-of-everyone-the-birth-maturity-and-renewal-of-public-health-at-u-of-t-2/.

87 J.W.S. McCullough, excerpt of the Editorial Section, *Canadian Public Health Journal* (August 1940): 395–6, Correspondence "F," A68-0006/045(06), UTARMS.

88 June Callwood, "The Miracle Factory That Began in a Stable," *Maclean's* 68, no. 22 (1 October 1955): 14.

89 Callwood, "Miracle Factory That Began," 88.

90 Rutty, "'Do Something!,'" 390. Another indication of the impression Connaught Labs (and the school) made on him is that he dedicated his dissertation to Andrew Rhodes (see vi).

91 T.O. Hecht, Continental Pharma Ltd, to G.D.W. Cameron, deputy minister of national health, 14 August 1957, file 311-P11-3, vol. 343, 85-86/248, RG29, LAC; quoted in Hecht to Cameron, 14 August 1957, 368.

92 Rutty, "'Do Something!,'" 368.

93 Rutty, "'Do Something!,'" 377–8.

94 Edwards, "Peacetime Munitions Plant," 5.

95 FitzGerald, *What Disturbs Our Blood*, 239.
96 Rutty, "Personality, Politics, and Canadian Public Health," 275.
97 Rutty, "Personality, Politics, and Canadian Public Health," 286.
98 Callwood, "Miracle Factory," 90.
99 Malcolm Burrows, "Canada's Greatest Impact Donation," All about Estates, 16 May 2019, https://www.allaboutestates.ca/canadas-greatest-impact-donation/. Also correspondence with James FitzGerald, 18 December 2019.
100 Burrows, "Canada's Greatest Impact Donation."
101 FitzGerald, "Troubled Healer," 92.
102 J.G. FitzGerald, "Report of the Director of the Connaught Antitoxin Laboratories," in *President's Report, for the Year Ending June 30, 1922*, 78.
103 J.G. FitzGerald, "Report of the Director of the Connaught Antitoxin Laboratories," in *President's Report, for the Year Ending June 30, 1923*, 76, 77.
104 "Medical Research Results in Important Discovery," *University of Toronto Monthly* 22, no. 8 (May 1922): 346.
105 "Medical Research Results in Important Discovery," 347.
106 FitzGerald, "Troubled Healer," 91.
107 F.G. Banting, "Address: 'The Story of Insulin,'" 5 March 1923, *Addresses Delivered before the Canadian Club of Toronto, Season of 1922–23* (Toronto: Warwick Bros & Rutter, 1923), 20, 234, 236.
108 Michael Bliss, *The Discovery of Insulin*, 25th anniversary ed. (Toronto: University of Toronto Press, 2011), 133.
109 File "Insulin, Pt 2," box 81, Robert Falconer, President's Papers, A67-0007, UTARMS. See undated set of nine pages with no cover letter, 2–4. (Note, box 81 is for the academic year 1922–23 and has three insulin files, parts 1 to 3.)
110 File "Insulin, Pt 2," 4–5.
111 File "Insulin, Pt 2," 9.
112 File "Insulin, Pt 2," 1.
113 File "Insulin, Pt 2," 2.
114 File "Insulin, Pt 2," 2–3.
115 File "Insulin, Pt 2," 4.
116 File "Insulin, Pt 2," 8.
117 File "Insulin, Pt 2," 9.
118 Newton W. Rowell to F.A. Mouré, 29 January 1923, file "Insulin, Pt 3," box 81, Robert Falconer, President's Papers, A67-0007, UTARMS.
119 J.G. FitzGerald to Falconer, 18 June 1923, file "Correspondence, Fitzgerald, John G., Director Connaught Research Labs, June 1923–May 1924," box 83a, Robert Falconer, President's Papers, A67-0007, UTARMS.
120 *University of Toronto Report of the Board of Governors for the Year Ending 30th June 1924*, 13–14, UTARMS.
121 Friedland, *University of Toronto: A History*, 2nd ed., 291–2.
122 Minutes of the meeting of 1 September 1922, 1, file 1, "Original Minutes of the Insulin Committee," box 044, Insulin Committee, Board of Governors, A82-0001, UTARMS. (Minutes are signed by the chair, Col. Gooderham.)
123 6 May 1922, 6, box 76 (also classified as Banting Collection box 37), ms coll. 00232, Frederick Banting papers, Thomas Fisher Rare Book Library, University of Toronto.
124 Folder 1, "FGB's Account of the Discovery," 9. (Note, the pages are not consecutive. Typewritten p. 9 follows handwritten p. 11.)

125 J.T.H. Connor, *Doing Good: The Life of Toronto General Hospital* (Toronto: University of Toronto Press, 2000), 207.
126 *For the Common Good, Superintendent's Report, Toronto General Hospital,* 1923, 5.
127 Bator and Rhodes, *Within Reach of Everyone,* 1:13.
128 Bator and Rhodes, *Within Reach of Everyone,* 1:29–30.
129 Geoffery O. Storey and Heather Smith, "George Newman (1870–1948)," *Journal of Medical Biography* 13, no. 1 (February 2005): 31–8.
130 *Globe*, "Commencement Day Begins with Opening of Hygiene Building," 9 June 1927, 1. Note, the other Toronto newspapers did not give the opening the same billing, some not even mentioning it. Sir George was also receiving an honorary degree, and all mentioned that.
131 *Globe*, "School of Hygiene Draws High Praise from Visitor," 19 April 1927, 14.
132 "The Opening of the New School of Hygiene, University of Toronto," *Public Health Journal* 18, no. 7 (July 1927): 320.
133 FitzGerald, *What Disturbs Our Blood*, front cover overleaf.
134 Rutty, "'Do Something!,'" 390.
135 FitzGerald, "Sins of the Fathers," 72.
136 "Interview with Dr G.H. Beaton, August 20, 1985, Reel 1," 4, transcript, School of Hygiene History Project, B89-0009, UTARMS.
137 Interview with G.H. Beaton.
138 Interview with G.H. Beaton, 51:43, 20 August 1985, digitized audio recording, School of Hygiene History Project, B1989-0009_05S, UTARMS.
139 Alison Li, "Expansion and Consolidation: The Associate Committee and the Division of Medical Research of the NRC, 1938–1959," *Scientia Canadensis* 15, no. 2 (1991): 95.
140 Henry Etzkowitz and Chunyan Zhou, *The Triple Helix: University-Industry-Government Innovation and Entrepreneurship*, 2nd ed. (New York: Routledge, 2017), 3.
141 Transcript, 2, School of Hygiene History Project, B89-0009, UTARMS. See also audiocassette #6/6, side 1.
142 For information on the organization of the Basel Institute, see Thomas Söderqvist, *Science as Autobiography: The Troubled Life of Niels Jerne*, trans. David Mel Paul (New Haven, CT: Yale University Press, 2003), 259–60.
143 Wright, *SickKids*, 360.
144 Paul Adolphus Bator, *Within Reach of Everyone: A History of the University of Toronto School of Hygiene and the Connaught Laboratories*, vol. 2, *1955 to 1975, with an Update to the 1990s* (Ottawa: Canadian Public Health Association, 1995), 41.
145 Bator, *Within Reach of Everyone*, 2:63–6.
146 G.D.W. Cameron, "The First Donald Fraser Memorial Lecture," *Canadian Journal of Public Health* 51, no. 9 (September 1960): 341–8.
147 See "Dr Robert D. Defries (1889–1975)," Museum of Health Care at Kingston," http://www.museumofhealthcare.ca/explore/exhibits/vaccinations/profiles.html. Bator and Rhodes note that in the 1930s, though FitzGerald was the titular head of the Department of Hygiene and Preventive Medicine, as the result of his responsibilities as dean of the faculty and his obligations to the International Health Board, League of Nations, and Dominion Council of

Health, Fraser "was the *de facto* head of the department." See *Within Reach of Everyone*, 1:51.

148 R.D. Defries to Sidney Smith, 31 January 1946, file "School of Hygiene," Office of the President, A68-0007/003(09), UTARMS. The other eight universities were Johns Hopkins, Harvard, Columbia, Yale, North Carolina, Michigan, Minnesota, and California.

149 Bator and Rhodes, *Within Reach of Everyone*, 1:48.

150 Bator and Rhodes, *Within Reach of Everyone*, 1:25.

151 Rutty, "'Do Something!,'" 381.

152 Rutty, "'Do Something!,'" 383, 390, 391.

153 Reich, *Selling Our Souls*, 4.

154 Rutty, "'Do Something!,'" 382.

155 Rutty, "'Do Something!,'" 382.

156 Rutty, "'Do Something!,'" 392–3.

157 Callwood, "Miracle Factory," 93.

158 Helen M. Carpenter, *A Divine Discontent: Edith Kathleen Russell – Reforming Educator* (Toronto: Faculty of Nursing, University of Toronto, 1982), 14.

159 See Farley, *To Cast Out Disease*, 230, 234. For some of the challenges of altering "deep-seated traditions" (hospital-based schools of nursing), the economic challenges (Great Depression), issues of public health nursing vs basic nursing education, see Carpenter, *Divine Discontent*, 15–18.

160 Carpenter, *Divine Discontent*, 14.

161 "Proposals Concerning: School of Hygiene and Connaught Laboratories," n.d. (though handwritten at the top is "From Dr FitzGerald"), file 1, 1919–1927, box 005, School of Nursing, A73-0053, UTARMS.

162 Carpenter, *Divine Discontent*, 14.

163 Farley, *To Cast Out Disease*, 230.

164 Farley, *To Cast Out Disease*, 231.

165 Natalie Nitia Riegler, "The Work and Networks of Jean I. Gunn, Superintendent of Nurses, Toronto General Hospital, 1913–1941: A Presentation of Some Issues in Nursing during Her Lifetime, 1882–1941" (PhD diss., University of Toronto, 1992), 276.

166 "A Conference on Social Hygiene," *Public Health Journal* 10, no. 8 (August 1919): 372.

167 See University of Toronto, "Curriculum for the Diploma in Public Health Nursing," *Calendar of the School of Hygiene, 1931–1932*, 17.

168 Riegler, "Work and Networks of Jean I. Gunn," 272–3.

169 Riegler, "Work and Networks of Jean I. Gunn," 278.

170 Riegler, "Work and Networks of Jean I. Gunn," 281.

171 Riegler, "Work and Networks of Jean I. Gunn," 277.

172 Joseph Flavelle to Robert Falconer, 10 November 1922, box 077, Correspondence 1922–23, Office of the President (Falconer), A1967-0007, UTARMS.

173 E.K. Russell, "Report of the Director of the School of Nursing," *President's Report, for the Year Ending 30th June 1940*, 104.

174 J.G. FitzGerald, "Gordon Bell Memorial Lecture: Some Aspects of Preventive Medicine," *Canadian Public Health Journal* 20, no. 2 (February 1929): 64.

175 Paul Adolphus Bator, "The Emergence of Public Health Education Programs in the University of Toronto: Some Comparisons with the United States" (paper for the Rockefeller Conference on the History of Education in Public

Health, Bellagio, Italy, 18 August 1987), 11, file 12, box 10, Andrew James Rhodes fonds, B2000-001, UTARMS.

176 See "The School of Nursing," *Calendar, School of Nursing, 1933–1934*, 7–9.

177 See "School of Nursing," 17, 26.

CHAPTER FOUR

1 J.G. FitzGerald, "A Plan for Instruction in Hygiene, Preliminary Medical Inspection of Students, and Free Dispensary or Hospital Treatment in Canadian Universities," *Public Health Journal* 8, no. 11 (November 1917): 305.

2 Bator and Rhodes, *Within Reach of Everyone*, 1:63.

3 J.G. FitzGerald et al., *An Introduction to the Practice of Preventive Medicine*, 2nd ed. (St Louis, MO: C.V. Mosby, 1926), 2–3. Note, these same statements appear (on the same pages) in an earlier edition of the book published in 1922.

4 J.G. FitzGerald, "Measures to Lessen Preventable Mortality and Morbidity (Address Delivered at the Annual Meeting of the Canadian Life Insurance Officers Association)," in *Collected Papers of J.G. FitzGerald*, [v.p.] [19–], 10. This is a collection of fifty-five original papers and addresses of FitzGerald from 1907 to 1938.

5 FitzGerald, "Gordon Bell Memorial Lecture," 69.

6 Conference on Medical Services in Canada, *Report of the Conference on the Medical Services in Canada, Held at Ottawa, December 18, 19, 20, 1924* (Ottawa: F.A. Acland, King's Printer, 1925), 7.

7 These included Drs M.M. Seymour and R.E. Wodehouse.

8 Conference on Medical Services in Canada, *Report*, 77.

9 Conference on Medical Services in Canada, *Report*, 80–7.

10 Conference on Medical Services in Canada, *Report*, 87–115.

11 Conference on Medical Services in Canada, *Report*, 58.

12 These included Drs A.G. Fleming, M.M. Seymour, and R.E. Wodehouse.

13 Canada, Department of Health, *Second Conference on Medical Services in Canada, House of Commons, March 28, 29, 30, 1927* (Ottawa: F.A. Acland, King's Printer, 1928), 12–13.

14 Canada, Department of Health, *Second Conference*, 71–2.

15 Canada, Department of Health, *Second Conference*, 150–1.

16 Dianne Dodd, "Advice to Parents: The Blue Books, Helen MacMurchy, MD, and the Federal Department of Health, 1920–34," *Canadian Bulletin of Medical History* 8 (1991): 205.

17 Canada, Department of Health, *Second Conference*, 21.

18 J.G. FitzGerald, "The Future of Public Health," *Public Health Journal* 19, no. 4 (April 1928): 155.

19 FitzGerald, "Gordon Bell Memorial Lecture," 70.

20 FitzGerald, "Gordon Bell Memorial Lecture," 71.

21 FitzGerald, "Gordon Bell Memorial Lecture," 72.

22 FitzGerald, "Gordon Bell Memorial Lecture," 73–4.

23 FitzGerald, "Gordon Bell Memorial Lecture," 75.

24 Canada, House of Commons, Select Standing Committee on Industrial and International Relations, *Report, Proceedings and Evidence of the Select Standing Committee on Industrial and International Relations upon the Question of Insurance against Unemployment, Sickness and Invalidity as Ordered by*

the House on the 14th of February, 1929 (Ottawa: F.A. Ackland, King's Printer, 1929); session of 14 March 1929, 32. (Note, this committee also looked at this question, sickness insurance, during the year before.)
25 Canada, House of Commons, Select Standing Committee on Industrial and International Relations, *Report*, 32–3.
26 Canada, House of Commons, Select Standing Committee on Industrial and International Relations, *Report*, 33.
27 J.G. Gibbon, *Medical Benefit: A Study of the Experience of Germany and Denmark* (Westminster: P.S. King and Son, 1912).
28 Canada, House of Commons, Select Standing Committee on Industrial and International Relations, *Report*, 33–4.
29 Canada, House of Commons, Select Standing Committee on Industrial and International Relations, *Report*, 34–5.
30 Canada, House of Commons, Select Standing Committee on Industrial and International Relations, *Report*, 37.
31 Canada, House of Commons, Select Standing Committee on Industrial and International Relations, *Report*, 37–9.
32 Canadian Medical Association and Department of Pensions and National Health, *Third Conference on the Medical Services in Canada ..., Ottawa, on November 21 and 22, 1929* (Ottawa: F.A. Acland, King's Printer, 1930), 3.
33 These were Drs A.G. Fleming, F.C. Middleton, and R.E. Wodehouse. See Canadian Medical Association and Department of Pensions and National Health, *Third Conference*, 3–4; and Bator and Rhodes, *Within Reach of Everyone*, 1:206–9. They all did quite well. Dr Middleton was deputy minister in the Saskatchewan Department of Public Health. Dr Wodehouse would become deputy minister in the Department of Pensions and National Health. Dr Fleming would become dean of medicine at McGill.
34 Canadian Medical Association and Department of Pensions and National Health, *Third Conference*, 17.
35 Canadian Medical Association and Department of Pensions and National Health, *Third Conference*. See 18–58 for health and the state, and 58–87 for medical education.
36 Canadian Medical Association and Department of Pensions and National Health, *Third Conference*, 95.
37 Canadian Medical Association and Department of Pensions and National Health, *Third Conference*, 111–12.
38 J.G. FitzGerald, "The Municipal Physician System in Operation in the Provinces of Manitoba and Saskatchewan," *University of Toronto Monthly* 33, no. 6 (March 1933): 191.
39 FitzGerald, "Municipal Physician System," 190.
40 J. Heurner Mullin, "Obituaries – Dr John Gerald FitzGerald – An Appreciation," *CMAJ* 43, no. 2 (August 1940): 192.
41 FitzGerald, "Municipal Physician System," 192.
42 FitzGerald, "Municipal Physician System," 193–4.
43 FitzGerald, "Municipal Physician System," 194.
44 For a list of the members and the report of the committee, see Report of the Committee of Economics, "A Plan for Health Insurance in Canada," in "Sixty-Fifth Annual Meeting of the Canadian Medical Association, Calgary, Alberta, June 18, 19, 20, 21, 22, 1934," supplement, *CMAJ* 31, no. 3 (September 1934): S25. The report is on S25–34. Note, there were thirty-one sections

on this topic in the supplement. They looked at the issue from many perspectives, including the initiatives of other countries, costs of care, provincial action, administration, benefits, payment of physicians, among others. There are three relevant sections on the topic for our immediate purposes. The first is the first three sections of the report, which provide an overivew. There was also "Part Two: The Situation in Canada" and "Part Three: The Canadian Medical Association's Plan for State Health Insurance in Canada." Note, there is no designated Part One (which comprises the first sixteen sections). The bibliography (S60–1) is a good source of historical literature on the topic. Also note, the designation *S* in front of the page numbers is my own, to differentiate the supplement pages (which are numbered differently) from those of the regular articles for that month in the journal.

45 Taylor, *Health Insurance and Canadian Public Policy*, 23.

46 Canadian Medical Association, "A Plan for Health Insurance in Canada, *CMAJ* 31, no. 3 (0000): S38.

47 Grauer was a Rhodes Scholar with a BA from the University of Southern California and another from Oxford, and a PhD from the University of California. He was hired as a lecturer in the Department of Political Science in 1930, became director of the Department of Social Science in 1936, and left in 1938 (see staff card, Albert Edward Grauer, UTARMS).

48 Canada, Royal Commission on Dominion-Provincial Relations, *Studies*, A.E. Grauer, "No. 7, Public Health" (Ottawa: King's Printer, 1939), 60.

49 Canada, Royal Commission on Dominion-Provincial Relations, *Hearings*, Ottawa, 26 May 1938, Health League of Canada, Dr Gordon Bates, 9273–4.

50 See Riegler, "Work and Networks of Jean I. Gunn," 417–20, 426–30, 466.

51 Jean I. Gunn, "Towards Action," *Canadian Nurse* 30, no. 9 (September 1934): 407, 411.

52 Canada, Royal Commission on Dominion-Provincial Relations, *Hearings*, Ottawa, 9 May 1938, presentation by Jean I. Gunn, chair, Health Insurance and Nursing Service Committee of the Canadian Nurses' Association, 8000.

53 Canada, Royal Commission, presentation by Gunn, 8003.

54 Canada, Royal Commission, presentation by Gunn, 8008.

55 Canada, Royal Commission, presentation by Gunn, 8008.

56 Canada, Royal Commission, presentation by Gunn, 8008.

57 Canada, Royal Commission, presentation by Gunn, 8008–9.

58 Canada, House of Commons, Select Standing Committee on Industrial and International Relations, *Report*, session of 12 March 1929, 23.

59 Canada, House of Commons, Select Standing Committee on Industrial and International Relations, *Report*, 23–4.

60 Canada, House of Commons, Select Standing Committee on Industrial and International Relations, *Report*, 24.

61 Canada, House of Commons, Select Standing Committee on Industrial and International Relations, *Report*, 25.

62 Canada, House of Commons, Select Standing Committee on Industrial and International Relations, *Report*, 26. Dr Fleming repeated the same point on 30.

63 A.E. Grauer, "Is Unemployment Insurance Enough?," *University of Toronto Quarterly* 4, no. 4 (July 1935): 523. Note, Grauer was the author of two of the "Red Books" of the Rowell-Sirois Commission.

64 Grauer, "Is Unemployment Insurance Enough?," 523.

65 F.R. Scott, "The Royal Commission on Dominion-Provincial Relations," *University of Toronto Quarterly* 7, no. 2 (January 1938): 150–1.

66 Bator and Rhodes, *Within Reach of Everyone*, 1:63.

67 For example, Fleming worked with Harry Cassidy in the latter's role in trying to implement health insurance in BC. He was one author of *Health and Unemployment*; see Leonard C. Marsh in collaboration with A. Grant Fleming and C.F. Blackler, *Health and Unemployment: Some Studies of Their Relationships* (Toronto: Oxford University Press, published for McGill University, 1938). In addition, he wrote a number of articles that dealt in whole or in part with the issue. See, for example, Grant Fleming, "The Relationship of Public Health to Medical Care," *Canadian Public Health Journal* 25, no. 10 (October 1934): 464–5; "Editorial: Unemployment Relief," *CMAJ* 29, no. 1 (July 1933): 71.

68 The information in the preceding two paragraphs is taken from "Dr Amyot Outlines Health Work in War," file "FitzGerald, John Gerald," Department of Graduate Records, A73-0026/103(66), UTARMS. See "Details of the Progress Made in Scandinavia," "Finds Scandinavian Hospitals the Best," "Co-operative Commonwealth Is Far Advanced in Democracy and Educational Institutions," "Denmark Shows Way to Medical World."

69 J.G. FitzGerald, "The Work of the Health Organisation of the League of Nations," *Canadian Public Health Journal* 24, no. 8 (August 1933): 368–72.

70 Selected clippings: "Dean of Medicine Will Study Abroad," "Finds Many Public Health Nurses in Europe Trained in Schools in Dominion," "Rockefeller Work Lauded by Doctor," ile: "FitzGerald, John Gerald," Department of Graduate Records, A73-0026/103(66), UTARMS.

71 Bator and Rhodes, *Within Reach of Everyone*, 1:47–8. For the full letter, see G. Ramon to J.G. FitzGerald, 3 November 1927, file "FitzGerald, John Gerald," box 107a, Office of the President, A67-007, UTARMS. The original of the letter was in French, and what was in the president's file was a translation. See also J.G. FitzGerald to E.F. Russell, 24 October 1927 for a letter to the Rockefeller Foundation about his visit, Paul A. Bator fonds, B90-0035/001(09), UTARMS.

72 President to J.G. FitzGerald, 18 February 1928, file "FitzGerald, John Gerald," box 107a, Office of the President, A67-007, UTARMS.

CHAPTER FIVE

1 Some very good material on such initiatives and the evolution of health insurance in the United States is on the Social Security Administration website. In 1969 Peter A. Corning, a journalist and PhD candidate at New York University, completed a contract with SSA's Office of Research and Statistics for a history of developments in health insurance leading up to the passage of Medicare in 1965. Corning's history is a very accessible, highly readable account of Medicare in the broader historical context of social insurance in America. For the entire history, called *The Evolution of Medicare*, see https://www.ssa.gov/history/corning.html. For a history of the interwar period, where several initiatives were floated, see "Chapter 2: The Second Round – 1927 to 1940," https://www.ssa.gov/history/corningchap2.html. For the history of a particularly fertile period, occurring just after the Second World War, see "Chapter 3: The Third Round 1943–1950," https://www.ssa.gov/history/corningchap3.html.

2 Ontario Hospital Association, *80 Years of Progress, 1924–2004* (Toronto: Ontario Hospital Association, [2005?]), 1.4.
3 "A Tribute to Dr Harvey Agnew," *Hospital Administration in Canada* 13, no. 11 (November 1971): 21.
4 "Obituaries, George Harvey Agnew," *Canadian Medical Association Journal* 105, no. 12 (18 December 1971): 1341.
5 G. Harvey Agnew, *Canadian Hospitals, 1920 to 1970: A Dramatic Half-Century* (Toronto: University of Toronto Press, 1974), 65. Note, Agnew signed his articles three different ways: G. Harvey Agnew, Harvey Agnew, and G.H.A. In all cases the way he signed his article is the way his name is cited.
6 G. Harvey Agnew, "After Twenty-Five Years …," *Canadian Hospital* 30, no. 7 (July 1953): 44.
7 Bator and Rhodes, *Within Reach of Everyone*, 1:143.
8 Agnew, "After Twenty-Five Years," 45.
9 Editorial Board, "The Passing of Two Pioneers," *Canadian Journal of Public Health* 44, no. 10 (October 1953): 375.
10 Canadian Medical Association, Department of Hospital Service; Canada, Department of Pensions and National Health, *A Directory of the Hospitals of Canada, with Maps, 1929* (Ottawa: F.A. Acland, King's Printer, 1929).
11 Canada, Department of Health, *A List of the Hospitals of Canada, with Map, 1925* (Ottawa: F.A. Acland, King's Printer, 1926). It was only sixteen pages long, with a single map. Its map legend showed only three different types of hospitals, whereas the 1929 version had twelve.
12 Agnew, "After Twenty-Five Years," 45.
13 G. Harvey Agnew, "The Department of Hospital Service," *Canadian Medical Association Journal* 20, no. 3 (March 1929): 294–5.
14 G. Harvey Agnew, "The Medical Survey of Canada," *Canadian Medical Association Journal* 24, no. 1 (January 1931): 123–9; the quote on health insurance appears on 126.
15 For more on this history of *Hospital World*, see Agnew, *Canadian Hospitals, 1920–1970*, 61.
16 Canada, House of Commons, *Debates*, Sixth Session, Seventeenth Parliament, vol. 2, 22 February 1935 (Ottawa: King's Printer, 1935), 1136–7.
17 Canada, House of Commons, *Debates*, Second Session, Eighteenth Parliament, vol. 1, 19 January 1937 (Ottawa: King's Printer, 1937), 101.
18 Canada, House of Commons, *Debates*, Fourth Session, Eighteenth Parliament, vol. 3, 17 April 1939 (Ottawa: King's Printer, 1939), 2884.
19 G.M. Weir, "A National Health Program," *Maclean's*, 15 March 1939, 12.
20 Weir, "National Health Program," 54.
21 Weir, "National Health Program," 56.
22 See the chapter "Health and Welfare Services," in Research Committee of the League for Social Reconstruction, *Social Planning for Canada* (1935; Toronto: University of Toronto Press, 1975), 389–406.

Irving notes that Cassidy's name was not listed among the authors of the book, because by the time it was published in 1935 he was the equivalent to a deputy minister in a Liberal government in BC, and it would not have been politically correct for his name to appear in a book that rejected many of the tenets of capitalism and openly favoured socialism. See Alan Irving, "Canadian Fabians: The Work and Thought of Harry Cassidy and Leonard Marsh, 1940–1945," *Canadian Journal of Social Work Education* 7, no. 1 (1981): 14.

23 Harry M. Cassidy, *Social Security and Reconstruction in Canada* (Toronto: Ryerson, 1943).
24 Harry Cassidy, *Public Health and Welfare Reorganization: The Postwar Problem in the Canadian Provinces* (Toronto: Ryerson, 1945).
25 Harry M. Cassidy, "School of Hygiene Lectures 1946–50," /64(03), B1972-022, Harry Morris Cassidy fonds, UTARMS.
26 This is also dealt with – differently, but overall in more detail – by Bator and Rhodes, *Within Reach of Everyone*, 1:83–7.
27 Harold J. Kirby, minister of health, to J.G. FitzGerald, 29 May 1939, file 05 "D," box 041 Correspondence, Office of the President (Cody), A68-0006, UTARMS.
28 R.D. Defries to Harold J. Kirby, minister of health, 22 June 1939, file 05 "D," box 041 Correspondence, Office of the President (Cody), A68-0006, UTARMS.
29 Ontario, Department of Health, *Fifteenth Annual Report of the Department of Health, Ontario, Canada, for the Year 1939* (Toronto: T.E. Bowman, King's Printer, 1940), 11.
30 Ontario, Department of Health, *Fifteenth Annual Report*, 47.
31 Ontario, Department of Health, *Sixteenth Annual Report of the Department of Health, Ontario, Canada, for the Year 1940* (Toronto: T.E. Bowman, King's Printer, 1941), 10.
32 Ontario, Department of Health, *Sixteenth Annual Report*, 10.
33 Bator and Rhodes, *Within Reach of Everyone*, 1:86–7.
34 Bator, *Within Reach of Everyone*, 2:40.
35 Bator and Rhodes, *Within Reach of Everyone*, 1:87.
36 Great Britain, *Interim Report on the Future Provision of Medical and Allied Services* (Dawson Report) (London: His Majesty's Stationery Office, 1920).
37 C. Rufus Rorem, *Capital Investment in Hospitals*, Committee on the Costs of Medical Care, no. 7 (Chicago: University of Chicago Press, 1930), 9.
38 Rorem, *Capital Investment*, 10.
39 Ontario, Royal Commission on Public Welfare, *Report* (Toronto: King's Printer, 1930), 13–14.
40 G.H. Agnew, "The Report of the Royal Commission on Public Welfare," *CMAJ* 24, no. 1 (January 1931), 105.
41 Agnew, *Canadian Hospitals, 1920 to 1970*, xiii.
42 Agnew, *Canadian Hospitals, 1920 to 1970*, 1.
43 Niles Carpenter, *Hospital Service for Patients of Moderate Means: A Study of Certain American Hospitals,* Committee on the Costs of Medical Care, no. 4 (Chicago: University of Chicago Press, 1930), 9–10.
44 Rockefeller Foundation, Committee on the Training of Hospital Executives, *Principles of Hospital Administration and the Training of Hospital Executives, April 1922, Report* [n.p., 1922], 19–28.
45 Rockefeller Foundation, Committee on the Training of Hospital Executives, *Principles of Hospital Administration*, 26.
46 Michael Davis, *Hospital Administration: A Career: The Need for Trained Executives for a Billion-Dollar Business, and How They May Be Trained* (New York: [n.p., 1929]), 58.
47 Davis, *Hospital Administration*, 73.
48 Davis, *Hospital Administration*, 2–3.
49 Davis, *Hospital Administration*, 4.

50 Committee on the Costs of Medical Care, *Final Report* (Chicago: University of Chicago Press, 1932), 143.
51 Committee on the Costs of Medical Care, *Final Report*, 144.
52 G.H.A, "Training in Hospital Administration," *Canadian Hospital* 17, no. 5 (May 1940): 27–9, 46, 48.
53 American Council on Education, "Table 2, Organization of the University Graduate Programs, 1953," *University Education for Administration in Hospitals* (Washington DC: American Council on Education, 1954), 12. Of the twelve programs, seven were located in Schools of Public Health, one in a Faculty of Medicine, two in business schools, and two in graduate schools.
54 American Council on Education, *University Education for Administration in Hospitals*, 63–72.
55 A recently released book on him goes into further detail; see Geoff Mynett, *Service on the Skeena: Horace Wrinch, Frontier Physician* (Vancouver: Ronsdale, 2019). See also "Wrinch, Horace Cooper," A73-0026/528(83), UTARMS, for press clippings on him, in particular a picture of the hospital he built in Hazelton, BC.
56 For a time, some of the federated colleges of the U of T had their own medical school. These were all consolidated within the university in the early 1900s.
57 Robert Lampard, "The Hoadley Commission (1932–34) and Health Insurance in Alberta," *Canadian Bulletin of Medical History* 26, no. 2 (Winter 2009): 440.
58 British Columbia, Royal Commission on State Health Insurance and Maternity Benefits, *Final Report* (Victoria, BC: Charles F. Banfield, King's Printer, 1932), 23.
59 Cassidy was good friends with Dr Charles Fielding, dean of divinity at Trinity College.
60 See, for example, Cassidy, *Social Security and Reconstruction in Canada*.
61 Harvey Agnew, "The Proposed Formation of a Canadian Hospital Council," *Canadian Medical Association Journal* 25, no. 4 (October 1931): 458.
62 Agnew, "Proposed Formation," 459.
63 G.H.A., "The Canadian Hospital Council," *Canadian Medical Association Journal* 25, no. 5 (November 1931): 608–9. See also Agnew, *Canadian Hospitals, 1920 to 1970*, 258, 259.
64 "The Second Session of the Canadian Hospital Council," *Canadian Medical Association Journal* 29, no. 2 (August 1933): 201–2.
65 "Editorial Board," *Canadian Hospital* 15, no. 4 (April 1938): 6. See also "A Tribute to Dr Harvey Agnew," *Hospital Administration in Canada* 13, no. 11 (November 1971): 21.
66 Bator and Rhodes, *Within Reach of Everyone*, 1:145.
67 Ontario Blue Cross, *Fifty Year Anniversary, 1941–1991* (Toronto: Ontario Blue Cross, 1991), 5–6.
68 Agnew, *Canadian Hospitals, 1920 to 1970*, 89.
69 Agnew, *Canadian Hospitals, 1920 to 1970*, 88–9.
70 Henry J. Cody, "The Contribution a Hospital May Make to Its Community," *Canadian Hospital* 17, no. 1 (January 1940): 11.
71 Cody, "Contribution a Hospital May Make," 11, 14.
72 Cody, "Contribution a Hospital May Make," 12–14.
73 "Administrators Talk It Over," *Canadian Nurse* 35, no. 1 (January 1939): 30.

74 "Successful Refresher Course in Hospital Administration Held at University of Toronto School of Nursing," *Canadian Hospital* 16, no. 1 (January 1939): 36.
75 *University of Toronto Calendar: School of Nursing 1938–1939*, 27.
76 *University of Toronto Calendar: School of Nursing 1938–1939*, 30.
77 *University Of Toronto Calendar: School of Nursing 1939–1940*, 31.
78 "Hospital Administration Course at the University of Toronto," *Canadian Hospital* 17, no. 1 (January 1940): 14.
79 Meeting of 26 November 1940, file "Teaching Staff Minutes 1940–44," box 001, Teaching Staff Minutes, School of Nursing, A73-0053, UTARMS.
80 *University of Toronto Calendar: School of Nursing 1941–1942*, 32–3. See also the calendar for 1942–43, 34; 1943–44, 34; 1944–45, 27.
81 Carpenter, *Divine Discontent*, 38.
82 See *University of Toronto Calendar: School of Nursing 1945–1946*, 34–5.
83 "Hospital Administration Course at the University of Toronto," *Canadian Hospital* 17, no. 1 (January 1940): 14.
84 Malcolm T. MacEachern, "Fundamental Principals and Trends in Hospital Administration, Part I," *Canadian Hospital* 16, no. 1 (January 1939): 14.
85 Malcolm T. MacEachern, "Fundamental Principals and Trends in Hospital Administration, Part II," *Canadian Hospital* 16, no. 2 (February 1939): 20.
86 MacEachern, "Fundamental Principals and Trends in Hospital Administration, Part II," 20.

CHAPTER SIX

1 G. Harvey Agnew, "The Possible Effect of Health Insurance upon Our Hospitals," *Bulletin of the American Hospital Association* 5, no. 10 (October 1931): 36.
2 Agnew, "Possible Effect of Health Insurance," 41.
3 Agnew, "Possible Effect of Health Insurance," 42.
4 G. Harvey Agnew, "The Possible Effect of Health Insurance upon Hospitals," *Canadian Medical Association Journal (CMAJ)* 26, no. 2 (February 1932): 182.
5 Agnew, "Possible Effect of Health Insurance upon Hospitals," 182
6 Agnew, "Possible Effect of Health Insurance upon Hospitals," 183.
7 Agnew, "Possible Effect of Health Insurance upon Hospitals," 184–5.
8 Harvey Agnew, "Health Insurance and Hospitals," *Canadian Hospital* (December 1934): 6.
9 Agnew, "Health Insurance and Hospitals," 5.
10 Harvey Agnew on Canadian Hospital Council letterhead to "Mr Chairman and Members of the Royal Commission on Dominion-Provincial Relations," 29 December 1937, Robarts Library, University of Toronto.
11 Harvey Agnew, secretary, Canadian Hospital Council, "Brief Submitted to the Royal Commission on Federal-Provincial Relations by the Canadian Hospital Council," *Canadian Hospital* 15, no. 2 (February 1938): 32–3.
12 Canadian Hospital Association, brief to the Royal Commission on Dominion-Provincial Relations, Toronto, 1937, 2. Note, the "brief," while bound in the U of T library, is really a four-page letter on CHA letterhead from Dr Agnew to the chair and members of the Royal Commission, 29 December 1937.
13 Canadian Hospital Association, ["Brief"], 4.
14 Canadian Hospital Association, ["Brief"], 4.

15 Harvey Agnew, "An Observer Looks at Group Hospitalization," *Canadian Hospital* 15, no. 2 (February 1938), 14–15.
16 Editorial Section, "A Public Health Charter for Canada," *Canadian Public Health Journal* 33, no. 7 (July 1942): 344–6.
17 Ronald Hare, P.A. Creelman, R.O. Davison, Grant Fleming, A.R. Foley, and J.J. McCann, "Resolutions Adopted at the Thirty-First Annual Meeting of the Canadian Public Health Association Held in Toronto, June 1–3, 1942," *Canadian Public Health Journal* 33, no. 7 (July 1942): 347.
18 F.W. Jackson, "The Integration of Preventive and Curative Medicine in Health Insurance," *CJPH* 35, no. 3 (March 1944): 104–8. Note, the *CJPH* had various nomenclatures. It was the *Canadian Public Health Journal* from 1928 to 1943 (see note above), after which it became the *CJPH*. From its inception in 1910 until 1928 it was known as the *Public Health Journal*.
19 "Memorandum on Health Insurance Presented to Parliamentary Committee," *Canadian Hospital* 20, no. 5 (May 1943): 15–19, 42–6.
20 Canada, House of Commons, Special Committee on Social Security, *Minutes of Proceedings and Evidence*, no. 6, 9 April 1943, 171.
21 Canada, House of Commons, Special Committee on Social Security, *Minutes of Proceedings and Evidence*, no. 6, 9 April 1943, 173–4.
22 Canada, House of Commons, Special Committee on Social Security, *Minutes of Proceedings and Evidence*, no. 6, 9 April 1943, 176.
23 Canada, House of Commons, Special Committee on Social Security, *Minutes of Proceedings and Evidence*, no. 6, 9 April 1943, 175–9.
24 Canada, House of Commons, Special Committee on Social Security, *Minutes of Proceedings and Evidence*, no. 6, 9 April 1943, 179–80.
25 Canada, House of Commons, Special Committee on Social Security, *Minutes of Proceedings and Evidence*, no. 6, 9 April 1943, 181.
26 Canada, House of Commons, Special Committee on Social Security, *Minutes of Proceedings and Evidence*, no. 6, 9 April 1943, 183.
27 George Harvey Agnew, "State Aid for Hospitals Urged by Toronto Doctor," *Toronto Telegram*, 26 September 1939.
28 Canada, House of Commons, Special Committee on Social Security, *Minutes of Proceedings and Evidence*, no. 12, 21 May 1943, 342, 356–7.
29 Canada, House of Commons, Special Committee on Social Security, *Minutes of Proceedings and Evidence*, no. 12, 21 May 1943, 342.
30 Canada, House of Commons, Special Committee on Social Security, *Minutes of Proceedings and Evidence*, no. 12, 21 May 1943, 344.
31 Canada, House of Commons, Special Committee on Social Security, *Minutes of Proceedings and Evidence*, no. 12, 21 May 1943, 344–7.
32 Canada, House of Commons, Special Committee on Social Security, *Minutes of Proceedings and Evidence*, no. 12, 21 May 1943, 348–9.
33 Canada, House of Commons, Special Committee on Social Security, *Minutes of Proceedings and Evidence*, no. 12, 21 May 1943, 356.
34 Bator and Rhodes, *Within Reach of Everyone*, 1:71.
35 Defries, *First Forty Years*, 151–96.
36 R.D. Defries, "Report of the Director of the School of Hygiene," *President's Report for the Year Ending 30th June 1940*, 36.
37 R.D. Defries, "Report of the Director of the School of Hygiene," *President's Report for the Year Ending 30th June 1941*, 45.

38 R.D. Defries, "Report of the Director of the School of Hygiene," *President's Report for the Year Ending 30th June 1943*, 38.
39 R.D. Defries, "Report of the Director of the School of Hygiene," *President's Report for the Year Ending 30th June 1944*, 40.
40 R.D. Defries, "Report of the Director of the School of Hygiene," *President's Report for the Year Ending 30th June 1946*, 52. Enrolment for 1944–5 was 483, for 1945–6 was 1138.
41 Canada, House of Commons, Special Committee on Social Security, *Minutes of Proceedings and Evidence, No. 13*, 25 May 1943 (Ottawa: King's Printer, 1943). See also Canada, House of Commons, Special Committee on Reconstruction and Re-establishment, *Minutes of Proceedings and Evidence*, No. *16*, 25 May 1943 (Ottawa: King's Printer, 1943), 409–23, for the identical text.
42 Trish Reay, Elizabeth Goodrick, and Bob Hinings, "Institutionalization and Professionalization," in *The Oxford Handbook of Health Care Management*, ed. Ewan Ferlie, Kathleen Montgomery, and Anne Reff Pedersen, 27–30 (New York: Oxford University Press, 2016).

CHAPTER SEVEN

1 Leigh J. Crozier, "The Hospital: Keynote to National Health," *Canadian Hospital* 24, no. 9 (September 1947): 39.
2 Guenter B. Risse, *Hospital Life in Enlightenment Scotland: Care and Teaching at the Royal Infirmary of Edinburgh* (Cambridge: Cambridge University Press, 1986), 279; quoted in Connor, *Doing Good*, 260.
3 C. Ian Kyer, *Lawyers, Families, and Businesses: The Shaping of a Bay Street Law Firm, Faskens 1863–1963* (Toronto: Published for the Osgoode Society for Canadian Legal History by Irwin Law, 2013), 119. See also 291n125.
4 "David Fasken, Excelsior Life President, Dead," *Toronto Daily Star*, 2 December 1929.
5 Kyer, *Lawyers, Families, and Businesses*, 172.
6 Harvey Agnew, "Graduate Training in Hospital Administration," *Canadian Hospital* 24, no. 10 (October 1947): 29.
7 See Committee on the Costs of Medical Care, specifically Ray Lyman Wilbur, "Foreword," in *The Costs of Medical Care: A Summary of Investigations on the Economic Aspects of the Prevention and Care of Illness*, publication no. 27 (Chicago: University of Chicago Press, 1933), v.
8 We have spoken of these reports earlier. They are not devoted exclusively to health, but health figures in each of them. They are the Rowell-Sirois Report, and Heagerty, Marsh, and Cassidy Reports.
9 Commission on Hospital Care, *Hospital Care in the United States* (New York: Commonwealth Fund, 1947), 65.
10 Canada, Department of National Health and Welfare, *Hospital Care in Canada: Trends and Developments, 1948–1962* (Ottawa: Queen's Printer, 1964), 3. The exact figures depict the gross operating expenditures for all classes of hospital, going from $210 million in 1948 to $930 million in 1961.
11 Crozier, "Hospital – Keynote," 39.
12 George Campbell Gosling, *Payment and Philanthropy in British Healthcare, 1918–48* (Manchester: Manchester University Press, 2017), 5.
13 Adam D. Reich, *Selling Our Souls: The Commodification of Hospital Care in the United States* (Princeton, NJ: Princeton University Press, 2014), 1.

14 Bator, *Within Reach of Everyone*, 2:191.
15 Bator and Rhodes, *Within Reach of Everyone*, 1:134.
16 *President's Report, for the Year Ending 30th June 1941*, Toronto: University of Toronto Press, 1941, p. 45.
17 *President's Report, for the Year Ending 30th June 1941*, 4.
18 *President's Report, for the Year Ending 30th June 1940*, 36.
19 "William Mosley," in "The Canadian Public Health Association, Annual Report, 1971–1972, June 1972," supplement, CJPH 63 (1972): S12–13.
20 *President's Report, for the Year Ending 30th June 1941*, 45.
21 *President's Report, for the Year Ending 30th June 1942* (Toronto: University of Toronto Press, 1942), 41.
22 Bator and Rhodes, *Within Reach of Everyone*, 1:86.
23 This is also known as the Emergency Medical Service, though, to be accurate, this was a later and distinct aspect, which denoted the medical staff and medical activities of the Service. Each organized hospitals and medical staff respectively into a national system. Related services such as lab services for blood typing, pathology, and public health (to diagnose epidemic disease) were also included.
24 For a very good overview of the Emergency Hospital Service, see the Titmuss work on British social policy during the war: chapter 5, "Preparations: The Emergency Medical Service," 54–86; chapter 11, "Hospitals in Transition: September 1939–May 1940," 183–202; and chapter 22, "Hospitals in Demand," 442–505, in Titmuss, *Problems of Social Policy.*
25 Webster, *National Health Service*, 7.
26 Webster, *National Health Service*, 6.
27 Great Britain, Ministry of Health, *Statement Relating to the Emergency Hospital Organization, First Aid Posts and Ambulances* (London: HMSO, 1939), 4.
28 Great Britain, Ministry of Health, *Statement*, 6.
29 Eleanor G. Kinney, *The Affordable Care Act and Medicare in Comparative Context* (New York: Cambridge University Press, 2015), 371.
30 Webster, *National Health Service*, 17.
31 Titmuss, *Problems of Social Policy*, 504.
32 Titmuss, *Problems of Social Policy*, 504.
33 See NHS Scotland, "Emergency Hospital Service (EHS)," http://www.our nhsscotland.com/history/birth-nhs-scotland/emergency-hospital-service.
34 Great Britain, Ministry of Health, *On the State of the Public Health During Six Years of War: Report of the Chief Medical Officer of the Ministry of Health* (London: HMSO, 1946), 136. For an account of the inception of the EHS, see *On the State of the Public Health: Annual Report of the Chief Medical Officer of the Ministry of Health for the Year 1938* (London: HMSO, 1939), 57–69.
35 Great Britain, House of Commons, *Debates*, 9 October 1941, vol. 374, coll. 1116.
36 Great Britain, House of Commons, *Debates*, 9 October 1941, vol. 374, coll. 1119.
37 Great Britain, House of Commons, *Debates*, 21 October 1941, vol. 374, coll. 1677.
38 Great Britain, House of Commons, *Debates*, 21 October 1941, vol. 374, coll. 1682.

39 This column continued after the war years and was still featured in 1952 (which appears to have been its last year).
40 See "With the Hospitals in Britain," *Canadian Hospital* 19, no. 9 (September 1942): 25, 48, 50. For other references to the EHS, see the same column, March 1943, 43; also November 1943, 35.
41 For a sense of this heightened interest, see Taylor, *Health Insurance and Canadian Public Policy*; A.W. Johnson, *Dream No Little Dreams: A Biography of the Douglas Government of Saskatchewan, 1944–1961* (Toronto: University of Toronto Press, 2004); and Nancy Christie, *Engendering the State: Family, Work, and Welfare in Canada* (Toronto: University of Toronto Press, 2000), chap. 7.
42 Webster, *National Health Service*, 7.
43 Titmuss, *Problems of Social Policy*, 474.
44 See the section "The Idea of Social Citizenship" (77–8) and "The Internationalization of Social Security and Diffusion beyond Europe and the New World: The Role of the ILO" (78–9) in the chapter by Stein Kuhnle and Anne Sander, "The Emergence of the Western Welfare State" (61–80) in *The Oxford Handbook of the Welfare State*, ed. Francis G. Castles, Stephan Leibried, Jane Lewis, Herbert Obinger, and Christopher Pierson (Oxford: Oxford University Press, 2010).
45 Kuhnle and Sander, "Emergence of the Western Welfare State," table 5.1, which shows social security schemes prior to 1945 in selected ILO member countries (including Canada), 70–4.
46 See Frank Nullmeier and Franz-Xaver Kaufmann, "Post War Welfare State Development," in Castles et al., *Oxford Handbook of the Welfare State*, 84.
47 Canada, House of Commons, *Debates*, Fourth Session, Twentieth Parliament, vol. 4, 14 May 1948 (Ottawa: King's Printer, 1948), 3931.
48 See Barnett, *Audit of War*. (Chapter 1, "The Dream of New Jerusalem," is very relevant for our purposes, especially 14–32.)
49 Julian Huxley, "Health for All," *Picture Post* 10, no. 1, 4 January 1941, 32.
50 Barnett, *Audit of War*, 21.
51 Barnett, *Audit of War*, 22.
52 Timmins, *Five Giants*, 23.
53 Cédric Guinand, "A Pillar of Economic Integration: The ILO and the Development of Social Security in Western Europe," in *Networks of Global Governance: International Organizations and European Integration in a Historical Perspective*, ed. Lorenzo Mechi, Guia Migani, and Francesco Petrini (Newcastle: Cambridge Scholars Publishing, 2014), 116.
54 See Nadja van Ginneken, Simon Lewin, and Virginia Berridge, "The Emergence of Community Health Worker Programmes in the Late Apartheid Era in South Africa: An Historical Analysis," *Social Science and Medicine* 71, no. 6 (September 2010): 1110.
55 Timmins, *Five Giants*, 25.
56 Webster, *National Health Service*, 8.
57 Handwritten note from "Office of the Chairman, Committee on Reconstruction," acc. 0000-0028, C6, MG1017 (Frank Cyril James), McGill University Archives.
58 High commissioner for Canada to secretary of state for external affairs, 10 December 1942, 1–2, acc. 0000-0028, C6, MG1017 (Frank Cyril James),

McGill University Archives. For a portion of this, see also Christie, *Engendering the State*, 274.

59 See Canada, House of Commons, Special Committee on Social Security, *Minutes of Proceedings and Evidence*, no. 13, 25 May 1943 (Ottawa: King's Printer, 1943), 365–79.

60 Editorial (R.D. Defries, editor), "The Beveridge Report: A Stimulus to Canadian Thinking," *Canadian Journal of Public Health* 33, no. 12 (December 1942): 600.

61 "Select Committee to Consider Federal Social Insurance," *Canadian Hospital* 20, no. 3 (March 1943): 25.

62 Editorial (R.D. Defries, editor), "Implementing Social Security Plans in Great Britain," *Canadian Journal of Public Health* 39, no. 8 (August 1948): 345–7.

63 José Harris, *William Beveridge: A Biography*, 2nd ed. (Oxford: Clarendon, 1997), 425–6.

64 Harris, *William Beveridge*, 425–6.

65 *Time*, "Cradle to Grave to Pigeonhole," 41, no. 12 (22 March 1943): 13.

66 *Time*, "'Thirty Years Late,'" 41, no. 21 (24 May 1943): 18.

67 *Time*, "Four and Twelve," 41, no. 23 (7 June 1943): 22.

68 Fraser, *Evolution of the British Welfare State*, 228.

69 Fraser, *Evolution of the British Welfare State*, 230.

70 Fraser, *Evolution of the British Welfare State*, 228–30.

71 Paul Addison, *The Road to 1945: British Politics and the Second World War*, rev. ed. (London: Jonathan Cape, 1994), 131.

72 Richard M. Titmuss, *Problems of Social Policy* (London: His Majesty's Stationery Office and Longman's, Green, 1950), 506. Chapter 25, from which this quote is taken, provides a very good overview of government involvement in health (see 506–38).

73 F.R. Davis, "The Importance of the Voluntary Hospital to the Community," *Canadian Hospital* 18, no. 8 (August 1941): 21.

74 Davis, "Importance of the Voluntary Hospital," 21.

75 G.H.A., "Three Proposals for Social Advancement Offered to the British People," *Canadian Hospital* 20, no. 1 (January 1943): 18–19, 42.

76 See United States, Social Security Administration, "Social Security History, The Evolution of Medicare, Chapter 3: The Third Round 1943–1950," https://www.ssa.gov/history/corningchap3.html.

77 G.H.A., "Health Insurance Imminent in Canada," *Hospitals* 17, no. 5 (May 1943): 67–8.

78 G. Harvey Agnew, "Health Insurance Proposal That Has Hospital Support," *Hospitals* 17, no. 11 (November 1943): 81.

79 Thomas Parran, "More Heath Care Inevitable," *Hospitals* 17, no. 10 (October 1943): 48–51.

80 Great Britain, Ministry of Health, *A National Health Service. Presented by the Minister of Health and the Secretary of State for Scotland to Parliament by Command of His Majesty, February 1944* (London: H.M. Stationery Office, 1944), 6.

81 Great Britain, Ministry of Health, *National Health Service*, 6.

82 Great Britain, Ministry of Health, *National Health Service*, 3–5.

83 Great Britain, Ministry of Health, *National Health Service*, for example, 12, 52.

84 Saskatchewan Health Services Survey Commission, *Report of the Commis-*

sioner, presented to the minister of public health, 4 October 1944 (Regina: Thos H. McConica, King's Printer, 1944).

85 Some very good material on the evolution of health insurance in the United States is on the Social Security Administration website. For the history of events we are speaking about, see "The Evolution of Medicare, Chapter 3, The Third Round, 1943–1950." For the entire history, see Corning, *History of Medicare*. For all social security history, see Social Security, https://www.ssa.gov/history/index.html.

86 Agnew, *Canadian Hospitals, 1920 to 1970*, 168.

87 United States, *Statutes at Large* 60, pt 1, 1946, 79th Congress, Second Session (Washington: Government Printing Office, 1947), 1043.

88 Harry Perlstadt, "The Development of Hill-Burton Legislation: Interests, Issues and Compromises," *Journal of Health and Social Policy* 6, no. 3 (1995): 78.

89 United States Congress, Senate, Committee on Education and Labor, *Hospital Construction Act, Hearings before the Committee on Education and Labor, United States Senate, Seventy-Ninth Congress, First Session, on S. 191, a Bill to Amend the Public Health Service Act to Authorize Grants to the States for Surveying Their Hospitals and Public Health Centers and for the Planning Construction of Additional Facilities, and to Authorize Grants to Assist in Such Construction*, 12 March 1945, Dr Frederick D. Mott (Washington: U.S. Government Printing Office, 1945), 180. See 179–96 for all of Mott's testimony.

90 United States Congress, Senate, Committee on Education and Labor, *Hospital Construction Act, Hearings*.

91 United States Congress, Senate, Committee on Education and Labor, *National Health Program, Hearings before the Committee on Education and Labor, United States Senate, Seventy-Ninth Congress, Second Session, on S. 1606, a Bill to Provide for a National Health Program, Part One*, 2 April 1946, Opening Session, National Health Program (Washington: US Government Printing Office, 1946), 1–8.

92 United States Congress, Senate, Committee on Education and Labor, *National Health Program … Part Three*, 25 April 1946, Frederick D. Mott, 1181 (see 1178–1210 for all of Mott's testimony).

93 United States Congress, Senate, Committee on Education and Labor, *National Health Program … Part Three*, 1181.

94 United States Congress, Senate, Committee on Education and Labor, *National Health Program … Part Three*, 1185.

95 Bator and Rhodes, *Within Reach of Everyone*, 1:137.

96 Bator and Rhodes, *Within Reach of Everyone*, 1:138.

97 Bator and Rhodes, *Within Reach of Everyone*, 1:138–9.

98 Berridge, *Public Health*, 69.

99 R.B. Jenkins, "The Place of the Hospital in Public Health Work in Canada," *Canadian Hospital* 16, no. 11 (November 1939): 28–9, 49–50.

100 Canada, House of Commons, *Debates*, Third Session, Twentieth Parliament, 6 February 1947 (Ottawa: Edmond Cloutier, King's Printer, 1947), 1:177. See 177–84 for the complete discussion.

101 Great Britain, House of Commons, *Debates*, 15 August 1945, vol. 413 (London: His Majesty's Stationery Office, 1945), coll. 56.

102 Ontario, Legislative Assembly, *Debates*, 6 March 1947, Twenty-Second Legislature, vol. 1, no. 1 (Toronto: King's Printer, 1947), 7.
103 Ontario, Legislative Assembly, *Debates*, 11 March 1947, vol. 1, no. 4, 72.
104 Ontario, Legislative Assembly, *Debates*, 27 March 1947, vol. 1, no. 15, 540. Hospitals were discussed in detail on 539–43 of that session.
105 Commission on Hospital Care, *Hospital Care in the United States* (New York: Commonwealth Fund, 1947), 3.
106 A.L. Swanson and Harvey Agnew, "Lack of Hospital Facilities Stressed in Memorandum to Dominion Council on Health," *Canadian Hospital* 24, no. 6 (June 1947): 25–6.
107 "Minutes, 51st Meeting, May 14–16, 1947," appendix D, 3, Department of Public Health, Dominion Council of Health, R-1367, SAB.
108 "Minutes, 52nd meeting, October 15–17, 1947," 9, Department of Public Health, Dominion Council of Health, R-1367, SAB.
109 Taylor, *Health Insurance and Canadian Public Policy*, 163.
110 Taylor, *Health Insurance and Canadian Public Policy*, 205.
111 Canada, House of Commons, *Debates*, Fourth Session, Twentieth Parliament, vol. 4, 14 May 1948 (Ottawa: King's Printer, 1948), 3934.
112 Canada, House of Commons, *Debates*, Fourth Session, Twentieth Parliament, 4:3935.
113 Canada, Department of National Health and Welfare, *National Health Grants, 1948–1961* (Ottawa: Roger Duhamel, Queen's Printer, 1962), 9.
114 "Minutes, 54th Meeting, June 7–8, 1948," Department of Public Health, Dominion Council of Health, R-1367, SAB.
115 See Taylor, *Health Insurance and Canadian Public Policy*, 163.
116 Agnew, *Canadian Hospitals, 1920 to 1970*, 169.
117 Canada, Department of National Health and Welfare, *National Health Grants, 1948–1961*, 42.
118 "Minutes, 54th Meeting, June 7–8, 1948," 53–4.
119 Agnew, *Canadian Hospitals, 1920 to 1970*, 169.
120 "Minutes, 54th Meeting, June 7–8, 1948," 95.
121 "Minutes, 54th Meeting, June 7–8, 1948," 105.
122 Canada, Department of National Health and Welfare, *National Health Grants, 1948–1961*, 20.
123 See, Canada, Department of National Health and Welfare, *National Health Grants*, 23.
124 Bator and Rhodes, *Within Reach of Everyone*, 1:137.
125 Bator and Rhodes, *Within Reach of Everyone*, 1:138.
126 Bator and Rhodes, *Within Reach of Everyone*, 1:137–8. Regarding Dr Jackson, see also R.D. Defries to Sidney Smith, 9 June 1950, "Hygiene," July 1949–June 1950, Office of the President, A68-0007/064(06), UTARMS.
127 Webster, *National Health Service*, 38.
128 Webster, *National Health Service*, 29.
129 Webster, *National Health Service*, 29.
130 George Godber, *The Health Service: Past, Present, and Future* (London: Athlone, 1975), 24.
131 Douglas Black, "Obituary: Sir George Godber," *Guardian*, 11 February 2009, https://www.theguardian.com/society/2009/feb/11/sir-george-godber-obituary. Sir Douglas Black was another CMO and the author of the famous Black Report (1980).

132 Webster, *National Health Service*, 38.
133 Ontario, Department of Health, Hospitals Division, *The Hospitals of Ontario: A Short History* (Toronto: Herbert H. Ball, King's Printer, 1934), 20. It noted that in the 1870s provincial grants to hospitals were $27,880, in the early 1900s $110,000. By 1932 this had increased to $1.2 million.
134 Jeanne Kisacky, *Rise of the Modern Hospital: An Architectural History of Health and Healing, 1870–1940* (Pittsburgh: University of Pittsburgh Press, 2017), 257, 259.
135 Kisacky, *Rise of the Modern Hospital*, 248.
136 Kisacky, *Rise of the Modern Hospital*, 248.
137 Kisacky, *Rise of the Modern Hospital*, 293.
138 Wright, *SickKids*, 198–9.
139 Lesley Marrus Barsky, *From Generation to Generation: A History of Toronto's Mount Sinai Hospital* (Toronto: McClelland & Stewart, 1998), 53, 62.
140 Cosbie, *Toronto General Hospital*, 283–90.
141 David Blumenthal, "Academic Health Centers: Current Status, Future Challenges," in *The Academic Health Center: Leadership and Performance*, ed. Don E. Detmar and Elaine B. Steen (Cambridge: Cambridge University Press, 2005), 14–15.
142 The term is used by George Campbell Gosling in a chapter of the same name in *Payment and Philanthropy in British Healthcare, 1918–48* (Manchester: Manchester University Press), 120–56. Gosling actually does not mean it in the sense used here. He means it as a kind of private medicine practised in British hospitals that was seen as a threat to "the charitable nature of the institution" (120).
143 See, for example, Laurinda Abreu and Sally Sheard, eds, *Hospital Life: Theory and Practice from the Medieval to the Modern* (Bern: Peter Lang, 2013); or Christopher Bonfield, Jonathan Reinarz, and Teresa Huguet-Termer, eds, *Hospitals and Communities, 1100–1960* (Bern: Peter Lang, 2013).
144 David Gagan and Rosemary Gagan, *For Patients of Moderate Means: A Social History of the Voluntary Public General Hospital in Canada* (Montreal and Kingston: McGill-Queen's University Press, 2002), ix–x.
145 The University of Toronto Gerstein Library collection gives some indication of the import of hospitals. There is shelf upon shelf with books on hospitals from various countries. For example, the RA 983 section has books published on numerous Canadian hospitals. It has an even more extensive section (RA 986–8) on British hospitals and one on U.S. hospitals (RA 982, where the hospitals section begins). It continues to RA 989 with hospitals of other countries, an estimated 800 books in total.
146 H.E. MacDermot, *History of the School of Nursing of Montreal General Hospital* (Montreal: Alumnae Association, 1940), 1.
147 Bob Bell, deputy minister, Health and Long-Term Care, University of Toronto, IHPME GSU Lunch & Learn, 18 May 2017. I was in the audience.

CHAPTER EIGHT

1 R.D.D., "Planning Graduate Course in Hospital Administration at University of Toronto," *Canadian Hospital* 24, no. 5 (May 1947): 32. Note R.D.D. is almost certainly R.D. Defries, director of the School of Hygiene at the time.
2 "Council Meeting School of Hygiene, February 25, 1947," 1–3, file 6, box 19, "Office of the President," A1968-0007, UTARMS.

3 Graham L. Davis, director, Division of Hospitals, Kellogg Foundation, to R.D. Defries, 6 January 1947, "Hygiene," file 6, box 19, A68-0007, UTARMS.
4 Commission on Hospital Care, "Hospitals and Health Departments," *Hospital Survey News Letter*, August 1946, 2, 4, file 6, box 19, A68-0007, UTARMS.
5 Council Meeting, School of Hygiene, 25 February 1947, file 6, box 19, A68-0007, UTARMS.
6 Sidney Smith to Emory Morris, 25 March 1947, file 6, box 19, "Office of the President," A1968-0007, UTARMS.
7 Defries to Sidney Smith, 8 April 1947; and Sidney Smith to Davis, 12 April 1947, file 6, box 19, "Office of the President," A1968-0007, UTARMS.
8 Emory W. Morris, president and general director, Kellogg Foundation, to Sidney Smith, 22 April 1947, file 6, box 19, "Office of the President," A1968-0007, UTARMS.
9 Statute 1837, "Respecting the Diploma in Hospital Administration and the Course of Instruction Leading Thereto," 11 April 1947, Statute Numbers 1481–1999, Statutes, 3 June 1940–9 December 1949, Senate, series II, box 146, Office of the Chief Accountant, A73-0005/146, UTARMS.
10 "Information Relating to the Recommendation of the Council of the School of Hygiene That a Post-Graduate Course in Hospital Administration Be Established," 1, attached to Statute 1837, Statute Numbers 1481–1999, Statutes, 3 June 1940–9 December 1949, Senate, series II, box 146, Office of the Chief Accountant, A73-0005/146, UTARMS.
11 "Information Relating to the Recommendation," 1–2.
12 "Information Relating to the Recommendation," 2.
13 President to R.D. Defries, 7 May 1947; and R.D. Defries to Sidney Smith, 4 June 1947, with enclosures of poster and course brochure, file 6, box 19, "Office of the President," A1968-0007, UTARMS.
14 Minutes, 8 May 1947, 63, Minutes of Board of Governors, 1947–48, A1970-0024/034(01b), UTARMS.
15 Minutes, 8 May 1947, 66.
16 Minutes, 29 May 1947, 77, Minutes of Board of Governors, 1947–48, A1970-0024/034(01b), UTARMS.
17 Minutes, 29 May 1947, 135. The salary was $5,400 as associate professor of hospital administration and $1,100 as associate in public health administration.
18 *President's Report, for the Year Ending June 1947*, 50. See also School of Hygiene, University of Toronto, *Twenty-Second Annual Report, 1946–1947*, 7, 9.
19 "Hygiene, July '46–June '47," and "Resolution (1)," file 6, box 19, "Office of the President," A1968-0007, UTARMS.
20 "Memorandum: Proposed Course in Hospital Administration in the University of Toronto," file 6, box 19, "Office of the President," A1968-0007, UTARMS.
21 "Oral History Interviews, University of Toronto, Faculty of Medicine, Dr Milton Brown," 22 February 1980, 67–8, vol. 4, B87-0044, UTARMS.
22 *President's Report, for the Year Ending June 1947*, 50.
23 W.K. Kellogg Foundation, *The First Twenty-Five Years: The Story of a Foundation [1930–1955]* (Battle Creek, MI: [Foundation, 1955 or 6]), 108, 109, 211, 255. Dr Agnew is noted on 239.

24 W.K. Kellogg Foundation, *The First Half Century, 1930–1980: Private Approaches to Public Needs* (Battle Creek, MI: [Foundation, 1980]), 92, 138.

25 "Interview with Dr Andrew Rhodes," 23 July 1985, side 2, tape 4/6, audiocassette, School of Hygiene History Project, B890009(04), UTARMS. For a partial account of the interview, see "Transcript, Recorded Interview with Dr Andrew J. Rhodes," 23 July 1985, 2.

26 Letters from R.D. Defries to Sidney Smith, one regarding the study visit dated 28 May 1947, the other as payment for the lectures delivered by the deputy minister dated 7 May 1947, file 6, box 19, "Office of the President," A1968-0007, UTARMS.

27 For a brief (and the most complete) synopsis of G. Harvey Agnew's professional life, as well as tributes from prominent administrators in the field, see "A Tribute to Dr Harvey Agnew," *Hospital Administration in Canada* 13, no. 11 (November 1971): 20–5. Note the title of the article in the body of the magazine is "A Tribute to the Grand Old Man of Canada's Hospital System," which differs from the table of contents.

For other tributes, see A.F., "Tribute to the Late G. Harvey Agnew," *Canadian Hospital* 48, no. 11 (November 1971): 62–3, which also has a different title within the magazine: "G. Harvey Agnew, MD: A Tribute to the Man." See also "Obituaries, George Harvey Agnew," *Canadian Medical Association Journal*, 105, no. 12 (18 December 1971): 1341.

28 G. Harvey Agnew, "An Explanation of Canada's Health Insurance Proposal That Has Hospital Support," *Hospitals* 17, no. 11 (November 1943): 82.

29 G. Harvey Agnew, "An Explanation of Canada's Health Insurance Proposal That Has Hospital Support," in *Hospital Trends and Developments, 1940–1946*, ed. Arthur C. Bachmeyer and Gerhard Hartman, 767–71 (New York: Commonwealth Fund, 1948). He had also written articles in a 1943 publication of the Commonwealth Fund, with the same two editors, *The Hospital in Modern Society*.

30 *Bulletin*, December 1947, 7, UTARMS.

31 Sidney Smith, "Report of the President," *President's Report, for the Year Ending June 1948*, 25.

32 *University of Toronto, Calendar, School of Hygiene, 1947–1948*, 4.

33 School of Hygiene, "Post-Graduate Course in Hospital Administration, School of Hygiene, University of Toronto, 1947–1948," file 6, box 19, "Office of the President," A1968-0007, UTARMS.

34 Educational Policies Committee, American College of Hospital Administrators, *The Administrative Residency in the Hospital* (Chicago: American College of Hospital Administrators, 1954), 5.

35 Louis Horlick, *They Built Better Than They Knew: Saskatchewan's Royal University Hospital, A History: 1955–1992* (Saskatoon: Royal University Hospital Foundation, 2001), 285.

36 Horlick, *They Built Better Than They Knew*, 280. Note, neither Earl nor the deputy minister (J. Graham Clarkson) was a DHA graduate; however, Earl was a very well-respected administrator, an originator of the *Canadian Hospital Accounting Manual*, and did mentor DHA grads. I consulted him from time to time on hospital matters.

37 Valerie A. Rakow, *A Fifty-Year Retrospective, 1947–1997, University of Toronto Department of Health Administration* ([Toronto]: Ruth Corbin, Decision Resources Inc., 1998), 4.

38 School of Hygiene, *Twenty-Third Annual Report, 1947–1948*, 25.
39 Mynett, *Service on the Skeena*, 240, 415.
40 School of Hygiene, *Twenty-Third Annual Report, 1947–1948*, 26.
41 R.D.D., "Planning Graduate Course in Hospital Administration at University of Toronto," *Canadian Hospital* 24, no. 5 (May 1947): 32. Note, R.D.D. is almost certainly R.D. Defries, director of the School of Hygiene at the time.
42 Harvey Agnew, "The Role of the Hospital on Medical Economics," CMAJ 56, no. 5 (May 1947): 558.
43 Agnew, "Role of the Hospital on Medical Economics," 562.
44 "Graduate Course in Hospital Administration at the University of Toronto," *Canadian Hospital* 24, no. 6 (June 1947): 31.
45 "University of Toronto, School of Hygiene, Post Graduate Course in Hospital Administration," *Canadian Hospital* 24, no. 6 (June 1947): 84.
46 "To Teach Hospital Administration," *Canadian Hospital* 24, no. 7 (July 1947): 34.
47 Harvey Agnew, "Graduate Training in Hospital Administration," *Canadian Hospital* 24, no. 10 (October 1947): 29.
48 "Administration Course at Toronto," *Hospitals* 22, no. 2 (February 1948): 112.
49 Rakow, *Fifty-Year Retrospective*, 4–5. The seven original members were Columbia University, Johns Hopkins University, Northwestern University, University of Chicago, University of Minnesota, University of Toronto, and Yale University.
50 School of Hygiene, *Twenty-Fourth Annual Report, 1948–1949*, 26.
51 School of Hygiene, *Thirtieth Annual Report, 1954–1955*, 18.
52 R.D. Defries, "Report of the Director of the School of Hygiene," *President's Report for the Year Ending June 1949*, 57.
53 R.D. Defries, "Report of the Director of the School of Hygiene," *President's Report for the Year Ending June 1952*, 84.
54 School of Hygiene, *Twenty-Eighth Annual Report, 1952–1953*, 10.
55 R.D. Defries, "Report of the Director of the School of Hygiene," *President's Report for the Year Ending June 1955*, 105.
56 Edwin V. Wahn, "A Plan for an Integrated Hospital System in Saskatchewan" (DHA thesis, University of Toronto, 1950), 3.
57 "Institute for Hospital Administrators Exceeds Expectations," *Canadian Hospital* 23, no. 12 (December 1946): 44–5.
58 "Fourth Western Canadian Institute Proves Unqualified Success," *Canadian Hospital* 26, no. 11 (November 1949): 37–8.
59 Agnew, *Canadian Hospitals, 1920 to 1970*, 85.
60 Taylor, *Health Insurance and Canadian Public Policy*, 198.
61 "Notes about People," *Canadian Hospital* 39, no. 7 (July 1962): 28.
62 See "People," *Canadian Hospital* 47, no. 11 (September 1970): 21.
63 "People," *Canadian Hospital* 45, no. 5 (May 1968): 28.

CHAPTER NINE

1 J.A. McNab, "A Tribute to Eugenie M. Stuart, Professor Emeritus Hospital Administration, University of Toronto, October 25, 1971," 2–3, Department of Health Administration, A1998-0023/002, UTARMS; contained in a leather-bound album presented to Stuart, dated 25 October 1971.
2 "A Tribute, First Annual W.D. Piercey Memorial Lecture," Department of Health Administration, A1998-0023/002, UTARMS. Miss Stuart delivered this

lecture, and a short bio of her was included in the program brochure. It is contained in the leather-bound album presented to Miss Stuart.

3 McNab, "Tribute to Eugenie M. Stuart." See also first interview with Burns Roth, 16 July 1985, digitized audio recording, School of Hygiene History Project, B89-0009_01S, UTARMS.

4 "A Tribute, First Annual W.D. Piercey Memorial Lecture."

5 Riegler, *Jean I. Gunn*, 213.

6 Eugenie M. Stuart, "Pooling Resources," one of five papers in "A Symposium: Regional Approach to Nursing Administration in Small Hospitals," *Canadian Hospital* 31, no. 3 (March 1954): 38–9. These papers were presented at the Ontario Hospital Association Convention in October 1953.

7 Bator and Rhodes, *Within Reach of Everyone*, 1:152.

8 Jean I. Gunn, chair, Health Insurance and Nursing Service Committee of the Canadian Nurses' Association, presentation, *Hearings*, 9 May 1938, Ottawa, Royal Commission on Dominion-Provincial Relations (Rowell-Sirois Commission), 7998.

9 An example is the index for 1952, which has a number of articles by graduates, such as R.B. Ferguson, J. Lee, and E.V. Wahn. See "Author Index," *Canadian Hospital* 29, no. 12 (December 1952): 100–1.

10 Malcolm Taylor, "Hospital Utilization and Costs under Compulsory Prepaid Coverage, Part 1," *Canadian Hospital* 27, no. 1 (January 1950): 31.

11 Malcolm Taylor, "Hospital Utilization and Costs under Compulsory Prepaid Coverage, Part 2," *Canadian Hospital* 27, no. 2 (February 1950): 60.

12 F.B. Roth, "Government Plan in Saskatchewan," *Canadian Hospital* 30, no. 9 (September 1953): 38.

13 Roth, "Government Plan in Saskatchewan," 76.

14 Meeting 29 March 1949, "Participation in Short Courses in Hospital Administration," 1, file "School of Hygiene Council Minutes," box 002, School of Hygiene, A1975-0029, UTARMS.

15 Meeting 29 March 1949, 2.

16 Harvey Agnew, "Training of Hospital Administrators," *Canadian Hospital* 27, no. 7 (July 1950): 84. See also 58, 27–9. Note, on page 29 there is a picture of the third class in the DHA program in front of the School of Hygiene Building as it was then known (now called the FitzGerald Building). The caption notes they had completed their nine months of academic work and were about to embark on their administrative residencies. The hospitals they were going to were noted next to their names.

17 "Discussion Outline of Proposals for a Canadian Hospital Council Course in Hospital Administration," 1, 4, file 4, "Hygiene, July '50–June '51," box 77, "Office of the President," A1968-0007, UTARMS.

18 "Discussion Outline of Proposals," 2–3.

19 R.D. Defries to Sidney Smith, 28 December 1950, file 4, "Hygiene, July '50–June '51," box 77, "Office of the President," A1968-0007, UTARMS.

20 "Item 7, Report of Arrangements with the Canadian Hospital Council," Meeting 21 May 1951, 3, file "Minutes, Council of the School of Hygiene," box 002, School of Hygiene, A1975-0029, UTARMS.

21 *President's Report, for the Year Ending June 1952*, 84.

22 "Item 6, Report on Hospital Administration Course," Meeting 21 May 1951, 2, file "Minutes, Council of the School of Hygiene," box 002, School of Hygiene, A1975-0029, UTARMS.

23 W.K. Kellogg Foundation, *First Twenty-Five Years*, 163.
24 They provided expertise in areas such as administration, accounting, nursing and other health professions, purchasing, etc.
25 Andrew Boehm was a member of the H.O.M. graduating class of 1962; see "H.O.M. Course Completes Successful Year," *Canadian Hospital* 39, no. 9 (September 1962): 67; see also "Hospital Organization and Management – Summer Session," *Canadian Hospital* 38, no. 9 (September 1961): 70. I still remember his enthusiasm of being at the four-week intensive, of being at the University of Toronto, and the city itself. I didn't know it at the time, but from pictures he brought back and because I was later a don there, they were billeted at New College, then the only university residence that was air-conditioned.
26 "Saskatchewan H.O.M. Alumni," *Canadian Hospital* 39, no. 9 (September 1962): 68.
27 There is a brief mention of his time at the Charles Camsell Hospital in Charles Camsell History Committee, *The Camsell Mosaic: The Charles Camsell Hospital, 1945–1985* (Altona, MB: D.W. Friesen, for the Charles Camsell History Committee, 1985), 53.
28 "Preceptor-Staff Meetings to 1970," box 09, Department of Health Administration, 1956–1977, UA1986-0034, UTARMS; see various Preceptor-Staff Meeting minutes.
29 "Preceptor-Staff Meetings to 1970"; see an undated list of preceptors, facility, and students. Though undated, judging from some of the administrators involved it was the early 1950s.
30 "Preceptor-Staff Meetings to 1970"; memo from Elwood W. Camp, director of education, American College of Hospital Administrators requesting list for 11th Congress, 8–10 February 1968, with attached list of Canadian preceptors.
31 "Personnel Management – Mr G. Turner" and "1622 – Advanced Planning Seminars 9/5/75, Long Range Planning – G. Turner, T. Freedman," box 010, Department of Health Administration, 1956–1977, A1986-0034, UTARMS. There is no date specified for when the courses were taught.
32 Personal conversation with the author, 20 May 2016.
33 *Department of Political Economy*, A1976-0025, UTARMS. The Finding Aid notes final marks for a class for Department of Hospital Administration students from 1950–51 through 1954–55.
34 F.R. Crocombe to D.I. MacLean, 9 November 1950, listing students and marks, file 11, box /042, Department of Political Economy, A76-0025, UTARMS.
35 Eugenie M. Stuart to H.A. Innis, 9 January 1952, noting the two courses and two students who had withdrawn, file 15, box /047, Department of Political Economy, A76-0025, UTARMS.
36 Letter to J.H. Sword, 30 May 1953, listing students and their final marks, file 24, box /052, Department of Political Economy, A76-0025, UTARMS; file 03, Department of Hospital Administration, correspondence, box /060; memo from Eugenie M. Stuart to C.A. Ashley, 23 September 1953, listing the students involved in taking Economics 1a. A description of the course is in *University of Toronto, Calendar, Faculty of Arts, 1953–54*, 118.
37 See, for example, file 22, Department of Hospital Administration, third-year marks 1954–55, box /065, Department of Political Economy, A76-0025, UTARMS; and file 23, Department of Hospital Administration Examinations, 1954–55.

38 Meeting with the author, 20 May 2016.
39 *University of Toronto Directory: Staff and Students of the University and the Federated Colleges, 1955–1956*, 87.
40 *University of Toronto Calendar, School of Hygiene, 1953–1955*, 32.
41 *University of Toronto Calendar, School of Graduate Studies, 1955–1956*, 99.
42 Bator, *Within Reach of Everyone*, 2:68.
43 Bator and Rhodes, *Within Reach of Everyone*, 1:134.
44 F.W. Jackson to Sidney Smith, 12 February 1946; Sidney Smith to F.W. Jackson, 14 February 1946; and F.W. Jackson to Sidney Smith, 20 February 1946, School of Hygiene, file (09), box /003, President's Office, A68-0007, UTARMS.
45 See correspondence from Sidney Smith to W.E. Phillips (29 April), to Defries (3 May), from Brook Claxton (18 May), and to Claxton (21 May 1946), School of Hygiene, file (09), box /003, President's Office, A68-0007, UTARMS.
46 Ontario, *Report of the Ontario Health Survey Committee*, [Toronto, 1950–52], 1:18.
47 Ontario, *Report of the Ontario Health Survey Committee*, 1:7.
48 Agnew, "Training of Hospital Administrators," 27–8.
49 "Fifth Western Canada Institute – Another Bang-up Success," *Canadian Hospital* 27, no. 11 (November 1950): 42–4, 58.
50 "University Atmosphere and Facilities Contribute to Successful Western Canada Institute," *Canadian Hospital* 28, no. 7 (July 1951): 44–5, 96, 104.
51 "Bigger and Better – Western Canada Institute," *Canadian Hospital* 29, no. 7 (July 1952): 37–40, 68, 70, 72, 97.
52 "Saskatchewan Plays Host to Western Canada Institute," *Canadian Hospital* 30, no. 7 (July 1953): 50–2.
53 "Winnipeg Welcomes Western Institute," *Canadian Hospital* 31, no. 11 (November 1954): 42–5, 84.
54 "Edmonton Plays Host to Tenth Western Canada Institute," *Canadian Hospital* 32, no. 7 (July 1955) 48–52, 60, 62, 64, 66.
55 See University of Saskatchewan, "Honorary Degrees," https://library.usask.ca/archives/campus-history/honorary-degrees.php. See also, "Notes about People, U. of Sask. Honours Several People in the Health Field," *Canadian Hospital* 32, no. 5 (May 1955): 12, 16.
56 See "Notes about People: E.V. Wahn Accepts Position at University of Saskatchewan Hospital," *Canadian Hospital* 30, no. 2 (February 1953): 66.
57 W. Douglas Piercey, "Obiter Dicta, Featuring University Hospital, Saskatoon," 35. The other articles were A.L. Swanson, "Canada's Newest Teaching Hospital," 37–8; E.J. Gilbert, "An Architect's Tour," 39–48; T.E. Hunt, "Rehabilitation Medicine," 49–51; Charlotte Paxton, "Dietary Facilities and Services," 52–4, 68; J.L. Summers, "Pharmaceutical Services," 55–6, 108, 110; and E.L. Casey, "Mechanizing Business Office Procedures," 58–60, 102. All articles in *Canadian Hospital* 32, no. 9 (September 1955).
58 *The Hospital in Tomorrow's World: A Symposium, "Changing Emphasis in the Functional Role of the Hospital,"* 4, Tommy Douglas Papers, XIV.564, R-33.1, SAB.
59 "Notes about People, U. of Sask. Honours Several People in the Health Field," *Canadian Hospital* 32, no. 5 (May 1955): 16.
60 "University of Toronto Announces Research Program in Hospital Administration," *Canadian Hospital* 32, no. 7 (July 1955): 12. See also R.D. Defries,

"School of Hygiene," *President's Report for the Year Ending June 1955*, 191; and D.L. MacLean, "Report of the Director of the School of Hygiene," *President's Report for the Year Ending June 1956*, 177.

61 "Education for Hospital Administration," *Canadian Hospital* 34, no. 4 (April 1957): 102.

62 School of Hygiene, University of Toronto, *Practical Studies in Education for Hospital Administration*, rev. ed. (Toronto: University of Toronto Press, 1960), iii, v.

63 Agnew, *Canadian Hospitals, 1920 to 1970*, 133.

64 Correspondence with Michel Champagne, archiviste, Division de la gestion de documents et des archives, Université de Montréal, 4 May 2018.

65 Sister Jeanne Mance Bertrand, "Education in Hospital Administration" (DIIA thesis, University of Toronto, 1954).

66 Gérald La Salle, "L'administration hospitalière," *Relations* 13, no. 152 (August 1953): 212.

67 Information obtained through correspondence with Michel Champagne, archiviste, Université de Montréal, 3 May 2018.

68 G. Harvey Agnew, "Report: Inspection of Graduate Program in Hospital Administration, School of Hygiene, University of Montreal," May 1959, Institut supérieur d'administration hospitalière, Fonds du Secrétariat général (D0035) C21, 20, Division de la gestion de documents et des archives, Université de Montréal.

69 William C. Hibbert, "Certification of Hospital Administrators," *Canadian Hospital* 33, no. 9 (September 1956): 72–6.

70 Taylor, *Health Insurance and Canadian Public Policy*, 234.

71 Statistics Canada, *Historical Statistics of Canada*, series B189–236, "Patient Days (Adult and Children) in Reporting Hospitals, Canada, 1932 to 1975, Public, Total General and Allied Special." See https://www150.statcan.gc.ca/n1/en/pub/11-516-x/pdf/5500093-eng.pdf?st=IlftPNY_.

72 Taylor, *Health Insurance and Canadian Public Policy*, table 15, 235.

73 Canada, *Proceedings of the Conference of Federal and Provincial Governments, Ottawa, December 4–7, 1950* (Ottawa: Edmond Cloutier, King's Printer, 1951), 43.

74 Canada, *Proceedings of the Federal-Provincial Conference 1955, Ottawa, October 3rd, 1955* (Ottawa: Edmond Cloutier, King's Printer, 1955), 10–11. Note, Premier Douglas responded to the federal proposal at 86–8.

75 Ontario, *Legislature of Ontario Debates*, First Session, Twenty-Fifth Legislature (Toronto: Queen's Printer, 1956), session 5 March 1956, 726.

76 Ontario, *Legislature of Ontario Debates*, First Session, Twenty-Fifth Legislature, 7 March 1956, 831, 849.

77 Ontario, *Legislature of Ontario Debates*, First Session, Twenty-Fifth Legislature, 7 March 1956, 831.

78 Ontario, *Legislature of Ontario Debates*, Third Session, Twenty-Fifth Legislature (Toronto: Queen's Printer, 1957), session 27 February 1957, 645.

79 Canada, House of Commons, *Debates*, Fifth Session, Twenty-Second Parliament, vol. 3, 1957 (Ottawa: Queen's Printer, 1957), beginning 2644. See Stanley Knowles response, both supporting the legislation and indicating where it fell short, 2648–9.

80 Canada, *Dominion-Provincial Conference 1957, Ottawa, November 25th and 26th, 1957* (Ottawa: Edmond Cloutier, King's Printer, 1958), 10. Premier Douglas responded to the federal proposal at 84–5.
81 Canada, House of Commons, *Debates*, First Session, Twenty-Fourth Parliament (Ottawa: Queen's Printer, 1958), 1:181.
82 Kathryn Leslie and Elizabeth Bruce, "Hospitals ... the Changing Scene," *Canadian Hospital* 33, no. 12 (December 1956), 48–50, 52, 80.
83 H.E. Goldsborough and Edwina King, "A Year of Challenge: Trends in Hospital Design," *Canadian Hospital* 34, no. 12 (December 1957): 46.
84 Goldsborough and King, "Year of Challenge," 48.
85 Goldsborough and King, "Year of Challenge," 49.
86 "O.H.A. Section Meetings," *Canadian Hospital* 34, no. 12 (December 1957): 68.
87 Harriett Goldsborough and Barbara Sinkins, "'Here's to Tomorrow!' Hospital Careers," *Canadian Hospital* 35, no. 12 (December 1958): 48.
88 See Murray Ross, "Saskatchewan Hospitals Convene," *Canadian Hospital* 35, no. 12 (December 1958): 58–9.
89 Kathryn Leslie and Elizabeth Bruce, "Hospitals ... the Changing Scene," *Canadian Hospital* 33, no. 12 (December 1956): 82.
90 Goldsborough and King, "Year of Challenge," 52.
91 Harriett Goldsborough and Barbara Sinkins, "Here's to Tomorrow! Hospital Careers," *Canadian Hospital* 35, no. 12 (December 1958): 51.
92 See F.B. Roth, "Focus on Hospital Insurance: How a Plan Administrator Sees It," *Canadian Hospital* 34, no. 2 (February 1957): 34.
93 Malcolm G. Taylor, "The Hospital Challenge of the Future," *Canadian Hospital* 34, no. 1 (January 1957): 33. The article notes Taylor at that time was a faculty member at U of T.
94 Taylor, "Hospital Challenge of the Future," 33.
95 Taylor, "Hospital Challenge of the Future," 33.
96 Taylor, "Hospital Challenge of the Future," 76.
97 See "Editorial Board," *Canadian Hospital* 34, no. 1 (January 1957): 6.
98 Where, when referring to a DHA student, next to an individual's name the term "class of" and the year is used rather than DHA and the year it is because the individual did not receive the diploma. This usually meant the individual attended classes but did not complete the thesis and therefore did not receive the diploma. The year stated is the year of the end of the program, so the class of 1955 would have started in 1953.
99 "Notes about People," *Canadian Hospital* 39, no. 8 (August 1962): 26.
100 "Notes about People," *Canadian Hospital* 36, no. 3 (March 1959), 16.
101 See "Former Administrator of LV hospital, George Riesz Dies," *Las Vegas Review-Journal*, 15 August 2007, https://www.reviewjournal.com/news/former-administrator-of-lv-hospital-george-riesz-dies/.
102 "SHA Studies Small Hospital Closure and Amalgamation," *Canadian Hospital* 46, no. 2 (February 1969): 37.
103 Craig McInnes, *The Mighty Hughes: From Prairie Lawyer to Western Canada's Moral Compass: A Biography of E.N. "Ted" Hughes* (Victoria: Heritage House, 2017), 86–9. He would write a number of articles on hospital trusteeship. See, for example, Judge E.N. Hughes, "A Trustee Looks at Trustee-Administrator Relationships," *Canadian Hospital* 45 no. 3 (March 1968): 56–9.

104 Peter was in the class of 1953–55 but did not submit his thesis in time to graduate with his class.
105 "Notes about People," *Canadian Hospital* 34, no. 2 (February 1957): 12.
106 "Obituary," *Winnipeg Free Press*, 26 July 2016.
107 "Obituary," *Winnipeg Free Press*.
108 Box 6 (1953–55), Department of Hospital Administration, A1986-0033, UTARMS.
109 Box 6 (1953–55), Department of Hospital Administration.
110 There is ample evidence of this. Former Deputy Provincial Treasurer Al Johnson says, "Always we relied heavily upon the nomination or recommendations of professors known to us," in *Dream No Little Dreams: A Biography of the Douglas Government of Saskatchewan, 1944–1961* (Toronto: University of Toronto Press, 2004), 197. He discusses the issue of recruitment and training in detail on 196–8. There is a very brief discussion in his dissertation (on which the book is based). See Albert Wesley Johnson, "Biography of a Government: Policy Formulation in Saskatchewan 1944–1961" (PhD diss., Harvard University, 1963), 553–4.

Former premier Alan Blakeney said, "The Douglas government attached great importance to recruiting a corps of young, able public servants. It combed Canada's universities to find people who were interested in designing and administering new government programs." Alan Blakeney and Stanford Borins, *Political Management in Canada: Conversations on Statecraft* (Toronto: University of Toronto Press, 1998), 147.

Speaking of the Saskatchewan civil service, Ken Rasmussen notes, "It began with the recruitment of the most promising graduates … from the political science, economics, or commerce departments of the University of Saskatchewan, and from the University of Toronto, Queen's University, and Carlton University – plus, of course, applicants from other universities." See "'Super Diplomat and Super Expediter': Wes Bolstad as Cabinet Secretary in Saskatchewan, 1973–79," in *Searching for Leadership: Secretaries to Cabinet in Canada*, ed. Patrice Dutil (Toronto: University of Toronto Press, 2008), 190.
111 Box 6 (1953–55).

CHAPTER TEN

1 First interview with Burns Roth, digitized audio recording, 1:34:08.
2 *School of Hygiene, University of Toronto, Thirtieth Annual Report, 1965–1955*, 18, file "Annual Report: School of Hygiene, 1941–1955," S013.002, UTARMS.
3 Taylor, *Health Insurance and Canadian Public Policy*, 111. Chapter 3 of this book is devoted to the establishment of hospital insurance in Ontario.
4 Taylor, *Health Insurance and Canadian Public Policy*, 109.
5 Malcolm Taylor, "Report on Health Insurance, Concise Summary," Office of the Provincial Economist, Department of the Provincial Treasurer, 22 December 1954, 1, B292341, 122-G, Premier Leslie M. Frost, General Correspondence, RG 3-23, Archives of Ontario.
6 Taylor, *Health Insurance and Canadian Public Policy*, 123.
7 Ontario, Legislative Assembly, *Debates*, March 23, 1955, Twenty-Fourth Legislature, vol. 1, no. 34 (Toronto: Queen's Printer, 1955), 1147.
8 Ontario, Legislative Assembly, *Debates*, 5 March 1956, Twenty-Fifth Legislature, First Session, vol. 1, no. 23 (Toronto: Queen's Printer, 1956), 726.

9 Ontario, Legislative Assembly, Standing Committee on Health, *Stenographic Report of the Meetings of the Standing Committee on Health with Respect to Hospital Insurance in Ontario* (Toronto: Baptist Johnston, Queen's Printer, 1956), 23 March 1956, 137.
10 *Stenographic Report*, 25 March 1956, 177.
11 *Stenographic Report*, 16 March 1956, 38–9.
12 He had taught in epidemiology and biometrics (1933–43) and public health administration (1941–55); see Bator and Rhodes, *Within Reach of Everyone*, 1:222.
13 "News Notes," *Canadian Journal of Public Health* 51, no. 6 (June 1960): 250. He also taught at the School in the Department of Public Health Administration (1949–55); see Bator and Rhodes, *Within Reach of Everyone*, 1:218.
14 Ontario, Legislative Assembly, *Debates*, 28 January and 21 February 1957, Twenty-Fifth Legislature, Third Session, vol. 1, no. 1 and no. 19 (Toronto: Queen's Printer, 1957), 5, 543.
15 Ontario, *Hospital Care Insurance for Ontario: The Proposal of the Ontario Government* (Toronto: Baptist Johnston, Queen's Printer, 1957), 4.
16 Arthur J. Swanson, "The Ontario Commission and Its Hospital Insurance Program: Looking Inside the Commission," *Canadian Hospital* 35, no. 1 (January 1958): 39.
17 A.J. Rhodes, "Report of the Director of the School of Hygiene," in *President's Report, for the Year Ending June 1958*, 73, UTARMS.
18 Ontario, Legislative Assembly, *Debates*, 7 January 1959, Twenty-Fifth Legislature, Fifth Session, vol. 1, no. 1 (Toronto: Queen's Printer, 1959), 4.
19 Ontario, Legislative Assembly, *Debates*, 7 January 1959, 4.
20 Agnew, *Canadian Hospitals, 1920 to 1970*, 89.
21 Taylor, *Health Insurance and Canadian Public Policy*, 157.
22 Agnew, *Canadian Hospitals, 1920 to 1970*, 89.
23 "Preceptor-Staff Meetings to 1970," box 09, Department of Health Administration, 1956–77, A1986-0034, UTARMS; see an undated list of preceptors and students that mentions A.J. Swanson from Toronto Western Hospital. Though undated, judging from Swanson's name, it was the early 1950s, as he left TWH in 1955.
24 Taylor, *Health Insurance and Canadian Public Policy*, 157.
25 Taylor, *Health Insurance and Canadian Public Policy*, 114, 116.
26 Taylor, *Health Insurance and Canadian Public Policy*, 158–9.
27 Taylor, "Report on Health Insurance, Concise Summary," 2.
28 Taylor to J.R. Simpson, 2 August 1956, M.G. Taylor Correspondence, file 12, box /073, Department of Political Economy, A76-0025, UTARMS.
29 Taylor to government employee (name withheld), 4 February 1957, M.G. Taylor Correspondence, file 12, box /073, Department of Political Economy, A76-0025, UTARMS.
30 Student (name withheld) to Taylor, A.W. Johnson to Taylor, 22 March 1955, M.G. Taylor Correspondence, file 04, box /065, Department of Political Economy, A76-0025, UTARMS.
31 Telegram from Johnson, 11 March 1955, and a handwritten response for a telegram back, M.G. Taylor Correspondence, file 04, box /065, Department of Political Economy, A76-0025, UTARMS.
32 Bator and Rhodes, *Within Reach of Everyone*, 1:224.

33 Malcolm Taylor, *The Administration of Health Insurance in Canada* (Toronto: Oxford University Press, 1956).
34 Student (name withheld) to Taylor, Taylor to F.W. Jackson, copied to R.D. Defries, 22 February 1955, M.G. Taylor Correspondence, file 04, box /065, Department of Political Economy, A76-0025, UTARMS.
35 A.J. Rhodes to President C.T. Bissell, re: Council of the School of Hygiene, 1959–60, 21 August 1959, file "School of Hygiene, Office of the President," A71-0011/032(03), UTARMS.
36 Malcolm G. Taylor, "What Remains for Voluntary Effort?," *Canadian Hospital* 36, no. 7 (July 1959): 58–60.
37 *University of Toronto Calendar, School of Hygiene, 1953–1955*, 32–4, UTARMS,. There were actually six public health administration courses, but one was veterinary public health practice (and so not applicable).
38 A. Paul Williams, "In Tribute to Malcolm Gordon Taylor, 1915–1994," *Health and Canadian Society* 3, nos 1 & 2 (1995): 9–12.
39 Keith Brownsey, "The House Frost Built: Institutional Change and the Department of the Treasury, 1943–1961," in *The Guardian: Perspectives on the Ministry of Finance of Ontario*, ed. Patrice Dutil (Toronto: University of Toronto Press, 2011), 28, 32. He also notes on page 28 that the Department of Economics and Gathercole were "given the most critical and sensitive policy files of the government." Dutil notes that those who work in budget offices have been referred to as "the guardians," a zealous and self-effacing lot "whose role was to defend the public purse" and "fiercely dedicated to protecting its Minister and indeed the citadel of the state's finance" (4). See 4–5 for a description of the guardian's role.
40 Taylor, "Report on Health Insurance, Concise Summary," 518–19n53.
41 Taylor, "Report on Health Insurance, Concise Summary," 519n67.
42 Brownsey, "House Frost Built," 28.
43 "U of T Professor Is Chosen to Head New Alberta University," clipping from *Globe and Mail*, 18 January 1960, file "Taylor, Malcolm G.," Press Clippings Individuals, UTARMS.
44 Malcolm G. Taylor, "The Saskatchewan Hospital Services Plan: A Study in Compulsory Health Insurance" (PhD diss., University of California, mimeographed for limited distribution by the Saskatchewan Health Services Planning Commission, Regina, 1949).
45 T.K. Shoyama to chairman and members, Economic Advisory and Planning Board, "Economic Advisory and Planning Board, Minutes, January 1946–June 1953," memorandum, 17 September 1951, 4, file IV 144(4–7), R-33.1, SAB.
46 W. Douglas Piercey, "The Hospital as Meeting Place," *Canadian Hospital* 34, no. 4 (April 1957): 40–1. Piercey was appointed superintendent, Ottawa Civic Hospital, 28 May 1942 (see *Ottawa Journal*, 28 May 1942, 12). He had been assistant superintendent before that. He became associate professor, Hospital Administration, DOHA, 1954–65, and during the same period served as executive director, Canadian Hospital Association, and editor, *Canadian Hospital*.
47 A.T. Story, "A Building with a Future," *Canadian Hospital* 34, no. 4 (April 1957): 53.
48 Sister Mary James, "Holy Family School and Residence," *Canadian Hospital* 33, no. 4 (April 1956): 47–8.

49 David McLennan, *Our Towns: Saskatchewan Communities from Abbey to Zenon Park* (Regina: University of Regina, Canadian Plains Research Centre, 2008), 322.
50 A.J. Rhodes, "Report of the Director of the School of Hygiene," in *President's Report, for the Year Ending June 1958*, 73.
51 Rhodes, "Report of the Director of the School of Hygiene" ... *Year Ending June 1958*. Note, it is not clear that Mr McLaren received his DHA. The *President's Report* says he was a graduate, but *Finding Aid*, 5, A1986-0033, UTARMS, notes he did not submit a thesis. One explanation is that he would have been completing his program (to be receiving his degree in November 1958) when the *President's Report* went to press, so it is possible that it was anticipated he would be a graduate.
52 A.J. Rhodes, "The Director of the School of Hygiene," in *President's Report, for the Year Ending June 1961*, 81.
53 A.J. Rhodes, "The Director of the School of Hygiene," in *President's Report, for the Year Ending June 1959*, 74.
54 Rhodes, "Director of the School of Hygiene," in *President's Report, for the Year Ending June 1959*, 74.
55 A.J. Rhodes, "The Director of the School of Hygiene," in *President's Report, for the Year Ending June 1960*, 75.
56 Burns Roth, "Hospital Plans in Western Canada, S.H.S.P.: A Partnership," *Canadian Hospital* 36, no. 1 (January 1959): 39n, unnumbered.
57 Roth, "Hospital Plans in Western Canada, S.H.S.P.," 40n, unnumbered.
58 Roth, "Hospital Plans in Western Canada, S.H.S.P.," 40n, unnumbered.
59 Roth, "Hospital Plans in Western Canada, S.H.S.P.," 40n, unnumbered.
60 Roth, "Hospital Plans in Western Canada, S.H.S.P.," 40–1n, unnumbered.
61 Roth, "Hospital Plans in Western Canada, S.H.S.P.," 41n, unnumbered, 76n, unnumbered.
62 Roth, "Hospital Plans in Western Canada, S.H.S.P.," 76n, unnumbered.
63 Roth, "Hospital Plans in Western Canada, S.H.S.P.," 76n, unnumbered.
64 Roth, "Hospital Plans in Western Canada, S.H.S.P.," 90n, unnumbered.
65 Roth, "Hospital Plans in Western Canada, S.H.S.P.," 91n, unnumbered.
66 T.H. McLeod, dean of commerce, to Harvey Agnew, 8 October 1952, Hospital Administration Program, box 1, 1111-141, RG 2077, College of Commerce fonds, University Archives & Special Collections, University of Saskatchewan; see also Eugenie M. Stuart to Dean McLeod, 19 January 1953; G. Harvey Agnew to Dean McLeod, 11 October 1957.
67 Dean McLeod to Andrew Patullo, 18 January 1960, Hospital Administration Program, box 1, 1111-141, RG 2077, College of Commerce fonds, University Archives & Special Collections, University of Saskatchewan. Note the names are not specified in the letter but on the basis of accompanying correspondence it is obvious who the correspondents are.
68 G.M. Goodspeed, acting dean of commerce, to A. Patullo, 18 May 1961, Hospital Administration Program, box 1, 1111-141, RG 2077, College of Commerce fonds, University Archives & Special Collections, University of Saskatchewan.
69 UTARMS Finding Aid, A1986-033, for the Department of Health Administration, 2, notes Silversides did not graduate.
70 "Review of Health Care Administration Program, April 14, 1987," 1, Hospital Administration Program, box 1, 1111-141, RG 2077, College of Com-

merce fonds, University Archives & Special Collections, University of Saskatchewan.

71 See "Saskatchewan H.O.M. Alumni," *Canadian Hospital* 39, no. 9 (September 1962): 68. See also "Summer Seminar Students at the University of Saskatchewan," *Canadian Hospital* 38, no. 9 (September 1961): 90.

72 See "Saskatchewan H.O.M. Alumni," 69.

73 See Saskatchewan, Hospital Survey Committee, *Saskatchewan Hospital Survey and Master Plan 1961, Part I*, [Regina, 1962], 316.

74 Personal correspondence with his daughter, Sharon Gaudet (née Veillet), 23 June 2017.

75 Rhodes, "Report of the Director of the School of Hygiene," ... *Year Ending June 1961*, 80–1. See also, Rhodes, "Report of the Director of the School of Hygiene,"... *Year Ending June 1960*, 76.

76 A.J. Rhodes, "Report of the Director of the School of Hygiene," in *President's Report, for the Year Ending June 1963*, 113.

77 Harvey Agnew, "Foreword," in University of Toronto, Department of Hospital Administration, *The Program in Hospital Administration: Past, Present and Future*, [Toronto] 1961, iii, UTARMS.

78 *The Program in Hospital Administration: Past, Present and Future*, June 1961, 8, Department of Health Administration, A1998-0023/002, UTARMS.

79 See 181–94.

80 *Program in Hospital Administration*, 247–52.

81 Claude Bissell, "Report of the President," in *President's Report, for the Year Ending June 1962*, 19.

82 *Staff Bulletin*, July–August 1967, 20, UTARMS. His topic was "Changing Objectives in the Hospital World."

83 "People," *Canadian Hospital* 45, no. 1 (January 1968), 31.

84 See, "People," *Canadian Hospital* 47, no. 9 (September 1970): 21.

85 "Appointments," *Hospital Administration in Canada* 20, no. 1 (January 1978): 11.

86 Box 12, Department of Hospital Administration, A1986-033, UTARMS.

87 Box 13, Department of Hospital Administration.

88 W. Harding le Riche, *University of Toronto Medical School and School of Hygiene: Historical Comments 1959–1980* (self-pub., 1993), 54–7, UTARMS.

89 During the 1930s and 1940s, the journal was known as the *Canadian Hospital.* One wonders if the title was modelled on that of the British journal, the *Hospital.* At that time it would have been a possibility, as Canada had strong ties to Britain. Indeed the school had adopted the British nomenclature for its degree label.

90 Some examples: See an article by R.B Ferguson on pharmacists in small hospitals (*Canadian Hospital* 32, no. 5 [1955]). Volume 37 (1960) has articles by Ron McQueen on hospital planning (37, nos 1 and 2), and Gerry Turner on control of infections (37, no. 6). There are also articles by faculty in this volume and by individuals from the Saskatchewan Department of Public Health. Another example is an article by E.N. Stefaniuk (DHA, 1960) on comparing provincial hospital plans (47, no. 3 [1970]), and by Peter Carruthers on the personnel function in hospitals (47, no. 5).

91 Claus Wirsig, "Opinion: New Editorial Team at Your Service," *Hospital Administration in Canada* 8, no. 10 (October 1966): 4.

92 See journal masthead, *Hospital Administration and Construction* 3, no. 1

(January 1961): 4. See also "Robert Ferguson Resigns," *Hospital Administration in Canada* 4, no. 1 (January 1962): 4.

93 See journal masthead, *Hospital Administration in Canada* 4, no. 9 (September 1962): 7.

94 "The Provinces Report," *Hospital Administration and Construction* 1, no. 1 (June 1959): 21. The table is on 22–3, 24–5, 26–7. At the time PEI and Quebec did not have a plan in operation.

95 D.M. McNabb, "Did You Ever Think of Data Processing?," *Hospital Administration and Construction* 1, no. 1 (June 1959): 28–32. Note the title is different in the table of contents where it is listed as "Did You Ever Consider Punch Card Accounting?"

96 See "The Progressive Patient Care Issue," *Hospital Administration and Construction* 2, no. 6 (November 1960): 22–35.

97 "Small Hospital Problems," *Hospital Administration in Canada* 7, no. 1 (January 1965): 34–5. See also "Small Hospital Problems," *Hospital Administration in Canada* 7, no. 2 (February 1965): 35–7; and "Small Hospital Problems," *Hospital Administration in Canada* 7, no. 3 (March 1965): 43–6.

98 E.V. Wahn, "Your Hospital and the Law," *Hospital Administration in Canada* 8, no. 3 (March 1966): 8–9. Wahn's biography appears on 9.

99 One example was Gary Chatfield, "Buying Drugs: One Hospital's Decision," *Hospital Administration and Construction* 3, no. 1 (January 1961): 21–3. For the period from its inception to 1976 there were many other grads with articles.

100 See A.L. Swanson and E.V. Wahn, "From the Administrator's Point of View," *Hospitals* 35, no. 18 (16 September 1961): 59.

101 "Editorial Notes: The Canadian Experiment," *Hospitals* 35, no. 18 (16 September 1961): 41.

102 Swanson and Wahn, "From the Administrator's Point of View," 53–9.

103 W. Douglas Piercey, "The Present Picture," *Hospitals* 35, no. 18 (16 September 1961): 46–52. He was an associate professor in what was then the Department of Hospital Administration.

104 William McKillop, "A Canvass of Opinion," *Hospitals* 35, no. 18 (16 September 1961): 70–8. Burns Roth was deputy minister in Saskatchewan; Douglas Peart, administrator, Ottawa Civic; Peter Swerhone, assistant administrator, Winnipeg General; and G.B. Rosenfeld, administrator, Victoria General. Note: Roth and Rosenfeld are listed as "class of" rather than stating their degree. This is because, as Roth notes, he did not graduate (see first interview with Burns Roth, digitized audio recording; also first interview with Burns Roth, 16 July 1985, partial transcript of interviews, 3, School of Hygiene History Project, B89-0009, UTARMS). The UTARMS Finding Aid, A1986-033, for the Department of Health Administration, 3, notes Rosenfeld did not graduate.

105 See School of Hygiene, *Calendar, 1961–1962*, 28, on Sharp's position in the Department of Hospital Administration.

106 There is a very interesting history of both the British journal and the association in "History," Institute of Healthcare Management, https://ihm.org.uk/about-us/history/.

107 "Personal," *Hospital* 46, no. 2 (February 1950): 92.

108 Hjalmar Cederström, "The Söder Hospital, Stockholm: Its Planning and Shaping, 1 – Studies of Principles," *Hospital* 43, no. 1 (January 1947): 11–17;

Cederström, "The Söder Hospital, Stockholm: Its Planning and Shaping, 2 – Medical and Technical Considerations," *Hospital* 43, no. 2 (February 1947): 87–96.

109 "The Caroline Hospital, Stockholm," *Hospital* 45, no. 1 (January 1949): 25–8. The Swedish name for the hospital is the Karolinska Sjukhuset, affiliated with the state medical school, the Karolinska Institutet.

110 Malcolm G. Taylor, "The Historical Stream," *Hospitals* 35, no. 18 (16 September 1961): 44.

111 Taylor, "Historical Stream," 122.

112 Taylor, "Historical Stream," 122.

113 See J.A. Monaghan, "Alberta Blue Cross Forges Ahead," *Canadian Hospital* 30, no. 1 (January 1953): 50–1, 86.

114 Taylor, "Historical Stream," 45.

115 Taylor, "Historical Stream," 120

116 Taylor, "Historical Stream," 122.

117 See Agnew, *Canadian Hospitals, 1920 to 1970*, 172.

118 Jessie Fraser, "They Were Invited to Follow the Herd," *Canadian Hospital* 35, no. 11 (November 1958): 48–51, 90, 92, 94. The quote is taken from 48.

119 Jessie Fraser, "All Roads Lead to Winnipeg," *Canadian Hospital* 36, no. 10 (October 1959): 60–5, 126, 130.

120 Lawrence L. Wilson, "Setting Our Sights on the Sixties: 15th Western Canada Institute for Hospital Administrators and Trustees," *Canadian Hospital* 37, no. 10 (October 1960): 64–7.

121 Jessie Fraser, "Western Canada Institute," *Canadian Hospital* 38, no. 8 (August 1961): 38–41, 62–4.

CHAPTER ELEVEN

1 Ontario Hospital Services Commission, *Annual Report 1963 (Statistical Supplement)*, table 21, 67.

2 I was one of the administrative staff at TGH in the 1980s.

3 Ontario Hospital Services Commission, *Annual Report 1963*, table 21, 67.

4 Ontario Hospital Services Commission, *Annual Report 1964 (Statistical Supplement)*, x.

5 Ontario Hospital Services Commission, *Annual Report 1964*, 1.

6 First interview with Burns Roth, digitized audio recording.

7 First interview with Burns Roth, digitized audio recording.

8 "Interview with Dr. Burns Roth, Reel #1," 1–2.

9 Obituary on F.B. Roth, *Toronto Star*, 11 February 1987.

10 K.S. Coates and W.R. Morrison, *The Alaska Highway in World War II: The U.S. Army of Occupation in Canada's Northwest* (Norman: University of Oklahoma Press, 1992), 182, 184. This was subsequently also published by the University of Toronto Press (1992).

11 *Globe and Mail*, "Toronto Doctor Sees Success of Medicare," 5 July 1962.

12 First interview with Burns Roth, digitized audio recording.

13 "News," *Canadian Journal of Public Health* 43, no. 2 (February 1952): 93.

14 "Biographical Sketch," F.B. (Burns) Roth fonds, Yukon Archives. See these fonds as well for a picture of Burns Roth with hospital staff at the Whitehorse General Hospital, on the steps of the Nurses Residence that was next door to the hospital.

15 *Whitehorse Heritage Buildings: A Walking Tour of Yukon's Capital* (White-

horse: Yukon Historical and Museums Association, 1983), 33. See http://parkscanadahistory.com/publications/north/whitehorse-heritage-bldgs.pdf.

16 Ken S. Coates and William R. Morrison, *Land of the Midnight Sun: A History of the Yukon*, 3rd ed. (Montreal and Kingston: McGill-Queen's University Press, 2017), 253.

17 Coates and Morrison, *Land of the Midnight Sun*, 254.

18 Coates and Morrison, *Alaska Highway in World War II*, 192.

19 William D. Church, "The North Atlantic Area," in *Preventive Medicine in World War II*, ed. Ebbe Curtis Hoff (Washington: Office of the Surgeon General, Department of the Army, 1976), 8:168–9. See 8:168–73 for an overview of the public health issues encountered by the US Army in Whitehorse and area.

20 To give a further sense of the time, an article notes the "town was ill-equipped to cope with the influx," that "men slept in shifts in hotel rooms," that "the small cottage hospital that had served the town before the war became inadequate. A modern addition was quickly built to more than double the capacity." See Michael Gates, "Post-war Whitehorse Heralded Dramatic Change," *Yukon News*, 8 March 2018, https://www.yukon-news.com/opinion/post-war-whitehorse-heralded-dramatic-change/.

21 Obituary on F.B. Roth, *Toronto Star*.

22 First interview with Burns Roth, digitized audio recording.

23 First interview with Burns Roth, digitized audio recording.

24 Interview with Burns Roth, audiocassette #1/6. For a partial transcript of the cassette that deals with this, see "Interview with Dr Burns Roth, Reel #1," 3.

25 Interview with Burns Roth, audiocassette #1/6; "Interview with Dr Burns Roth, Reel #1," 3.

26 Interview with Burns Roth, audiocassette #1/6.

27 F.B. Roth, "Division of Hospital Administration and Standards," *Annual Report 1950–51, for the 15 Months Ending March 31, 1951* (Regina: Thos. H. McConica, Queen's Printer, 1952), 80.

28 First interview with Burns Roth, digitized audio recording.

29 "Introduction," *Annual Report 1950–51, for the 15 Months Ending March 31, 1951*, 9.

30 F. Burns Roth, "S.H.S.P.: A Partnership," *Canadian Hospital* 36, no. 1 (January 1959): 39.

31 F.B. Roth, "The Health Officer and Hospital Regionalization," *Canadian Journal of Public Health* 43, no. 11 (November 1952): 467–73.

32 F.B. Roth, M.S. Acker, M.I. Roemer, and G.W. Meyers, "Some Factors Influencing Hospital Utilization in Saskatchewan," *Canadian Journal of Public Health* 46, no. 8 (August 1955): 303–23.

33 F. Burns Roth, Glyn W. Meyers, Frederick Mott, and Leonard Rosenfeld, "The Saskatchewan Experience in Payment for Hospital Care," *American Journal of Public Nations Health* 43, no. 6, pt 1 (June 1953): 752–6.

34 Second interview with Dr Burns Roth, 18 July 1985, digitized audio recording, School of Hygiene History Project, B89-0009_02S, UTARMS.

35 T.C. Douglas to Paul Martin, 22 and 30 April 1947, Department of National Health and Welfare, T.C. Douglas papers, file XXIII. 737a(23-16), coll. R-33.1, SAB.

36 "Interview with Dr Burns Roth, Reel #2," 18 July 1985, 3, transcript, School of Hygiene History Project, B89-0009, UTARMS. See also interview with Dr

Burns Roth, audiocassette #2/6, side 2, School of Hygiene History Project, B89-0009, UTARMS.

37 Interview with Dr Andrew Rhodes, 23 July 1985, side 2, tape 4/6, audiocassette, School of Hygiene History Project, B89-0009(04), UTARMS. For a partial account of the interview, see "Transcript, Recorded Interview with Dr Andrew J. Rhodes," 23 July 1985, 2.

38 "Interview with Dr Burns Roth, Reel #2," 3. See also interview with Burns Roth, audiocassette #2/6, side 2.

39 Interview with Burns Roth, audiocassette #2/6, side 2.

40 For further information on the Douglas government see another former deputy provincial treasurer, A.W. Johnson, *Dream No Little Dreams: A Biography of the Douglas Government of Saskatchewan, 1944–1961* (Toronto: University of Toronto Press, 2004), based on his PhD dissertation. Johnson was a Saskatchewanian hired out of university who rose through the ranks of the provincial government.

41 "Burns Roth to Head 'Health Administration,'" 15 May 1967, Roth, F. Burns, Department of Graduate Records, A73-0026/388(23), UTARMS. Note this background is taken not from when he was appointed head of the Department of *Hospital* Administration in 1962, but rather from the announcement of when he was going to head the *Hospital* Administration and Public Health Administration Departments in a combined *Health* Administration Department in 1967.

42 Interview with Burns Roth, audiocassette #2/6, side 2.

43 "Interview with Dr Burns Roth, Reel #2," 4; also interview with Burns Roth, audiocassette #2/6, side 2.

44 Interview with Dr Andrew Rhodes, side 2, audiocassette #5/6, School of Hygiene History Project, B89-0009(02), UTARMS.

45 Interview with Dr Andrew Rhodes, 23 July 1985, side 1, tape 5/6, audiocassette, School of Hygiene History Project, B89-0009(04), UTARMS. For a partial account of the interview, see "Transcript, Recorded Interview with Dr Andrew J. Rhodes," 23 July 1985, 3.

46 F. Burns Roth, "Health," in *Canadian Annual Review for 1969*, ed. John T. Saywell (Toronto: University of Toronto Press, 1970), 371. A portion of this quote is in Bator, *Within Reach of Everyone*, 2:11.

47 Roth, "Health," 377.

48 F. Burns Roth, "Current Developments on the Canadian scene," *Medical Care* 8, no. 1 (January–February 1970): 1–2.

49 F. Burns Roth, "Training for Administration," *Canadian Public Health Journal* 55, no. 10 (October 1964): 445–9.

50 J.E. Hodgetts, *The Canadian Public Service: A Physiology of Government, 1867–1970* (Toronto: University of Toronto Press, 1973), 42.

51 Canada, House of Commons, *Debates*, Fourth Session, Twentieth Parliament, vol. 4, 14 May 1948, 3932. The prime minister opened the day's session with an announcement of the health services grants (see 3931–5). He also noted the capacity being built within the Department of Health and Welfare with a division for health insurance studies, a research division of the department "actively engaged in this field," and "specialists of outstanding ability" asked "to undertake more specific assignments" (3932).

52 Canada, House of Commons, *Debates*, Fourth Session, Twentieth Parliament, vol. 4, 30 June 1948, 6172–74. The MP speaking to this point was Joseph

William Burton, CCF member for Humboldt, Saskatchewan. Prior to going to Ottawa Mr Burton had been the only Catholic MLA in the Saskatchewan Legislative Assembly.

53 File "S. of H. Council 1957–62, School of Hygiene Council Minutes 1956–66," Box 004, School of Hygiene, A1975-0029, UTARMS.

54 See the records of the president, Claude Bissell, and the files for Medicine or Hygiene, each in box A71-0011/061.

55 Telegram (with signatures) to H.D. Dalgleish, M.R. McCharles, Woodrow Lloyd, n.d., file "Medicare in Saskatchewan with Relevant Newspaper Clippings," 1985-0041/22-6, box 22, F2006, G.M.A. and Gwenyth Grube fonds, University of Toronto, Trinity College Archives.

56 *Globe and Mail*, "MDs' Strike Deplored by Toronto Group," 17 July 1962, 1.

57 *Toronto Daily Star*, "Toronto Citizens Urge End to Doctors' Strike," 17 July 1962, 15, 18.

58 File "Medicare in Saskatchewan with Relevant Newspaper Clippings." See also Hastings fonds (B2002-0014) and Rhodes fonds (B2000-001), UTARMS.

59 A.J. Rhodes, "Report of the Director of the School of Hygiene," in *President's Report, for the Year Ending June 1964*, 112–13.

60 *Bulletin*, January 1965, 16, University of Toronto, UTARMS. The title of his talk was "Problems of Health and Welfare in East Africa."

61 *President's Report, for the Year Ending June 1965*, 106.

62 Richard Titmuss, "The Exhausting Road to Great Thoughts," address at the 1964 Fall Convocation, *Varsity Graduate* 11, no. 4 (February 1965): 36.

63 A.J. Rhodes, "Report of the Director of the School of Hygiene," in *President's Report, for the Year Ending June 1966*, 144.

64 A.J. Rhodes, "Report of the Director of the School of Hygiene," in *President's Report, for the Year Ending June 1967, Part One*, 156.

65 Rhodes, "Report of the Director of the School of Hygiene," ... *Year Ending June 1966*, 142.

66 Rhodes, "Report of the Director of the School of Hygiene," ... *Year Ending June 1966*, 143.

67 Rhodes, "Report of the Director of the School of Hygiene," ... *Year Ending June 1967, Part One*, 156.

68 Rhodes, "Report of the Director of the School of Hygiene," ... *Year Ending June 1967, Part One*, 157.

69 A.J. Rhodes, "Report of the Director of the School of Hygiene," in *President's Report, for the Year Ending June 1968, Part Two*, 75.

70 "Dr F. Burns Roth A.U.P.H.A. President," *Canadian Hospital* 46, no. 7 (July 1969): 15.

71 Bernard Bucove, "Report of the Director of the School of Hygiene," in *President's Report, for the Year Ending June 1971, Part Two*, 79.

72 Bucove, "Report of the Director of the School of Hygiene," ... *Year Ending June 1971, Part Two*, 79–80.

73 Second interview with Burns Roth, 18 July 1985, digitized audio recording, 0:56:25. For the same interview, see also with Burns Roth, audiocassette #2/6, side 2.

74 Second interview with Burns Roth, digitized audio recording, 1:01:05.

75 "Western Canada Institute, Regina Program Attracts 1200," *Canadian Hospital* 42, no. 10 (October 1965): 39, 42, 44.

76 "21st Western Canada Hospital Institute, Western Institute Delegates Urged

Not to Go Overboard on Facilities," *Canadian Hospital* 43, no. 8 (August 1966): 25–8.

77 In contrast the OHA annual convention in 1968 attracted 7,680 people and the AHA annual convention in the same year attracted 1,400. See "OHA Convention Grows and Grows," *Canadian Hospital* 46, no. 1 (January 1968): 30; and "Alberta Hospital Association Marks 50th Year," in the same issue, 31.

78 "Canada's Last Western Institute Hits 2,500 mark," *Canadian Hospital* 44, no. 8 (August 1967): 21–4. The quote is taken from 21.

79 Ontario, Legislative Assembly, *Debates*, 26th Legislature, 4th Session (Toronto: Queen's Printer, 1962), 1304.

80 A.L. Swanson, "Some Effects of 'Medicare' on Hospitals in Saskatchewan, Part 1," *Canadian Hospital* 42, no. 11 (November 1965): 53; Swanson, "Some Effects of 'Medicare' on Hospitals in Saskatchewan, Part 2," *Canadian Hospital* 42, no. 12 (December 1965): 42, 44–5.

81 Canada, *Federal-Provincial Conference, Ottawa, July 19–22, 1965* (Ottawa: Roger Duhamel, Queen's Printer, 1968), 15.

82 From the UTARMS clippings file, "Cameron, George Donald West," A73-0026/048(70). He served in England and France during the last few months of the First World War. On his return to Canada he entered U of T, then transferred to Queen's to study medicine. He came back to U of T for his DPH. At Connaught he rose to become assistant to the farm director, then in 1939 joined the Department of Pensions and National Health as chief of the Laboratory of Hygiene. In 1944 he succeeded J.J. Heagerty (who had done much work on health insurance) as director of health services. In 1946 he was appointed deputy minister of national health. He was a Fellow in the Royal College of Physicians (London) and the American College of Hospital Administrators.

83 Swanson, "Some Effects of 'Medicare' on Hospitals in Saskatchewan, Part 1."

84 Swanson, "Some Effects of 'Medicare' on Hospitals in Saskatchewan, Part 2."

85 R.B. Ferguson, "A Hospital Administrator Views Health Programs in the Canadian Economy," *Canadian Hospital* 46, no. 7 (July 1968): 69.

86 Roy Romanow, "My Experience in the Medicare Battle and the Woods Commission," *Canadian Bulletin of Medical History* 26, no. 2 (2009): 539. This article was subsequently published under the same title in *Making Medicare: New Perspectives on the History of Medicare in Canada*, ed. Gregory P. Marchildon, 288–9 (Toronto: University of Toronto Press, 2012).

87 Romanow, "My Experience in the Medicare Battle," 289.

88 Gregory P. Marchildon, "Canadian Medicare: Why History Matters," in Marchildon, *Making Medicare*, 15.

89 See *It Begins Here, 2006–2016: Report to the Community, School of Public Health, University of Alberta* (Edmonton: School of Public Health, University of Alberta, 2016), 4–5. See also "Our History: Visionary Leadership (1966–1995)," issuu, https://issuu.com/sphuofa/docs/it_begins_here_report_final_websm/8.

90 *It Begins Here, 2006–2016*, 5.

91 See Carl Alexander Meilicke, "The Saskatchewan Medical Care Dispute of 1962: An Analytic Social History" (PhD diss., University of Minnesota, 1967).

92 Walter H. Johns to J.W.T. Spinks, 11 September 1967, file "College of Commerce," Health Care Administration, 1967–68, University of Saskatchewan Archives.

93 L.I. Barber to R.W. Beg [principal, University of Saskatchewan], 29 March 1968, memorandum, file "College of Commerce," Health Care Administration, University of Saskatchewan Archives.
94 F.H. Silversides to Dean L.I. Barber, 5 February 1968, memorandum, file "College of Commerce," Health Care Administration, University of Saskatchewan Archives.
95 K.M. Smith to Faculty of the College of Commerce, 7 May 1984, memorandum, file "College of Commerce," Health Care Administration Certificate Program, University of Saskatchewan Archives.
96 "Review of Health Care Administration Certificate Program," 14 April 1987, 1, file "College of Commerce," Health Care Administration Certificate Program, University of Saskatchewan Archives.
97 Bator, *Within Reach of Everyone*, 2:69.
98 *Staff Bulletin*, October 1967, 14, UTARMS.
99 *Calendar, School of Hygiene, 1968–69*, 8, UTARMS.
100 "Interview with Dr Burns Roth, Reel #3," 23 July 1985," 23 July 1985, 1, transcript, School of Hygiene History Project, B89-0009, UTARMS.
101 "Extract from Letter sent to Dr J.D. Hamilton, Vice-President (Health Sciences), University of Toronto, 3rd March, 1967," 1, file "Hygiene," Office of the President, A75-0021/062, UTARMS.
102 "Extract from Letter sent to Dr J.D. Hamilton," 2.
103 "Extract from Letter sent to Dr J.D. Hamilton," 2–3.
104 Rakow, *Fifty-Year Retrospective*, 8.
105 For a list of the faculty in each section, see *University of Toronto, Calendar, School Of Hygiene, 1968–69*, 40–2.
106 Rhodes, "Director of the School of Hygiene," ... *Year Ending June 1967, Part One*, 157.
107 A.J. Rhodes, "School of Hygiene, Proposal to Amalgamate Departments of Hospital Administration and Public Health to Form New Department of Health Administration," 17 March 1967, file "Hygiene," Office of the President, A75-0021/062, UTARMS.
108 Claude Bissell to A.J. Rhodes, 6 April 1967, file "Hygiene," Office of the President, A75-0021/062, UTARMS.
109 Rhodes, "Director of the School of Hygiene," ... *Year Ending June 1967, Part One*, 156.
110 Bator, *Within Reach of Everyone*, 2:69.
111 "Interview with Dr Burns Roth, Reel #3."
112 "Interview with Dr Burns Roth, Reel #2," 5. See also interview with Burns Roth, audiocassette #3/6, side 1.
113 "Interview with Dr Burns Roth, Reel #2," 5. See also interview with Burns Roth, audiocassette #3/6, side 1.
114 Interview with Dr Burns Roth, audiocassette #3/6, side 1.
115 Rhodes, "Director of the School of Hygiene," ... *Year Ending June 1968, Part Two*, 76.
116 Bator, *Within Reach of Everyone*, 2:70.
117 Bator, *Within Reach of Everyone*, 2:70.
118 Rhodes, "Director of the School of Hygiene," ... *Year Ending June 1967, Part One*, 156.
119 Johnson, "Biography of a Government," 340.
120 Johnson, *Dream No Little Dreams*, 146–7.

121 See Frederick D. Mott and Milton I. Roemer, *Rural Health and Medical Care* (New York: McGraw-Hill Book, 1948).

122 There is very little good biographical information on Mott, perhaps because, as Grey notes, Mott caught the ire of the AMA because of his stance on health insurance. For example *JAMA* notes only his death, with no background on his life or career. There is nothing in either of the journals of the American or Canadian Public Health Associations. Grey's book does have some good information on him, which is supplemented by members of the Mott family I spoke to while compiling the information. See Michael R. Grey, *New Deal Medicine: The Rural Health Programs of the Farm Security Administration* (Baltimore, MD: Johns Hopkins University Press, 1999).

Mott was part of a family dedicated to human welfare. His father, John Raleigh Mott, was the pioneer YMCA missionary leader and 1946 Nobel Peace Prize co-winner, who received an honorary degree from U of T in 1944 (see A68-0006/063[05], UTARMS).

One scholar who has explored the Canadian part of Mott's career is J.T.H. Connor. For a list of some of his work, see Connor, "'One Simply Doesn't Arbitrate Authorship of Thoughts': Socialized Medicine, Medical McCarthyism, and the Publishing of *Rural Health and Medical Care* (1948)," *Journal of the History of Medicine and Allied Sciences* 72, no. 3 (July 2017): 27n103.

One brief biographical sketch is in the *Canadian Journal of Public Health* when he was given an honorary membership in the Canadian Public Health Association. See "Frederick Dodge Mott," *Canadian Journal of Public Health* 65, no. 2 (March/April 1974): 136–7.

123 Frederick D. Mott, "Some Aspects of the Case for State Medicine," *McGill Medical Undergraduate Journal* 1 (January 1932): 4.

124 Mott, "Some Aspects of the Case for State Medicine," 4.

125 Mott, "Some Aspects of the Case for State Medicine," 4.

126 Mott, "Some Aspects of the Case for State Medicine," 5.

127 "Health and Medical Care: Goals, Status and Trends, Proposals and Recommendations, March 1960: A Background Report prepared by F.D. Mott, M.D., for Governor G. Mennon Williams' Conference on Health and Medical Care," 62, "Thompson Papers, Advisory Planning Committee on Medical Care," MG 17, University of Saskatchewan Archives.

128 *Staff Bulletin*, February 1967, 18, UTARMS.

129 Rhodes, "Report of the Director of the School of Hygiene," … *Year Ending June 1961*, 80 UTARMS.

130 Canada, Royal Commission on Health Services, *Hearings*, vol. 17, January 22 1962, held at Regina, SK, appearance of Department of Public Health, Saskatchewan.

131 File "Canada, Royal Commission on Health Services: Brief Prepared by School of Hygiene," 6, box 18, Milton Herbert Brown fonds (B77-0047), UTARMS. (For information presented at the hearings by the school, see also, Canada, Royal Commission on Health Services, "*Hearings*, vol. 52, The School of Hygiene, University of Toronto," 14 May 1962, 9957–10005.)

132 File "Canada, Royal Commission on Health Services: Brief Prepared by School of Hygiene," 3–5.

133 File "Canada, Royal Commission on Health Services: Brief Prepared by School of Hygiene," 54.

134 Bator, *Within Reach of Everyone*, 2:38–9.

135 J.K.W. Ferguson, Connaught Medical Research Laboratories, University of Toronto, Submission to the Royal Commission on Health Services, "Recommendations for the Provision of Drugs under Medical Care Insurance Plans," [Toronto, 1960], ii (note, the introductory pages are not numbered). See also Canada, Royal Commission on Health Services, "*Hearings*, vol. 51, Connaught Laboratories, University of Toronto," 11 May 1962, 9820–38.
136 Ontario, Legislative Assembly, *Debates*, 25 April 1963, Twenty-Sixth Legislature, no. 46 (Toronto: Queen's Printer, 1963), 2776. For the full discussion of the bill see 2769–2800.
137 Ontario, Legislative Assembly, *Debates*, 25 April 1963. Goldberg received his PhD in political economy from the University of Toronto in 1962. His dissertation was "Trade Union Interest in Medical Care and Voluntary Health Insurance: A Study of Two Collectively Managed Programmes" (PhD diss., University of Toronto, 1962).
138 Goldberg, "Trade Union Interest," frontispiece.
139 See W.P. Thompson, *Medical Care: Programs and Issues* (Toronto: Clarke, Irwin, 1964), 54–5, 95–6.
140 Ted Goldberg to W.P. Thompson, 27 June 1963, "W.P. Thompson, Personal Papers, Medical Care, Correspondence: a) Doctor's Appraisal of Medicare to f) Correspondence on Book on Medicare, 1963–65," MG 17, University of Saskatchewan Archives.
141 See Antonia Maioni, *Parting at the Crossroads: The Emergence of Health Insurance in the United States and Canada* (Princeton, NJ: Princeton University Press, 1998), 130n48.
142 Ontario, Legislative Assembly, *Debates*, 1 June 1965, Twenty-Seventh Legislature, Third Session, no. 114 (Toronto: Queen's Printer, 1965), 3535. The *Globe and Mail* article referred to was 14 May 1965.
143 Ontario, Legislative Assembly, *Debates*, 27 April 1966, Twenty-Seventh Legislature, Fourth Session, no. 89 (Toronto: Queen's Printer, 1966), 2737.
144 Ontario, Legislative Assembly, *Debates*, 28 April 1966, 2759–60.
145 Canada, Royal Commission on Health Services, *Studies*, J.E.F. Hastings and W. Mosley, *Organized Community Health Services* (Ottawa: Queen's Printer, 1966), 69.
146 Canada, Royal Commission on Health Services, *Studies*, 43. See also 82.
147 Canada, Royal Commission on Health Services, *Studies*, 82.
148 Bator, *Within Reach of Everyone*, 2:39.
149 Rhodes, "Report of the Director of the School of Hygiene," ... *Year Ending June 1965*, 131–2.
150 Rhodes, "Report of the Director of the School of Hygiene," ... *Year Ending June 1965*, 133.
151 Rhodes, "Report of the Director of the School of Hygiene," ... *Year Ending June 1965*, 133–4.
152 A.J. Rhodes, "Report of the Director of the School of Hygiene," in *President's Report, for the Year Ending June 1970, Part Two*, 53.
153 Bator, *Within Reach of Everyone*, 2:37–8.
154 Rhodes, "Director of the School of Hygiene," ... *Year Ending June 1961*, 80.
155 Rhodes, "Report of the Director of the School of Hygiene," ... *Year Ending June 1970, Part Two*, 51–2.
156 Rhodes, "Report of the Director of the School of Hygiene," ... *Year Ending June 1970, Part Two*, 50–1.

157 See Ontario, Committee on the Healing Arts, *Report*, vol. 2, 1970. The reference from Mott's article, "Patterns of Medical Care," is on 18. Ken Clute's book, *The General Practitioner*, is referenced on 22, 81, 94, 228, 240, and 291. Hastings's Hall Commission study is on 5 and 19.
158 See Ontario, Committee on the Healing Arts, *Report*, vol. 3. A paper by F.B. Roth, "The Hospital and Health Services of the Future," is referenced on 124. Ken Clute's *The General Practitioner* is referenced on 136, 170, and 190.
159 See John E.F. Hastings, "The Report of the Ontario Committee on the Healing Arts," *Canadian Journal of Public Health* 61, no. 5 (September/October 1970): 367–9.
160 See Ontario, Committee on the Healing Arts, Study, R.D. Fraser, *Selected Economic Aspects of the Health Care Sector in Ontario* (Toronto: Queen's Printer, 1970). The references from Mott and Milton Roemer's *Rural Health and Medical Care* appear on 196, 198, and 202. Ken Clute's *The General Practitioner* is referenced on 47, 56, 62, 93, 96, 102, 103, and 198. Hastings's study, noted in the previous section, is on 199. The reference to Clute and Mott on physicians' rural practice is on 196.
161 See Ontario, Committee on the Healing Arts, *Report*, vol. 3 (Toronto: Queen's Printer, 197), 242.
162 See Ontario, Ministry of Health, Health Planning Task Force, 1974, 15.
163 Claude Bissell, "Report of the President," in *President's Report, for the Year Ending June 1963*, 39.
164 Claude Bissell, "Report of the President," in *President's Report, for the Year Ending June 1967, Part One*, 53.
165 *Staff Bulletin*, February 1968, 19, UTARMS. See also *Staff Bulletin*, November 1967, 23, UTARMS.
166 Bissell, "Report of the President," ... *Year Ending June 1967, Part One*, 48–9.
167 Bissell, "Report of the President," ... *Year Ending June 1967, Part One*, 40.
168 See "People," *Canadian Hospital* 47, no. 9 (September 1970): 21.
169 See J.A. McNab, "A Tribute to Eugenie M. Stuart, Professor Emeritus Hospital Administration, University of Toronto, October 25, 1971," Department of Health Administration, University of Toronto, A1998-0023/002, UTARMS; contained in a leather-bound album presented to Miss Stuart, dated 25 October 1971.
170 Agnew, *Canadian Hospitals, 1920 to 1970*, 133.
171 See Department of Health Administration, University of Toronto, A1998-0023/002, UTARMS. These pictures, letters, and telegrams were gathered in the leather-bound album presented to Miss Stuart, dated 25 October 1971.
172 I attended many of these functions while at TGH.
173 Kathryn J. Ellis, "Dagnone, Antonio," *Encyclopedia of Saskatchewan* (Regina: Canadian Plains Research Centre, University of Regina, 2005), 233.
174 Horlick, *They Built Better Than They Knew*, 285. For more on Tony's career, see the index entry on 365.
175 "People," *Canadian Hospital* 50, no. 12 (December 1973): 17.
176 "People," *Canadian Hospital* 47, no. 4 (April 1970): 21.
177 David W. Corder, "Operating Room Technicians: Their Role and Functions as Seen by Operating Room Supervisors" (DHA thesis, School of Hygiene, University of Toronto, 1970), ii.
178 See Chris Dooley, "End of the Asylum (Town): Community Responses to the Depopulation and Closure of the Saskatchewan Hospital, Weyburn," *Histoire*

Sociale/Social History 44, no. 88 (November 2011): 335. The article deals with its economic impact on the Weyburn area, the mental health reforms of the Douglas era, and its eventual closure in 1971.

179 "People," *Canadian Hospital* 44, no. 1 (January 1967): 32.

180 Jeannine Girard, "The Four-Day Work Week and the Hospital" (DHA thesis, School of Hygiene, University of Toronto, 1972). (Mrs) I. Dombrs, Interlibrary loan librarian to chairperson, Department of Hospital Administration, Department of Hygiene, University of Toronto, 28 June 1977, noting Mr O. Sijbrandij, National Ziekenhuisinst, Utrecht, Netherlands, wished a copy of the thesis. The letter is stapled to the flyleaf of the thesis.

181 Edwin V. Wahn, Press Clippings File, University of Saskatchewan Archives; see *Toronto Telegram*, "Hospital Planning Director Quits Post," 17 March 1971; *Globe and Mail*, "Hospital Council Head Resigns to Join WHO," 3 October 1972.

182 E.V. Wahn, "The Integration of Hospital Facilities and Services in the North-Western Area of Metropolitan Toronto: Some Recommended Future Developments Based on the Findings of a Study Conducted under the Direction of the District No. 2 Ad Hoc Hospital Planning Committee," Toronto Metropolitan Toronto Hospital Planning Council, April 1970, 7, 19.

183 Bator, *Within Reach of Everyone*, 2:72.

184 *Finding Aid*, 3, Phyllis E. Jones fonds, B2008-009, UTARMS.

185 Phyllis Edith Jones, "The Family Physician and the Public Health Nurse: An Investigation of One Method of Collaboration" (MSc thesis, University of Toronto, 1969), ii.

186 Phyllis E. Jones fonds, B2008-009, UTARMS. See box 1, file 01, "Manuscripts of Presentations 1967–1972" for those made to the School of Hygiene. See file 02, "Manuscripts of Presentations 1973–1976" for "Interpretation of the Hastings Report, March 26, 1973," and "The Nurse Practitioner: Community Health Worker of the Future, Presentation to the Inaugural Symposium, Community Health, October 23, 1975."

187 Claus Wirsig, "Opinion," "New Editorial Team at Your Service," *Hospital Administration in Canada* 8, no. 10 (October 1966), 4.

188 "Appointments," *Hospital Administration in Canada* 19, no. 3 (March 1977): 8.

189 See *Toronto Star*, "Claus Wirsig Guest Book," 15 July 2017, https://www.legacy.com/obituaries/thestar/obituary.aspx?n=claus-wirsig&pid=186095975. See also "Appointment: Claus A. Wirsig to Assistant Editor *Hospital Administration and Construction,*" *Hospital Administration and Construction* 3, no. 1 (January 1961): 39.

190 See "Appointments," *Hospital Administration in Canada* 19, no. 10 (October 1977): 10.

191 See WUSC, "Remembering Claus Wirsig (1933–2017)," 21 July 2017, https://wusc.ca/remembering-claus-wirsig-1933–2017/.

192 "Appointment: Claus A. Wirsig," 39.

193 Claus A. Wirsig, "Management Initiative in the Organization and Staffing of the Patient Care Unit: Old Problems, New Trends and Opportunities" (DHA thesis, School of Hygiene, University of Toronto, 1968), ii.

194 Wirsig, "Management Initiative."

195 Wirsig, "Management Initiative," iii.

196 See Claus A. Wirsig, "John Thomas Law, 1917–1977: A Tribute," *Hospital Administration in Canada* 20, no. 2 (February 1978): 35–6.
197 Wright, *SickKids*, 246.
198 Boxes /016 and /015, A1986-0033, UTARMS.
199 A1986-0033/017, UTARMS.
200 Boxes /018 and /019, A1986-0033, UTARMS.
201 Personal correspondence between the author and Don Carley, received 18 April 2019 (note sent to Don by Al).
202 Personal correspondence between the author and Don Carley received 18 April 2019 (information forwarded to Don by Ken).
203 Personal correspondence between the author and Don Carley received 18 April 2019 (note to Don from Dick).

CHAPTER TWELVE

1 Harold Averill, "Biographical Note," *Finding Aid*, Hastings (John E.F.) Family fonds, B2002-0014, June 2004, 3–4, UTARMS.
2 Averill, "Biographical Note," 4–5.
3 Averill, "Biographical Note," 5.
4 Averill, "Biographical Note," 6–7.
5 Paul Bator, interview with Dr John Hastings, 10 June 1993; quoted in Bator, *Within Reach of Everyone*, 2:150.
6 John Browne, personal meeting with the author, 25 August 2016.
7 See "Saskatchewan Health Services Survey Commission," B2002-0014/034 (09), John E.F. Hastings Family fonds, UTARMS.
8 Hastings to Defries on Department of Public Health letterhead, 29 July 1954, "Experience in Saskatchewan Department of Public Health – Summer 1954 – Corresp.," B2002-0014/023(10), Hastings (John E.F.) Family fonds, UTARMS.
9 G.H. Hatcher to A.F.W. Peart, 29 June 1954, 1, "Western Canadian Trip, Aug–Sept 1954, Notebook, Letter," B2002-0014/023(08), Hastings (John E.F.) Family fonds, UTARMS. The letter also has a tentative itinerary.
10 Stenographer's notebook with handwritten title "Notes on Western Trip, August–September 1954," B2002-0014/023(08), Hastings (John E.F.) Family fonds, UTARMS.
11 Averill, "Biographical Note," 16.
12 Hatcher to Peart, 29 June 1954, 2.
13 For further information on the department at that time, see F.B. Roth and R.D. Defries, "The Saskatchewan Department of Public Health," *CJPH* 49, no. 7 (July 1958): 276–85.
14 See Saskatchewan, Department of Public Health, *Annual Report, April 1, 1954 to March 31, 1955* (Regina: Lawrence Amon, Queen's Printer, 1956), 4. See 12 for the organization chart of the department.
15 Saskatchewan, Department of Public Health, *Annual Report*, 130.
16 Saskatchewan, Department of Public Health, *Annual Report*, 130.
17 For a brief bio on Roemer, see Emily K. Abel, Elizabeth Fee, and Theodore M. Brown, "Milton I. Roemer, Advocate of Social Medicine, International Health, and National Health Insurance," *American Journal of Public Health* 98, no. 9 (September 2008): 1596–7.
18 Deputy minister of public health to provincial auditor, memorandum, 19 August 1954, "Experience in Saskatchewan Department of Public Health – Summer 1954 – Corresp."

19 Hastings to Defries, 29 July 1954.
20 Hatcher to Peart, 29 June 1954.
21 "Finding Aid," 1, V.L. Matthews fonds, University of Saskatchewan Archives.
22 Hatcher to Peart, 29 June 1954.
23 See, Saskatchewan, Department of Public Health, *Annual Report, April 1, 1954 to March 31, 1955*, 20–63, for the section on regional health services, and 24–5 for information on the Swift Current plan. Note that headings and pagination in table of contents do not correspond with the text.
24 Saskatchewan, Department of Public Health, *Annual Report, April 1, 1954 to March 31, 1955*, 20.
25 Saskatchewan, Department of Public Health, *Annual Report, April 1, 1953 to March 31, 1954* (Regina: Lawrence Amon, Queen's Printer, 1955), 97.
26 For further information on the Douglas government, see the work mentioned earlier of one of the civil servants who ended up at Harvard twice, for a master's and doctorate. Al Johnson was a wunderkind hired by the Douglas government. He was put through the Budget Bureau, which was the Douglas government's informal proving ground for promising new civil servants. He rose to become deputy provincial treasurer at a very young age. He was one of the "Saskatchewan mafia" who moved on to the federal government after the defeat of the NDP in 1964.

For some specifics on where Saskatchewan civil servants ended up, see Johnson, *Dream No Little Dreams*, 198. See also Gregory P. Marchildon, "Saskatchewan Mafia," *Encyclopedia of Saskatchewan*, https://esask.uregina.ca/entry/saskatchewan_mafia.jsp.
27 Personal conversation with the author. Galbraith was Brownstone's PhD supervisor.
28 See Canada, Department of National Health and Welfare, *A New Perspective on the Health of Canadians: A Working Document* (Lalonde Report), Ottawa, 1974.
29 John Browne, personal correspondence with the author, 11 August 2016.
30 Browne, personal correspondence with the author, 11 August 2016.
31 John Browne, personal meeting with the author, 25 August 2016.
32 For a bit of insight into H.L. (Bert) Laframboise, see Kenneth Kernaghan, "Speaking Truth to Academics: The Wisdom of the Practitioners," *Canadian Public Administration* 52, no. 4 (December 2009): 503–23. There is a paragraph on him on 510, but he is mentioned at various points throughout the article. Kernaghan calls him a "scholarly practitioner" and groups him along with the likes of A.W. Johnson, Gordon Robertson, Arthur Kroeger, and others. Over the course of his career Laframboise published a number of articles in academic journals.
33 H.L. Laframboise, "Health Policy: Breaking the Problem Down into More Manageable Segments," *CMAJ* 108, no. 3 (3 February 1973): 393.
34 H.L. Laframboise, "Administrative Reform in the Federal Public Service: Signs of a Saturation Psychosis," *Canadian Public Administration* 14, no. 3 (3 February 1973): 303–25.
35 Berridge, *Public Health*, 98.
36 Meeting 30 May 1950, "Post-Graduate Degrees, Diplomas and Certificates in Public Health and Hospital Administration," 2–3, file "School of Hygiene Council Minutes," box 002, A1975-0029, School of Hygiene, UTARMS.

37 A.J. Rhodes, "Diplomas or Master's Degrees: Patterns of Postgraduate Education in Public Health," *CJPH* 52, no. 4 (April 1961): 142.
38 Rhodes, "Report of the Director of the School of Hygiene," ... *Year Ending June 1961*, 79.
39 President's Committee on the School of Graduate Studies, *Graduate Studies in the University of Toronto: Report of the President's Committee on the School of Graduate Studies, 1964–1965*. See 38–41 for discussion of the diploma courses. The school made two submissions to the committee (see 140).
40 John Browne, personal correspondence with the author, 11 August 2016.
41 Jay Cassel, "Public Health in Canada," in *The History of Public Health and the Modern State*, ed. Dorothy Porter (Amsterdam: Editions Rodopi B.V., 1994), 305.
42 Quebec, Commission of Inquiry on Health and Social Welfare (Castonguay-Nepveu Report), *Report*, vol. 4, tome 1, "Health," 1970, 30, para. 78 (at this time Gerard Nepveu was the chairman).
43 Quebec, Commission of Inquiry on Health and Social Welfare (Castonguay-Nepveu Report), *Report*, vol. 1, "Health Insurance," 1967, 117 (at this time Claude Castonguay was the chairman).
44 Quebec, Commission of Inquiry on Health and Social Welfare, *Report*, vol. 1, "Health Insurance," 36–7.
45 See Quebec, Commission of Inquiry on Health and Social Welfare, *Report*, vol. 1, "Health Insurance," 40–2.
46 Quebec, Commission of Inquiry on Health and Social Welfare, *Report*, vol. 4, tome 2, "Health," 1970, 38–44.
47 Quebec, Commission of Inquiry on Health and Social Welfare, *Report*, vol. 4, tome 2, "Health," 1970, 59.
48 Quebec, Commission of Inquiry on Health and Social Welfare, *Report*, vol. 1, "Health Insurance," 70.
49 Interview with Burns Roth, audiocassette #4/6, side 1. See also "Interview with Dr Burns Roth, Reel #4," 24 July 1985, 2, transcript, School of Hygiene History Project, B89-0009, UTARMS.
50 See Rakow, *Fifty-Year Retrospective*, 9.
51 John Browne, personal correspondence with the author, 10 August 2017.
52 Browne, personal correspondence with the author, 10 August 2017.
53 Browne, personal correspondence with the author, 10 August 2017.
54 Browne, personal correspondence with the author, 10 August 2017.
55 See Rakow, *Fifty-Year Retrospective*, 9–10.
56 John Browne, personal correspondence with the author, 11 August 2016.
57 Browne, personal correspondence with the author, 11 August 2016.
58 John Browne, personal meeting with the author, 25 August 2016.
59 A1986-0033, UTARMS. See the *Finding Aid* that lists the students by year (1947–80).
60 See Barbara Mann Wall, *Unlikely Entrepreneurs: Catholic Sisters and the Hospital Marketplace, 1865–1925* (Columbus: Ohio State University Press, 2005). By the same author, see *American Catholic Hospitals: A Century of Changing Markets and Missions* (New Brunswick, NJ: Rutgers University Press, 2011).
61 G.H. Beaton to Miss McNeely, 14 August 1969, 2, memorandum, "Law, John Thomas," School of Graduate Studies, A2002-0013/081, UTARMS.

62 Wright, *SickKids*, 258. See also Beaton to McNeely, 14 August 1969, basically Law's resumé, though it is not labelled as such.
63 Beaton to McNeely, 14 August 1969, 2.
64 Wright, *SickKids*, 258.
65 School of Graduate Studies, A2002-0013/081, UTARMS; and personal correspondence with Tys Klumpenhouwer, 15 October 2018, UTARMS. See also Wright, *SickKids*, 259.
66 Wright, *SickKids*, 259.
67 Wright, *SickKids*, 259–60.
68 Wright, *SickKids*, 266.
69 Law, "Impact of the Canadian Federal-Provincial Hospital Program on the Voluntary Hospital," in "Canadian-American Conference on Hospital Programs," supplement, *Medical Care* 7, no. 6 (November–December 1969): S34–5.
70 Law, "Impact of the Canadian Federal-Provincial Hospital Program," S34.
71 Law, "Impact of the Canadian Federal-Provincial Hospital Program," S35.
72 Law, "Impact of the Canadian Federal-Provincial Hospital Program," S41.
73 John Thomas Law, "Present and Future Roles of Hospital Boards of Trustees in Ontario" (MSc thesis, University of Toronto, 1974).
74 "Law, John Thomas," School of Graduate Studies, roll 22, A1984-0032, UTARMS. Also meetings 17 and 19 October 2018, and personal correspondence 18 October 2018 with Tys Klumpenhouwer.
75 See Will Rooen, "Stan Martin: Man with a Mission," *Canadian Hospital* 46, no. 4 (April 1969): 47.
76 Law, "Present and Future Roles," 15–16.
77 Law, "Present and Future Roles," 11.
78 John T. Law, "Autonomy's Strong Men," *Canadian Hospital* 41, no. 2 (February 1964): 40. Note the title is different in the table of contents, "Where Do We Go from Here?"
79 F. Burns Roth to G.H. Beaton, "Law, John Thomas," 29 January 1973, memorandum from School of Graduate Studies, A2002-0013/081, UTARMS. See also Bernard Bucove to M.F. McNeely, 7 February 1973; and M.F. McNeely to B. Bucove, 28 February 1973.
80 Ontario, Ontario Hospital Services Commission, "Report of the Commission," *Annual Report 1970* (Toronto: Ontario Hospital Services Commission, 1971), 3.
81 Ontario, Ontario Hospital Services Commission, "Report of the Commission," 3.
82 Beaton to Miss Mceely, 14 August 1969, 1.

CHAPTER THIRTEEN

1 J.E.F. Hastings, John W. Browne, William R. Mindell, and Janet H. Barnsley, "The Canadian Health Administrators Study," *Canadian Journal of Public Health* 72, no. 2, Supplement One (March/April 1981): S1–60.
2 "Chapter 1: The Context and Approach of the Canadian Health Administrator Study," *Canadian Journal of Public Health* 72, no. 2, Supplement One (March/April 1981): S12. The supplement was published as a separate issue with its own cover and binding.
3 "Chapter 1: Context and Approach," S12.

4 Canada, Department of National Health and Welfare, *The Community Health Centre in Canada*, vol. 1, *Report of the Community Health Centre Project to the Health Ministers* (Ottawa: Information Canada, 1972), ii–iii.
5 Correspondence with John Browne, 23 July 2017.
6 Correspondence with John Browne, 24 July 2017.
7 Correspondence with Browne, 23 July 2017.
8 "Progress Report, November 30, 1971," B2002-0014/039(15), Hastings (John E.F.) Family fonds, UTARMS. The quotes are taken from a fourth (unnumbered) page.
9 "Progress Report, November 30, 1971," II-2.
10 "Progress Report, November 30, 1971," II-7.
11 "Progress Report, November 30, 1971," II-8.
12 "CHC Project, Administrative Memos, 1971–72," B2002-0014/039(03), Hastings (John E.F.) Family fonds, UTARMS. See Joan Hollobon, "Radical Changes in Health Care to e stuSdied," *Globe and Mail*, 9 December 1971.
13 For topics and people involved, see Canada, Department of National Health and Welfare, *The Community Health Centre in Canada*, vol. 1: commissioned papers, C-1 to C-7; briefs, C-10 to C-19; visits and discussions, C-20 to C-31.
14 Community Health Centre Project, "A Commissioned Paper to the Community Health Project," pt 31–62; A.S. Haro, "The Health Care System in Finland: Description of Non-Quantifiable Aspects" (Ottawa: Canadian Public Health Association, [1974?]), 3–5.
15 The notes of and the papers presented at the seminars take up almost an entire box in the archives. See B2002-0014/040(05-15), Hastings (John E.F.) Family fonds, UTARMS, for the files on the proceedings. For a list of the people involved in each seminar, see Canada, Department of National Health and Welfare, *The Community Health Centre in Canada*, vol. 1, C-32 to C-49.
16 Canada, Department of National Health and Welfare, *Community Health Centre in Canada*, vol. 1, C-8 to C-9.
17 Canada, Department of National Health and Welfare, *Community Health Centre in Canada*, vol. 1, i.
18 Canada, Department of National Health and Welfare, *Community Health Centre in Canada*, vol. 1, 1.
19 Canada, Department of National Health and Welfare, *The Community Health Centre in Canada*, vol. 2, A.P. Ruderman, *Economic Characteristics of Community Health Centres* (Ottawa: Information Canada, 1973), i. Note: A.P. Ruderman received a BS from Harvard, an MBA from the University of Chicago, and PhD in economics from Harvard. He came to the department in 1967 and left in 1975 to become dean of administrative studies at Dalhousie University.
20 John Browne, personal correspondence with the author, 9 October 2016.
21 Canada, Department of National Health and Welfare, *The Community Health Centre in Canada*, vol. 3, Anne Crichton, "Conclusions," *Community Health Centres: Health Care Organization of the Future?* (Ottawa: Information Canada, 1973), 19-10.
22 Crichton, "Conclusions," 19–9.
23 Browne, personal correspondence with the author, 9 October 2016.
24 See Crichton, "Canadian Objective and Health Care," *Community Health Centres*, 9-6 to 9-9.

25 See Crichton, "Canadian Objective and Health Care," 9-10 to 9-15.
26 See Crichton, "Ten Main Issues: A Personal View," *Community Health Centres*, 1, 2.
27 See "Special Supplement: Report of the Community Health Centre Project to the Conference of Health Ministers," CMAJ 107, no. 4 (19 August 1972): S361–80.
28 "Association News – Hastings II: Where Your Association Stands re the CHC Project Report," CMAJ 107, no. 7 (7 October 1972): 677.
29 The second volume cited a report by Hastings, Mott, Barclay, and Hewitt on prepaid practice in Sault Ste Marie. See Canada, Department of National Health and Welfare, *The Community Health Centre in Canada*, vol. 2, A.P. Ruderman, *Economic Characteristics of Community Health Centres*, 28.
30 In the third volume, which was written by Anne Crichton at the University of British Columbia, Mott was cited a number of times. F.B. Roth's article on the relationship of hospitals to community health facilities was noted. Palin was referenced on the centralization of services. See Canada, Department of National Health and Welfare, *The Community Health Centre in Canada*, vol. 3, Anne Crichton, *Community Health Centres: Health Care Organization of the Future?* (Ottawa: Information Canada, 1973). For Hastings and Mott, see 10-32. For Mott, see 2-3, 6-14, 10-32, and 12-17. For Roth, see 3-4, 4-11, 5-13, 12-9, and 13-8. For Palin see 5-10
31 Canada, Department of National Health and Welfare, *The Community Health Centre in Canada*, vol. 3, Anne Crichton, *Community Health Centres: Health Care Organization of the Future?* 9-10, 10-15.
32 Barbara J. Fenn, "The Regina Community Clinic: A Comparison with the Hastings Model for Community Health Centres in Canada" (thesis, Diploma of Public Health, University of Toronto, 1981), 30, 39–41. There is a table comparing the Regina Community Clinic with the Hastings model on 31–7.
33 Fenn, "Regina Community Clinic," 93–4.
34 Fenn, "Regina Community Clinic," 103–4.
35 J.E.F. Hastings, F.D. Mott, A. Barclay, and D. Hewitt, "Prepaid Group Practice in Sault Ste Marie, Ontario: Part I: Analysis of Utilization Records," *Medical Care* 11, no. 2 (March–April 1973): 91. See also John E.F. Hastings, F.D. Mott, D. Hewitt, and A. Barclay, "An Interim Report on the Sault Ste Marie Study: A Comparison of Personal Health Services Utilization: A Joint Canada–World Health Organization Project," CJPH 61, no. 4 (July/August 1970): 289–96.
36 F.D. Mott, J.E.F. Hastings, and A.T. Barclay, "Prepaid Group Practice in Sault Ste Marie, Ontario: Part II: Evidence from the Household Survey," *Medical Care* 11, no. 3 (May–June 1973): 173.
37 John Browne, personal correspondence with the author, 9 October 2016.
38 "Conference of Deputy Ministers of Health and Canadian Schools of Public Health, 1971," B2002-0014/042(01), Hastings (John E.F.) Family fonds, UTARMS.
39 "The Ditchley Foundation: Conference on Development of Health Services and Medical Care, 8–11.12.1972," B2002-0014/42(02), Hastings (John E.F.) Family fonds, UTARMS.
40 Harold Averill, "Biographical Note," *Finding Aid*, Hastings (John E.F.) Family fonds, B2002-0014, June 2004, 7 UTARMS.

41 Averill, "Biographical Note," 22.
42 For the Planning Committee members, see "Planning Committee for the Symposium," in *Papers: Health and Society: Emerging International and Canadian Trends: Addresses to the Anniversary Symposium of the School of Hygiene, University of Toronto, April 13 and 14, 1973*, ed. Kenneth F. Clute ([Toronto] School of Hygiene, University of Toronto, 1973), iv. For the department faculty listing, see *University of Toronto, Calendar, School Of Hygiene, 1972–73*, 50–1.
43 Kenneth F. Clute to George Ignatieff, 4 July 1973, "Speech Notes: School of Hygiene Anniversary Symposium Hart House, 'Changing Social and Political Scene,'" file 44-26, series 8 – Speeches, box 44, George Ignatieff fonds, F2020, University of Toronto, Trinity College Archives. It is difficult to know how the connection to Dr Ignatieff was made. In the archives there is correspondence with Omand Solondt (Correspondence January–August 1972) and Dr R.M. Morgan, chair, Department of Preventive Medicine (Correspondence December 1972–31 May 1973) on other matters, and these could have been possible connections. The correspondence with Dr Morgan was to establish a United Nations University in Toronto.
44 Note, the Pan American Health Organization at that time was known as the Pan American Sanitary Bureau. Faculty members from Hygiene, including FitzGerald and Defries, were active in it.
45 Marc Lalonde, "The Changing Philosophic Context," in Clute, *Papers: Health and Society*, 5–6, 11–15.
46 Lalonde, "Changing Philosophic Context," 5–6.
47 John Brotherston, "The United Kingdom: New Trends and Issues," in Clute, *Papers: Health and Society*, 31–42.
48 George Ignatieff, "The Changing Social and Political Scene," in Clute, *Papers: Health and Society*, 67.
49 David M. Grenville, "Omond McKillop Solandt: A Biographical Sketch," in *Perspectives in Science and Technology: The Legacy of Omond Solandt: Proceedings of a Symposium Held at the Donald Gordon Centre, Queen's University at Kingston, Ontario, 8–10 May 1994*, ed. C.E. Law, G.R. Lindsay, and D.M. Grenville ([Kingston]: Queen's Quarterly, [1995]), 5, 11.
50 Jason Sean Ridler, *Maestro of Science: Omond McKillop Solandt and Government Science in War and Hostile Peace, 1939–1956* (Toronto: University of Toronto Press, 2015),127–8.
51 Bator, *Within Reach of Everyone*, 2:65.
52 See *Corporate Name Authority*, August 1988, U-77 UTARMS; also a conversation with Harold Averill, 15 September 2017. The U of T Faculty of Arts established a Department of Physiology in 1892. In 1921 it moved from Arts to the Faculty of Medicine. In 1906 a Department of Physiological Chemistry was established. Its name changed in 1909–10 to the Department of Biochemistry. The School of Hygiene established a Department of Physiological Hygiene in 1924–25 at the same time as the school was established. It encompassed both physiology and environmental health, and its name was changed to Environmental Health in November 1970. This was the department located in the FitzGerald Building, where Charles Best had his lab.
53 Bator, *Within Reach of Everyone*, 2:37.
54 *University of Toronto, Calendar, School of Hygiene, 1935–36*, 17.

55 *University of Toronto, Calendar, School of Hygiene, 1935–36*, 26.
56 File 31, Interview Summary, Solandt, Omond, p. 1, part 1, box 4, David Morgan Grenville fonds, B2009-0046, UTARMS.
57 Audiotape 041S, box 4, David Morgan Grenville fonds, B2009-0046, UTARMS. Note, the list of audiotapes is listed in the finding aid, 15–18.
58 Ridler, *Maestro of Science*, 35.
59 G.D.W. Murphy, L.B. Jaques, T.S. Perrett, and C.H. Best, "Heparin and the Thrombosis of Veins Following Injury," in Charles Herbert Best, *Selected Papers of Charles H. Best* (Toronto, University of Toronto Press, 1963), 644.
60 Omond M. Solandt, "The Impact of Science on Health," in Clute, *Papers: Health and Society*, 71.
61 Solandt, "Impact of Science on Health," 71.
62 Solandt, "Impact of Science on Health," 73–5.
63 Solandt, "Impact of Science on Health," 71–2.
64 Solandt, "Impact of Science on Health," 75–6.
65 Solandt, "Impact of Science on Health," 78.
66 Omond Solandt, "Message to the Symposium," in Law et al., *Perspectives in Science and Technology: The Legacy of Omond Solandt*, xiii.
67 Bernard Bucove, "Concluding Remarks," in Clute, *Papers: Health and Society*, 111.

CHAPTER FOURTEEN

1 Bator, *Within Reach of Everyone*, 2:171–3.
2 Arthur Allen, *Vaccine: The Controversial Story of Medicine's Greatest Lifesaver* (New York: W.W. Norton, 2007), 428.
3 Allen, *Vaccine*, 428.
4 John Hastings, "A Postscript by Dr John Hasting: Part B Public Health/ Community Health as a Discipline," in Bator, *Within Reach of Everyone*, 2:165.
5 Hastings, "Postscript by Dr John Hasting," 2:164.
6 Hastings, "Postscript by Dr John Hasting," 2:164.
7 See, for example, Bator, *Within Reach of Everyone*, 2:137.
8 Rhodes, "Report of the Director of the School of Hygiene," ... *Year Ending June 1970, Part Two*, 52.
9 "A Tribute to Bernard Bucove," *American Journal of Public Health* 64, no. 1 (January 1974): 87–9.
10 Interview with Dr Andrew Rhodes, 23 July 1985, side 1, tape 5/6, audiocassette, School of Hygiene History Project, B89-0009(04), UTARMS. For a partial account of the interview, see "Transcript, Recorded Interview with Dr Andrew J. Rhodes," 23 July 1985, 3.
11 Rhodes, "Directors of the School of Hygiene," ... *Year Ended June 1970, Part Two*, 52. Note, this report of the school is labelled as "directors," as Dr Bucove also submitted a report.
12 Bernard Bucove, "The Directors of the School of Hygiene," *President's Report for the Year Ended June 1970, Part Two*, 55.
13 Personal interview with the author, 2 November 2016.
14 Interview with Dr Andrew Rhodes, 26 July 1985, tape 6/6, audiocassette, School of Hygiene History Project, B89-0009, UTARMS. For a partial account of the interview, see "Transcript, Recorded Interview with Dr Andrew J. Rhodes," 26 July 1985, 4.

15 John Browne, personal correspondence with the author, 11 August 2016.
16 Interview with Burns Roth, audiocassette #3/6, side 1.
17 Interview with Burns Roth, audiocassette #4/6, side 1.
18 Interview with Dr Burns Roth, 24 July 1985.
19 See Bator, *Within Reach of Everyone*, 2:139–41.
20 G.H. Beaton, "Community Health: A New Approach at the University of Toronto," *Canadian Journal of Public Health* 65, no. 6 (November/December 1974): 463.
21 W. Harding le Riche, *The Memoirs of Dr W. Harding le Riche*, vol. 2, *Canada over the Years* (self-pub., 1993), 277.
22 Personal correspondence with the author, 24 August 2017.
23 John Browne concurs with these author's conclusions. See personal correspondence with the author, 24 August 2017.
24 John Browne, personal correspondence with the author, 11 August 2016.
25 *Finding Aid, Department of Health Administration, A1986-0033*, 2, 5, UTARMS.
26 Bator, *Within Reach of Everyone*, 2:160.
27 Bator, *Within Reach of Everyone*, 2:160.
28 Bator, *Within Reach of Everyone*, 2:161.
29 See Shaun Murphy, "The Early Days of the MRC Social Medicine Research Unit," *Social History of Medicine* 12, no. 3 (1999): 389–406.
30 See Roy M. Acheson and David Hewitt, "Oxford Child Health Survey: Stature and Skeletal Maturation in the Pre-School Child," *British Journal of Preventive and Social Medicine* 8, no. 2 (1954): 59–65.
31 I. Oransky, "Obituary: Roy M. Acheson," *Lancet* 362, no. 9379 (19 July 2003): 253.
32 Great Britain, Department of Health, *Independent Inquiry into Inequalities in Health*, Acheson Report, London: Stationery Office, 1998.
33 Bator, *Within Reach of Everyone*, 2:161.
34 Bator, *Within Reach of Everyone*, 2:154.
35 Bator, *Within Reach of Everyone*, 2:151.
36 W.H. le Riche to C.T. Bissell, 2 September 1966; Claude Bissell to W.H. le Riche, 12 October 1966, file "Hygiene," Office of the President, A75-0021/062, UTARMS.
37 John Browne, correspondence with the author, 11 August 2016.
38 John Browne, correspondence with the author, 18 October 2016.

CHAPTER FIFTEEN

1 Rakow, *Fifty-Year Retrospective*, 11.
2 Interview with Vayda, 11 July 2016.
3 Personal correspondence with John Browne, January 13, 2020.
4 Personal correspondence with John Browne, January 14, 2020.
5 Bator, *Within Reach of Everyone*, 2:153.
6 Larry Wayne Richards, *University of Toronto: An Architectural Tour* (New York: Princeton Architectural Press, 2009), 61–2.
7 Interview with Dr Vayda, 11 July 2016.
8 Bator, *Within Reach of Everyone*, 2:153–4; also interview with Vayda.
9 "Gerry Turner," file (unnumbered), A1998-0023/002, Department of Health Administration, UTARMS; see letters and attachments from J. Hastings and G. Turner for December 1975 through August 1976.

10 I was a member of that first class. Through his relationship with the Saskatchewan deputy minister of health, Milton Orris also arranged for the Saskatchewan government to provide a bursary to me to partially cover costs.
11 I recall that one of the biggest challenges in this construction was material. The oil companies and the hospitals were competing with each other for material. There was a big shortage of plasterboard for walls. The oil companies usually won out (they could pay more), so the shortages were felt in the public sector and it slowed the pace of construction.
12 During the first practicum I recall a director in the Alberta department telling me that my career should be in teaching hospitals. As it turned out, that is what happened.
13 The term "core courses" is used within quotation marks, as it is specific rather than generic. It was a term used by faculty and students for many years referring to three courses common to students in all five streams.
14 Second interview with Burns Roth, digitized audio recording, 1:29:56.
15 Second interview with Burns Roth, digitized audio recording, 1:34:38.
16 I was a student in that first core class.
17 John Browne, correspondence with the author, 11 August 2016.
18 University of Toronto, School of Graduate Studies, *Calendar 1979–1980*, 128. Note, the 1978–79 calendar, the first for the new degree program, did not list the classes for the MHSC degree.
19 Interview with the author 11 July 2016.
20 Bator, *Within Reach of Everyone*, 2:47–9.
21 Bator, *Within Reach of Everyone*, 2:154.
22 Bator, *Within Reach of Everyone*, 2:154–5.
23 Correspondence with Gene Vayda, 18 August 2017.
24 Rakow, *Fifty-Year Retrospective*, 11.
25 Correspondence by the author with Rhonda Cockerill, 30 August 2017.
26 See Manitoba, Information Services Branch, "Health Sciences Centre Study to Be Launched," 15 February 1974, http://news.gov.mb.ca/news/archives/1974/02/1974-02-15-health_sciences_centre_study_to_be_launched.pdf.
27 "University of Toronto School of Hygiene History Project: A Report to the Dean, Faculty of Medicine, University of Toronto, with an Application for Further Funding," 8 March 1987, 3–5, B90-0035/002(10), Paul Adolphus Bator fonds, UTARMS.
28 Paul Adolphus Bator, "'Saving Lives on the Wholesale Plan': Public Health Reform in the City of Toronto" (PhD diss., University of Toronto, 1979).
29 Bator and Rhodes, *Within Reach of Everyone*, 1:vii–viii.
30 See Charles W. Birkett, "Privatization and Health Care: The Case of Ontario Nursing Homes," *CMAJ* 146, no. 1 (1 January 1992): 16; Eugene Vayda, "Dr Vayda responds," 16.
31 Eugene Vayda, "Private Practice in the United Kingdom: A Growing Concern," *Journal of Public Health Policy* 10, no. 3 (Autumn 1989): 373.
32 Eugene Vayda, "Universal Health Insurance in Canada: Are There Lessons for the United States?," *Vital Speeches of the Day* 54, no. 23 (15 September 1988): 716.
33 Correspondence with the author, 12 April 2017.
34 Correspondence with the author, 12 April 2017.

CHAPTER SIXTEEN

1 Andrew Pattullo, "Introduction," in *Unmet Needs: Education for Health Services Administration in Canada, Proceedings of a Conference Sponsored by the W.K. Kellogg Foundation* (Ottawa: Canadian College of Health Executives, 1978), 1.
2 Pattullo, "Introduction," 1.
3 Robert A. DeVries, "Concluding Remarks," Commission on Education for Health Administration, *Report of the Commission on Education for Health Administration*, vol. 3, *A Future Agenda* (Ann Arbor, MI: Health Administration, 1977), 171–3.
4 W. Harding le Riche, *The Memoirs of Dr W. Harding le Riche*, vol. 3, *Up to the Eighties* (self-pub., 1993), 375, UTARMS.
5 In some of the work we did together, Don arranged for students in my basic income class to attend special functions, such as meeting with Hugh Segal, former Canadian senator, master of Massey College, and an expert on basic income. As well Don took on a student in an independent study course I coordinated at Trinity.
6 B.A.T. Pederson to W.V. Stoughton, memorandum, 15 November 1982, with Telemedicine for Ontario program attached, dated 10 September 1982, file "Education, Continuing," A96-0004/012(02), Office of the Dean, Faculty of Medicine, UTARMS.
7 F.B. Fallis to Dr F. Lowy, memorandum, 1 October 1982, file "Telemedicine 82/83," A96-0004/012(03), Office of the Dean, Faculty of Medicine, UTARMS.
8 File "Education: Continuing 85/86," *Telemedicine for Ontario: News*, 1, no. 8 (May 1986), A94-0012/011, Office of the Dean, Faculty of Medicine, UTARMS.
9 File "Education: Continuing 85/86," Telemedicine for Ontario Presents Part II of Its TV Series.
10 E.A. Lindsay, D.A. Davis, F. Fallis, D.B. Willison, and J. Biggar, "Continuing Education through Telemedicine for Ontario," *CMAJ* 137, no. 6 (15 September 1987): 503–6.
11 Dr D. Davis, memorandum, 12 February 1990, file "Telemedicine Canada," A96-0011/007, Office of the Dean, Faculty of Medicine, UTARMS.
12 Correspondence from Gerard Mercer, 27 February 2017.
13 Meeting with the author 2 August 2017, and correspondence 6 August 2017.
14 *Graduate Education in Community Health, 1981–82*, 1, Division of Community Health, Faculty of Medicine, University of Toronto, UTARMS.
15 See Chandrakant Shah and L.A. Boehm, "Telemedicine: The New Frontier," in *Hospital-Based Ambulatory Care*, ed. Emil F. Pascarelli, 447–58 (Norwalk, CT: Appleton-Century-Crofts, 1982).
16 Department of Health Administration, Division of Community Health, Faculty of Medicine, University of Toronto, "Ontario Health Administrator Survey," October 1976; 2–3 for general, 4 for Canada, 5 for United States on education for health administrators.
17 "Ontario Health Administrator Survey," 90.
18 "Ontario Health Administrator Survey," 90–2.
19 John M. Phin, "Canadian College of Health Service Executives," in "The Canadian Health Administrators Study," Supplement 1, *Canadian Journal of Public Health* 72 (March/April 1981): S3.

20 "Summary" in "The Canadian Health Administrators Study," S11.
21 "Issues and Trends in Canadian Health Care" in "The Canadian Health Administrators Study," S58–60.
22 "The Canadian Health Administrators Study," S60.
23 See "Sidney Liswood Papers," http://data2.archives.ca/pdf/pdf001/p000000348.pdf
24 Ken Tremblay, "Conversations in the Executive Suite: Hume Martin," *Healthcare Quarterly* 8, no. 4 (2005): 34. Hume received the Robert Wood Johnson Award in 1981.
25 I was the young student who did a practicum with him in 1979.
26 William Boyd and William Anderson, *Boyd's Pathology for the Surgeon*, 8th ed. (Philadelphia: W.B. Saunders, 1967).
27 Letter and brief to Robert Baker, 6 January 1976, file "Gerald Turner," Department of Health Administration, University of Toronto, A1998-0023/002, UTARMS. See also J.E.F. Hastings to G.P. Turner, 15 December 1975.
28 Turner from Ron McQueen, 9 March 1988, file "Gerald Turner," Department of Health Administration, University of Toronto, A1998-0023/002, UTARMS.
29 External Advisory Committee, Minutes, meeting of 9 March 1979, file "Gerald Turner," Department of Health Administration, University of Toronto, A1998-0023/002, UTARMS.
30 Diploma in Hospital Administration (the name of the committee is not noted), meeting of 6 May 1975, 4, file "Gerald Turner," Department of Health Administration, University of Toronto, A1998-0023/002, UTARMS.
31 *The Memoirs of Dr W. Harding le Riche*, 3:366, le Riche, UTARMS.
32 Goldberg, "Trade Union Interest in Medical Care and Voluntary Health Insurance," ii.
33 Bator, *Within Reach of Everyone*, 2:155.
34 "In Memoriam," *University of Toronto Bulletin*, 26 October 1987, 7.
35 Grey, *New Deal Medicine*, 179.
36 Grey, *New Deal Medicine*, 224n13.
37 Theodore Goldberg, "Book Review: Derek Bok, *Higher Learning*," in *Teaching Secrets: The Technology in Social Work Education*, ed. Ruth Middleman and Gale Goldberg Wood, 129–30 (Binghamton, NY: Haworth, 1991). Note this was also published in the *Journal of Teaching in Social Work* 5, no. 2 (January 1992): 129–32 (the page numbers are the same in the book and the journal).
38 Goldberg, "Book Review: Derek Bok, *Higher Learning*." 130–1.
39 Ted Goldberg to Dean Lowy, 21 August 1984 and 7 August 1984, file "Department of Health Administration," A94-0012/006, Office of the Dean, Faculty of Medicine, UTARMS.
40 Peggy Leatt to John Krauser, 25 January 1985, file "Department of Health Administration," A94-0012/006, Office of the Dean, Faculty of Medicine, UTARMS.
41 File (not numbered), "Undergraduate Program," A1998-0023/001, School of Hygiene, UTARMS; see T. Goldberg, memorandum, 11 June 1986 with attached "Proposal for a Programme Leading to a Bachelor of Health Administration Degree," 1.
42 "Proposal for a Programme Leading to a Bachelor of Health Administration Degree," 2.
43 Correspondence with the author, 19 September 2016.

44 Roy M. Acheson to P. Bator, 20 May 1987, file 12, "Bator, Dr Paul, 1986–1987," box 10, Andrew James Rhodes fonds, B2000-001, UTARMS. See 3 in particular.

45 Acheson to Bator, 20 May 1987. In the file see Bator's presentation "The Emergence of Public Health Education Programs in the University of Toronto," 7.

46 Bator, "Emergence of Public Health Education Programs in the University of Toronto," 10–12.

47 Bator, "Emergence of Public Health Education Programs in the University of Toronto," 13–14.

48 See Elizabeth Fee and Roy Acheson, eds, *A History of Education in Public Health: Health That Mocks the Doctors' Rules* (Oxford: Oxford University Press, 1991). The conference is noted in the "Acknowledgements."

49 Because the Thatcher government tried to suppress the report, only 260 copies were mimeographed. However it was subsequently published in Douglas Black [et al.]; *Inequalities in Health: The Black Report, the Health Divide*, ed. Peter Townshend and Nick Davidson (London: Penguin Books, 1982).

50 Correspondence with Gene Vayda, 29 August 2017.

51 Frederick H. Lowy, *Dean's End-of-Term Report, 1987*, [Toronto]: Faculty of Medicine, University of Toronto, [1987], 33–5.

52 Lowy, *Dean's End-of-Term Report, 1987*, 21. For the connection to the subsequent class, see the subsection on the partnership with UTM during the term of Louise Lemieux-Charles (the class I developed).

53 Cynthia MacDonald, "A New Life after Loss," *U of T Magazine* 45, no. 2 (Winter 2018): 44–6.

54 John Oliver, "MP John Oliver Will Not See Re-election," *Oakville News*, 27 February 2019, https://oakvillenews.org/mp-john-oliver-re-election/.

55 Tanya Talaga and Prithi Yelaja, "Dr. Sheela Basrur, 51: Guided City through SARS," *Toronto Star*, 3 June 2008, https://www.thestar.com/news/obituaries/2008/06/03/dr_sheela_basrur_51_guided_city_through_sars.html.

56 See Public Health Ontario, https://www.publichealthontario.ca/en/education-and-events/sheela-basrur-centre.

CHAPTER SEVENTEEN

1 File (not numbered) "Community Health: Task Force to Review Comm. Health" (Hannah Report), A96-0011/012, Office of the Dean, Faculty of Medicine, UTARMS; W.J. Hannah to J.H. Dirks, 3 February 1988.

2 John Browne, correspondence with the author, 21 October 2016.

3 File (not numbered) "Community Health: Task Force to Review Comm. Health" (Hannah Report), "Task Force to Review Community Health, Final Report, February 1988," 57, A96-0011/012, Faculty of Medicine, Office of the Dean, UTARMS. See 45 for the task force membership.

4 "Task Force to Review Community Health," 53.

5 "Task Force to Review Community Health," 55.

6 "Task Force to Review Community Health," 56–7.

7 Bator, *Within Reach of Everyone*, 2:141. Note, Bator references the two editorials by Last in the *CJPH*.

8 John M. Last, "Editorial: The Need for Schools of Public Health in Canada," *Canadian Journal of Public Health* 79, no. 4 (July/August 1988): 220.

9 Last, "Editorial: Need for Schools of Public Health in Canada," 219.

10 John M. Last, "Editorial: The Future of Higher Education for Public Health – 2," *Canadian Journal of Public Health* 79, no. 6 (November/December 1988): 411.
11 "Letters: The Future Need for Schools of Public Health in Canada," *Canadian Journal of Public Health* 79, no. 6 (November/December 1988): 466–70.
12 Comment by Adalstein Brown after having read a draft of this section, 13 March 2017.
13 John Browne, meeting with the author, 25 August 2016.
14 Bator, *Within Reach of Everyone*, 2:165.
15 Bator, *Within Reach of Everyone*, 2:164.
16 Bator, *Within Reach of Everyone*, 2:164.
17 Interview with Dr Goel, 2 November 2016. See Friedland, *University of Toronto: A History*, 1st ed., 580.
18 Friedland, *University of Toronto: A History*, 2nd ed., xiv.
19 Peggy Leatt, "Reflections," in Rakow, *Fifty-Year Retrospective*, 24.
20 Rakow, *Fifty-Year Retrospective*, 17.
21 Rakow, *Fifty-Year Retrospective*, 17.
22 "Peggy Leatt," file (unnumbered), A1998-0023/002, Department of Health Administration, UTARMS; see "Statement to the External Review by Peggy Leatt, PhD Chair Department of Health Administration, October 1997," 4.
23 Interview with Dr Goel, 2 November 2016.
24 See P. Leatt, memorandum to members of the department, 2 February 1998, with the five-year review report attached, file (unnumbered), A1998-0023/002, Department of Health Administration, UTARMS. The quote is on second page of the report.
25 P. Leatt, memorandum.
26 P. Leatt, memorandum, 6.
27 P. Leatt, memorandum, 12.
28 Rakow, *Fifty-Year Retrospective*, 19.
29 Rakow, *Fifty-Year Retrospective*, 15.
30 While researching this book I once passed by her office and she called me in to say she saved some old files for me in case they were of use for the book. One was a collection of Christmas song sheets. Raisa could recite from memory a number of the phrases on the sheets. I asked her how she could do this. She demurred. In researching another part of the book I found a reference to Raisa and the fact that many years at the department/institute Christmas party the students would sing a Christmas tune with recast lyrics into ones that poked fun at both themselves and faculty. I went back to Raisa that what she didn't say initially is that the reason she could recite lines from many of them by memory was that she wrote almost all of them herself (personal conversations between her and me; 4 and 10 April 2017).
31 Correspondence with P. Williams, 13 April 2018.
32 I was in the audience.
33 Letters to Michael Dector, Jay Kaufman, and Margaret Mottershead, all dated 24 August 1993, personal files of Raisa Deber.
34 I was one practitioner who did this from the early 1980s onward.
35 Meeting between the author and P. Williams, 3 July 2018. Correspondence between the author and P. Williams, 4 July 2018.
36 "Evaluate Your Programs, 21st Annual Refresher Course, March 3–5, 1980," brochure, personal files, Raisa Deber.

37 Barry received the Robert Wood Johnson Award for 1974.
38 Ontario, *Looking Back, Looking Forward: The Ontario Health Services Restructuring Commission (1996–2000), A Legacy Report*, [Toronto]: The Commission, 2000, p. iv.
39 Duncan Sinclair, Mark Rochon, and Peggy Leatt, *Riding the Third Rail: The Story of Ontario's Health Services Restructuring Commission, 1996–2000* (Montreal: Institute for Research on Public Policy, 2005).
40 "Reconnect: Alumni Profiles: Shirlee Sharkey, CEO Saint Elizabeth Healthcare, MHSC," *IHPME Connect*, August 2017, P2–P4.
41 "The City Is Her Patient," *U of T Magazine* 45, no. 2 (Winter 2018): 81.
42 See http://www.mi2health.com.

CHAPTER EIGHTEEN

1 Interview with Dr Goel, 2 November 2016.
2 Correspondence with Vivek Goel, 17 October 2017.
3 Correspondence with Goel, 18 October 2017.
4 Connor, *Doing Good*, 232–3.
5 Mariana Ionova, "Sick Kids Honours Donor Peter Gilgan for $40 Million Donation," *Toronto Star*, 26 August 2013.
6 Wright, *SickKids*, 358, 360.
7 See Nicola Davis, "Francis Crick's £700 Million Altar to Biomedical Science," *Guardian*, 17 February 2016, https://www.theguardian.com/science/2016/feb/17/francis-crick-institute-biomedical-science-research. See Oliver Wainwright, "Francis Crick Institute: Cathedral of Science 'Looks Better from 1,000 Feet,'" *Guardian*, 2 September 2016, https://www.theguardian.com/artanddesign/2016/sep/02/francis-crick-institute-review-it-looks-better-from-1000-feet.
8 See "Working Ventures, Hospital Form Fund," *Globe and Mail*, 26 January 1999, B7.
9 Technology Partnerships Canada, *Moving Forward: Annual Report, 1998–1999* (Ottawa: Industry Canada, 1999), 6.
10 Comment made by Dr Alberto Martin at an address at Trinity College, University of Toronto, 21, March 2017.
11 See Sanofi, "Our Toronto Site Boasts a Proud Legacy of Innovations in Public Health," 2019, https://www.sanofi.ca/en/about-us/sanofi-pasteur.
12 See Sanofi, "Our Toronto Site Boasts a Proud Legacy of Innovations in Public Health."
13 See facebook, "Pasteur Canada Centenary," https://www.facebook.com/SanofiPasteurCanada100/photos/a.569769476402479.1073741859.520495177996576/569769903069103/?type=3&size=800%2C529&fbid=569769903069103.
14 Correspondence with City of Toronto Archives (CTA), 6 January 2018. It notes the street was named on 12 July 2004. Also a conversation with CTA on the same date notes a reference 66M-2411, which the archivist says is likely a plan number that is likely linked to a document in City of Toronto Roads Transportation and/or the Provincial Registry Office. Gerry Fitzgerald Drive links Steeles Avenue West to Dufferin Street.
15 See "Naming of Public Lanes in Blocks Bounded by Dupont Street, Bathurst Street, Bloor Street West and Christie Street – Seaton Village (Ward 20)," agenda item TE30.6, Minutes, 25 February 2014, Toronto and East York

Community Council, City of Toronto; also Toronto Bylaw 196-2014, "To Authorize the Naming of a Public Lane Located South of Barton Avenue Extending between Christie Street and Clinton Street as 'Crestfallen Lane,'" Enacted and Passed February 25, 2014." See also Robyn Doolittle, "'Crestfallen Lane' May Celebrate Bit of Local Lore," *Toronto Star*, 15 February 2014, GT1, GT6; or the web version, "'Crestfallen Lane' May Soon Commemorate Piece of Seaton Village history," https://www.thestar.com/news/gta/2014/02/15/crestfallen_lane_may_soon_commemorate_piece_of_seaton_village_history.html. Finally, correspondence 5 January 2018 from Sylvia Lassam, Trinity archivist, who sent the link for Seaton Village's LaneNaming Project, http://kleinosky.com/domains/svlanes/2303.php, alerted me to the fact there was also naming activity in downtown Toronto and prompted sleuthing to uncover the historical record for Crestfallen Lane.

16 Ontario, *Vaccines: The Best Medicine, 2014 Report of the Chief Medical Officer of Health of Ontario to the Legislative Assembly of Ontario*, http://www.health.gov.on.ca/en/common/ministry/publications/reports/cmoh_14_vaccines/docs/cmoh_14_vaccines.pdf.

17 Ontario Hospital Association, "A Foreword from the OHA," *The Hospital Report '99: A Balanced Scorecard for Ontario Acute Care Hospitals* (Toronto: University of Toronto, Department of Health Administration, 1999), 2.

18 Ontario Hospital Association, *The Hospital Report '98: A System-Wide Review of Ontario's Hospitals* (Toronto: Ontario Hospital Association, 1998), 1.

19 Ontario Hospital Association, *Hospital Report '99*, cover.

20 Ontario Hospital Association, *Hospital Report '99*, 3–6; appendix 4, 14–18.

21 See G. Ross Baker, Dalla Lana School of Public Health, http://ihpme.utoronto.ca/faculty/g-ross-baker/. Also correspondence between the author and Ross Baker, 31 July 31, 2018.

22 DLSPH, "View Our History," "Next Generation," "Better Health at a Lower Cost," http://www.dlsph.utoronto.ca/history/. Also correspondence between the author and Ross Baker, 31 July 2018.

23 Shorter, *Partnership for Excellence*, 617.

24 Mark J. Dobrow, Vivek Goel, and R.E.G. Upshur, "Evidence-Based Health Policy: Context and Utilisation," *Social Science and Medicine* 58, no. 1 (2004), 207–17.

25 Vivek Goel, "Building Public Health Ontario: Experience in Developing a New Public Health Agency," *Canadian Journal of Public Health* 103, no. 4 (July 2012): 268.

26 Goel, "Building Public Health Ontario," 269.

27 Larry Wayne Richards, *The Campus Guide, University of Toronto*, 2nd ed. (New York: Princeton Architectural, 2019), 241–2.

28 File "Buildings: Health Sciences Building," Press Clippings, UTARMS.

29 Raisa B. Deber, "Delivering Health Care: Public, Not-for-Profit, or Private?," in *Romanow Papers*, vol. 1, *The Fiscal Sustainability of Health Care in Canada*, ed. Gregory P. Marchildon, Tom McIntosh, and Pierre-Gerlier Forest, 233–96 (Toronto: University of Toronto Press, 2004).

30 Gail Tomblin Murphy and Linda O'Brien-Pallas, "How Do Human Resource Policies and Practices Inhibit Change in Health Care? A Plan for the Future," in *Romanow Papers*, vol. 2, *Changing Health Care in Canada*, ed. Pierre-Gerlier Forest, Gregory P. Marchildon, and Tom McIntosh, 150–82 (Toronto: University of Toronto Press, 2004).

31 Colleen M. Flood and Sujit Choudhry, "Strengthening the Foundations: Modernizing the Canada Health Act," in *Romanow Papers*, vol. 3, *The Governance of Health Care in Canada*, ed. Tom McIntosh, Pierre-Gerlier Forest, and Gregory P. Marchildon, 346–87 (Toronto: University of Toronto Press, 2004).
32 For a video of his presentation, see "The Romanow Commission: Toronto, May 31, 2002," cpac, http://www.cpac.ca/en/programs/public-record/episodes/90004687/episode-still-from-media-server-7434/.
33 "Romanow Commission: Toronto, May 31, 2002."
34 "Romanow Commission: Toronto, May 31, 2002," 17:10.
35 For a video of her presentation see http://www.cpac.ca/en/programs/public-record/episodes/90004687/episode-still-from-media-server-7434/, 20:17.
36 "Romanow Commission: Toronto, May 31, 2002," 24:34
37 "Romanow Commission: Toronto, May 31, 2002," 25:21
38 "Romanow Commission: Toronto, May 31, 2002," 29:32
39 "Romanow Commission: Toronto, May 31, 2002," 33:50
40 "Romanow Commission: Toronto, May 31, 2002," 36:11
41 Correspondence with Louise Lemieux-Charles, 16 October 2017.
42 See, for example, *Summary Report: National Workshop on Research Leadership and Management*, December 2005, 13.
43 They were heading up research administration at the following teaching hospitals respectively: University Health Network, Mount Sinai Hospital, the Addiction Research Foundation, and Sunnybrook Health Sciences Centre. Some had separately incorporated or named research institutes.
44 As it turned out this was a completely chance encounter. Andreas, a young Cambridge doctoral student at the time, was seeking directions. His query turned into a discussion of his research and a common interest between us in commercialization, which continues to this day. Andreas is now on faculty at Imperial College, London.
45 See Andreas B. Eisingerich and Leslie Boehm, "Hospital Visitors Ask for More Shopping Outlets," *Harvard Business Review* 87, no. 5 (May 2009): 21; and https://hbr.org/2009/05/hospital-visitors-ask-for-more-shopping-outlets; and Eisingerich and Boehm, "Group Analysis: Why Some Regional Clusters Works Better Than Others," *Wall Street Journal* and MIT *Sloan Management Review* (jointly published), 15 September 2007, https://www.wsj.com/articles/SB118841858437012520.
46 See L. Boehm, "Let's Boldly Go," *Health Research & Innovation* 1, no. 1 (Spring 2012): 12–13. See also Simon Haley, "A New Magazine for a New Era," in the same issue, 5.
47 Martin French and Fiona Alice Miller, "Leveraging the 'Living Laboratory': On the Emergence of the Entrepreneurial Hospital," *Social Science & Medicine* 75, no. 4 (August 2012): 717–24.
48 Correspondence between Dr Brownstone and the author, 6 June 2016.
49 See "Life Support: Medicare's Mid-Life Crisis," CBC, *The Sunday Edition*, 27 September 2015, http://www.cbc.ca/radio/thesundayedition/yogi-berra-medicare-on-life-support-alice-in-wonderland-at-150–1.3243374/life-support-medicare-s-mid-life-crisis-1.3244234.
50 David L. Buckeridge and Vivek Goel, "Health Informatics Education: An Opportunity for Public Health in Canada," *CJPH* 92, no. 3 (May–June 2001): 233.
51 Correspondence with the author, 30 September 2016.

52 See Stephen Strauss, "Canadian Medical Schools Slow to Integrate Health Informatics into Curriculum," CMAJ 182, no. 12 (7 September 2010): E551–2. See also CMAJ 182, no. 18 (2010), https://www.cmaj.ca/content/182/18.

53 Friedland, *University of Toronto*, 2nd ed., 579.

54 Bator, "Emergence of Public Health Education Programs in the University of Toronto," 12.

55 James FitzGerald, "A New Era in Public Health," *U of T Magazine* 36, no. 2 (Winter 2009): 31.

56 Government of Canada, National Advisory Committee on SARS and Public Health, *Learning from SARS* (Ottawa: Health Canada, 2003), 214, recommendation 12B.1; 217, recommendation 12B.8.

57 "A Canadian Agency for Public Health: If Not Now, When?," editorial, CMAJ 169, no. 8 (14 October 2003): 741.

58 FitzGerald, "New Era in Public Health," 31.

59 University of Toronto, Faculty of Medicine, "A Message from David Naylor," in *Public Health Sciences at the University of Toronto*, n.d. [2004?], 3. It is surmised that this was a fund-raising document because of its orientation but also the last page, which was titled "How You Can Help." In addition to saying U of T "was a leader in the public health revolution of the 20th century." it said it "is preparing to lead the way with its vision for a School of Public Health." It then listed financial goals and ended with "Please join as we create knowledge, educate the next generation of public health professionals, and keep Canadians healthy longer" (see 18).

60 "The Legacy: Public Health at U of T," in *Public Health Sciences at the University of Toronto*, 4.

61 "Keeping People Healthy Longer: A Message from Harvey Skinner, Chair, Public Health Sciences," in *Public Health Sciences at the University of Toronto*, 5.

62 Niamh McGarry, "Jack Mandel and His Vision for Public Health Renewal," *UToronto Medicine* 5, no. 1 (December 2008): 7.

63 See University of Toronto, Faculty of Medicine, "Report on the Deliberations of the Dalla Lana School of Public Health and the Institute of Health Policy, Management and Evaluation Steering Committee," 2, http://docs.google.com/viewerng/viewer?url=http://ihpme.utoronto.ca/wp-content/uploads/2014/06/Steering-Committee-DLSPH-IHPME.pdf.

64 Steering Committee to Develop a Plan for a School of Public Health, "Proposal to Establish a School of Public Health at the University of Toronto" (Mustard Report), 18 December 2006, 3, Adalsteinn Brown, personal files, Faculty of Medicine, University of Toronto,.

65 Steering Committee, "Proposal to Establish a School of Public Health," 4–5.

66 Steering Committee, "Proposal to Establish a School of Public Health," 8.

67 Steering Committee, "Proposal to Establish a School of Public Health," 23.

68 For a pictorial and textual history of U of T involvement in this area, see Christopher J. Rutty, "Within Reach of Everyone: The Birth, Maturity & Renewal of Public Health at the University of Toronto," http://www.dlsph.utoronto.ca/history/.

CHAPTER NINETEEN

1 University of Toronto, Institute of Health Policy, Management and Evaluation, "Thought Leadership," IHPME *Annual Highlights: A Year of Good Outcomes, 2015 Annual Highlights*, 10.
2 University of Toronto, Institute of Health Policy, Management and Evaluation, "IHPME Research," *IHPME 2015 Annual Highlights*, 4–5.
3 University of Toronto, Institute of Health Policy, Management and Evaluation, "IHPME Programs," *IHPME: Our First Seventy Years, 2017 Annual Highlights*, 36.
4 University of Toronto, Institute of Health Policy, Management and Evaluation, "Practicum Placements," IHPME *Annual Highlights: Five-Year Progress Report, 2016 Annual Highlights*, 37.
5 University of Toronto, Institute of Health Policy, Management and Evaluation, "Practicum Placements," IHPME: *Our First Seventy Years, 2017 Annual Highlights*, 37.
6 See Adalsteinn Brown, "Transferring Research from Research to Knowledge Users: The Importance of Relationships and Getting Them Right," *Journal of Health Services Research and Policy* 21, no. 2 (2016): 134–6; Adalsteinn Brown and Jonathan Lomas, "Research and Advice Giving: A Functional View of Evidence-Informed Policy Advice in a Canadian Ministry of Health," *Milbank Quarterly* 87, no. 4 (2009): 903–26.
7 University of Toronto, Dalla Lana School of Public Health, "Dean's Message," *Annual Report 2014–2015: The Beauty of What We Pursue*, 2.
8 Catherine Whiteside, "Why Is the Faculty of Medicine Focusing on Global Health?," *U of T Medicine* (Fall 2013): 2.
9 Howard Hu, "A Roadmap for Global Health," *U of T Medicine* (Fall 2013): 3.
10 Christopher J. Rutty, Dalla Lana School of Public Health, "Within Reach of Everyone: The Renewal of Public Health at the University of Toronto," historical poster series, 2014, http://www.dlsph.utoronto.ca/history/.
11 University of Toronto, Dalla Lana School of Public Health, "Dean's Message," *Annual Report 2014–2015*, 2.
12 See "U of T Public Health Ranked Fifth Globally in 2017 Shanghai Rankings," 19 July 2017, http://www.dlsph.utoronto.ca/2017/07/u-of-t-public-health-ranked-fifth-globally-in-2017-shanghai-rankings/. See also Academic Ranking of World Universities, http://www.shanghairanking.com/ShanghairankingSubject-Rankings/public-health.html.
13 University of Toronto, Faculty of Medicine, "Report on the Deliberations of the Dalla Lana School of Public Health and the Institute of Health Policy, Management and Evaluation Steering Committee," 1.
14 University of Toronto, Dalla Lana School of Public Health, "Dean's Message," *Annual Report 2014–2015*, 3.
15 University of Toronto, Dalla Lana School of Public Health, "Making a Greater Collective Impact on Public Health," *Annual Report 2014–2015*, 21.
16 University of Toronto, Faculty of Medicine, "Report on the Deliberations of the Dalla Lana School of Public Health and the Institute of Health Policy, Management and Evaluation Steering Committee," 4.
17 University of Toronto, Dalla Lana School of Public Health, "Dean's Message," *Annual Report 2014–2015*, 2, 22.

18 Meeting between the author and Geoff Anderson, 22 January 2020.
19 For further information see a programming brochure, IHPME, "System Leadership & Innovation," https://ihpme.utoronto.ca/wp-content/uploads/2016/05/IHPME-SLI-Brochure-2016.pdf
20 "System Leaders, Innovative Thinkers. First Cohort of MSc SLI Students Graduate," *IHPME Connect*, 8 November 2018, http://ihpme.utoronto.ca/2018/11/system-leaders-innovative-thinkers-first-cohort-of-msc-sli-students-graduate/.
21 See "MHI Health Informatics," http://ihpme.utoronto.ca/academics/pp/mhi/.
22 Correspondence with Julie Zarb and the author, 30 September 2016.
23 Correspondence between P. Williams and the author, 23 April 2018.
24 Correspondence between P. Williams and the author, 23 April 2018.
25 For a list of such collaborations, see "Research Centres & Initiatives," http://ihpme.utoronto.ca/research/research-centres-initiatives/.
26 See ichr, http://www.ichr.ca.
27 ichr, http://www.ichr.ca, 11.
28 ichr, http://www.ichr.ca, 24.
29 Conversation with the author, 7 September 2017.
30 Conversation with the author, 20 September 2017.
31 University of Toronto, Dalla Lana School of Public Health, "High-Cost Health-Care Users," *Annual Report 2015–2016: Diversity and Partnerships in an Evolving Health Landscape*, 11.
32 Walter P. Wodchis, Peter C. Austin, and David A. Henry, "A 3-Year Study of High-Cost Users of Health Care," *CMAJ* 188, no. 3 (16 February 2016): 182–8.
33 University of Toronto, Dalla Lana School of Public Health, "Improving Infectious Outbreak Reporting," *Annual Report 2015–2016*, 23.
34 University of Toronto, Institute of Health Policy, Management and Evaluation, *IHPME Annual Highlights: A Year of Good Outcomes, 2015 Annual Highlights*, 38.
35 University of Toronto, Institute of Health Policy, Management and Evaluation, *IHPME Annual Highlights … 2015 Annual Highlights*, 39.
36 University of Toronto, Institute of Health Policy, Management and Evaluation, *IHPME Annual Highlights … 2015 Annual Highlights*, 40.
37 For Martin's own account of the exchange, see Danielle Martin, "Dr Martin Goes to Washington," *Better Now: Six Big Ideas to Improve Health Care for All Canadians* ([Toronto]: Allen Lane, 2017), 9–15. See, in particular, 11–13.
38 See the video clip of the exchange between Martin and Burr on C-SPAN, 11 March 2014, http://www.c-span.org/video/?c4486962/dr-danielle-martin-senator-richard-burr.
39 For a sampling of the coverage, see Michael Bolen, "Canadian Doctor Gives U.S. Senator a Clinic on Public Health Care," Huffpost, 13 March 2014, http://www.huffingtonpost.ca/2014/03/13/canadian-doctor-us-senator-health-care_n_4956468.html. See also Alexander Manetta, "Political Offers Pour In for Toronto Doctor Who Defended Canada's Medicare," CTV News, 5 April 2014, http://www.ctvnews.ca/canada/political-offers-pour-in-for-toronto-doctor-who-defended-canada-s-medicare-1.1762306.
40 See Canada, House of Commons, Standing Committee on Health, 18 April 2016, http://www.parl.gc.ca/HousePublications/Publication.aspx?Language=e&Mode=1&Parl=42&Ses=1&DocId=8197723.

41 See Canada, House of Commons, Standing Committee on Health, 6 June 2016, http://www.parl.gc.ca/HousePublications/Publication.aspx?Language=e&Mode=1&Parl=42&Ses=1&DocId=8332768.
42 See Canada, House of Commons, Standing Committee on Health, 6 June 2016.
43 See "Health and Retirement Security Research," HOOPP, 9 December 2016, https://hoopp.com/en/Home/article-details/health-and-retirement-security-research. See also "Health and Retirement Security Research," HOOPP, October 2016, https://hoopp.com/docs/default-source/newsroom-library/research/hrsr_public.pdf.
44 See Rob Carrick, "Longer Lifespans for Women Make Retirement Planning All the More Crucial," *Globe and Mail*, 8 December 2016, http://www.theglobeandmail.com/globe-investor/retirement/retire-planning/longer-lifespans-make-retirement-planning-all-the-more-crucial-for-women/article33275797/.

CHAPTER TWENTY

1 Marcia Kaye, "For This Syrian Grad Student, a Fresh Start," *U of T Magazine* 45, no. 1 (Autumn 2017): 36–7.
2 Meeting with Julia Zarb, 5 October 2017.
3 Meeting with Julia Zarb, 5 October 2017.
4 Meeting with Rebecca Biason. Also meeting with Rhonda Cockerill. Both meetings 28 September 2017.
5 Meeting with Rebecca Biason, 28 September 2017.
6 Kaye, "For This Syrian Grad Student, a Fresh Start," 37.
7 Meeting with Julia Zarb, 5 October 2017.
8 Hayden Rodenkirchen, "'Tell the Truth,'" *Varsity* 136, no. 16 (8 February 2016): 7. Note, this article was revised and also appeared on the *Varsity* website, as the original version implied it was Johnston, not Wald, who experienced a bout of depression, which was the instance that led to a breakthrough for Wald and an epiphany for Johnston. See https://thevarsity.ca/2016/02/08/tell-the-truth/.
9 Richard Florida and Joshua Gans, "Trump's Gift to Canada: As the American Global Brand Wanes, Canada Has a Real Opportunity to Attract the World's Brightest Minds," *Globe and Mail*, 9 October 2017, A9. Also appears on the *Globe* website as "The Trump Effect: It's Canada's Moment to Win the Global Race for Talent," https://beta.theglobeandmail.com/opinion/the-trump-effect-its-canadas-moment-win-the-global-race-for-talent/article36521255/?ref=http://www.theglobeandmail.com&.
10 See Khaled Almilaji, as told to Nicholas Hune-Brown, "The Exile," *Toronto Life* 51, no. 9 (September 2017): 48–9.
11 Meeting with Julia Zarb, 5 October 2017.
12 "Khaled Almilaji Awarded Governor General's Meritorious Service Medal," IHPME *Connect*, January 2018, 2.
13 Correspondence (22 August 2016) from A. Moorehouse, program assistant, IHPME, based on the student lists for the five years from fall 2010 to 2015.
14 "U of T Helps Launch Health Informatics Program for Nurses in Israel," IHPME *Connect*, May 2018, P3–P4.
15 Institute of Health Policy, Management and Evaluation, Shandong University Partnership, *Annual Report 2018, Reaching across Silos: Toward Collaborative Change*, University of Toronto, 2018, 22.

16 University of Toronto, Institute of Health Policy, Management and Evaluation, "2017 Doctorates," *IHPME: Our First Seventy Years, 2017 Annual Highlights*, 24.
17 See http://ihpme.utoronto.ca/community/post-doctoral-fellows/ for the list and also a brief bio on the individuals.
18 "Introducing the HSR Alumni Mentorship Program," *IHPME Connect*, 4. Also, "Program Outline: IHPME Alumni Mentorship Program (Health Services Research – MSc/PhD), October 2017," included as part of correspondence with Julia Ho, 11 October 2017.
19 Correspondence with the author, 16 October 2017.
20 See "Former CFL Player Now IHPME Alumnus Works to Inspire Youth to Consider Careers in Health Systems and Public Health," *IHPME Connect*, 10 January 2019, https://ihpme.utoronto.ca/2019/01/former-cfl-player-now-ihpme-alumnus-is-working-to-inspire-youth-to-consider-careers-in-health-systems-and-public-health/.
21 See Stephanie Y. Zhou, "How Underprivilege Made Me a Better Doctor," *Star*, 25 August 2017, https://www.thestar.com/opinion/commentary/2017/08/25/how-underprivilege-made-me-a-better-doctor.html.
22 Stephanie Y. Zhou, "Underprivilege as Privilege," *JAMA* 318, no. 8 (August 2017): 705. For excerpts, see "A Personal History," *University of Toronto Magazine*, Spring 2019, 73. For an interview after her article went viral, see Carolyn Morris, "U of T's Stephanie Zhou on the Response to Her Essay about Fitting In at Medical School," *U of T News*, 26 November 2018, https://www.utoronto.ca/news/u-t-s-stephanie-zhou-huge-response-her-essay-about-fitting-medical-school.
23 Zhou, "Underprivilege as Privilege," 706.
24 See Power Unit Youth Organization, https://power-unit.org.

CHAPTER TWENTY-ONE

1 See Jon Gertner, *The Idea Factory: Bell Labs and the Great Age of American Innovation* (New York: Penguin, 2012).
2 C.B. Farrar, "I Remember J.G. FitzGerald," *American Journal of Psychiatry* 120 (July 1963): 52n4. This article provides a very good biographical sketch of FitzGerald's career by a lifelong friend who knew him from the very beginning of his career.
3 Farrar, "I Remember J.G. FitzGerald," 52.
4 Farrar, "I Remember J.G. FitzGerald," 50–1.
5 Farrar, "I Remember J.G. FitzGerald," 51.
6 Farrar, "I Remember J.G. FitzGerald," 51.
7 Farrar, "I Remember J.G. FitzGerald," 52.
8 Major J.G. FitzGerald and Major J.W.S. McCullough, "Sanitation in Some Canadian Barracks and Camps," *American Journal of Public Health* 7, no. 8 (August 1917): 660.
9 FitzGerald and McCullough, "Sanitation in Some Canadian Barracks and Camps," 659.
10 FitzGerald, *What Disturbs Our Blood*, 263.
11 Bator and Rhodes, *Within Reach of Everyone*, 1:21.
12 Friedland, *University of Toronto*, 1st ed., 266.
13 File "Amyot, John Andrew," Department of Graduate Records, A73-0026/007(35), UTARMS; "Dr Amyot Outlines Health Work in War," *Globe*, 11 March 1929.

14 Robert Davies Defries, *The First Forty Years, 1914–1955, Connaught Medical Research Laboratories* (Toronto: University of Toronto Press, 1968), 24. The antitoxin was supplied at $0.34. Previously $1.35 had been charged by a U.S. supplier per dose.
15 Andrew MacPhail, *Official History of the Canadian Forces in the Great War, 1914–1919: The Medical Services* (Ottawa: F.A. Acland, King's Printer, 1925), 106–7.
16 MacPhail, *Official History of the Canadian Forces in the Great War*, 105. He notes that the total British casualty rate was 55.99 per cent, but this includes those killed, died of disease, wounded, missing, and prisoners.
17 Shorter, *Partnership for Excellence*, 60.
18 George Dana Porter, *Crusading against Tuberculosis: The Memoirs of George Dana Porter* (Ottawa: Canadian Tuberculosis Association, 1953), 27. This is also quoted in Bator and Rhodes, *Within Reach of Everyone*, 1:48.
19 FitzGerald, "Gordon Bell Memorial Lecture," 68.
20 FitzGerald, "Gordon Bell Memorial Lecture," 69.
21 University of Toronto, *Calendar of the School of Hygiene, 1928–1929*, 14.
22 University of Toronto, *Calendar, School of Hygiene, 1935–1936*, 15, 21.
23 FitzGerald, "Gordon Bell Memorial Lecture," 62.
24 Tina Saryeddine, "What Disturbs Our Blood: From Bestseller List to Handbook?," *Healthcare Quarterly* 16, no. 3 (2013): 57.
25 Saryeddine, "What Disturbs Our Blood."
26 Saryeddine, "What Disturbs Our Blood." The heading in the article is "A Glorious Tradition of Research."
27 All of the points in this paragraph taken from Saryeddine, "What Disturbs Our Blood," 58. The three headings under which these appear are "The Evolution of a Research Institute," "The Relationship between Public Health and Healthcare," and "The Development of World-Class Organizations."
28 R.D. Defries, "Report of the Director of the School of Hygiene," *President's Report for the year ending 30th June 1941* (Toronto: University of Toronto Press, 1941), 45.
29 See University of Toronto, *School of Hygiene, Calendar, 1945–1946*, 24.
30 FitzGerald, *What Disturbs Our Blood*, 238–9. See also "What's New: Within Reach of Everyone: The Birth, Maturity and Renewal of Public Health at U of T," 1 May 2014, http://www.dlsph.utoronto.ca/2014/05/within-reach-of-everyone-the-birth-maturity-and-renewal-of-public-health-at-u-of-t-2/.
31 FitzGerald, *What Disturbs Our Blood*, 240.
32 FitzGerald, *What Disturbs Our Blood*, 240–1.
33 See Etzkowitz, *Triple Helix*.
34 See Great Britain, *Lambert Review of Business-University Collaboration*.
35 See Michael L. Dertouzos, Richard K. Lester, and Robert M. Solow, *Made in America: Regaining the Productive Edge* (Cambridge, MA: MIT Press, 1989). See also Suzanne Berger, *Making in America: From Innovation to Market* (Cambridge, MA: The MIT Press, 2013).
36 FitzGerald, *What Disturbs Our Blood*, 267.
37 FitzGerald, *What Disturbs Our Blood*, 269.
38 FitzGerald, *What Disturbs Our Blood*, 292.
39 FitzGerald, *What Disturbs Our Blood*, 293.
40 FitzGerald, "Troubled Healer," 93. James FitzGerald also notes two other notable achievements of Connaught: the control of diphtheria and its role with the World Health Organization in eradicating smallpox.

41 Vivek Goel, "Opinion: There's No Magic Bullet, No Single Path to Innovation," *Globe and Mail, Report of Business*, 4 August 2016, B4.
42 "Medicine Is a Calling, Not a Business: Henry Mintzberg," CBC *Radio, Sunday Edition*, 4 February 2018. See recording and transcript at http://www.cbc.ca/radio/thesundayedition/the-sunday-edition-february-4-2018-1.4516513/medicine-is-a-calling-not-a-business-henry-mintzberg-1.4516553.
43 FitzGerald, "Troubled Healer," 93.
44 Linda McQuaig, *The Sport & Prey of Capitalists: How the Rich Are Stealing Canada's Public Wealth* (Toronto: Dundurn, 2019), 143.
45 McQuaig, *Sport & Prey of Capitalists*, 132–3.
46 McQuaig, *Sport & Prey of Capitalists*, 136.
47 McQuaig, *Sport & Prey of Capitalists*, 135.
48 C.K. Clarke, "Report of the Dean of the Faculty of Medicine," *President's Report, for the Year Ending 30th June 1915*, 14.
49 Bator and Rhodes, *Within Reach of Everyone*, 1:21.
50 MacPhail, *Official History of the Canadian Forces in the Great War*, 106–7.
51 Harold Averill, Marnee Gamble, and Loryl MacDonald, *We Will Do Our Share: The University of Toronto and the Great War, Exhibition by the University of Toronto Archives* (Toronto: Thomas Fisher Rare Book Library, 2014), 56–7.
52 Bator and Rhodes, *Within Reach of Everyone*, 1:18, 21.
53 Gordon Bates, "Lowering the Cost of Life-Saving: How the University of Toronto Is Performing Active Public Service," *Maclean's Magazine*, August 1915, 14.
Bates was the founder and director of the Health League of Canada, editor-in-chief of *Health*, and also for a time editor of the *Public Health Journal* (later renamed the *Canadian Journal of Public Health*). For more on Bates and *Health* magazine, see multiple index entries on each in Catherine Carstairs, Bethany Philpot, and Sara Wilmshurst, *Be Wise! Be Healthy! Morality and Citizenship in Canadian Public Health Campaigns* (Vancouver: UBC Press, 2018).
54 Bates, "Lowering the Cost of Life-Saving," 16.
55 FitzGerald, "Gordon Bell Memorial Lecture," 77.
56 "Within Reach," *Economist* 427, no. 9089 (28 April–4 May 2018): cover page and 9. There is also a twelve-page "Special Report" on universal health care after 42. I want to credit one of my U of T, Trinity College students, Norene Lach, for bringing the article to my attention.
57 Bates, "Lowering the Cost of Life-Saving," 16.
58 Bates, "Lowering the Cost of Life-Saving," 104.
59 J.G. FitzGerald to President Falconer, 2 December 1915, file 083, "FitzGerald, John Gerald, Sept, 1915–Jan. 1916," box 083a, correspondence, Office of the President, A670007, UTARMS. I am grateful to Loryl MacDonald, university archivist and department head UTARMS, who, in a conversation with me, remembered the letter and searched the records of an exhibit she had helped curate on the First World War (January to May 2014) in which there was a reference to FitzGerald and found its citation, which I was able to use to track down the actual letter.
60 Bates, "Lowering the Cost of Life-Saving," 104.
61 Bates, "Lowering the Cost of Life-Saving," 15–16.

62 Bates, "Lowering the Cost of Life-Saving," 104.
63 McQuaig, *Sport & Prey of Capitalists*, 136.
64 Badgley had done important work in preventive health and was also the co-author of a book on the doctors' strike in Saskatchewan. The preventive health work was part of an initiative of Wendal Macleod, the first dean of the College of Medicine at the University of Saskatchewan. The college was one of Tommy Douglas's accomplishments, and Macleod's initiative was connected to Douglas's objective of preventive medicine.
65 Bator and Rhodes, *Within Reach of Everyone*, 1:134.
66 Bator and Rhodes, *Within Reach of Everyone*, 1:21.
67 Major John L. Todd, "The Meaning of Rehabilitation," *Annals of the American Academy of Political Science* 80, no. 1 (November 1918): 5. Also quoted in Desmond Morton, "Military Medicine during and after the First World War: Precursor of Universal Public Health Care in Canada," *Canadian Defence Quarterly* 13, no. 1 (Summer 1983): 34.
68 Morton, "Military Medicine during and after the First World War," 38.
69 Morton, "Military Medicine during and after the First World War," 38.
70 Morton, "Military Medicine during and after the First World War," 41; my emphasis.
71 Thomas Parran, "Health Security," *American Journal of Public Health and the Nation's Health* 26, no. 4 (April 1936): 329–35.
72 See David B. Evans, Justine Hsu, and Ties Boerma, "Universal Health Coverage and Universal Access," *Bulletin of the World Health Organization*, 2013, http://www.who.int/bulletin/volumes/91/8/13-125450/en/.
73 Correspondence with Sylvia Lassam, Trinity College Archives, 13 February 2018.
74 Canon Cody, "The University of Toronto as a Public Servant," 12 December 1927, *Addresses Delivered before the Canadian Club of Toronto, Season of 1927–28* (Toronto: Warwick Bros. & Rutter, 1928), 25:143.
75 Cody, "University of Toronto as a Public Servant," 143–4.
76 McQuaig, *Sport & Prey of Capitalists*, 136–7.
77 Correspondence between the author and Adalesteinn Brown, 20 January 2020.
78 FitzGerald, "Work of the Health Organisation of the League of Nations," 368.
79 FitzGerald, "Work of the Health Organisation of the League of Nations," 369.
80 FitzGerald, "Work of the Health Organisation of the League of Nations," 370.
81 Esylit W. Jones, "Health and Nation through a Transnational Lens: Radical Doctors and the History of Medicare in Saskatchewan," in *Within and Without the Nation: Canadian History as Transnational History*, ed. Karen Dubinsky, Adele Perry, and Henry Yu (Toronto: University of Toronto Press, 2015), 293.
82 Jones, "Health and Nation," 296, 305.
83 "Association News," "Sixty-Third Annual Meeting of the American Public Health Association, Pasadena, California, 1934, New Officers of APHA," *American Journal of Public Health* 23, no. 11 (November 1933): 1175. See also "American Public Health Association Year Book, 1933–1934," supplement, *American Journal of Public Health* 24, no. 2 (February 1934): S19.
84 Rockefeller Foundation, *Annual Report 1935*, xi.
85 "Building Brains," 14 January 2013, 38:53 CBC Radio, *Ideas*. See http://www.cbc.ca/radio/ideas/building-brains-1.2913273.
86 Correspondence and material from American Philosophical Society, 13 February

2018, Dr J.G. FitzGerald to Dr Simon Flexner, 17 October 1917, file "FitzGerald, J.G.," B:F365, Simon Flexner Papers, APS Library. Note the APS is the oldest learned society in the United States, established by Benjamin Franklin in 1743.

87 File "Flexner, Simon," box 047a, Correspondence, Office of the President (Falconer), A67-0007, UTARMS, what appears to be the template for a letter to invited guests of the President, dated 15 October 1917.

88 "Dr Flexner Lectures on Surgical Progress in the Present War," *Varsity* 37, no. 14 (29 October 1917): 1. As noted above, the *Globe* also reported on Dr Flexner's lecture. Its coverage was almost the same as that in the *Varsity* (or perhaps this should read the other way round, given the *Globe*'s coverage was three days ahead of that in the *Varsity*). See "Surgery's Fight with Infection: Dr Simon Flexner of New York Tells of Work of Doctors on War Front," *Globe*, 26 October 1917, 8. The *Telegram* had a very short report on the talk, about one-quarter the length of that in the *Varsity* and the *Globe*. See "Surgeon's Good Work," *Telegram*, 26 October 1917, 11.

89 Ibid.

90 "Able to Check Dread Gas Bacilli, Chemists Have Solved One of the Costliest Problems of the War, Great Good to Result, Dr Flexner Tells of Experiments at Rockefeller Institute," *Mail and Empire*, 26 October 1917, 4. This report was the longest and most detailed of the Toronto media.

91 *Toronto Daily News*, "Scientists Work for Fighting Men," 26 October 1917, 3.

92 F.P. Gay to J.G. FitzGerald , 3 November 1922, file 039, FitzGerald, John Gerald, Correspondence 1922–23, box 77, Office of the President (Falconer), A1967-0007, UTARMS.

93 Wicliffe Rose to Dr FitzGerald, 14 November 1922, file 039, FitzGerald, John Gerald, Correspondence 1922–23, box 77, Office of the President (Falconer), A1967-0007, UTARMS.

CHAPTER TWENTY-TWO

1 Howard Hu, "Dean's Message," in *Dalla Lana School of Public Health, Annual Report, 2014–2015*, ed. Nicole Bodnar, 2.

2 See Dalla Lana School of Public Health, *Healthy Lives for All: The Campaign for the Dalla Lana School of Public Health*, [n.d.], the first two chapters, "A Leader from the Beginning" and "Institute of Health Policy, Management and Evaluation," 4–9 and 10–13 respectively.

3 Adalsteinn Brown, "Message from the Director," *IHPME Annual Highlights: Five-Year Progress Report, 2016*, 2.

4 "University of Toronto School of Hygiene History Project: A Report to the Dean, Faculty of Medicine, University of Toronto, with an Application for Further Funding," 8 March 1987, 1, B90-0035/002(10), Paul Adolphus Bator fonds, UTARMS.

5 Bator and Rhodes, *Within Reach of Everyone*, 1:ix.

6 Bator, in his 1987 report to the dean noted previously, talks of two stages (establishing the labs and the school). Bator and Rhodes speak of three stages, the third being "founding the School of Hygiene as one of the Rockefeller Schools of Public Health" (*Within Reach of Everyone*, 1:ix).

7 R.D. Defries, "Report of the Director of the School of Hygiene," *President's Report for the Year Ending 30th June 1940*, 34.

8 J.G. FitzGerald, "Report of the Director of the School of Hygiene," *President's Report for the Year Ending 30th June 1938*, 46.
9 FitzGerald, "Report of the Director of the School of Hygiene," ... *Year Ending 30th June 1938*.
10 R.D. Defries, "Report of the Director of the School of Hygiene," *President's Report for the Year Ending 30th June 1939*, 38.
11 Defries, "Report of the Director of the School of Hygiene," ... *Year Ending 30th June 1939*, 38.
12 Bator, *Within Reach of Everyone*, 2:58.
13 Bator, *Within Reach of Everyone*, 2:58.
14 Interview with Dr Andrew J. Rhodes, 26 July 1985, 4, transcript, School of Hygiene History Project, B89-0009, UTARMS.
15 Bator and Rhodes, *Within Reach of Everyone*, 1:134.
16 Bator, *Within Reach of Everyone*, 2:58.
17 Saskatchewan, Legislative Assembly, *Debates*, 25 February 1948, http://docs.legassembly.sk.ca/legdocs/Legislative%20Assembly/Hansard/10L5S/480225Debates.pdf. Note, in Hansard his name is given as Hanes, rather than Hames.
18 "Finding Aid," p. 1, V.L. Matthews fonds, University of Saskatchewan Archives.
19 James FitzGerald, "Fitzgerald, John Gerald," *Dictionary of Canadian Biography*, vol. 16, published 12 September 2018, http://biographi.ca/en/bio/fitzgerald_john_gerald_16F.html.
20 FitzGerald, "Fitzgerald, John Gerald."
21 R.D. Defries, "Obituary: John Gerald FitzGerald," *Science* 92, no. 2381 (16 August 1940): 141.
22 *Toronto Star*, "Two Crusaders at the Connaught," 15 December 1990. For a picture of Dr Defries with former president Truman, see Bator and Rhodes, *Within Reach of Everyone*, 1:178.
23 Bator, "'Saving Lives on the Wholesale Plan.'" It is interesting that Bator's dissertation, which deals with public health reform at the provincial and Toronto levels, does not deal with the public health activities underway at U of T under FitzGerald and how these might have supported or did support what was happening at the provincial and Toronto levels. There is only one reference to the School of Hygiene (vol. 2, p. 340). A question for Bator, especially given his subsequent *Within Reach of Everyone*, would be, from at least 1913 onward, how much FitzGerald and FitzGerald's public health activities should be factoring into his story. In other words, how much was FitzGerald a part of the public health reform that Bator describes was happening in Ontario and Toronto? How did they interrelate?
24 Bator, "'Saving Lives on the Wholesale Plan,'" 2:334. See 2:333–40 for reasons why.
25 See Bator, "'Saving Lives on the Wholesale Plan,'" 2:333.
26 Bator, "'Saving Lives on the Wholesale Plan,'" 2:336.
27 Bator, "'Saving Lives on the Wholesale Plan,'" 2:339.
28 "Report of the Department of Hospital Service," in "Business Report of the Fifty-Ninth Annual Meeting of the Canadian Medical Association Held in Charlottetown, P.E.I., June 18–23, 1928," supplement, *CMAJ* 19, no. 3 (September 1928): Sxxx.
29 "Report of the Department of Hospital Service," Sxxxiii.

30 FitzGerald, *What Disturbs Our Blood*, 324–5.
31 Donald T. Fraser, "John Gerald FitzGerald (1882–1940)," *Proceedings and Transactions of the Royal Society of Canada*, vol. 35 (Ottawa: Royal Society of Canada, 1941), 115. See 113–15 for the biographical entry on FitzGerald. FitzGerald was elected a Fellow of the RSC in 1920. He was president of Section V of the RSC in 1932–3 (see 25). IHPME faculty member Raisa Deber was elected to the RSC in 2018.
32 Michael Bliss, "Book Review: What Disturbs Our Blood: A Son's Quest to Redeem the Past," *Canadian Bulletin of Medical History* 28, no. 2 (Winter 2011): 404–5.
33 Bliss, "Book Review: What Disturbs Our Blood," 404. Bliss's reference is to James FitzGerald's family but it is clear that it is to his grandfather.
34 Farrar, "I Remember J.G. FitzGerald," 52.
35 FitzGerald, *What Disturbs Our Blood*, 325. Note, the phrase James uses is "the stress of his crowded life," and he is referring to Banting, but the phrase could equally apply to his grandfather.
36 FitzGerald, *What Disturbs Our Blood*, 327.
37 Bliss, "Book Review: What Disturbs Our Blood," 405.
38 Bliss, "Book Review: What Disturbs Our Blood," 405.

CHAPTER TWENTY-THREE

1 See G. Ross Baker and Jean-Louis Denis, *A Comparative Study of Three Transformative Healthcare Systems: Lessons for Canada* (Ottawa: Canadian Health Services Research Foundation, 201).
2 Dr Bob Bell, deputy minister, Health and Long-term Care, IHPME GSU Lunch & Learn, 18 May 2017.
3 See G. Ross Baker and Renata Axler, *Creating a High Performing Healthcare System for Ontario: Evidence Supporting Strategic Changes in Ontario*, sponsored by the Ontario Hospital Association, 2015.
4 Correspondence between the author and Adalstein Brown and Ross Baker, 3 May 2017.
5 See "Alison Paprica," Dalla Lana, http://ihpme.utoronto.ca/faculty/alison-paprica/.
6 See "Patient-Oriented Health Research 2016–17 Seminar Series," Institute of Health Policy, Management & Evaluation, http://ihpme.utoronto.ca/wp-content/uploads/2016/09/OSSU-Seminar-Series-Fall-2016-Lineup-Poster-FINAL-vSeptember-27–2016.pdf.
7 Correspondence with Fiona Miller, 10 and 11 March 2017.
8 Correspondence with Vivek Goel, 18 October 2017.
9 See https://www.ryerson.ca/crncc/.
10 Correspondence with the author, 4 April 2018.
11 Gregory P. Marchildon, "Introduction to the 2012 Edition: Community Clinics and Stan Rand's Struggle for the Transformation of Health Care in Canada," in Stan Rands, *Privilege and Policy: A History of Community Clinics in Saskatchewan*, ed. Gregory P. Marchildon and Catherine Leviten-Reid, rev. ed. (Regina: Canadian Plains Research Centre, 2012), vii.
12 Marchildon, "Introduction," vii.
13 Marchildon, "Introduction," xii.
14 HAD 5020 class session, 12 April 2018.

15 Fernand Braudel, *Civilization and Capitalism, 15th–18th Century*, volume 3, *The Perspective of the World* (New York: Harper and Row, 1984), 26–7.
16 Bator and Rhodes, *Within Reach of Everyone*, 1:65.
17 See Ontario, Premier's Highly Skilled Workforce Expert Panel, *Building the Workforce of Tomorrow: A Shared Responsibility*, June 2016, 25–9.
18 The first chapter of this report sets out the rationale for experiential learning. See *Community-Connected Experiential Learning*, 2016, http://www.ontla.on.ca/library/repository/mon/30001/333493.pdf.
19 See Ontario, Ministry of Colleges and Universities, "Career Ready Fund," http://www.tcu.gov.on.ca/pepg/programs/careerreadyfund.html. It notes that practicums are an example of experiential learning.
20 See Cheryl Regehr, "Career Ready Fund for Experiential Learning Opportunities," 8 September 2017, https://memos.provost.utoronto.ca/career-ready-fund-for-experiential-learning-opportunities-pdadc-12/.
21 See the Council of Ontario Universities approach in *Partnering for a Better Future*, 2017, 14–15.
22 Hayden Rodenkirchen, "'Tell the Truth,'" *Varsity* 136, no. 16, 8 February 2016, 7.
23 Lewis Auerbach, "Introduction," in George Wald, *Therefore Choose Life: The Found Massey Lectures* (Toronto: Anansi, 2017). xviii.
24 See "Research Centres & Initiatives," Dalla Lana, http://ihpme.utoronto.ca/research/research-centres-initiatives/.
25 Correspondence between the author and G. Marchildon, 23 July 2018.

CHAPTER TWENTY-FOUR

1 Reed et al., *Building Healthier Communities*.
2 Bator and Rhodes, *Within Reach of Everyone*, 1:ix–x.
3 Bator and Rhodes, *Within Reach of Everyone*, 1:1.
4 R.D. Defries, *The Connaught Medical Research Laboratories, 1914–1949* [Toronto: Connaught Medical Research Laboratories, University of Toronto, 1950?], 1.
5 Defries, *Connaught Medical Research Laboratories*, 9.
6 Simon Szreter, "Introduction," in Simon Szreter, *Health and Wealth: Studies in History and Policy* (Rochester, NY: University of Rochester Press, 2005), 18–19.
7 Simon Szreter, "The Population Health Approach in Historical Perspective," in Szreter, *Health and Wealth*, 29–30.
8 Szreter, "Population Health Approach in Historical Perspective," 35.
9 See Connor, *Doing Good*, text beneath the picture of PMH on the illustration page (unnumbered) before 117; see also 227–8.
10 See "About the School," Dalla Lana, http://www.dlsph.utoronto.ca/about/; and "Within Reach of Everyone," http://www.dlsph.utoronto.ca/history/. The historian involved in the history section of the website is Christopher J. Rutty.
11 See "About the School," Dalla Lana.
12 "Meet IHPME's New Acting Director," *IHPME Connect*, August 2017, P1.
13 See "University of Toronto, Department of Health Administration, 1956–1977," case studies and HOM (Hospital Organization and Management) topics, A1986-0034, UTARMS.
14 Bator, *Within Reach of Everyone*, 2:160, 2:58.

15 Dr H.J. Cody, "One of Toronto's Best Assets," 16 April 1934, *Addresses Delivered before the Canadian Club of Toronto, Season of 1933–34, vol. 31* (Toronto: Warwick Bros & Rutter, 1934), 397.
16 Advertisement, "The University of Toronto," *University of Toronto Monthly* 27, no. 8 (May 1927): 391. Note, this ad appeared in a number of issues of vol. 27.
17 Though I altered the terms a bit, the credit for the assessment-action and assessment-action-evaluation ideas needs to be given to John Browne (correspondence of 17 August 2017).
18 "CEHCR MSc/PhD," *IHPME Annual Highlights: Five-Year Progress Report, 2016*, 39.
19 Dean Dirks to A.R. Ten Cate, 23 February 1990, A1996/0011/0018 (4), UTARMS; quoted in Shorter, *Partnership for Excellence*, 616.
20 University of Toronto, Faculty of Medicine, *Plan 2000–4*, 68–69; *MedEmail*, 25 May 1998, quoted in Shorter, *Partnership for Excellence*, 617.

CHAPTER TWENTY-FIVE

1 See Converge3, https://converge3.ca.
2 Adalsteinn Brown files, *Ontario Transfer Payment Agreement – Institute of Health, Policy, Management and Evaluation (IHPME) – Centre for Evidence and Health in All Policies, Ministry Grant #0444*, "Schedule 'C' – Program Description and Timelines," 21–8.
3 Correspondence with the author, 13 June 2018.
4 The preceding three paragraphs on genesis taken from correspondence with Adalsteinn Brown, 8 July 2018.
5 See "NAO: North American Observatory on Health Systems and Policies," Dalla Lana, 2019, http://ihpme.utoronto.ca/research/research-centres-initiatives/nao/.
6 Romanow address at the launch of the NAO at the University of Toronto, 6 February 2017 (I was in attendance). See also a text of the speech (provided to me by Dr Gregory Marchildon).
7 See http://www.hspm.org/mainpage.aspx.
8 Meeting with Marchildon, 7 March 2017.
9 Romanow address at the launch of the NAO.
10 Gregory Marchildon files, "North American Observatory on Health Systems and Policies," included in correspondence with the author, 1 February 2016.
11 Ibid.
12 Greg Marchildon, "Series Editor's Foreword," in Katherine Fierlbeck, *Nova Scotia: A Health System Profile* (Toronto: University of Toronto Press, 2018), xiii.
13 See Fierlbeck, *Nova Scotia*.
14 See Quebec, Commission of Inquiry on Health and Social Welfare, *Report*, vol. 1.
15 Meeting between the author and P. Williams, 3 July 2018.
16 See "Bill n°67: Autonomy Insurance Act," http://www.assnat.qc.ca/en/travaux-parlementaires/projets-loi/projet-loi-67-40-1.html.
17 See Québec, Ministère de la santé et des services sociaux, *Autonomy for All: White Paper on the Creation of Autonomy Insurance* (Quebec: Santé et services sociaux, 2013).
18 *North American Observatory on Health Systems and Policies*, Fall 2018, 6.

19 *North American Observatory*, 9.
20 Tsung-Mei Cheng, "Taiwan's Single Payer National Health Insurance: Experience So Far and Future Challenges," University of Toronto, IHPME, NAO Lecture, 13 February 2019.
21 Meeting between the author and Grace Harn, 13 February 2019, and correspondence between the author and Grace Harn, 19 and 21 February 2019.
22 Her grandfather started the hospital in Peikang in 1944, during the Japanese occupation. When he completed medical school, he wanted to go back to his hometown in the countryside to start a hospital. He knew the people were very poor and that many suffered from liver disease and he wanted to help. He became well known in the country for treating liver abscesses using percutaneous drainage.
23 Meeting at the DLSPH, 12 June 2019.
24 Tsung-Mei Cheng, "Taiwan and Other Advanced Asian Economies," in *Bending the Cost Curve in Health Care: Canada's Provinces in International Perspective*, ed. Gregory P. Marchildon and Livio Matteo (Toronto: University of Toronto Press, 2015), 448–9. See also Gregory P.Marchildon and Livio Matteo, "Introduction and Overview," in the same work, xxvi.
25 Meeting between the author and Greg Marchildon, 13 February 2019.
26 Correspondence with Greg Marchildon, 14 February 2019.
27 The material for this section is taken from an interview with Mark Dobrow, 15 December 2017.
28 Meeting between Greg Marchildon and the author, 27 August 2019.
29 For history, see, for example, Gregory P. Marchildon, "Canadian Medicare: Why History Matters," in *Making Medicare: New Perspectives on the History of Medicare in Canada*, ed. Marchildon (Toronto: University of Toronto Press, 2012), 17n10, 17n14; George McGovern, "The Historian as Policy Analyst," *Public Historian* 11, no. 2 (Spring 1989): 37–8; Simon Szreter, "History, Policy and the Social History of Medicine," *Social History of Medicine* 22, no. 2 (2009): 235–8; John Tosh, *Why History Matters* (London: Palgrave Macmillan, 2008). For political science: Nicole F. Bernier and Carole Clavier, "Public Health Policy Research: Making the Case for a Political Science Approach," *Health Promotion International* 26, no. 1 (March 2011): 109–16.
30 Meeting between Greg Marchildon and the author, 22 August 2018.
31 Meeting between Greg Marchildon and the author, 22 August 2018.
32 Correspondence with Greg Marchildon, 22 January 2020. See European Observatory on Health Systems and Policies, "Health System Reviews [HiT Series]), http://www.euro.who.int/en/about-us/partners/observatory/publications/health-system-reviews-hits.
33 Correspondence between the author and Greg Marchildon, 25 August 2018.
34 Inderjeet Parmar, *Think Tanks and Power in Foreign Policy: A Comparative Study of the Role and Influence of the Council on Foreign Relations and the Royal Institute of International Affairs, 1939–1945* (New York: Palgrave Macmillan, 2004), 29–30.
35 Canadian Institute of International Affairs, *The Canadian Institute of International Affairs: Its Organization, Objects, and Constitution* (Montreal: Southam, 1929), 14.
36 Canadian Institute of International Affairs, *Canadian Institute of International Affairs*, 16, 24.
37 Harold Averill, "Series 6, Other Activities," *Finding Aid*, Hastings (John E.F.)

Family fonds, B2002-0014, June 2004, UTARMS. For the reference to his staying there with his family, see 25. For his other King's Fund activities, see 58, 59, 61, and 63.

38 *The Health Service Administrator: Innovator or Catalyst*, ed. with commentaries by Leslie Paine, foreword by Robert Maxwell (London: King Edward's Hospital Fund for London, 1978), 187, 189. At the time, Boyd McAuley was executive director of Toronto Western Hospital, and Peter Carruthers president and CEO of Greater Niagara General Hospital. Other Canadian participants are listed in the "Members" section (n.p.), and those who presented papers on 187–9. For mention of the Canadian contribution, see especially the "Current Health Care Scenes" (3–17) and "Summary and Conclusion" (179–86).

39 Correspondence between the author and John Brown, 4 August 2018.

40 One could argue it always did work with practitioners; its practicum classes necessitated that it work.

41 Meeting with Dr Marchildon, 12 July 2018.

42 Gordon Martel, "From *Round Table* to *New Europe:* Some Intellectual Origins of the Institute of International Affairs," in *Chatham House and British Foreign Policy 1919–1945: The Royal Institute of International Affairs during the Inter-war Period*, ed. Andrea Bosco and Cornelia Navari (London: Lothian Foundation, 1994), 1.

43 Arnold J. Toynbee, *A Study of History*, 12 vols. (Oxford: Oxford University Press, 1934–61).

44 Frank Prochaska, "The King's Fund: A Century of Hospital charity," *Lancet* 349, no. 9049 (8 February 1997): 425.

45 In relation to the RIIA, see Paul Williams, "A Commonwealth of Knowledge: Empire, Intellectuals and the Chatham House Project, 1919–1939," *International Relations* 17, no. 1 (March 2003): 55, where, in regard to the RIIA, he notes "an image of expertise and intellectual authority based on applying what they saw as the scientific method to the study of international affairs."

46 James G. McGann, *The Fifth Estate: Think Tanks, Public Policy, and Governance* (Washington, DC: Brookings Institution Press, 2016), 1. For the quote from the Duke University academic, see Craufurd D. Goodwin and Michael Nacht, *Beyond Government: Extending the Public Debate in Emerging Democracies* (Boulder, CO: Westview), 12.

47 For a study on policy institutes in Canada, see Evert Anthony Lindquist, "Behind the Myth of Think Tanks: The Organization and Relevance of Canadian Policy Institutes" (PhD diss., University of California–Berkeley, 1989). Interestingly he also does not deal with the RIIA (or the CIIA) or its US counterpart, the CFR.

48 The Department of History, also Economics and Political Science (as it was then called), and Trinity College had close ties to it and it was housed there for many years.

49 John W. Holmes, *The CIIA and Canadian Foreign Policy: Hits and Myths: An Address to the Canadian Institute of International Affairs at Its 50th Jubilee Banquet, Toronto, 10 June 1978* (Toronto: Canadian Institute of International Affairs, 1978), 4, file 7, box 13, F2260, John W. Holmes fonds, University of Toronto, Trinity College Archives.

50 William Wallace, "Afterword: Soft Power, Global Agendas," in Diane Stone

and Andrew Denham, *Think Tank Traditions: Policy Research and the Politics of Ideas*, (Manchester: Manchester University Press, 2004), 289.
51 Meeting between Dr Brown and the author, 29 May 2018.
52 Meeting between the author and M. Dobrow, another between the author and S. Allin, both on 30 January 2019.
53 Meeting between the author and Allie Peckham, 17 July 2018.
54 John W. Holmes, "First Draft, CIIA Jubilee Dinner, Toronto, 10 June 1978," 1, file 7, box 13, F2260, John W. Holmes fonds, University of Toronto, Trinity College Archives.
55 Holmes, "First Draft, CIIA Jubilee Dinner," 1.
56 Holmes, "First Draft, CIIA Jubilee Dinner," 4.
57 Canada, House of Commons, *Debates*, First Session, Twenty-Eighth Parliament, vol. 1, 12 September 1968, 8.
58 R.S. Ritchie, *An Institute for Research on Public Policy: A Study and Recommendations* (Ottawa: Information Canada, 1971), 90. Interestingly he does not deal with the RIIA (or the CIIA) or its US counterpart the CFR. Each was among the first policy institutes and would have been considered important at the time. The RIIA and CFR still exist and with stellar reputations.
59 Ritchie, *Institute for Research on Public Policy*, 3, 4.
60 Conversation with the author, 9 March 2017.
61 *Description and Finding Aid: John W. Holmes fonds*, F2260 Archives, Trinity College in the University of Toronto. For an overview of the people involved, see "Miscellaneous Correspondence" (113–35) and "Personal Correspondence" (162–5) sections, which are alphabetized and list the individuals by name.
62 Royal Institute of International Affairs, "Memorandum on Important Changes in the Labour Situation and Social Conditions in Great Britain since the Outbreak of War," document no. 17, Conference on North Atlantic Relations, 4–9 September 1941, 17.
63 Christopher Brewin, "Arnold Toynbee and Chatham House," in *Chatham House and British Foreign Policy 1919–1945: The Royal Institute of International Affairs during the Inter-war Period*, ed. Andrea Bosco and Cornelia Navari (London: Lothian Foundation, 1994), 138.
64 Barnett, *Audit of War*, 20.
65 See General Assembly of the United Nations, "Moving Together to Build a Healthier World."
66 See, for example, Jeremy Youde, *Globalization and Health* (Lanham, MD: Rowman and Littlefield, 2020), 39–47; see also chap. 1, "The Globalization of Health," 5–27.

CHAPTER TWENTY-SIX

1 Correspondence between the author and A. Brown, 15 June 2018.
2 See "Health and Care Explained," King's Fund, https://www.kingsfund.org.uk/health-care-explained.
3 Meeting between the author and R. Cockerill, 17 July 2018.
4 See "North American Observatory on Health Systems and Policies," YouTube, https://www.youtube.com/channel/UCKNpWxikdbl31bLhOLUoMrA.
5 Donald T. Fraser and George D. Porter, *Canadian Health Book* (Toronto: Copp Clark, 1925, 1926).

6 Donald T. Fraser and George D. Porter, authorized by the Minister of Education, *Ontario Public School Health Book* (Toronto: Copp Clark, 1925). The price of the book, printed on the cover, was twenty-five cents.
7 Fraser and Porter, *Ontario Public School Health Book*, 1.
8 Donald T. Fraser, "Science: Protection against Disease," *Canadian Forum* 7, no. 82 (July 1927): 300–2.
9 A.L. McKay and Donald T. Fraser, "Radio Talks: The Prevention of Diphtheria and Scarlet Fever," *Public Health Journal* 16, no. 11 (November 1925): 521–4. This was the seventeenth in a series of talks under the auspices of the Canadian Social Hygiene Council, of which Dr Gordon Bates was Secretary (see 521).
10 Adalsteinn Brown, dean DLSPH, and Robert Steiner, director, Munk School Fellowship in Global Journalism, e-mail to the DLSPH community, 25 July 2018.
11 "Certificate in Health Impact," Dalla Lana, http://www.dlsph.utoronto.ca/programs/certificate-in-health-impact/.
12 Brown and Steiner to the DLSPH community.
13 See "Certificate in Health Impact."
14 Adalsteinn Brown, "Journalism Training for Health Research Impact: Proposal for 'Research Impact' Grant – Vice-President, Research, University of Toronto," co-investigators Robert Steiner and Adalsteinn Brown, 11.
15 Brown, "Journalism Training for Health Research Impact," 3.
16 Brown, "Journalism Training for Health Research Impact," 3.
17 Brown, "Journalism Training for Health Research Impact," 4–6.
18 Brown, "Journalism Training for Health Research Impact," 2–3.
19 Correspondence between the author and John Browne, 4 August 2018.
20 British Institute of International Affairs, *Gift of No. 10 St James Square to the British Institute of International Affairs* (Suffolk: Richard Clay and Sons, 1923[?]), 8–9.
21 British Institute of International Affairs, *Gift of No. 10 St James Square*, 8–9.
22 United States, Interdepartmental Committee to Coordinate Health and Welfare Activities, *Proceedings of the National Health Conference* (Washington: Government Printing Office, 1938), 144.
23 United States, Interdepartmental Committee to Coordinate Health and Welfare Activities, *Proceedings*, 144.
24 United States, Interdepartmental Committee to Coordinate Health and Welfare Activities, *Proceedings*, 132–3.
25 Council of the Royal Society, *The Public Understanding of Science: Report of a Royal Society Ad Hoc Group Endorsed by the Council of the Royal Society (Bodmer Report)* (London: Royal Society, 1985), 9.
26 Nicholas Russell, *Communicating Science: Professional, Popular, Literary* (Cambridge: Cambridge University Press, 2010), 72.
27 Russell, *Communicating Science*, 85. See also Great Britain, House of Lords, Third Report of the House of Lords Select Committee on Science and Technology, *Science and Society*, 23 February 2000.
28 "Certificate in Health Impact," Dalla Lana.".
29 Meeting with Adalsteinn Brown, 31 July 2018, and follow-up correspondence, 10 August 2018.
30 The material for this section was obtained in a meeting with Adalsteinn Brown, 31 July 2018, and through follow-up correspondence, 10 August 2018.

31 See "Health System Impact Fellowships (for Doctoral Trainees and Post-Doctoral Fellows) – Profiles of Host Partner Organizations," Canadian Institutes of Health Research, http://www.cihr-irsc.gc.ca/e/50612.html.
32 See UK Research and Innovation, https://www.ukri.org, and a webpage called "Excellence with Impact," https://www.ukri.org/innovation/excellence-with-impact/.
33 For Oxford, see "Research Impact," https://www.ox.ac.uk/research/research-impact?wssl=1, and for Cambridge, see "Research Impact," https://www.cam.ac.uk/research/impact.
34 See "Investing for Impact," Medical Research Council, https://mrc.ukri.org/successes/investing-for-impact/.
35 See "Chief Scientific Advisers, GOV.UK, https://www.gov.uk/government/groups/chief-scientific-advisers.
36 See Government Office for Science, GOV.UK, https://www.gov.uk/government/organisations/government-office-for-science.
37 See "Broader Impacts Review Criterion," National Science Foundation, https://www.nsf.gov/pubs/2007/nsf07046/nsf07046.jsp.
38 Correspondence with Adelsteinn Brown, 4 September 2018.
39 Correspondence with Adelsteinn Brown, 5 September 2018.
40 Dr. Brown to Annette Paul and the author, 10 August 2018.
41 Adalsteinn Brown, "Leading Edge Options of Public Health," opening address at the Boehm Lectures, 29 November 2018, YouTube, https://www.youtube.com/watch?v=5bS9IF0BgTg.
42 Robert N. Ruesch, *In The Warmth of the Shadow* (Meadville, PA: Christian Faith Publishing, 2017), explores growing up in a vacation world high in the Colorado Rockies through the eyes of a child.
43 Meeting between the author and Annette Paul, 16 August 2018.
44 CFTR, 21 October 2017, 9:05 a.m.
45 I was in the audience.
46 Colin Freeze, "Sanders Lauds Canadian Health-Care System in Speech," *Globe and Mail*, 30 October 2017, A4.
47 Theresa Boyle and Alex McKeen, "'We Need Your Help,' Sanders Tells Canada," *Toronto Star*, 30 October 2017, A2.
48 See Margot Sanger-Katz, "What Did Bernie Sanders Learn in His Weekend in Canada?," *New York Times*, 2 November 2017, https://mobile.nytimes.com/2017/11/02/upshot/bernie-sanders-went-to-canada-and-learned-a-few-things.html.
49 Jack O. Denton, "'Be a Little Bit Louder,'" *Varsity* 138, no. 8, 30 October 2017, 3. See also 1. The web version of the article has an additional section on student reaction to the event; see Denton, "Bernie Sanders Speaks at Con Hall," https://thevarsity.ca/2017/10/30/bernie-sanders-speaks-at-con-hall/.
50 My notes. Also reported in the *Toronto Star* article mentioned above.
51 See https://online-learning.harvard.edu/course/justice.
52 See "Michael J. Sandel: Bio," Harvard University, https://scholar.harvard.edu/sandel/sandel/bio.
53 Correspondence between the author and Dr Brown, 3 April 2018.
54 See "Public Engagement," Medical Research Council, https://mrc.ukri.org/research/public-engagement/.
55 See, for example, United Kingdom, Minister of State for the Cabinet Office and Paymaster General, *Open Data White Paper: Unleashing the Potential* (London: HM Stationery Office, 2012). See also United Kingdom, Report on

the Working Group on Expanding Access to Published Research Findings, *Accessibility, Sustainability, Excellence: How to Expand Access to Research Publications* (Finch Report), June 2012.

56 For GO-Science and Foresight, see https://www.gov.uk/government/organisations/government-office-for-science.

57 See "Events," Dalla Lana," https://mrc.ukri.org/research/public-engagement/.

58 See "How We Engage the Public," Wellcome, https://wellcome.ac.uk/what-we-do/our-work/public-engagement; and "Public Engagement Fund (Closed)," Wellcome, https://wellcome.ac.uk/funding/public-engagement-fund.

59 See National Co-ordinating Centre for Public Engagement, http://www.publicengagement.ac.uk; and "The Engaged University: A Manifesto for Public Engagement," https://www.publicengagement.ac.uk/sites/default/files/publication/manifesto_for_public_engagement_final_january_2010.pdf.

CHAPTER TWENTY-SEVEN

1 Correspondence with the author, 15 March 2017.

2 Correspondence with the author, 5 April 2017.

3 He delivered a talk on this topic at IHPME, 16 March 2017.

4 Arnold Toynbee, *Acquaintances* (London: Oxford University Press, 1967), 165.

5 Here is a very incomplete list: Jim McNab, Peter Lewis, Carl Hunt, Gerry Turner, Ted Friedman, Jeannine Girard-Pearlman, Joe Mapa, Les Boehm, Elizabeth and Michael McCartney, Vytas Mickevicius, and Sally Brown.

6 Barbara Lazenby Craig and Ronald K. MacLeod, *A Separate and Special Place: An Appreciative History of Toronto's Queen Elizabeth Hospital on the Occasion of its 110th anniversary* (Toronto: Queen Elizabeth Hospital, 1984), 102. See 100–2 regarding the process of securing the site. See also Barsky, *From Generation to Generation: A History of Toronto's Mount Sinai Hospital*, 148.

7 Connor, *Doing Good: The Life of Toronto General Hospital*, 249. See also E.A. McCulloch, *The Ontario Cancer Institute: Successes and Reverses at Sherbourne Street* (Montreal and Kingston: McGill-Queen's University Press, 2003), 172.

8 Meeting of author with Building Identification Office, 30 October 2018.

9 See MaRS, "Place Matters," https://placematters.marsdd.com.

10 See UTEST, http://utest.to.

11 See "Entrepreneurship," University of Toronto, http://entrepreneurs.utoronto.ca.

12 Joseph Orozco, "It's Time to Bring Innovators out of the Garage," *Globe and Mail, Report on Business*, 27 December 2017, B4.

13 Jennifer Robinson, "University Ranked among Top 30 Public Institutions Worldwide by Reuters," *U of T News*, 27 September 2017, https://www.utoronto.ca/news/u-t-named-canada-s-most-innovative-university.

14 A number of media sources have used the term. Knowledge@Wharton is one: see Wharton, "The Next Silicon Valley? Why Toronto Is a Contender," https://knowledge.wharton.upenn.edu/article/the-next-silicon-valley-why-toronto-is-a-contender/.

15 See the cover of *Toronto Life*, October 2017, with picture and caption "The New Silicon Valley: Inside Toronto's Tech Revolution." See also the cover story, "The Incredible, Unstoppable Rise of Tech: 30 Reasons Why Toronto Is the New Silicon Valley," *Toronto Life* 51, no. 10, October 2017, 49–68.

16 See https://placematters.marsdd.com.

17 André Picard, "Record $100-Million CAMH Donation Marks Shift on Mental Health," *Globe and Mail*, 12 January 2018, A1, A17. See also the web version "Record $100-million Donation to CAMH Underscores Cultural Shift on mental health," 11 January 2018, https://www.theglobeandmail.com/opinion/columnists/record-100-million-donation-to-camh-underscores-cultural-shift/article37571805/.

18 Joseph Hall, "A $100 Million 'Injection of Hope' for Mental Health," *Toronto Star*, 12 January 2018, A1, A12. See also the web version "A Donor Is Giving a Record $100 Million to CAMH – and Doesn't Want to Be Named," *Toronto Star*, 11 January 2018, https://www.thestar.com/news/gta/2018/01/11/a-donor-is-giving-a-record-100-million-to-camh-and-doesnt-want-to-be-named.html.

19 Hall, "$100 Million 'Injection of Hope,'" A12. See also the web version.

20 Marcia Kaye, "Make No Mistake: Can a Group of Toronto Hospitals Eliminate Medical Errors?," *U of T Magazine* 45, no. 2, Winter 2018, 57–60.

21 In a by no means exhaustive list, at the Rotman School people like Richard Florida, or at the Munk School, Shiri Breznitz, Dan Breznitz, David Wolfe, at IHPME, Fiona Miller.

22 Anthony Lacavera, *How We Can Win: And What Happens to Us and Our Country if We Don't* (Toronto: Random House Canada, 2017), 176. See chapter 6, from which this is taken, "Sometimes It *Is* Rocket Science," 175–211.

23 C.P. Snow, "The Rede Lecture, 1959," in *The Two Cultures* (1959; Cambridge: Cambridge University Press, 1993).

24 "Oral History Interviews, University of Toronto, Faculty of Medicine, Dr C.H. Hollenberg," 3 February 1983, 147–8, vol. 21, B87-0044, UTARMS.

25 Taylor, *Health Insurance and Canadian Public Policy*, 413; Quebec, Commission of Inquiry on Health and Social Welfare, *Report*, vol. 1.

26 Reed et al., *Building Healthier Communities*; also David Maguire, "The Economic Influence of the NHS at the Local Level" (London: King's Fund, 16 January 2020), https://www.kingsfund.org.uk/publications/economic-influence-nhs-local-level.

27 Claire Greszczuk, ed., *Implementing Health in All Policies: Lessons from around the World* (London: Health Foundation, August 2019).

28 Tim Elwell-Sutoon, Adam Tinson, Claire Greszczuk, David Fimch, Erica Holt-White, Grace Everest, Nadya Mihaylova, Suzanne Wood, and Jo Bibby, *Creating Healthy Lives: A Whole-Government Approach to Long-Term Investment in the Nation's Health* (London: Health Foundation, September 2019), 2.

29 Elwell-Sutoon et al., *Creating Healthy Lives*, 26.

30 Visiting the Chatham House website reveals policy forums and briefings on aspects of UHC. There is also a report they undertook with the WHO; see Allison Beattie, Robert Yates, and Douglas Noble, *Accelerating Progress Towards Universal Health Coverage for Women and Children in South Asia, East Asia and the Pacific* (Kathmandu: UNICEF South Asia and Chatham House, October 2016).

31 For a list of all OHA board chairs, see Ontario Hospital Association, *80 Years of Progress, 1924–2004*, 8.4. I wish to acknowledge Tessa Dundas at the OHA who loaned me her personal copy.

32 Ontario Hospital Association, *80 Years of Progress*, 1.21.
33 Ontario Hospital Association, *80 Years of Progress*, 1.28.
34 Ontario Hospital Association, *80 Years of Progress*, 1.29.
35 Correspondence between the author and M. Rochon, 27 and 28 August 2019.
36 Ontario Hospital Association, *80 Years of Progress*, 1.15.
37 Correspondence with the author, 28 May 2019.
38 World Bank Group, *The Evolution of the Canadian Pension Model: Practical Lessons for Building World-Class Pension Organizations* (Washington: International Bank for Reconstruction and Development / The World Bank, 2017), 2.
39 World Bank Group, *The Evolution of the Canadian Pension Model*, ix.
40 World Bank Group, *The Evolution of the Canadian Pension Model*, 1.
41 Ontario Hospital Association, *80 Years of Progress*, 1.26.
42 Correspondence with the author, 29 May 2019.
43 Ontario Hospital Association, *80 Years of Progress*, 5.30.
44 J.G. FitzGerald, "Report of the Director of the Antitoxin Laboratory," *President's Report, for the Year Ending June 30, 1914*, 25.
45 These were Saskatchewan Government Telephones, Saskatchewan Power Corporation, and the Saskatchewan Government Insurance Office.
46 Other examples (by no means an exhaustive list) are Canadian National Railway, Ontario Hydro, as well as companies set up by a successor to Douglas (Alan Blakeney) in potash, oil, and uranium. Blakeney also set up a sovereign wealth fund in Saskatchewan. There are numerous other examples from other provinces.
47 See, for example, articles by Freedman, Gerring, Gamble, and Monaghan, in "Annual Author/Subject Index," *Leadership in Health Services* 1, no. 6 (November/December 1992): 38.
48 Dr Bob Bell, deputy minister, Health and Long-term Care, IHPME GSU Lunch & Learn, 18 May 2017. I was in the audience.
49 See, for example, "Active Trustees Mean a Better Hospital," with a piece by E.P. McGavin of the Ontario Hospital Association and another by Judge Hughes, *Canadian Hospital* 45, no 7 (July 1968): 67–8.
50 See "Directors Education Program," Institute of Corporate Directors / Institut des administrateurs de sociétés, https://www.icd.ca/Courses/Directors-Education-Program.aspx.

CHAPTER TWENTY-EIGHT

1 Meetings and correspondence between the author and G. Marchildon, July 2018. Also correspondence of 6 August 2018.
2 See Jennifer Robinson, "New Global Ranking Places U of T in Top 10 in Seven Subjects," *U of T News*, 30 June 2017, https://www.utoronto.ca/news/new-global-ranking-places-u-t-top-10-seven-subjects.
3 Correspondence with Rebecca Biason, re: Ahmed Bayoumi, 13 February 2018.
4 Correspondence with Rebecca Biason, re: Ahmed Bayoumi.
5 Correspondence with Rebecca Biason, re: Wendy Ungar, 13 February 2018.
6 "Programs in Progress," *IHPME Annual Highlights: Five-Year Progress Report, 2016 Annual Highlights*, 32.
7 Correspondence between Gene Vayda and L. Boehm, 18 June 2019.

8 David Johnston and Tom Jenkins, *Ingenious: How Canadian Innovators Made the World Smarter, Smaller, Kinder, Safer, Healthier, Wealthier, and Happier* (Toronto: Signal, 2017), 59.
9 Taylor, *Health Insurance and Canadian Public Policy*, 490–1.
10 Goel, "Opinion," B4.

Index